Management of Infections in the Immunocompromised Host

Brahm H. Segal
Editor

Management of Infections in the Immunocompromised Host

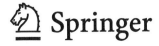 Springer

Editor
Brahm H. Segal
Departments of Medicine and Immunology
Roswell Park Comprehensive Cancer Center
Buffalo, NY, USA

Department of Medicine
University at Buffalo Jacobs School of Medicine
and Biomedical Sciences
Buffalo, NY, USA

ISBN 978-3-319-77672-9   ISBN 978-3-319-77674-3   (eBook)
https://doi.org/10.1007/978-3-319-77674-3

Library of Congress Control Number: 2018943702

Printed on acid-free paper

This Springer imprint is published by the registered company Springer International Publishing AG part of Springer Nature.
The registered company address is: Gewerbestrasse 11, 6330 Cham, Switzerland

To my wife, Stephanie, and to our children, Joshua and Emily.

Preface

"Now inflammation as understood in man and the higher animals is a phenomenon that almost always results from the intervention of some pathogenic microbe. So it is held that the afflux of mobile cells towards points of lesion shows the organism's reaction against foreign bodies in general and against infectious microbes in particular. On this hypothesis, disease would be a fight between the morbid agent, the microbe from outside, and the mobile cells of the organism itself. Cure would come from the victory of the cells and immunity would be the sign of their acting sufficiently to prevent the microbial onslaught" (Ilya Mechnikov, Nobel lecture, 1908). Mechnikov's conclusions were based on his seminal experiments involving the application of splinters to larvae of the starfish, Bipinnaria, that led to the discovery of phagocytosis as a critical factor in host defense. In the same lecture, Mechnikov noted that individuals have different susceptibility to infections: "It is often seen that in households where all members are exposed to the same danger, or again in schools or troops where everyone lives the same life, disease does not strike everyone indifferently."

The overriding theme of this textbook – that our immune system must sense pathogens, migrate to sites of infection, and kill pathogens or at least limit their growth to avoid disease, and that disorders of the immune system predispose to infection – is echoed in Mechnikov's prescient statements made 110 years ago. The progress made in our understanding of the immune system and development of novel immunotherapies for infectious diseases, cancer, autoimmunity, and other disorders has been extraordinary. The challenge of this textbook is to link knowledge about host defense to assist clinicians in a practical fashion in the care of patients with suspected or known immunodeficiencies and infectious diseases. In addition to practical knowledge applied at the bedside, we also aim to provide an understanding of gaps in knowledge, cutting-edge technology in immunotherapy, and future directions of research.

Because of the importance in understanding the normal immune system as a prerequisite for understanding immunodeficiencies, this textbook provides detailed overviews of phagocyte biology, complement, cytokines, and other soluble mediators of immunity, mucosal immunity, and T-cell and B-cell immunity. The next section of the textbook is focused on primary immunodeficiencies. Indeed, hundreds of primary immunodeficiencies have been described, the majority resulting from defects in single genes. From these patients, we learn that our immune system has redundant pathways for host defense, and deficits in specific genes lead to susceptibility to specific pathogens.

The majority of immunodeficiencies are acquired rather than inherited. The major acquired immunodeficiencies include HIV infection, cancer, transplantation, and immunosuppressive therapy for autoimmune diseases. Among this large group of patients with acquired immunodeficiencies, important differences in infection risk are observed, and even within these patient groups, substantial heterogeneity exists regarding the underlying disease and intensity of immunosuppressive therapy. Severely immunocompromised patients can have substantial exposure to antibacterial, antifungal, and antiviral agents, both as prophylaxis and as treatment. In addition, these patients are frequently hospitalized and are at risk for nosocomial infections. It is therefore important to understand the growing trends in antimicrobial resistance and judicious use of antibacterial, antifungal, and antiviral agents to guide appropriate therapy. Chapters written by expert clinicians provide practical evidence-based approaches to prevention, diagnosis, and treatment of infectious complications in these patient populations.

The last chapters address standard and novel approaches for enhancing host defense in immunocompromised patients. They include vaccination of patients and household members and immunoglobulin therapy. Finally, dedicated chapters on stem cell transplantation for patients with primary immunodeficiencies, adoptive cellular immunotherapy, and gene therapy will provide readers with insight into these rapidly evolving and cutting-edge therapies.

I hope that this textbook will be of value to a broad readership, from trainees to clinicians and scientists interested in the fields of infectious diseases and immunology. I want to extend my gratitude to the expert authors who contributed chapters to this textbook. Needless to say, the success of this textbook is a direct result of their knowledge and effort. I also want to thank the staff at Springer for their helpful suggestions, efficiency, and commitment to the project.

Buffalo, NY, USA   Brahm H. Segal

Contents

Contributors

Alessandro Aiuti San Raffaele Telethon Institute for Gene Therapy (TIGET), San Raffaele Scientific Institute, Milan, Italy

Pediatric Immunohematology and Bone Marrow Transplantation Unit, IRCCS San Raffaele Scientific Institute, Milan, Italy

Vita-Salute San Raffaele University, Milan, Italy

Nikolaos G. Almyroudis Jacobs School of Medicine and Biomedical Sciences, State University of New York at Buffalo, Division of Infectious Diseases, Roswell Park Comprehensive Cancer Center, Buffalo, NY, USA

Ella J. Ariza-Heredia Department of Infectious Diseases, Infection Control and Employee Health, The University of Texas MD Anderson Cancer Center, Houston, TX, USA

Thomas Baker Department of Infectious Diseases, Weill Cornell Medicine, New York, NY, USA

Catherine M. Bollard Program for Cell Enhancement and Technologies for Immunotherapy, Sheikh Zayed Institute for Pediatric Surgical Innovation, and Center for Cancer and Immunology Research, Children's National Health System, Washington, DC, USA

Claire Booth Department of Paediatric Immunology, Great Ormond Street Hospital, London, UK

R. Douglas Bruce Yale University School of Medicine, Cornell Scott-Hill Health Center, New Haven, CT, USA

Agostinho Carvalho Life and Health Sciences Research Institute (ICVS), School of Medicine, University of Minho, Braga, Portugal

ICVS/3B's – PT Government Associate Laboratory, Braga/Guimarães, Portugal

Srinjoy Chakraborti Division of Infectious Diseases and Immunology, Department of Medicine, University of Massachusetts Medical School, Worcester, MA, USA

Roy F. Chemaly Department of Infectious Diseases, Infection Control and Employee Health, The University of Texas MD Anderson Cancer Center, Houston, TX, USA

Maria Pia Cicalese San Raffaele Telethon Institute for Gene Therapy (TIGET), San Raffaele Scientific Institute, Milan, Italy

Pediatric Immunohematology and Bone Marrow Transplantation Unit, IRCCS San Raffaele Scientific Institute, Milan, Italy

Morton J. Cowan Allergy, Immunology, and Blood and Marrow Transplant Division, Department of Pediatrics, University of California, San Francisco, CA, USA

Cristina Cunha Life and Health Sciences Research Institute (ICVS), School of Medicine, University of Minho, Braga, Portugal

ICVS/3B's – PT Government Associate Laboratory, Braga/Guimarães, Portugal

Frank R. DeLeo Laboratory of Bacteriology, Rocky Mountain Laboratories, National Institute of Allergy and Infectious Diseases, National Institutes of Health, Hamilton, MT, USA

Morna J. Dorsey Allergy, Immunology, and Blood and Marrow Transplant Division, Department of Pediatrics, University of California, San Francisco, CA, USA

Firas El Chaer Department of Infectious Diseases, Infection Control and Employee Health, The University of Texas MD Anderson Cancer Center, Houston, TX, USA

Abdul Aziz Elkadri Medical College of Wisconsin, Milwaukee, WI, USA

Alison G. Freifeld Internal Medicine, Division of Infectious Diseases, University of Nebraska Medical Center, Omaha, NE, USA

Lee Ann Garrett-Sinha Department of Biochemistry, Center of Excellence in Bioinformatics and Life Sciences, State University of New York at Buffalo, Buffalo, NY, USA

Samuel M. Gonçalves Life and Health Sciences Research Institute (ICVS), School of Medicine, University of Minho, Braga, Portugal

ICVS/3B's – PT Government Associate Laboratory, Braga/Guimarães, Portugal

Steven M. Holland Laboratory of Clinical Infectious Diseases, National Institute of Allergy and Infectious Diseases, NIH, Bethesda, MD, USA

Shahid Husain Division of Infectious Diseases, Department of Medicine, University of Toronto, and Multi-organ Transplant Program, University Health Network, Toronto, ON, Canada

Aspasia Katragkou Transplantation-Oncology Infectious Diseases Program, Division of Infectious Diseases, Department of Medicine, Pediatrics, and Microbiology & Immunology, Weill Cornell Medicine, Henry Schueler Foundation Scholar, New York, NY, USA

Shalu Sharma Kharkwal Department of Microbiology and Immunology, Albert Einstein College of Medicine, Bronx, NY, USA

Scott D. Kobayashi Laboratory of Bacteriology, Rocky Mountain Laboratories, National Institute of Allergy and Infectious Diseases, National Institutes of Health, Hamilton, MT, USA

Jana P. Lovell Laboratory of Clinical Infectious Diseases, National Institute of Allergy and Infectious Diseases, NIH, Bethesda, MD, USA

Lawrence G. Lum Cellular Therapy and Stem Cell Transplant Program, Emily Couric Cancer Center, University of Virginia, Charlottesville, VA, USA

Natalia Malachowa Laboratory of Bacteriology, Rocky Mountain Laboratories, National Institute of Allergy and Infectious Diseases, National Institutes of Health, Hamilton, MT, USA

Matthew W. McCarthy Department of Infectious Diseases, Weill Cornell Medicine, New York, NY, USA

Aleixo Muise The Hospital for Sick Children, Inflammatory Bowel Disease Center, Toronto, Canada

Tyler Nygaard Laboratory of Bacteriology, Rocky Mountain Laboratories, National Institute of Allergy and Infectious Diseases, National Institutes of Health, Hamilton, MT, USA

Onyema Ogbuagu Section of Infectious Diseases, Yale University School of Medicine, New Haven, CT, USA

Neil U. Parikh University of Central Florida, Orlando, FL, USA

Steven A. Porcelli Department of Microbiology and Immunology, Albert Einstein College of Medicine, Bronx, NY, USA

Paratosh Prasad Division of Infectious Diseases, University of Rochester Medical Center, Rochester, NY, USA

Sanjay Ram Division of Infectious Diseases and Immunology, Department of Medicine, University of Massachusetts Medical School, Worcester, MA, USA

Emmanuel Roilides Infectious Disease Unit, 3rd Department of Pediatrics, Faculty of Medicine, Aristotle University School of Health Sciences, Hippokration Hospital, Thessaloniki, Greece

Coleman Rotstein Division of Infectious Diseases, Department of Medicine, University of Toronto, and Multi-organ Transplant Program, University Health Network, Toronto, ON, Canada

Mark F. Sands Division of Allergy, Immunology & Rheumatology, Department of Medicine, University at Buffalo, Buffalo General Medical Center, Buffalo, NY, USA

Michael J. Satlin Department of Infectious Diseases, Weill Cornell Medicine, New York, NY, USA

Stanley A. Schwartz Division of Allergy Immunology & Rheumatology, Department of Medicine, University at Buffalo, Buffalo General Medical Center, Buffalo, NY, USA

Juliana Silva Department of Bone Marrow Transplantation, Great Ormond Street Hospital, London, UK

John Treanor Division of Infectious Diseases, University of Rochester Medical Center, Rochester, NY, USA

Paul Veys Department of Bone Marrow Transplantation, Great Ormond Street Hospital, London, UK

Thomas J. Walsh Department of Infectious Diseases, Weill Cornell Medicine, New York, NY, USA

Departments of Pediatrics, Microbiology and Immunology Weill Cornell Medicine, New York, NY, USA

Andrea J. Zimmer Internal Medicine, Division of Infectious Diseases, University of Nebraska Medical Center, Omaha, NE, USA

Phagocytes

Tyler Nygaard, Natalia Malachowa,
Scott D. Kobayashi, and Frank R. DeLeo

Abbreviations

APC	Antigen-presenting cell
BMCP	Basophil-MC progenitor cell
BPI	Bactericidal/permeability-increasing protein
CCL2	CC-chemokine ligand 2
cDC	Classical DC
CDP	Common DC progenitor
CLP	Common lymphoid progenitor
CMP	Common myeloid progenitor
CXCL8	CXC-chemokine ligand 8 (IL-8)
DAMP	Damage-associated molecular pattern
DC	Dendritic cell
EPC	Embryonic progenitor cell
ESL1	E-selectin ligand 1
ET	Extracellular trap
GAG	Glycosaminoglycan
GMP	Granulocyte-macrophage progenitor
H_2O_2	Hydrogen peroxide
HMGB1	High-mobility group box 1
HNP	Human neutrophil peptide
HOCl	Hypochlorous acid
HSC	Hematopoietic stem cell
ICAM-1	Intercellular adhesion molecule 1
iNOS	Inducible nitric oxide synthase
JAM-A	Junctional adhesion molecule A
JAM-C	Junctional adhesion molecule C
LMPP	Lymphoid-myeloid multipotent progenitor
LPS	Lipopolysaccharide
MDP	Macrophage-DC progenitor
MEP	Megakaryocyte-erythrocyte progenitor
MHC	Major histocompatibility complex
MPO	Myeloperoxidase
MPP	Multipotent progenitor
NET	Neutrophil extracellular trap
PAMP	Pathogen-associated molecular pattern
pDC	Plasmacytoid DC
PECAM-1	Platelet-endothelial cell adhesion molecule-1 (CD31)
PMN	Polymorphonuclear leukocyte (or neutrophil)
PRR	Pattern recognition receptor
PSGL1	P-selectin glycoprotein ligand 1
RNS	Reactive nitrogen species
ROS	Reactive oxygen species
SYK	Spleen tyrosine kinase
TCR	T cell receptor
TEM	Transendothelial cell migration
TNF	Tumor necrosis factor
VCAM-1	Vasculature intercellular adhesion molecule 1
VLA-4	Very late antigen 4

T. Nygaard · N. Malachowa · S. D. Kobayashi
F. R. DeLeo (✉)
Laboratory of Bacteriology, Rocky Mountain
Laboratories, National Institute of Allergy and
Infectious Diseases, National Institutes of Health,
Hamilton, MT, USA
e-mail: fdeleo@niaid.niaid.nih.gov

Origin and Development of Phagocytes

Phagocytic leukocytes are important for innate and acquired immunity. These cells are also involved in the initiation and resolution of the inflammatory response, and they maintain tissue homeostasis in the steady state. There are multiple types of phagocytes, and each can contribute uniquely to the maintenance of human health and the defense against microorganisms. Phagocytes originate from self-renewing and multipotent hematopoietic stem cells in bone marrow or during embryogenesis from yolk sac and/or fetal liver stem cells [1–3]. In the traditional model of hematopoiesis, multipotent progenitor (MPP) cells differentiate into common lymphoid progenitor (CLP) and common myeloid progenitor

(CMP) cells (Fig. 1.1). CLPs differentiate ultimately into B cells, T cells, and natural killer cells. The CMPs give rise to granulocyte-macrophage progenitors (GMPs), which can then differentiate ultimately into phagocytes, including granulocytic phagocytes (neutrophils, eosinophils, and mast cells), and mononuclear phagocytes (monocytes, macrophages, and dendritic cells) [1].

Recent findings indicate that MPPs can differentiate into a lymphoid-myeloid multipotent progenitor cell (rather than a direct differentiation of MPPs to CLPs as described above), which in turn gives rise to GMPs, CLPs, or early thymic precursors (Fig. 1.1) [4]. Differentiation to phagocytes from GMPs in this model is similar to that in the traditional model. It is also noteworthy that dendritic cells and monocytes/macrophages can

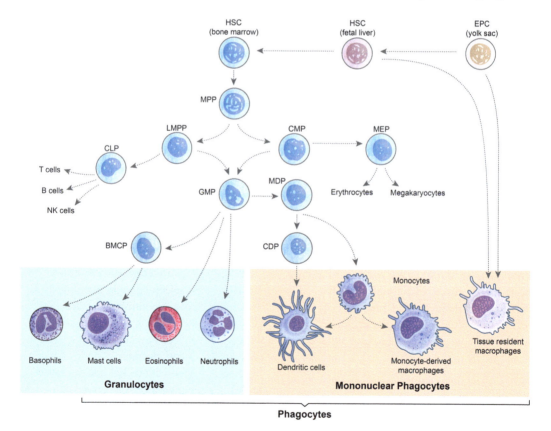

Fig. 1.1 Hematopoiesis and production of phagocytes. Leukocytes originate from embryonic progenitor cells in the fetal yolk sac, multipotent hematopoietic stem cells in bone marrow, and/or fetal liver stem cells. BMCP basophil/mast cell progenitor, CDP common dendritic cell, CLP common lymphoid progenitor, CMP common myeloid progenitor, DC dendritic cell, EPC embryonic progenitor cell, GMP granulocyte-macrophage progenitor, HSC hematopoietic stem cell, LMPP lymphoid-primed multipotent progenitor, MDP macrophage-dendritic cell progenitor, MEP megakaryocyte-erythrocyte progenitor, MPP multipotent progenitor

be derived from reprogramming of CLPs by specific cytokines [1, 5]. Therefore, the current model of hematopoiesis is not absolute and will need revision and updating as new discoveries are made.

Not all phagocytic leukocytes are produced during hematopoiesis in bone marrow. Based on studies in mice, a significant proportion of tissue-resident macrophages are now known to originate from stem cells during embryogenesis (Fig. 1.1) [2, 3]. These tissue macrophages develop from embryonic progenitor cells in the yolk sac or fetal liver and then self-renew and are thus maintained independent of blood monocytes [2, 6]. This is a major deviation from the traditional model of bone marrow hematopoiesis and the process of myeloid cell differentiation, from which all mononuclear phagocytes were thought to be derived [7]. A detailed review of hematopoiesis and phagocyte development is beyond the scope of this chapter, and we refer the reader to relevant articles on the topic [1–4, 8–15]. Instead, we highlight a few features of phagocyte development that are important for our understanding of the function of each cell type.

Mononuclear Phagocytes

Monocytes, macrophages, and dendritic cells (DCs) comprise cells of the mononuclear phagocyte system [16]. These cells are important for innate and adaptive immunity, and they play a key role as antigen-presenting cells and in maintaining immune system homeostasis. In humans, monocytes comprise ~10% of all leukocytes in blood (considerable variability between individuals exists), and production (as determined by turnover) is on the order of 7×10^6 cells/h/kg body weight [17–19]. There are ~3 times more monocytes in the marginal pool than in circulation in blood (~2×10^5 cells/ml) [17, 18]. The half-life for monocytes in human blood is ~1–2 days, although there is considerable variance among individuals [17, 19]. Hematopoiesis maintains steady-state production of monocytes that originate initially from a CMP and, then more proximally, from a recently described progenitor cell known as a macrophage-dendritic

cell progenitor (MDP) [20, 21]. MDPs can differentiate to monocytes or to classical or plasmacytoid DCs via an intermediate known as a common DC progenitor cell (CDP) (Fig. 1.1) [22]. Human monocytes are characterized by cytochemistry, nuclear morphology, and surface expression of selected receptors. For example, monocyte subsets can have high, intermediate, and low surface expression of CD14. Those with comparatively high levels of CD14 on the cell surface represent the vast majority of monocytes in healthy humans and are known as classical monocytes [22]. More recent studies have shown that monocytes can be segregated further into distinct subsets based on high or low surface expression of CD16 [23], or those with high or low expression of CX3CR1, the fractalkine receptor [24]. Fractalkine (CX3CL1) has a number of functions, including stimulation of adhesion of leukocytes to activated endothelial cells. Depending on the stimulus or condition, a subset of monocytes can differentiate further to monocyte-derived dendritic cells or monocyte-derived macrophages in tissues (Fig. 1.1) [3]. For example, during severe inflammation or inflammation-related injuries, macrophages are replenished by blood-derived monocytes [3]. In mice, monocytes with high expression of CX3CR1 differentiate into long-term persisting tissue-resident phagocytes, whereas those with comparatively low CX3CR1 expression are inflammatory monocytes that serve as precursors for antigen-presenting cells [24]. Importantly, monocytes are innate immune effector cells that phagocytose (ingest) and kill a wide range of microbes, such as bacteria and fungi.

Tissue-resident mononuclear phagocytes are diverse and include macrophages (e.g., microglia, osteoclasts, Kupffer cells, Langerhans cells, and monocyte-derived macrophages) and DCs (classical DCs, plasmacytoid DCs, and monocyte-derived DCs) [3, 9, 25]. Like monocytes, these cells are defined by morphology, phenotype (cell surface markers), and function. Macrophages maintain steady-state tissue homeostasis by phagocytosing and removing dead cells and debris. During infection, they ingest and kill microbes and produce many different chemokines and cytokines that contribute to the acute inflammatory response. Tissue-resident macrophages are well-known for their ability to function as antigen-presenting cells and thus serve as a bridge between innate and acquired immunity. Historically, activated macrophages have been categorized as classic (M1) and alternative (M2), so named to reflect the prototypical Th1 and Th2 mouse strains from which they were isolated [26, 27]. In accordance with this nomenclature, M1 macrophages are those activated by interferon gamma and Toll-like receptor ligands (e.g., lipopolysaccharide) or tumor necrosis factor (TNF-α), whereas M2 macrophages are activated by IL-4, IL-10, IL-13, or IL-33 [26–29]. M1 macrophages are proinflammatory and produce reactive nitrogen or reactive oxygen intermediates and cytokines such as IL-1, IL-6, and TNF-α [28, 29]. By comparison, M2 macrophages have been characterized by production of polyamines and IL-10 and IL-12, regulate wound healing, and in general suppress immune responses [28, 29]. Inasmuch as macrophage activation is complex and varied among mammals, and there is inconsistent use of defining features for macrophage activation, the M1-M2 macrophage nomenclature has been brought into question recently, and new guidelines have been proposed [30]. Although it is widely acknowledged that a primary purpose of macrophages is to kill ingested microbes, these phagocytes are readily parasitized by a number of bacterial pathogens [31]. For example, *Brucella* spp., *Chlamydia pneumoniae*, *Coxiella burnetii*, *Francisella tularensis*, *Legionella pneumophila*, *Listeria monocytogenes*, *Mycobacterium tuberculosis*, and *Salmonella enterica* can replicate in macrophages [31]. This interesting topic has been reviewed recently by Price and Vance, and they suggest several factors contribute to the ability of bacteria to survive and replicate within macrophages [31]. These factors include intracellular access by phagocytosis, extended host cell lifespan, and nutrient availability [31]. It is also noteworthy that macrophages have limited bactericidal activity compared with neutrophils, which are infrequently parasitized by bacteria. Tissue-resident macrophages are maintained in steady state by self-renewal, and it is only under immune system duress, as with acute inflammatory processes, that monocytes are recruited to tissues to replenish tissue macrophages.

DCs have the capacity to phagocytose microbes and produce high levels of cytokines (depending on the type of DC), but their primary function is largely as antigen-presenting cells that activate naive T cells [8, 9, 32]. There are three or four subsets of DCs, depending on whether Langerhans cells are classified as macrophages or DCs. Langerhans cells were traditionally classified as DCs, but recent gene expression data and their origin from fetal liver precursor cells are more in line with characteristics of tissue macrophages [33, 34]. Regardless, Langerhans cells are abundant resident phagocytes in human skin and serve as sentinels of the immune system [35]. Classical DCs (cDCs; originally identified by Steinman and Cohn [36]) present antigen to T cells in the context of major histocompatibility complex (MHC) I and MHC II [37] molecules. These cells are present in many types of tissues and organs, and ultimately migrate (if necessary) to areas that promote interaction with T cells, such as the spleen or lymph nodes [37]. The lifespan of cDCs is relatively short (~1 week), and they are replenished by hematopoiesis from blood-borne CDPs [9]. Plasmacytoid DCs (pDCs) also originate from a CDP, but unlike cDCs, pDCs have a long lifespan and are involved in the response to viral infections [9]. Monocyte-derived or inflammatory DCs, such as TNF and iNOS-producing DCs, originate from monocytes during the inflammatory response [9, 38]. A more detailed discussion of DC subsets is outside the scope of this chapter, but there are several recent articles on this topic [35, 39].

Granulocytes

Polymorphonuclear leukocytes (PMNs or neutrophils) are the most numerous circulating leukocytes in humans and are the most prominent cellular defense against bacterial and fungal infections. Indeed, 60% of the cells in bone marrow are granulocytes or granulocyte precursors, and ~60% of white cells in human blood are neutrophils [40]. Neutrophils and eosinophils are identified readily by cytochemistry and phenotype (e.g., nuclear morphology). Under steady-state conditions, neutrophils develop in bone marrow for ~14 days (5–6 days excluding mitotic precursors), circulate in blood for a day, and then enter tissues, where they remain for another 1–2 days before undergoing apoptosis [40, 41]. Compared to mononuclear phagocytes, especially macrophages, the lifespan of mature neutrophils is short. They are terminally differentiated end cells. However, this short lifespan is offset by the tremendous number of cells produced during hematopoiesis. Neutrophil turnover in humans is approximately 10^{11} cells per day in an average healthy adult [41, 42]. Such turnover is remarkable, and a mechanism dependent on the mononuclear phagocyte system is in place to remove dead and dying neutrophils from tissues, thereby maintaining immune system homeostasis.

The myeloblast is an early neutrophil precursor cell and is followed in sequence by the promyelocyte, myelocyte, metamyelocyte, band cell, and mature neutrophil [40]. As neutrophils mature in bone marrow, they develop protein machinery and specialized organelles known as granules that are necessary for microbicidal activity. Azurophilic or primary granules (peroxidase-positive granules) appear first during granulopoiesis and contain numerous antimicrobial peptides and proteins, including myeloperoxidase, alpha defensins, elastase, cathepsin G, proteinase 3, and azurocidin [43, 44]. Azurophilic granules are synthesized largely during the promyelocyte stage of cell development. Specific granules, gelatinase granules, and secretory vesicles, which are peroxidase-negative, appear after azurophilic granules during neutrophil development in bone marrow [40]. The membranes of the specific and gelatinase granules and those of the secretory vesicles contain receptors and other membrane-bound proteins important for virtually all neutrophil functions. For example, at least 90% of neutrophil gp91*phox*/p22*phox* heterodimer (flavocytochrome b_{558}), which forms the nidus of the superoxide-generating NADPH oxidase in neutrophils, is located in the membranes of these granules [45, 46]. These organelles serve as storage compartments for the molecules required for neutrophil microbicidal activity, which is discussed below. Although mature neutrophils are fully equipped with the molecules required for PMN microbicidal activity, they retain some biosynthetic capacity [45]. Importantly, neutrophil production can be rapidly increased as needed, as, for example, during severe systemic bacterial or fungal infections. This process is known as emergency granulopoiesis [14, 47].

Basophils, eosinophils, and mast cells are granulocytes that participate in innate and acquired immunity. They are key cells in the response to allergens and function as antigen-presenting cells [29, 48, 49]. Basophils are not typically considered as phagocytes and will not be discussed further [48]. Eosinophils and mast cells can phagocytose microbes, but phagocytic capacity is either significantly less than that of other phagocytes or incompletely characterized and the role in vivo not fully understood [29, 49, 50]. The ability of eosinophils to kill bacteria has also been linked to extracellular release of cytotoxic molecules [51, 52]. These leukocytes, like basophils, are known historically for their role in the host defense against parasites, especially helminths [49, 53]. Mast cell precursors develop in bone marrow and then migrate to tissues, where they differentiate and mature (Fig. 1.1) [29, 54]. Mast cells are long-lived cells that have been reported to phagocytose and kill multiple bacterial species [55]. However, the in vivo significance of this direct bactericidal activity remains unknown, and these cells are more characterized for their ability to coordinate immune and allergic responses. For simplicity, much of the discussion of phagocyte function is based on studies with mononuclear phagocytes and neutrophils. For those interested in a more detailed review of basophils, eosinophils, and mast cells, we recommend specific articles on these cell types [29, 48–50, 53, 56, 57].

Recruitment, Chemotaxis, and Priming

The rapid recruitment of phagocytes to damaged tissue is critical for an effective inflammatory response. Circulating phagocytes must quickly

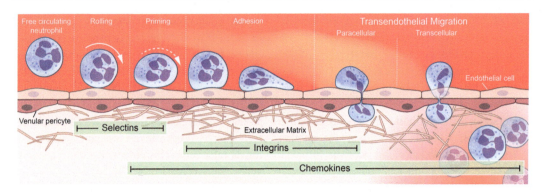

Fig. 1.2 Neutrophil chemotaxis and transmigration. Migration of neutrophils from blood to infected or injured tissues is characterized by four distinct stages: rolling, priming, adhesion, and transendothelial cell migration. Chemokines and other chemoattractants promote neutrophil rolling and priming, which in turn leads to integrin-dependent interactions. Selectins and integrins present on the endothelium and neutrophils promote neutrophil adhesion and transendothelial migration

recognize danger signals emanating from distressed host cells, efficiently breach the postcapillary venule wall, and immigrate to the site of tissue damage to successfully resolve host injury. Phagocyte extravasation, namely, the migration from circulation into extravascular tissue, follows a process referred to as the leukocyte adhesion cascade that can be divided into four primary events: rolling, priming, adhesion, and transendothelial cell migration (TEM) (Fig. 1.2) [58, 59]. These events are largely coordinated by a hierarchical chemokine gradient and through direct interactions with activated host cells that act in concert to sequentially recruit specific phagocyte subsets to the site of host insult [60–62]. Following extravasation, phagocytes are transformed from patrolling sentinel cells in circulation to fully activated effector cells that play critical roles in orchestrating subsequent immune responses, destroying pathogens, and removing unwanted debris.

Rolling

Circulating phagocytes appear to roll along the wall of postcapillary venules as they near the site of host tissue distress. This rolling motion is primarily mediated by the transient on and off binding of cell surface molecules called selectins under the shear-force conditions encountered in postcapillary venules [63]. There are three members of the selectin family, with the nomenclature of these molecules indicating the cell type in which they were first identified (E for endothelia, L for leukocytes, and P for platelets). Selectins bind to glycosylated proteins on the surface of adjacent host cells. Although P-selectin glycoprotein ligand 1 (PSGL1) was first identified as a ligand for P-selectin, this molecule is now known to be a primary ligand for all three selectins. E-selectin on endothelial cells also binds to E-selectin ligand 1 (ESL1) and glycosylated CD44 on the surface of phagocytes. Surface expression of selectins is varied among cell types and is dependent on the activation state of the cell. These expression attributes facilitate efficient targeting of phagocytes to specific sites of host tissue inflammation. The constitutive expression of L-selectin by circulating phagocytes largely mediates rolling at high velocities. In contrast, E-selectin is only expressed by activated endothelial cells early during the inflammatory response and acts to decrease the velocity of phagocytes as they near injured tissue. As the velocity of rolling phagocytes decreases, signals localized near the site of compromised host tissue enhance the activation state of these cells in a process referred to as priming.

Priming

Phagocytes in circulation detect relatively low concentrations of host- and/or microbe-derived signaling molecules, such as chemokines, cytokines, and bacterial N-formylated peptides, as they near the site of damaged tissue or infection. These molecules can "prime" phagocytes for enhanced function, and this phenomenon has been investigated extensively in neutrophils [64]. Priming of neutrophils was described originally as the ability of a primary agonist (at sub-stimulatory concentrations) to enhance or influence production of superoxide in response to a second stimulus [65, 66]. It is now known that priming enhances multiple neutrophil functions, including adhesion, phagocytosis, superoxide production, and degranulation [64, 67]. In general, neutrophil priming promotes the timely recruitment of these leukocytes to damaged and infected tissues and enhances capacity to destroy infectious microbes.

Many molecules that promote phagocyte priming contain molecular moieties that are normally absent or concealed in the healthy host but are exposed during infection and injury. For example, infectious agents generate structurally conserved molecules that display pathogen-associated molecular patterns (PAMPs) [68]. These molecules include lipopolysaccharide (LPS) or muramyl dipeptide specific to bacteria, double-stranded RNA that comprises the genome of certain viruses, or β-glucan located on the surface of fungi. Alternatively, sterile injury induces the release of damage-associated molecular patterns (DAMPs) that are normally confined within the cytosol of host cells [69]. High-mobility group box 1 (HMGB1) and cytosolic heat-shock proteins are examples of DAMPs released by necrotic cells [69]. PAMPs and DAMPs are recognized by a number of cell surface and cytosolic receptors that are collectively referred to as pattern recognition receptors (PRRs) [69]. These molecules include the Toll-like receptors, scavenger receptors [70], and C-type lectin receptors (e.g., the mannose receptor and Dectin-1) located on the cell surface or within endolysosomes, as well as the NOD-like receptors and RIG-like receptors that are only found within the cytosol and act to recognize infection by intracellular pathogens. Phagocytes generally express a large number of PRRs, and they play a major role in recognizing host injury, immune surveillance, and directing subsequent immune responses. Other resident tissue cells, such as endothelial cells and keratinocytes, express PRRs to a lesser degree and can also alert the immune system to tissue insult [71].

In addition to priming of recruited phagocytes, engagement of PRRs with corresponding ligands activates pathways that increase local cytokine concentrations. These molecules contribute to the ongoing inflammatory process, which includes continued recruitment of phagocytes and other leukocytes toward the site of tissue damage. In humans, CXC-chemokine ligand 8 (CXCL8 or IL-8) is a major cytokine that influences neutrophil recruitment and activation [60], while CC-chemokine ligand 2 (CCL2) plays an important role during monocyte recruitment to inflamed tissue [72]. Cytokines released by stimulated host cells bind to glycosaminoglycans (GAGs) such as heparin sulfate that are located on the surface of endothelial cells and attached to the extracellular matrix [59, 61]. As phagocytes travel through circulation, they encounter increasing concentrations of chemokines that are presented on the surface of vascular endothelium as they approach distressed tissue. These chemokines bind to cognate G-coupled-protein receptors on the surface of rolling phagocytes and induce very rapid cellular changes that result in arrest and firm adhesion to the postcapillary venule wall near the site of host injury.

Adhesion

The arrest and firm adhesion of circulating phagocytes in response to chemokines expressed at the site of distressed host tissue is mediated by the activation and binding of integrins. Integrins are a class of heterodimeric cell surface proteins consisting of α and β subunits. In mammals, 18 α subunits and 8 β subunits have been identified that give rise to at least 24 different types of integrins [73]. The binding of activated integrins expressed by phagocytes to immunoglobulin superfamily members on the surface of activated endothelial cells is imperative for firm adhesion of phagocytes to the vascular endothelium. Integrins and ligands that are important during this process include integrins $\alpha_M\beta_2$ (CD11b/CD18 or Mac-1) and $\alpha_L\beta_2$ (CD11a/CD18, also known as leukocyte function-associated antigen 1 or LFA-1), which bind to intercellular adhesion molecule 1 (ICAM-1) on endothelial cells, and $\alpha_4\beta_1$ (also known as very late antigen 4 or VLA-4) which binds vascular intercellular adhesion molecule 1 (VCAM-1) [73, 74]. In general, the integrins of unprimed circulating phagocytes are not in an active state. In a process termed inside-out signaling, the recognition of chemokines by G protein-coupled receptors on rolling phagocytes rapidly increases the avidity of integrins, resulting in almost immediate cell arrest via adhesion to adjacent activated endothelial cells [75].

The avidity of integrin-mediated adhesion is dependent upon the affinity of individual integrin molecules for their ligands and by the distribution of integrins on the cell surface [76]. Inactive integrins are diffusely spread on the cell membrane and hold a bent conformation with the binding region tightly pressed against the membrane surface, resulting in a low affinity for corresponding ligands. Inside-out signaling through activated G protein-coupled chemokine receptors quickly opens this bent conformation, exposing the integrin-binding domain to allow high-affinity interactions with ligands. Inside-out signaling also induces integrin clustering, further increasing the overall avidity of these molecules for ligands on the surface of endothelial cells.

When clustered integrins bind to corresponding ligands, changes are induced in the cytoplasmic domain of these molecules that activate intercellular tyrosine kinase-dependent signaling pathways in a process referred to as outside-in signaling [77]. Activation of these pathways leads to rearrangement of the phagocyte actin cytoskeleton that flattens the cell against the vessel wall, increasing surface area contact with the

vascular endothelium and enabling sustained adherence under sheer-flow conditions. In addition, outside-in signaling further primes phagocytes by mobilizing factors that are important for antimicrobial activity and TEM into the extravascular space.

Transendothelial Cell Migration

Primed phagocytes that are firmly adhered to activated vasculature endothelium must exit the capillary lumen to reach compromised host tissue and perform effector immune functions. As with previous steps in the leukocyte adhesion cascade, this process is largely directed by increasing concentrations of different chemotactic factors in conjunction with signals derived from direct interactions with activated host cells [78]. Collectively these cues orchestrate the migration of phagocytes between or even through activated endothelial cells lining the postcapillary venule wall, across the underlying endothelial basement membrane, and through the extravascular space to the site of distressed tissue.

Once phagocytes rolling through circulation have become firmly adhered to activated endothelium, they will often crawl in an amoeba-like fashion along the capillary lumen wall in search of suitable extravasation sites. Neutrophil and monocyte crawling requires interactions between integrin $\alpha_M\beta_2$ (Mac-1) with ICAM-1 on the surface of activated endothelium [59]. Forward cell displacement during crawling is dependent upon the reorganization of the phagocyte actin cytoskeleton and the polarization of intracellular signaling proteins, surface receptors, and adhesion molecules across the cell. On the leading edge of crawling phagocytes, new bonds are formed with adhesive molecules on the surface of activated vascular endothelium, while bonds at the trailing end are simultaneously broken. As phagocytes crawl, they extend pseudopods that probe the vessel wall for chemotactic factors and signals from underlying activated endothelial cells that indicate optimum sites for TEM.

The majority of phagocytes crossing the endothelial layer pass through the junctions between vascular endothelial cells in a process termed paracellular TEM [61]. A number of adhesion molecules expressed by both phagocytes and endothelial cells are important for paracellular TEM. These include platelet-endothelial cell adhesion molecule-1 (PECAM-1 or CD31), junctional adhesion molecules A and C (JAM-A and JAM-C), and CD99 [79]. VE-cadherin expressed by endothelial cells plays an important role in maintaining tight junctions between adjacent cells, and the expression of this molecule deters paracellular TEM [80]. Phagocytes can also pass directly through endothelial cells in a process referred to as transcellular TEM. In some instances recruited phagocytes prefer the transcellular path, such as TEM across brain vasculature endothelium that maintain very tight junctions between adjacent cells [61].

Migrating phagocytes that have crossed the vascular endothelium encounter the next major barrier during extravasation—the underlying basement membrane that ensheathes postcapillary venules. The basement membrane is composed of elongated mural cells termed venular pericytes imbedded in a complex layer of extracellular matrix proteins that include collagen IV, various laminins, and glycoproteins such as nidogens and perlecan [78]. Immigrating phagocytes preferentially breach the basement membrane between venular pericytes at areas where the density of extracellular matrix proteins is low. The expression of integrin ligands such as ICAM-1 by venular pericytes allows migrating phagocytes to use these cells as an adhesive substrate for traversing the basement membrane toward these extravasation hot spots [61]. Perivascular macrophages residing in the extravascular region adjacent to the basement membrane are thought to guide migrating phagocytes toward areas of optimal extravasation via the expression of chemokines such as CXCL1 and CXCL2 [78].

Once migrating phagocytes have breached the basement membrane, they crawl through the interstitial space toward increasing concentrations of so-called end-stage chemotactic factors [78, 80]. These molecules, which include formylated peptides and complement protein C5a, take precedence over other chemotactic factors and play a dominant role guiding phagocytes through the interstitial space directly to the site of host tissue injury.

Phagocytosis and Microbicidal Activity

The ability of phagocytes to ingest and subsequently kill invading microbial pathogens is paramount to maintenance of host health. Phagocytosis is functionally defined as the intracellular uptake of particles greater than 0.5 μm in diameter and is primarily executed by neutrophils and mononuclear phagocytes (monocytes, macrophages, and dendritic cells). Phagocytes have an enormous capacity for ingestion, and surface area can increase up to 300% for neutrophils and 600% for macrophages [81]. The process of phagocytosis is highly complex and can be conceptually divided into two different phases: recognition and binding and internalization.

Phagocytosis

Phagocyte recognition of invading microbial pathogens is mediated by receptors present on the outer surface of the host cell membrane. There are two primary types of receptors that are used to recognize microorganisms: (1) PRRs, which directly recognize microbial-derived structures, and (2) opsonic receptors, which recognize host proteins that are deposited on the microbial surface. Ligation of PRRs initiates a complex series of signal transduction cascades that modulate phagocyte effector functions such as enhanced phagocytosis, killing, and regulation of inflammation via cytokine production. Ligation of PRRs is generally insufficient to promote phagocytosis directly, but there are exceptions (e.g., Dectin-1 is a PRR that binds fungal β-glucans and promotes ingestion of bound fungi) [82–84]. Phagocytosis is most efficient in the presence of opsonins—soluble host molecules that promote uptake—of which specific IgG and complement are the major constituents and phagocyte recognition of these molecules directly mediates uptake (Fig. 1.3). IgG bound to the microbial surface activates the classical complement pathway and leads to deposition of complement C3 and derivatives. In addition, C3 can be deposited on the microbial surface following activation of the alternative pathway or the mannose-binding lectin pathway. Neutrophils and mononuclear phagocytes express distinct receptors for IgG (FcγRI, FcγRII, and FcγRIII) [85] and opsonic complement molecules C3b and C3bi (CR1, CR3, and CR4). Receptors that contribute to phagocytosis have varied affinities for target ligands. For example, FcγRI is a high-affinity receptor, whereas FcγRII and FcγRIII are constitutively expressed low- to moderate-affinity receptors. Integrins such as $\alpha_M\beta_2$ (CR3, CD11b/CD18, Mac-1), by contrast, dynamically equilibrate between conformational states on the cell surface—a closed conformation with low affinity and an open conformation with high affinity [86].

CR3 ligand affinity can increase following cell activation by inflammatory mediators such as tumor necrosis factor-α, LPS, and platelet-activating factor [87]. Efficient particle binding is enhanced by the engagement (simultaneous or sequential) of multiple receptors (of similar or differing types) on the phagocyte surface. In addition, elaboration of cellular extensions such as membrane ruffles [88] and macrophage filopodia [89] facilitate target binding by an actin-dependent mechanism [90], and membrane protrusions can be enhanced by stimulation of PRRs [88, 91].

Engagement of phagocyte receptors initiates a complex series of molecular signals that contribute to internalization of microbes or some other target object (e.g., debris) and is followed by complete activation of antimicrobial systems. There is inherent diversity in signaling between phagocyte receptors, and the variability in signals

Fig. 1.3 Neutrophil phagocytosis and microbicidal processes. Binding and ingestion of microbes (phagocytosis) are mediated optimally by host opsonins such as serum complement and antibody. Phagocytosis triggers fusion of cytoplasmic granules with the newly formed phagosome, thereby enriching the phagocytic vacuole with antimicrobial agents. Granule-phagosome fusion is followed by assembly and activation of NADPH oxidase. The NADPH oxidase produces superoxide ($O_2^{\bullet-}$), which in turn leads to the production of hypochlorous acid (HOCl) and other reactive oxygen species (ROS)

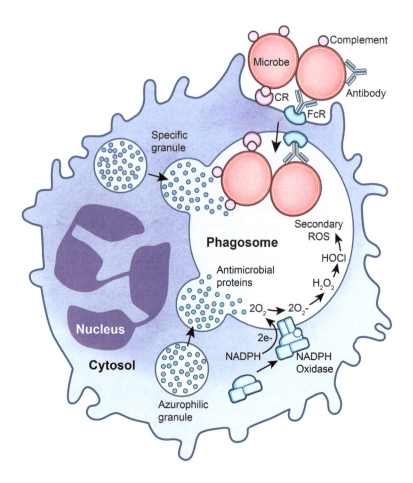

transduced extends to cell type-specific differences elicited by the same receptor. Although a detailed compendium on phagocyte receptor signal transduction is beyond the scope of this section (for reviews on the topic, see [92, 93]), we highlight features of FcR-mediated signaling elicited by a prototypical phagocytosis receptor. The complex signals govern cellular processes such as membrane reorganization and cytoskeletal remodeling that are required for phagocytosis. The cytosolic domain of the Fc receptor contains a region known as the immunoreceptor tyrosine-based activation motif (ITAM), which serves as a substrate for phosphorylation by tyrosine kinases of the Src family such as Lyn and Hck [94]. The signaling cascade is amplified by spleen tyrosine kinase (Syk), a cytosolic kinase essential for phagocytosis [95], and is followed by recruitment of adapter proteins and activation of lipid-modifying enzymes such as phosphatidylinositol 3-kinase and small GTPases [96]. Actin polymerization is requisite for phagocytosis and is facilitated by the Arp2/3 nucleator complex, a seven-protein complex that nucleates branched actin filaments. Actin polymerization, in conjunction with progressive FcR binding, provides the cytoskeletal framework to advance the phagocyte plasma membrane over the particle. Actin is concentrated at the tips of the advancing membrane cup during particle internalization, and depolymerization of actin occurs at the base of the cup. In addition, several classes of myosin, including myosin X, have been implicated in execution of FcR-mediated phagocytosis [97]. Although the final stage of particle internalization requires sealing of the opposing membrane leaflets to complete formation of the nascent vacuole, little is known about the mechanism of closure.

Maturation of Phagosomes

The newly formed phagosome lacks quintessential antimicrobial properties, and its lumen resembles the extracellular environment. To assemble microbicidal machinery and acquire antimicrobial properties, the nascent phagosome undergoes a dynamic process of maturation. In macrophages, this process starts immediately after the phagosome is sealed and is dependent on the endocytic pathway. In mononuclear phagocytes, nascent phagosomes fuse with early endosomes, followed by fusion with late endosomes and lysosomes, to yield a hybrid vacuole called phagolysosome. For simplicity, the terms phagosome and phagolysosome will be used interchangeably. Sequential early and late endosome-phagosome fusion events progressively acidify the lumen of the macrophage phagosome largely by incorporating vacuolar ATPase complexes (V-ATPases) [98]. This is followed by fusion of phagosomes with lysosomes, which, in turn, enrich the vacuole lumen with lysosomal proteases and other hydrolytic enzymes. The pH of the mature macrophage phagosome is ~5–6 [99–101], which is optimal for lysosomal protease activity [102]. In contrast to macrophages, the pH of the DC phagosome is near neutral, if not slightly alkaline (pH 7.0–7.6). This attribute of DCs is due to the comparatively limited phagosomal V-ATPase activity and sustained intraphagosomal production of superoxide by NADPH oxidase, a process that consumes protons [100]. More recent studies suggest NADPH oxidase alters the redox capacity of DC phagosomes and thereby controls proteolysis (of antigens) mediated by cysteine proteases [103]. In addition, DC lysosomes have reduced levels of proteases and associated proteolytic activity compared with those of macrophages [104]. From a functional standpoint, DC antigen processing and presentation are optimal in phagosomes that maintain near neutral/slightly basic pH and have limited lysosomal protease activity [100, 104, 105]. It is noteworthy that not all studies agree about the pH of the DC phagosome or the mechanism by which proteolysis is regulated [100, 103]. This may be a reflection of differences in DC subsets.

In contrast to mononuclear phagocytes [106], in which phagosome maturation involves the endocytic pathway to a significant extent, maturation of neutrophil phagosomes is based largely on fusion with specialized granules. Neutrophils can undergo granule exocytosis (also called degranulation), whereby the granules mobilize to and fuse with the plasma membrane, and release their contents into the extracellular space. Alternatively, granules fuse with forming phagosomes, and the lumen and membrane are enriched with granule proteins. In the resting state, human neutrophils in circulation have limited capacity to interface with the external environment, as there are relatively few proinflammatory receptors present on the cell surface. However, this attribute changes rapidly upon exposure to very low levels of host or microbe-derived proinflammatory molecules, such as chemokines or PAMPs. The cytoplasmic granules and secretory vesicles fuse with membranes in a hierarchy that is stimulus and calcium threshold dependent: secretory vesicles are mobilized first, followed by tertiary granules (gelatinase granules), secondary granules (specific or beta granules), and ultimately primary granules (azurophilic or alpha granules) [43]. Consistent with their ability to mobilize readily, secretory vesicles enrich the cell surface with receptors and other molecules needed for chemotaxis, transmigration, and microbicidal activity. The primary and secondary granules were known traditionally as peroxidase-positive and peroxidase-negative granules, respectively, nomenclature that reflects the presence and absence of myeloperoxidase (MPO). As indicated above, these granules contain antimicrobial peptides and enzymes required for oxygen-dependent and oxygen-independent killing of microbes by neutrophils. For a more comprehensive review of neutrophil granule synthesis, content, and mobilization, we refer the reader to excellent articles on the topic [43, 44, 107].

Compared with macrophages, there are fewer V-ATPase channels in neutrophil phagosome membranes early after ingestion, and the activity of these molecules is inhibited by reactive oxygen species [108, 109]. Notably, the pH of neutrophil phagosomes is near neutral (pH ~7.2) [99]. Although not all findings concur about the initial pH of neutrophil phagosomes, neutral pH in the phagocytic vacuole is needed for optimal bactericidal activity, and proton channel activity is required to offset charge differential caused by production of superoxide by NADPH oxidase

(see below) [99, 109–112]. Moreover, charge compensation in neutrophils is essential for optimal NADPH oxidase activity, and protons are needed for subsequent formation of hydrogen peroxide (H_2O_2) and hypochlorous acid (HOCl), each of which is important for oxygen-dependent killing of microbes [110]. In the end, multiple factors contribute to regulation of phagosome pH and function, including vesicle fusion events, production of superoxide, redox potential, recruitment of V-ATPases, and proton channel activity, each of which appears specific to phagocyte function and type [113].

Production of Reactive Oxygen Species

Professional phagocytes use oxygen-dependent and oxygen-independent processes to eliminate ingested microorganisms. Phagocytes have two main oxygen-dependent antimicrobial systems: NADPH oxidase and inducible nitric oxide synthase (iNOS). NADPH oxidase is a multicomponent enzyme complex that produces superoxide in activated cells. In unactivated cells, NADPH oxidase components are segregated in membrane and cytosolic compartments. Flavocytochrome b_{558} is a heterodimeric transmembrane protein comprised of gp91*phox* (NOX2) and p22*phox* subunits; it contains the electron transport machinery for the enzyme complex and forms the nidus of the assembling oxidase at the plasma or phagosome membrane. p47*phox*, p67*phox*, p40*phox*, and the small GTPase Rac (Rac1 or Rac2) are oxidase components located in the cytosol of resting cells. Upon phagocyte activation, p47*phox*, p67*phox*, and p40*phox* translocate to the plasma or phagosome membrane en bloc and interact directly with flavocytochrome b_{558}. Rac translocates to the membrane independent of the other cytosolic components and, in turn, associates with components (p67*phox* and flavocytochrome b_{558}) of the assembling enzyme complex [113]. NADPH oxidase catalyzes the transfer of electrons from cytosolic NADPH to molecular oxygen, thereby producing $O_2^{\bullet-}$. Although $O_2^{\bullet-}$ is weakly microbicidal, it is rapidly converted to other, more effective reactive oxygen species, including H_2O_2, hydroxyl radical, and HOCl (for more details see refs [45, 114]). For example, MPO catalyzes a reaction with H_2O_2 and chloride to generate HOCl, the main active ingredient in household bleach [115–117]. The high consumption of oxygen followed by generation of ROS is often termed "respiratory burst" [118, 119]. ROS cause damage to proteins, membrane lipids, and nucleic acids and are thus highly cytotoxic. Inasmuch as these ROS can cause non-specific damage to host tissues, production of ROS must be tightly regulated and contained within the confines of the phagosome. The NADPH oxidase is essential for competent host defense against bacterial and fungal infections. Chronic granulomatous disease is inherited defects in components of this enzyme system that predispose individuals to severe and/or fatal bacterial and fungal infections.

Production of Reactive Nitrogen Species

Compared with neutrophils, mononuclear phagocytes produce less NADPH oxidase-derived ROS. However, mononuclear phagocytes have the capacity to produce relatively high levels of reactive nitrogen species (RNS), which are generated by iNOS (NOS2). iNOS is one of the three isoforms of NOS present in mammalian cells (the other two isoforms are neural NOS and endothelial NOS). Unlike NADPH oxidase, which is assembled immediately upon appropriate signal transduction, proteins of the iNOS complex are synthesized de novo in phagocytes. Synthesis of iNOS requires signaling from pattern recognition receptors or stimulation from proinflammatory cytokines. iNOS catalyzes a two-step reaction in which L-arginine is transformed to NO• and citrulline in the presence of oxygen and NADPH [120, 121]. Nitric oxide and its derivatives (e.g., nitrogen dioxide, nitrosothiol, or nitrite) can inhibit bacterial DNA replication and bacterial respiration, and it additionally potentiates ROS-mediated killing [122]. The iNOS system is important for host defense against intracellular pathogens, such as mycobacteria and *Salmonella* [123, 124].

Oxygen-Independent Antimicrobial Systems

Oxygen-independent antimicrobial systems utilize antimicrobial peptides and enzymes to facilitate killing and degradation of ingested microbes. In neutrophils, antimicrobial peptides and proteins are stored largely in azurophilic granules (primary granules) and specific granules (secondary granules) [45]. For example, alpha defensins [125–127], bactericidal/permeability-increasing protein (BPI), azurocidin, cathepsin G, elastase, and proteinase 3 are contained within the azurophilic granules [128, 129], whereas lactoferrin, phospholipase A2, and the cathelicidin hCAP-18 [130] are stored in the specific granules [43]. Lysozyme, an antimicrobial enzyme well-known for its ability to degrade bacterial peptidoglycan, is contained within each of these granule subtypes. We discuss a few signature molecules that contribute to microbicidal functions of neutrophils.

Mature, processed human neutrophil alpha defensins are cationic peptides 30–33 amino acid residues in length (and 3–4 kDa) [131]. These peptides were originally named human neutrophil peptides 1–4 (HNP1–4), and HNP1–3 constitute up to 50% of the protein in azurophilic granules and 5–7% of protein in human neutrophils [131, 132]. It is estimated that the average adult produces 250 mg of alpha defensins each day to accommodate normal neutrophil turnover. Thus, they are abundant molecules. It is well-known that cationic peptides—including alpha defensins—disrupt bacterial membranes, which in turn kills the target microbe. In the context of bacteria, HNPs bind negatively charged components of the membrane, such as anionic phospholipids. That said, HNPs kill microbes by virtue of both cationic and hydrophobic properties, although the mechanism is varied depending on the specific microorganism [131]. It is worth noting that mouse neutrophils lack alpha defensins, thus underscoring differences between human and murine innate immune systems.

BPI is a cationic protein (~55 kDa) that binds LPS with high affinity, kills Gram-negative bacteria, and can opsonize bacteria for enhanced phagocytosis [128, 133, 134]. The interaction of BPI with the lipid A moiety of LPS ultimately causes membrane destruction, which in turn leads to bacterial death [133]. Moreover, LPS with bound BPI is not recognized by the innate immune system, and therefore, BPI neutralizes the host responses to LPS [133]. Functions of BPI extend beyond a role in innate immunity and are reviewed elsewhere [135].

Azurocidin, cathepsin G, elastase, and proteinase 3 are cationic serine proteases collectively known as serprocidins. They have microbicidal activity in vitro, contribute to host defense in vivo, and, except for azurocidin (also known as CAP37), have serine protease activity [136–142]. Serine protease activity is optimum at neutral or slightly basic pH, and the traditional view is that these molecules are kept inactive by the negatively charged proteoglycan matrix of the azurophil granule lumen [143]. This idea has been challenged recently, but no alternative regulatory mechanism has been reported [144]. Importantly, the serine proteases become active when they are released into the extracellular environment (and/or bound to the leukocyte surface) or the neutrophil phagosome following granule exocytosis or granule-phagosome fusion, respectively [137, 145]. Serine protease activity can contribute to breakdown of microbial proteins, such as the degradation of *Escherichia coli* outer membrane protein A by elastase, which kills the bacterium [136, 146]. These proteases are also important for the proteolytic processing of host molecules involved in host defense [145, 147–149]. For example, proteinase 3 enzymatically cleaves hCAP18, which is released from the lumen of specific granules, to generate the LL-37, a potent antimicrobial peptide [150]. In addition, IL-1β and IL-18 can be activated by neutrophil proteinase 3, processes previously ascribed uniquely to caspase-1 [151].

The antimicrobial activity of cathepsin G and elastase was originally reported as independent of serine protease activity [139, 152–154]. For example, *Neisseria gonorrhoeae* is readily killed by cathepsin G that has been rendered enzymatically inactive by diisopropyl fluorophosphate, a potent serine protease inhibitor [154]. The highly cationic nature of neutrophil serine proteases likely explains at least in part their ability to kill microbes independent of enzymatic activity [155].

Although neutrophil serine proteases contribute prominently to host defense, they can readily degrade host proteins and facilitate the breakdown of tissues and thereby play an important role in the pathogenesis of inflammatory diseases [145, 156]. This attribute highlights the need to have mechanisms in place to regulate neutrophil turnover and removal.

Extracellular Traps (ETs)

Extracellular traps (ETs) are decondensed strands of DNA that are extruded from leukocytes into the extracellular environment. These weblike structures were first identified with neutrophils and were therefore named neutrophil extracellular traps (NETs) [157]. More recently, mast cells [158], monocytes/macrophages [159, 160], DCs [161], basophils [162, 163], and eosinophils [51] have been shown to release ETs. ETs can be elicited by microbial products and/or a wide variety of microorganisms, including bacteria, fungi, protozoa, and viruses (Fig. 1.4). Host-derived molecules or pharmacological agents can also induce ETs. Inasmuch as there is a relatively large base of published works on the topic of NETs, here we use that information for the purpose of elaborating the role of ETs in host defense and disease.

NETs constitute a three-dimensional scaffold containing histones and antimicrobial proteins from granules and the cytoplasm. In general, NETs (and other ETs) ensnare microbes and thereby contribute to host defense [157, 164]. Whether there is significant killing of microbes by ETs versus binding/entrapping alone remains a topic of debate [165–167]. The bactericidal activity of ETs appears to be microbe-specific, and some microbes produce molecules that facilitate evasion of killing by these structures [157, 168–191]. In addition, formation of NETs is dictated by size of the microbe; i.e., microbes too large for phagocytosis elicit NETs [192]. NETs

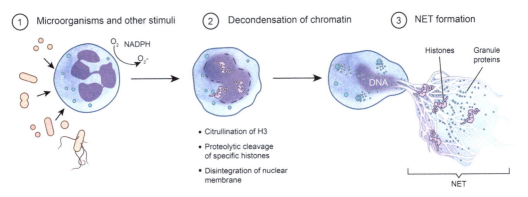

① Microorganisms and other stimuli ② Decondensation of chromatin ③ NET formation

O₂ NADPH
O₂⁻

Histones Granule proteins

DNA

• Citrullination of H3
• Proteolytic cleavage of specific histones
• Disintegration of nuclear membrane

NET

Fig. 1.4 Formation of NETs. Microorganisms and/or other stimuli or conditions can trigger formation of neutrophil extracellular traps (NETs). Formation of NETs has been associated with activation of NADPH oxidase, decondensation of chromatin, mixing of neutrophil granule proteins with nuclear DNA, and lysis of neutrophils. This process releases the DNA that forms NETs

were initially reported to form during a unique type of cell death named NETosis [193, 194]. During NETosis, neutrophil chromatin decondenses, and the nuclear membrane disintegrates [195], which, in turn, promotes association of cytosolic and granule proteins with DNA [193]. During this cell death process, neutrophil elastase translocates to the nucleus, where it facilitates proteolytic cleavage of specific histones, including core histone H4. This phenomenon leads directly to chromatin decondensation [194]. The chromatin decondensation process is enhanced by MPO and deimination of the histone H3 arginine residue to citrulline, which is catalyzed by peptidyl arginine deiminase type 4 (PAD4) [194, 196, 197]. It is important to note that NETs can also form from viable cells [198, 199], or alternatively, during non-specific osmotic lysis of neutrophils [200]. The mechanisms underlying these phenomena remain incompletely determined.

Although ETs can contribute to host defense, they are also associated with—or directly promote—host pathology [165, 201–204]. This is especially true for NETs, since lysis of neutrophils and release of cytotoxic molecules is known to cause non-specific host tissue damage. For example, NETs are associated with airway obstruction during inflammatory lung diseases and respiratory tract infections [205–208]. In addition, NETs have been implicated in the pathogenesis of Alzheimer's disease [209], atherosclerosis [210], rheumatoid arthritis [211, 212], cancer progression [213, 214], sickle-cell disease [215], thrombosis [216–218], and systemic lupus erythematosus [219–222]. Therefore, it is not surprising that precise mechanisms are in place to facilitate clearance of effete neutrophils and maintain immune system homeostasis, and these processes likely prevent or moderate NET-associated pathology.

Antigen Presentation

In addition to functions that are imperative for innate immunity, phagocytes play key roles in generating an effective adaptive immune response. In particular, the process of antigen presentation by DCs is critical for T cell activation and the initiation of adaptive immunity [223]. This process requires the capture and processing of antigen from insulted host tissue, migration through lymphatic vessels to secondary lymph tissue, and presentation of antigen to resting T cells via major histocompatibility complexes (MHCs). Additionally, DCs convey the nature of host insult corresponding to the antigen that is presented to T cells during the generation of an appropriate adaptive immune response [224–226].

Macrophages, DCs, and B cells are all considered professional antigen-presenting cells (APCs). However, DCs are the most potent APCs and are a major source of T cell activation.

Immature DCs are constantly examining the peripheral tissue lining the host-environment interface, such as the skin, gastrointestinal tract, and lung, for signals indicating a compromise of host integrity. These immune sentinels express high levels of PRRs that are used to identify a variety PAMPs and DAMPs present in impaired host tissue. The binding of specific PRRs and detection of cytokines that are associated with particular types of host tissue insult induce immature DCs to take specialized avenues of maturation. Antigen that is associated with the stimulus that caused DC activation is processed and prepared for presentation. Different types of host tissue distress drive corresponding DC maturation programs that direct appropriate T cell activation during antigen presentation.

The internalization of microbial antigens by DCs is accomplished through phagocytosis-, macropinocytosis-, and receptor-mediated endocytosis [227, 228]. As opposed to the highly proteolytic phagosome of neutrophils or macrophage, the antigen-processing compartments of activated DCs are optimized to generate partially digested peptides that are suitable for presentation to T cells (see above) [228, 229]. APCs present antigen-derived peptides on both MHC class I and MHC class II molecules that activate antigen-specific CD4+T cells and CD8+ T cells, respectively [230]. In general, processed antigen acquired from endogenous sources is presented on MHC class II molecules, while MHC class I molecules present antigen derived from intercellular sources that have undergone proteasome processing. However, peptides captured from the extracellular environment can also be loaded onto MHC class I molecules in a phenomenon known as cross-presentation [227, 231–234]. The CD8+ subset of DCs are particularly adept at cross-presentation of exogenous antigens on MHC class I molecules relative to CD8− DCs [232, 235].

Activated DCs migrate from peripheral tissue to secondary lymph tissue, transporting their antigen-derived peptide cargo to T cells for presentation. The mechanisms by which DCs exit peripheral tissue and migrate through afferent lymph vessels to the draining lymph node are not entirely understood [236]. However, it is known that the expression of chemokine receptor CCR7 by activated DCs is required for efficient migration and the expression of integrins such as $\alpha_M\beta_2$ (LFA-1) by DCs also play important roles in this process [237]. Mature DCs that have arrived in secondary lymph tissue present antigen-derived peptide loaded onto cell surface MHC molecules to naïve T cells. T cells with an antigen-specific T cell receptor (TCR) that recognizes presented antigen directly associate with these DCs and form what is termed the immunological synapse at the interface between these cells.

The association of the TCR with peptide presented by MHC molecules alone is insufficient for T cell activation. The binding of some T cell co-receptors with molecules on the surface of APCs can promote T cell activation, such as the association of the T cell co-receptor CD28 with CD80 expressed by DCs, while other T cell co-receptors can act to inhibit T cell activation [238]. The type of T cell activation program initiated by DCs largely depends upon stimulation from cytokines released at the immunological synapse. The DC maturation program initiated in response to specific host damage cues determines which cytokines these cells secrete during T cell antigen presentation. These cytokines induce different types of T cell maturation, directing an appropriate adaptive immune response for resolution of host tissue distress. The additional requirement of cytokine stimulation for T cell activation not only acts as a checkpoint to prevent immune dysfunction but also guides the T cell activation program to generate an appropriate adaptive immune response that will effectively target a specific microorganism.

Concluding Comments

Inasmuch as phagocytic leukocytes are essential for host defense against microorganisms, it is not surprising that defects in phagocyte production and function predispose individuals to a wide range of bacterial and fungal infections. These defects, such as reduced production of neutrophils, impaired leukocyte chemotaxis, or the inability of phagocytes to generate ROS, can be genetic or acquired. Significant progress has been made toward understanding the molecular and genetic basis of phagocyte defects and, in turn, the development of therapies for infections in patients with such defects.

Recent advances in genomics approaches and bioinformatics capabilities have enhanced the ability to identify complex polygenic defects and gene networks that impact phagocyte function and underlie susceptibility to infection. Indeed, recent whole-exome profiling studies of Alzheimer's patients identified rare coding variants in genes that are highly expressed in brain microglia cells [239]. These findings provide further support to the idea that microglia contribute to late-onset Alzheimer's disease. Single-cell genomics is a relatively new technology that has the ability to identify cells and cell states that would otherwise be missed using standard assays that analyze cells as a population [240]. For example, single-cell RNA sequencing has been used to reveal heterogeneity among pre-hematopoietic stems cells [241] and elucidate changes in the human macrophage transcriptome during interaction with bacteria (*Mycobacterium tuberculosis*) [242]. Notably, the latter studies used a high-throughput method to analyze transcriptomes from thousands of human macrophages individually. Although these approaches are still in varied stages of development, they serve as a springboard for future studies that will be directed to gain a better understanding of phagocytes and phagocyte responses during specific disease states.

Acknowledgments The authors thank Ryan Kissinger (National Institute of Allergy and Infectious Diseases) for preparation of illustrations. The authors are supported by the Intramural Research Program of the National Institute of Allergy and Infectious Diseases, National Institutes of Health.

References

1. Laiosa CV, Stadtfeld M, Graf T. Determinants of lymphoid-myeloid lineage diversification. Annu Rev Immunol. 2006;24:705–38.

2. Sieweke MH, Allen JE. Beyond stem cells: self-renewal of differentiated macrophages. Science. 2013;342:1242974.

3. Ginhoux F, Jung S. Monocytes and macrophages: developmental pathways and tissue homeostasis. Nat Rev Immunol. 2014;14:392–404.

4. Laslo P, Pongubala JM, Lancki DW, Singh H. Gene regulatory networks directing myeloid and lymphoid cell fates within the immune system. Semin Immunol. 2008;20:228–35.

5. Nimmo RA, May GE, Enver T. Primed and ready: understanding lineage commitment through single cell analysis. Trends Cell Biol. 2015;25:459–67.

6. Davies LC, Taylor PR. Tissue-resident macrophages: then and now. Immunology. 2015;144:541–8.

7. van Furth R, Cohn ZA. The origin and kinetics of mononuclear phagocytes. J Exp Med. 1968;128:415–35.

8. Guilliams M, Ginhoux F, Jakubzick C, Naik SH, Onai N, Schraml BU, et al. Dendritic cells, monocytes and macrophages: a unified nomenclature based on ontogeny. Nat Rev Immunol. 2014;14:571–8.

9. Geissmann F, Manz MG, Jung S, Sieweke MH, Merad M, Ley K. Development of monocytes, macrophages, and dendritic cells. Science. 2010;327:656–61.

10. Jenkins SJ, Hume DA. Homeostasis in the mononuclear phagocyte system. Trends Immunol. 2014;35:358–67.

11. Epelman S, Lavine KJ, Randolph GJ. Origin and functions of tissue macrophages. Immunity. 2014;41:21–35.

12. Ackermann M, Liebhaber S, Klusmann JH, Lachmann N. Lost in translation: pluripotent stem cell-derived hematopoiesis. EMBO Mol Med. 2015;7:1388–1402.

13. Pittet MJ, Nahrendorf M, Swirski FK. The journey from stem cell to macrophage. Ann N Y Acad Sci. 2014;1319:1–18.

14. Manz MG, Boettcher S. Emergency granulopoiesis. Nat Rev Immunol. 2014;14:302–14.

15. Alvarez-Errico D, Vento-Tormo R, Sieweke M, Ballestar E. Epigenetic control of myeloid cell differentiation, identity and function. Nat Rev Immunol. 2015;15:7–17.

16. van Furth R, Cohn ZA, Hirsch JG, Humphrey JH, Spector WG, Langevoort HL. The mononuclear phagocyte system: a new classification of macrophages, monocytes, and their precursor cells. Bull World Health Organ. 1972;46:845–52.

17. Meuret G, Hoffmann G. Monocyte kinetic studies in normal and disease states. Br J Haematol. 1973;24:275–85.

18. Dutta P, Nahrendorf M. Regulation and consequences of monocytosis. Immunol Rev. 2014;262:167–78.

19. Italiani P, Boraschi D. From Monocytes to M1/M2 Macrophages: phenotypical vs. functional differentiation. Front Immunol. 2014;5:514.

20. Yona S, Kim KW, Wolf Y, Mildner A, Varol D, Breker M, et al. Fate mapping reveals origins and

dynamics of monocytes and tissue macrophages under homeostasis. Immunity. 2013;38:79–91.

21. Fogg DK, Sibon C, Miled C, Jung S, Aucouturier P, Littman DR, et al. A clonogenic bone marrow progenitor specific for macrophages and dendritic cells. Science. 2006;311:83–7.

22. Mildner A, Yona S, Jung S. A close encounter of the third kind: monocyte-derived cells. Adv Immunol. 2013;120:69–103.

23. Passlick B, Flieger D, Ziegler-Heitbrock HW. Identification and characterization of a novel monocyte subpopulation in human peripheral blood. Blood. 1989;74:2527–34.

24. Geissmann F, Jung S, Littman DR. Blood monocytes consist of two principal subsets with distinct migratory properties. Immunity. 2003;19:71–82.

25. Wynn TA, Chawla A, Pollard JW. Macrophage biology in development, homeostasis and disease. Nature. 2013;496:445–55.

26. Martinez FO, Gordon S. The M1 and M2 paradigm of macrophage activation: time for reassessment. F1000Prime Rep. 2014;6:13.

27. Mills CD, Kincaid K, Alt JM, Heilman MJ, Hill AM. M-1/M-2 macrophages and the Th1/Th2 paradigm. J Immunol. 2000;164:6166–73.

28. Locati M, Mantovani A, Sica A. Macrophage activation and polarization as an adaptive component of innate immunity. Adv Immunol. 2013;120:163–84.

29. Galli SJ, Borregaard N, Wynn TA. Phenotypic and functional plasticity of cells of innate immunity: macrophages, mast cells and neutrophils. Nat Immunol. 2011;12:1035–44.

30. Murray PJ, Allen JE, Biswas SK, Fisher EA, Gilroy DW, Goerdt S, et al. Macrophage activation and polarization: nomenclature and experimental guidelines. Immunity. 2014;41:14–20.

31. Price JV, Vance RE. The macrophage paradox. Immunity. 2014;41:685–93.

32. Steinman RM, Witmer MD. Lymphoid dendritic cells are potent stimulators of the primary mixed leukocyte reaction in mice. Proc Natl Acad Sci U S A. 1978;75:5132–6.

33. Miller JC, Brown BD, Shay T, Gautier EL, Jojic V, Cohain A, et al. Deciphering the transcriptional network of the dendritic cell lineage. Nat Immunol. 2012;13:888–99.

34. Merad M, Manz MG, Karsunky H, Wagers A, Peters W, Charo I, et al. Langerhans cells renew in the skin throughout life under steady-state conditions. Nat Immunol. 2002;3:1135–41.

35. Merad M, Sathe P, Helft J, Miller J, Mortha A. The dendritic cell lineage: ontogeny and function of dendritic cells and their subsets in the steady state and the inflamed setting. Annu Rev Immunol. 2013;31:563–604.

36. Steinman RM, Cohn ZA. Identification of a novel cell type in peripheral lymphoid organs of mice. I. Morphology, quantitation, tissue distribution. J Exp Med. 1973;137:1142–62.

37. Mildner A, Jung S. Development and function of dendritic cell subsets. Immunity. 2014;40:642–56.

38. Serbina NV, Salazar-Mather TP, Biron CA, Kuziel WA, Pamer EG. TNF/iNOS-producing dendritic cells mediate innate immune defense against bacterial infection. Immunity. 2003;19:59–70.

39. Schlitzer A, McGovern N, Ginhoux F. Dendritic cells and monocyte-derived cells: two complementary and integrated functional systems. Semin Cell Dev Biol. 2015;41:9–22.

40. Bainton DF, Ullyot JL, Farquhar MG. The development of neutrophilic polymorphonuclear leukocytes in human bone marrow. J Exp Med. 1971;134:907–34.

41. Kennedy AD, DeLeo FR. Neutrophil apoptosis and the resolution of infection. Immunol Res. 2009;43:25–61.

42. Athens JW, Haab OP, Raab SO, Mauer AM, Ashenbrucker H, Cartwright GE, et al. Leukokinetic studies. IV. The total blood, circulating and marginal granulocyte pools and the granulocyte turnover rate in normal subjects. J Clin Invest. 1961;40:989–95.

43. Borregaard N, Sorensen OE, Theilgaard-Monch K. Neutrophil granules: a library of innate immunity proteins. Trends Immunol. 2007;28:340–5.

44. Faurschou M, Borregaard N. Neutrophil granules and secretory vesicles in inflammation. Microbes Infect. 2003;5:1317–27.

45. DeLeo FR, Nauseef WM. Granulocytic phagocytes. In: Bennett JE, Dolin R, Blaser MJ, editors. Mandell, Douglas, and Bennett's principles and practice of infectious diseases. 1. 8th ed. Philadelphia: Elsevier Saunders; 2014. p. 78–92.

46. Borregaard N, Heiple JM, Simons ER, Clark RA. Subcellular localization of the b-cytochrome component of the human neutrophil microbicidal oxidase: translocation during activation. J Cell Biol. 1983;97:52–61.

47. Nauseef WM, Borregaard N. Neutrophils at work. Nat Immunol. 2014;15:602–11.

48. Karasuyama H, Mukai K, Obata K, Tsujimura Y, Wada T. Nonredundant roles of basophils in immunity. Annu Rev Immunol. 2011;29:45–69.

49. Rothenberg ME, Hogan SP. The eosinophil. Annu Rev Immunol. 2006;24:147–74.

50. Taylor ML, Metcalfe DD. Mast cells in allergy and host defense. Allergy Asthma Proc. 2001;22:115–9.

51. Yousefi S, Gold JA, Andina N, Lee JJ, Kelly AM, Kozlowski E, et al. Catapult-like release of mitochondrial DNA by eosinophils contributes to antibacterial defense. Nat Med. 2008;14:949–53.

52. Persson T, Andersson P, Bodelsson M, Laurell M, Malm J, Egesten A. Bactericidal activity of human eosinophilic granulocytes against Escherichia coli. Infect Immun. 2001;69:3591–6.

53. Rosenberg HF, Dyer KD, Foster PS. Eosinophils: changing perspectives in health and disease. Nat Rev Immunol. 2013;13:9–22.

54. Ribatti D, Crivellato E. Mast cell ontogeny: an historical overview. Immunol Lett. 2014;159:11–4.

55. Feger F, Varadaradjalou S, Gao Z, Abraham SN, Arock M. The role of mast cells in host defense and their subversion by bacterial pathogens. Trends Immunol. 2002;23:151–8.

56. Dahlin JS, Hallgren J. Mast cell progenitors: origin, development and migration to tissues. Mol Immunol. 2015;63:9–17.

57. Nilsson G, Costa JJ, Metcalfe DD. Mast cells and basophils. In: Gallin JI, Snyderman R, editors. Inflammation: basic principles and clinical correlates. 1. 3rd ed. Philadelphia: Lippincott Williams & Wilkins; 1999. p. 97–117.

58. Butcher EC, Picker LJ. Lymphocyte homing and homeostasis. Science. 1996;272:60–6.

59. Ley K, Laudanna C, Cybulsky MI, Nourshargh S. Getting to the site of inflammation: the leukocyte adhesion cascade updated. Nat Rev Immunol. 2007;7:678–89.

60. Kolaczkowska E, Kubes P. Neutrophil recruitment and function in health and inflammation. Nat Rev Immunol. 2013;13:159–75.

61. Nourshargh S, Alon R. Leukocyte migration into inflamed tissues. Immunity. 2014;41:694–707.

62. Soehnlein O, Lindbom L. Phagocyte partnership during the onset and resolution of inflammation. Nat Rev Immunol. 2010;10:427–39.

63. Petri B, Phillipson M, Kubes P. The physiology of leukocyte recruitment: an in vivo perspective. J Immunol. 2008;180:6439–46.

64. Kobayashi SD, Voyich JM, Burlak C, DeLeo FR. Neutrophils in the innate immune response. Arch Immunol Ther Exp. 2005;53:505–17.

65. McPhail LC, Clayton CC, Snyderman R. The NADPH oxidase of human polymorphonuclear leukocytes. Evidence for regulation by multiple signals. J Biol Chem. 1984;259:5768–75.

66. Guthrie LA, McPhail LC, Henson PM, Johnston RB Jr. Priming of neutrophils for enhanced release of oxygen metabolites by bacterial lipopolysaccharide. Evidence for increased activity of the superoxide-producing enzyme. J Exp Med. 1984;160:1656–71.

67. Rigby KM, DeLeo FR. Neutrophils in innate host defense against *Staphylococcus aureus* infections. Semin Immunopathol. 2012;34:237–59.

68. Takeuchi O, Akira S. Pattern recognition receptors and inflammation. Cell. 2010;140:805–20.

69. Chen GY, Nunez G. Sterile inflammation: sensing and reacting to damage. Nat Rev Immunol. 2010;10:826–37.

70. Canton J, Neculai D, Grinstein S. Scavenger receptors in homeostasis and immunity. Nat Rev Immunol. 2013;13:621–34.

71. Nestle FO, Di Meglio P, Qin JZ, Nickoloff BJ. Skin immune sentinels in health and disease. Nat Rev Immunol. 2009;9:679–91.

72. Shi C, Pamer EG. Monocyte recruitment during infection and inflammation. Nat Rev Immunol. 2011;11:762–74.

73. Kinashi T. Intracellular signalling controlling integrin activation in lymphocytes. Nat Rev Immunol. 2005;5:546–59.

74. Arnaout MA. Biology and structure of leukocyte beta 2 integrins and their role in inflammation. F1000Res. 2016;5:2433.

75. Laudanna C, Kim JY, Constantin G, Butcher E. Rapid leukocyte integrin activation by chemokines. Immunol Rev. 2002;186:37–46.

76. Shattil SJ, Kim C, Ginsberg MH. The final steps of integrin activation: the end game. Nat Rev Mol Cell Biol. 2010;11:288–300.

77. Abram CL, Lowell CA. The ins and outs of leukocyte integrin signaling. Annu Rev Immunol. 2009;27:339–62.

78. Weninger W, Biro M, Jain R. Leukocyte migration in the interstitial space of non-lymphoid organs. Nat Rev Immunol. 2014;14:232–46.

79. Muller WA. Leukocyte-endothelial-cell interactions in leukocyte transmigration and the inflammatory response. Trends Immunol. 2003;24:327–34.

80. Nourshargh S, Hordijk PL, Sixt M. Breaching multiple barriers: leukocyte motility through venular walls and the interstitium. Nat Rev Mol Cell Biol. 2010;11:366–78.

81. Heinrich V. Controlled one-on-one encounters between immune cells and microbes reveal mechanisms of phagocytosis. Biophys J. 2015;109:469–76.

82. Brown GD, Gordon S. Immune recognition. A new receptor for beta-glucans. Nature. 2001;413:36–7.

83. Herre J, Marshall AS, Caron E, Edwards AD, Williams DL, Schweighoffer E, et al. Dectin-1 uses novel mechanisms for yeast phagocytosis in macrophages. Blood. 2004;104:4038–45.

84. Li X, Utomo A, Cullere X, Choi MM, Milner DA Jr, Venkatesh D, et al. The beta-glucan receptor Dectin-1 activates the integrin Mac-1 in neutrophils via Vav protein signaling to promote *Candida albicans* clearance. Cell Host Microbe. 2011;10:603–15.

85. Anderson CL, Shen L, Eicher DM, Wewers MD, Gill JK. Phagocytosis mediated by three distinct Fc gamma receptor classes on human leukocytes. J Exp Med. 1990;171:1333–45.

86. Springer TA, Dustin ML. Integrin inside-out signaling and the immunological synapse. Curr Opin Cell Biol. 2012;24:107–15.

87. Caron E, Self AJ, Hall A. The GTPase Rap1 controls functional activation of macrophage integrin alphaMbeta2 by LPS and other inflammatory mediators. Curr Biol. 2000;10:974–8.

88. Patel PC, Harrison RE. Membrane ruffles capture C3bi-opsonized particles in activated macrophages. Mol Biol Cell. 2008;19:4628–39.

89. Kress H, Stelzer EH, Holzer D, Buss F, Griffiths G, Rohrbach A. Filopodia act as phagocytic tentacles and pull with discrete steps and a load-dependent velocity. Proc Natl Acad Sci U S A. 2007;104:11633–8.

90. Flannagan RS, Harrison RE, Yip CM, Jaqaman K, Grinstein S. Dynamic macrophage "probing" is required for the efficient capture of phagocytic targets. J Cell Biol. 2010;191:1205–18.

91. Kheir WA, Gevrey JC, Yamaguchi H, Isaac B, Cox D. A WAVE2-Abi1 complex mediates CSF-1-induced F-actin-rich membrane protrusions and migration in macrophages. J Cell Sci. 2005;118:5369–79.

92. Freeman SA, Grinstein S. Phagocytosis: receptors, signal integration, and the cytoskeleton. Immunol Rev. 2014;262:193–215.

93. Levin R, Grinstein S, Schlam D. Phosphoinositides in phagocytosis and macropinocytosis. Biochim Biophys Acta. 1851;2015:805–23.

94. Wang AV, Scholl PR, Geha RS. Physical and functional association of the high affinity immunoglobulin G receptor (Fc gamma RI) with the kinases Hck and Lyn. J Exp Med. 1994;180:1165–70.

95. Jaumouille V, Farkash Y, Jaqaman K, Das R, Lowell CA, Grinstein S. Actin cytoskeleton reorganization by Syk regulates Fcgamma receptor responsiveness by increasing its lateral mobility and clustering. Dev Cell. 2014;29:534–46.

96. Swanson JA. Phosphoinositides and engulfment. Cell Microbiol. 2014;16:1473–83.

97. Cox D, Berg JS, Cammer M, Chinegwundoh JO, Dale BM, Cheney RE, et al. Myosin X is a downstream effector of PI(3)K during phagocytosis. Nat Cell Biol. 2002;4:469–77.

98. Lukacs GL, Rotstein OD, Grinstein S. Phagosomal acidification is mediated by a vacuolar-type H(+)-ATPase in murine macrophages. J Biol Chem. 1990;265:21099–107.

99. El Chemaly A, Nunes P, Jimaja W, Castelbou C, Demaurex N. Hv1 proton channels differentially regulate the pH of neutrophil and macrophage phagosomes by sustaining the production of phagosomal ROS that inhibit the delivery of vacuolar ATPases. J Leukoc Biol. 2014;95:827–839.

100. Savina A, Jancic C, Hugues S, Guermonprez P, Vargas P, Moura IC, et al. NOX2 controls phagosomal pH to regulate antigen processing during crosspresentation by dendritic cells. Cell. 2006;126:205–18.

101. Yates RM, Hermetter A, Russell DG. The kinetics of phagosome maturation as a function of phagosome/lysosome fusion and acquisition of hydrolytic activity. Traffic. 2005;6:413–20.

102. Claus V, Jahraus A, Tjelle T, Berg T, Kirschke H, Faulstich H, et al. Lysosomal enzyme trafficking between phagosomes, endosomes, and lysosomes in J774 macrophages. Enrichment of cathepsin H in early endosomes. J Biol Chem. 1998;273:9842–51.

103. Rybicka JM, Balce DR, Chaudhuri S, Allan ER, Yates RM. Phagosomal proteolysis in dendritic cells is modulated by NADPH oxidase in a pH-independent manner. EMBO J. 2012;31:932–44.

104. Delamarre L, Pack M, Chang H, Mellman I, Trombetta ES. Differential lysosomal proteolysis in antigen-presenting cells determines antigen fate. Science. 2005;307:1630–4.

105. Delamarre L, Couture R, Mellman I, Trombetta ES. Enhancing immunogenicity by limiting susceptibility to lysosomal proteolysis. J Exp Med. 2006;203:2049–55.

106. Mantegazza AR, Zajac AL, Twelvetrees A, Holzbaur EL, Amigorena S, Marks MS. TLR-dependent phagosome tubulation in dendritic cells promotes phagosome cross-talk to optimize MHC-II antigen presentation. Proc Natl Acad Sci U S A. 2014;111:15508–13.

107. Lominadze G, Powell DW, Luerman GC, Link AJ, Ward RA, McLeish KR. Proteomic analysis of human neutrophil granules. Mol Cell Proteomics. 2005;4:1503–21.

108. Jankowski A, Scott CC, Grinstein S. Determinants of the phagosomal pH in neutrophils. J Biol Chem. 2002;277:6059–66.

109. Morgan D, Capasso M, Musset B, Cherny VV, Rios E, Dyer MJ, et al. Voltage-gated proton channels maintain pH in human neutrophils during phagocytosis. Proc Natl Acad Sci U S A. 2009;106:18022–7.

110. Capasso M, DeCoursey TE, Dyer MJ. pH regulation and beyond: unanticipated functions for the voltage-gated proton channel, HVCN1. Trends Cell Biol. 2011;21:20–8.

111. Ramsey IS, Ruchti E, Kaczmarek JS, Clapham DE. Hv1 proton channels are required for high-level NADPH oxidase-dependent superoxide production during the phagocyte respiratory burst. Proc Natl Acad Sci U S A. 2009;106:7642–7.

112. Segal AW, Geisow M, Garcia R, Harper A, Miller R. The respiratory burst of phagocytic cells is associated with a rise in vacuolar pH. Nature. 1981;290:406–9.

113. Nunes P, Demaurex N, Dinauer MC. Regulation of the NADPH oxidase and associated ion fluxes during phagocytosis. Traffic. 2013;14:1118–31.

114. Babior BM. NADPH oxidase: an update. Blood. 1999;93:1464–76.

115. Wang G, Nauseef WM. Salt, chloride, bleach, and innate host defense. J Leukoc Biol. 2015;98:163–72.

116. Klebanoff SJ, Kettle AJ, Rosen H, Winterbourn CC, Nauseef WM. Myeloperoxidase: a front-line defender against phagocytosed microorganisms. J Leukoc Biol. 2013;93:185–98.

117. Eiserich JP, Hristova M, Cross CE, Jones AD, Freeman BA, Halliwell B, et al. Formation of nitric oxide-derived inflammatory oxidants by myeloperoxidase in neutrophils. Nature. 1998;391:393–7.

118. Sbarra AJ, Karnovsky ML. The biochemical basis of phagocytosis. I. Metabolic changes during the ingestion of particles by polymorphonuclear leukocytes. J Biol Chem. 1959;234:1355–62.

119. Baehner RL, Karnovsky ML. Deficiency of reduced nicotinamide-adenine dinucleotide oxidase in chronic granulomatous disease. Science. 1968;162:1277–9.

120. MacMicking J, Xie QW, Nathan C. Nitric oxide and macrophage function. Annu Rev Immunol. 1997;15:323–50.

121. Stuehr DJ. Mammalian nitric oxide synthases. Biochim Biophys Acta. 1999;1411:217–30.

122. Schapiro JM, Libby SJ, Fang FC. Inhibition of bacterial DNA replication by zinc mobilization during nitrosative stress. Proc Natl Acad Sci U S A. 2003;100:8496–501.

123. Bogdan C. Nitric oxide synthase in innate and adaptive immunity: an update. Trends Immunol. 2015;36:161–78.

124. Henard CA, Vazquez-Torres A. Nitric oxide and salmonella pathogenesis. Front Microbiol. 2011;2:84.

125. Ganz T, Selsted ME, Szklarek D, Harwig SS, Daher K, Bainton DF, et al. Defensins. Natural peptide antibiotics of human neutrophils. J Clin Invest. 1985;76:1427–35.

126. Selsted ME, Harwig SS, Ganz T, Schilling JW, Lehrer RI. Primary structures of three human neutrophil defensins. J Clin Invest. 1985;76:1436–9.

127. Ganz T. Extracellular release of antimicrobial defensins by human polymorphonuclear leukocytes. Infect Immun. 1987;55:568–71.

128. Elsbach P, Weiss J, Franson RC, Beckerdite-Quagliata S, Schneider A, Harris L. Separation and purification of a potent bactericidal/permeability-increasing protein and a closely associated phospholipase A2 from rabbit polymorphonuclear leukocytes. Observations on their relationship. J Biol Chem. 1979;254:11000–9.

129. Egesten A, Breton-Gorius J, Guichard J, Gullberg U, Olsson I. The heterogeneity of azurophil granules in neutrophil promyelocytes: immunogold localization of myeloperoxidase, cathepsin G, elastase, proteinase 3, and bactericidal/permeability increasing protein. Blood. 1994;83:2985–94.

130. Lehrer RI, Ganz T. Cathelicidins: a family of endogenous antimicrobial peptides. Curr Opin Hematol. 2002;9:18–22.

131. Lehrer RI, Lu W. Alpha-Defensins in human innate immunity. Immunol Rev. 2012;245:84–112.

132. Lehrer RI, Barton A, Daher KA, Harwig SS, Ganz T, Selsted ME. Interaction of human defensins with Escherichia coli. Mechanism of bactericidal activity. J Clin Invest. 1989;84:553–61.

133. Levy O. A neutrophil-derived anti-infective molecule: bactericidal/permeability-increasing protein. Antimicrob Agents Chemother. 2000;44:2925–31.

134. Krasity BC, Troll JV, Weiss JP, McFall-Ngai MJ. LBP/BPI proteins and their relatives: conservation over evolution and roles in mutualism. Biochem Soc Trans. 2011;39:1039–44.

135. Balakrishnan A, Marathe SA, Joglekar M, Chakravortty D. Bactericidal/permeability increasing protein: a multifaceted protein with functions beyond LPS neutralization. Innate Immun. 2013;19:339–47.

136. Belaaouaj A, Kim KS, Shapiro SD. Degradation of outer membrane protein A in Escherichia coli killing by neutrophil elastase. Science. 2000;289:1185–8.

137. Reeves EP, Lu H, Jacobs HL, Messina CG, Bolsover S, Gabella G, et al. Killing activity of neutrophils is mediated through activation of proteases by K+ flux. Nature. 2002;416:291–7.

138. Campanelli D, Melchior M, Fu Y, Nakata M, Shuman H, Nathan C, et al. Cloning of cDNA for proteinase 3: a serine protease, antibiotic, and autoantigen from human neutrophils. J Exp Med. 1990;172:1709–15.

139. Campanelli D, Detmers PA, Nathan CF, Gabay JE. Azurocidin and a homologous serine protease from neutrophils. Differential antimicrobial and proteolytic properties. J Clin Invest. 1990;85:904–15.

140. Morgan JG, Sukiennicki T, Pereira HA, Spitznagel JK, Guerra ME, Larrick JW. Cloning of the cDNA for the serine protease homolog CAP37/azurocidin, a microbicidal and chemotactic protein from human granulocytes. J Immunol. 1991;147:3210–4.

141. Hahn I, Klaus A, Janze AK, Steinwede K, Ding N, Bohling J, et al. Cathepsin G and neutrophil elastase play critical and nonredundant roles in lung-protective immunity against Streptococcus pneumoniae in mice. Infect Immun. 2011;79:4893–901.

142. Tkalcevic J, Novelli M, Phylactides M, Iredale JP, Segal AW, Roes J. Impaired immunity and enhanced resistance to endotoxin in the absence of neutrophil elastase and cathepsin G. Immunity. 2000;12:201–10.

143. Kolset SO, Tveit H. Serglycin—structure and biology. Cell Mol Life Sci. 2008;65:1073–85.

144. Niemann CU, Cowland JB, Klausen P, Askaa J, Calafat J, Borregaard N. Localization of serglycin in human neutrophil granulocytes and their precursors. J Leukoc Biol. 2004;76:406–15.

145. Pham CT. Neutrophil serine proteases: specific regulators of inflammation. Nat Rev Immunol. 2006;6:541–50.

146. Belaaouaj A, McCarthy R, Baumann M, Gao Z, Ley TJ, Abraham SN, et al. Mice lacking neutrophil elastase reveal impaired host defense against gram negative bacterial sepsis. Nat Med. 1998;4:615–8.

147. Scocchi M, Skerlavaj B, Romeo D, Gennaro R. Proteolytic cleavage by neutrophil elastase converts inactive storage proforms to antibacterial bactenecins. Eur J Biochem. 1992;209:589–95.

148. Meyer-Hoffert U. Neutrophil-derived serine proteases modulate innate immune responses. Front Biosci (Landmark Ed). 2009;14:3409–18.

149. Tongaonkar P, Golji AE, Tran P, Ouellette AJ, Selsted ME. High fidelity processing and activation of the human alpha-defensin HNP1 precursor by neutrophil elastase and proteinase 3. PLoS One. 2012;7:e32469.

150. Sorensen OE, Follin P, Johnsen AH, Calafat J, Tjabringa GS, Hiemstra PS, et al. Human cathelicidin, hCAP-18, is processed to the antimicrobial peptide LL-37 by extracellular cleavage with proteinase 3. Blood. 2001;97:3951–9.

151. Meyer-Hoffert U, Wiedow O. Neutrophil serine proteases: mediators of innate immune responses. Curr Opin Hematol. 2011;18:19–24.

152. Bangalore N, Travis J, Onunka VC, Pohl J, Shafer WM. Identification of the primary antimicrobial domains in human neutrophil cathepsin G. J Biol Chem. 1990;265:13584–8.

153. Shafer WM, Martin LE, Spitznagel JK. Cationic antimicrobial proteins isolated from human neutrophil granulocytes in the presence of diisopropyl fluorophosphate. Infect Immun. 1984;45:29–35.

154. Shafer WM, Onunka VC, Martin LE. Antigonococcal activity of human neutrophil cathepsin G. Infect Immun. 1986;54:184–8.

155. Zeya HI, Spitznagel JK. Cationic proteins of polymorphonuclear leukocyte lysosomes. II. Composition, properties, and mechanism of antibacterial action. J Bacteriol. 1966;91:755–62.

156. Kao RC, Wehner NG, Skubitz KM, Gray BH, Hoidal JR. Proteinase 3. A distinct human polymorphonuclear leukocyte proteinase that produces emphysema in hamsters. J Clin Invest. 1988;82:1963–73.

157. Brinkmann V, Reichard U, Goosmann C, Fauler B, Uhlemann Y, Weiss DS, et al. Neutrophil extracellular traps kill bacteria. Science. 2004;303:1532–5.

158. von Kockritz-Blickwede M, Goldmann O, Thulin P, Heinemann K, Norrby-Teglund A, Rohde M, et al. Phagocytosis-independent antimicrobial activity of mast cells by means of extracellular trap formation. Blood. 2008;111:3070–80.

159. Chow OA, von Kockritz-Blickwede M, Bright AT, Hensler ME, Zinkernagel AS, Cogen AL, et al. Statins enhance formation of phagocyte extracellular traps. Cell Host Microbe. 2010;8:445–54.

160. Boe DM, Curtis BJ, Chen MM, Ippolito JA, Kovacs EJ. Extracellular traps and macrophages: new roles for the versatile phagocyte. J Leukoc Biol. 2015;97:1023–35.

161. Loures FV, Rohm M, Lee CK, Santos E, Wang JP, Specht CA, et al. Recognition of Aspergillus fumigatus hyphae by human plasmacytoid dendritic cells is mediated by dectin-2 and results in formation of extracellular traps. PLoS Pathog. 2015;11:e1004643.

162. Yousefi S, Morshed M, Amini P, Stojkov D, Simon D, von Gunten S, et al. Basophils exhibit antibacterial activity through extracellular trap formation. Allergy. 2015;70:1184–8.

163. Morshed M, Hlushchuk R, Simon D, Walls AF, Obata-Ninomiya K, Karasuyama H, et al. NADPH oxidase-independent formation of extracellular DNA traps by basophils. J Immunol. 2014;192:5314–23.

164. Clark SR, Ma AC, Tavener SA, McDonald B, Goodarzi Z, Kelly MM, et al. Platelet TLR4 activates neutrophil extracellular traps to ensnare bacteria in septic blood. Nat Med. 2007;13:463–9.

165. Kaplan MJ, Radic M. Neutrophil extracellular traps: double-edged swords of innate immunity. J Immunol. 2012;189:2689–95.

166. Menegazzi R, Decleva E, Dri P. Killing by neutrophil extracellular traps: fact or folklore? Blood. 2012;119:1214–6.

167. Parker H, Albrett AM, Kettle AJ, Winterbourn CC. Myeloperoxidase associated with neutrophil extracellular traps is active and mediates bacterial killing in the presence of hydrogen peroxide. J Leukoc Biol. 2012;91:369–76.

168. Scharrig E, Carestia A, Ferrer MF, Cedola M, Pretre G, Drut R, et al. Neutrophil extracellular traps are involved in the innate immune response to infection with Leptospira. PLoS Negl Trop Dis. 2015;9:e0003927.

169. de Jong HK, Koh GC, Achouiti A, van der Meer AJ, Bulder I, Stephan F, et al. Neutrophil extracellular traps in the host defense against sepsis induced by Burkholderia pseudomallei (melioidosis). Intensive Care Med Exp. 2014;2:21.

170. Mejia SP, Cano LE, Lopez JA, Hernandez O, Gonzalez A. Human neutrophils produce extracellular traps against Paracoccidioides brasiliensis. Microbiology. 2015;161:1008–17.

171. Gunderson CW, Seifert HS. Neisseria gonorrhoeae elicits extracellular traps in primary neutrophil culture while suppressing the oxidative burst. MBio. 2015;6:e02452–14.

172. Juneau RA, Pang B, Armbruster CE, Murrah KA, Perez AC, Swords WE. Peroxiredoxin-glutaredoxin and catalase promote resistance of nontypeable Haemophilus influenzae 86-028NP to oxidants and survival within neutrophil extracellular traps. Infect Immun. 2015;83:239–46.

173. Shan Q, Dwyer M, Rahman S, Gadjeva M. Distinct susceptibilities of corneal Pseudomonas aeruginosa clinical isolates to neutrophil extracellular trap-mediated immunity. Infect Immun. 2014;82:4135–43.

174. Dohrmann S, Anik S, Olson J, Anderson EL, Etesami N, No H, et al. Role for streptococcal collagen-like protein 1 in M1T1 group A Streptococcus resistance to neutrophil extracellular traps. Infect Immun. 2014;82:4011–20.

175. Bonne-Annee S, Kerepesi LA, Hess JA, Wesolowski J, Paumet F, Lok JB, et al. Extracellular traps are associated with human and mouse neutrophil and macrophage mediated killing of larval Strongyloides stercoralis. Microbes Infect. 2014;16:502–11.

176. Liu P, Wu X, Liao C, Liu X, Du J, Shi H, et al. *Escherichia coli* and *Candida albicans* induced macrophage extracellular trap-like structures with limited microbicidal activity. PLoS One. 2014;9:e90042.

177. Thammavongsa V, Missiakas DM, Schneewind O. *Staphylococcus aureus* degrades neutrophil extracellular traps to promote immune cell death. Science. 2013;342:863–6.

178. Short KR, von Kockritz-Blickwede M, Langereis JD, Chew KY, Job ER, Armitage CW, et al. Antibodies mediate formation of neutrophil extracellular traps in the middle ear and facilitate secondary pneumococcal otitis media. Infect Immun. 2014;82:364–70.

179. Seper A, Hosseinzadeh A, Gorkiewicz G, Lichtenegger S, Roier S, Leitner DR, et al. Vibrio cholerae evades neutrophil extracellular traps by the activity of two extracellular nucleases. PLoS Pathog. 2013;9:e1003614.

180. Derre-Bobillot A, Cortes-Perez NG, Yamamoto Y, Kharrat P, Couve E, Da Cunha V, et al. Nuclease A (Gbs0661), an extracellular nuclease of *Streptococcus agalactiae*, attacks the neutrophil extracellular traps and is needed for full virulence. Mol Microbiol. 2013;89:518–31.

181. Lappann M, Danhof S, Guenther F, Olivares-Florez S, Mordhorst IL, Vogel U. In vitro resistance mechanisms of Neisseria meningitidis against neutrophil extracellular traps. Mol Microbiol. 2013;89:433–49.

182. Menten-Dedoyart C, Faccinetto C, Golovchenko M, Dupiereux I, Van Lerberghe PB, Dubois S, et al. Neutrophil extracellular traps entrap and kill Borrelia burgdorferi sensu stricto spirochetes and are not affected by Ixodes ricinus tick saliva. J Immunol. 2012;189:5393–401.

183. McDonald B, Urrutia R, Yipp BG, Jenne CN, Kubes P. Intravascular neutrophil extracellular traps capture bacteria from the bloodstream during sepsis. Cell Host Microbe. 2012;12:324–33.

184. Riyapa D, Buddhisa S, Korbsrisate S, Cuccui J, Wren BW, Stevens MP, et al. Neutrophil extracellular traps exhibit antibacterial activity against burkholderia pseudomallei and are influenced by bacterial and host factors. Infect Immun. 2012;80:3921–9.

185. Young RL, Malcolm KC, Kret JE, Caceres SM, Poch KR, Nichols DP, et al. Neutrophil extracellular trap (NET)-mediated killing of Pseudomonas aeruginosa: evidence of acquired resistance within the CF airway, independent of CFTR. PLoS One. 2011;6:e23637.

186. Abel J, Goldmann O, Ziegler C, Holtje C, Smeltzer MS, Cheung AL, et al. *Staphylococcus aureus* evades the extracellular antimicrobial activity of mast cells by promoting its own uptake. J Innate Immun. 2011;3:495–507.

187. Berends ET, Horswill AR, Haste NM, Monestier M, Nizet V, von Kockritz-Blickwede M. Nuclease expression by *Staphylococcus aureus* facilitates escape from neutrophil extracellular traps. J Innate Immun. 2010;2:576–86.

188. Urban CF, Reichard U, Brinkmann V, Zychlinsky A. Neutrophil extracellular traps capture and kill *Candida albicans* yeast and hyphal forms. Cell Microbiol. 2006;8:668–76.

189. Buchanan JT, Simpson AJ, Aziz RK, Liu GY, Kristian SA, Kotb M, et al. DNase expression allows the pathogen group A Streptococcus to escape killing in neutrophil extracellular traps. Curr Biol. 2006;16:396–400.

190. Sumby P, Barbian KD, Gardner DJ, Whitney AR, Welty DM, Long RD, et al. Extracellular deoxyribonuclease made by group A Streptococcus assists pathogenesis by enhancing evasion of the innate immune response. Proc Natl Acad Sci U S A. 2005;102:1679–84.

191. Lee MJ, Liu H, Barker BM, Snarr BD, Gravelat FN, Al Abdallah Q, et al. The fungal exopolysaccharide galactosaminogalactan mediates virulence by enhancing resistance to neutrophil extracellular traps. PLoS Pathog. 2015;11:e1005187.

192. Branzk N, Lubojemska A, Hardison SE, Wang Q, Gutierrez MG, Brown GD, et al. Neutrophils sense microbe size and selectively release neutrophil extracellular traps in response to large pathogens. Nat Immunol. 2014;15:1017–25.

193. Fuchs TA, Abed U, Goosmann C, Hurwitz R, Schulze I, Wahn V, et al. Novel cell death program leads to neutrophil extracellular traps. J Cell Biol. 2007;176:231–41.

194. Papayannopoulos V, Metzler KD, Hakkim A, Zychlinsky A. Neutrophil elastase and myeloperoxidase regulate the formation of neutrophil extracellular traps. J Cell Biol. 2010;191:677–91.

195. Neumann A, Berends ET, Nerlich A, Molhoek EM, Gallo RL, Meerloo T, et al. The antimicrobial peptide LL-37 facilitates the formation of neutrophil extracellular traps. Biochem J. 2014;464:3–11.

196. Wang Y, Li M, Stadler S, Correll S, Li P, Wang D, et al. Histone hypercitrullination mediates chromatin decondensation and neutrophil extracellular trap formation. J Cell Biol. 2009;184:205–13.

197. Li P, Li M, Lindberg MR, Kennett MJ, Xiong N, Wang Y. PAD4 is essential for antibacterial innate immunity mediated by neutrophil extracellular traps. J Exp Med. 2010;207:1853–62.

198. Yousefi S, Mihalache C, Kozlowski E, Schmid I, Simon HU. Viable neutrophils release mitochondrial DNA to form neutrophil extracellular traps. Cell Death Differ. 2009;16:1438–44.

199. Pilsczek FH, Salina D, Poon KK, Fahey C, Yipp BG, Sibley CD, et al. A novel mechanism of rapid nuclear neutrophil extracellular trap formation in response to *Staphylococcus aureus*. J Immunol. 2010;185:7413–25.

200. Malachowa N, Kobayashi SD, Freedman B, Dorward DW, DeLeo FR. *Staphylococcus aureus* leukotoxin GH promotes formation of neutrophil extracellular traps. J Immunol. 2013;191:6022–9.

201. Behnen M, Leschczyk C, Moller S, Batel T, Klinger M, Solbach W, et al. Immobilized immune complexes induce neutrophil extracellular trap release by human neutrophil granulocytes via FcgammaRIIIB and Mac-1. J Immunol. 2014;193:1954–65.

202. Lu T, Kobayashi SD, Quinn MT, Deleo FR. A NET Outcome. Front Immunol. 2012;3:365.

203. Simon D, Simon HU, Yousefi S. Extracellular DNA traps in allergic, infectious, and autoimmune diseases. Allergy. 2013;68:409–16.

204. Darrah E, Andrade F. NETs: the missing link between cell death and systemic autoimmune diseases? Front Immunol. 2012;3:428.

205. Cortjens B, de Boer OJ, de Jong R, Antonis AF, Sabogal Pineros YS, Lutter R, et al. Neutrophil extracellular traps cause airway obstruction during respiratory syncytial virus disease. J Pathol. 2016;238:401–411.

206. Grabcanovic-Musija F, Obermayer A, Stoiber W, Krautgar`tner WD, Steinbacher P, Winterberg N, et al. Neutrophil extracellular trap (NET) formation characterises stable and exacerbated COPD and correlates with airflow limitation. Respir Res. 2015;16:59.

207. Obermayer A, Stoiber W, Krautgartner WD, Klappacher M, Kofler B, Steinbacher P, et al. New aspects on the structure of neutrophil extracellular traps from chronic obstructive pulmonary disease and in vitro generation. PLoS One. 2014;9:e97784.

208. Marcos V, Zhou Z, Yildirim AO, Bohla A, Hector A, Vitkov L, et al. CXCR2 mediates NADPH oxidase-independent neutrophil extracellular trap formation in cystic fibrosis airway inflammation. Nat Med. 2010;16:1018–23.

209. Zenaro E, Pietronigro E, Della Bianca V, Piacentino G, Marongiu L, Budui S, et al. Neutrophils promote Alzheimer's disease-like pathology and cognitive decline via LFA-1 integrin. Nat Med. 2015;21:880–6.

210. Warnatsch A, Ioannou M, Wang Q, Papayannopoulos V. Inflammation. Neutrophil extracellular traps license macrophages for cytokine production in atherosclerosis. Science. 2015;349:316–20.

211. Spengler J, Lugonja B, Jimmy Ytterberg A, Zubarev RA, Creese AJ, Pearson MJ, et al. Release of active peptidyl arginine deiminases by neutrophils can explain production of extracellular citrullinated autoantigens in rheumatoid arthritis synovial fluid. Arthritis Rheumatol. 2015;67:3135–45.

212. Wright HL, Moots RJ, Edwards SW. The multifactorial role of neutrophils in rheumatoid arthritis. Nat Rev Rheumatol. 2014;10:593–601.

213. Cools-Lartigue J, Spicer J, Najmeh S, Ferri L. Neutrophil extracellular traps in cancer progression. Cell Mol Life Sci. 2014;71:4179–94.

214. Cools-Lartigue J, Spicer J, McDonald B, Gowing S, Chow S, Giannias B, et al. Neutrophil extracellular traps sequester circulating tumor cells and promote metastasis. J Clin Invest. 2013;123:3446–3458

215. Chen G, Zhang D, Fuchs TA, Manwani D, Wagner DD, Frenette PS. Heme-induced neutrophil extracellular traps contribute to the pathogenesis of sickle cell disease. Blood. 2014;123:3818–27.

216. Martinod K, Wagner DD. Thrombosis: tangled up in NETs. Blood. 2014;123:2768–76.

217. Demers M, Krause DS, Schatzberg D, Martinod K, Voorhees JR, Fuchs TA, et al. Cancers predispose neutrophils to release extracellular DNA traps that contribute to cancer-associated thrombosis. Proc Natl Acad Sci U S A. 2012;109:13076–81.

218. Fuchs TA, Brill A, Duerschmied D, Schatzberg D, Monestier M, Myers DD Jr, et al. Extracellular DNA traps promote thrombosis. Proc Natl Acad Sci U S A. 2010;107:15880–5.

219. Dorner T. SLE in 2011: deciphering the role of NETs and networks in SLE. Nat Rev Rheumatol. 2012;8:68–70.

220. Lande R, Ganguly D, Facchinetti V, Frasca L, Conrad C, Gregorio J, et al. Neutrophils activate plasmacytoid dendritic cells by releasing self-DNA-peptide complexes in systemic lupus erythematosus. Sci Transl Med. 2011;3:73ra19.

221. Garcia-Romo GS, Caielli S, Vega B, Connolly J, Allantaz F, Xu Z, et al. Netting neutrophils are major inducers of type I IFN production in pediatric systemic lupus erythematosus. Sci Transl Med. 2011;3:73ra20.

222. Hakkim A, Furnrohr BG, Amann K, Laube B, Abed UA, Brinkmann V, et al. Impairment of neutrophil extracellular trap degradation is associated with lupus nephritis. Proc Natl Acad Sci U S A. 2010;107:9813–8.

223. Kambayashi T, Laufer TM. Atypical MHC class II-expressing antigen-presenting cells: can anything replace a dendritic cell? Nat Rev Immunol. 2014;14:719–30.

224. Guermonprez P, Valladeau J, Zitvogel L, Thery C, Amigorena S. Antigen presentation and T cell stimulation by dendritic cells. Annu Rev Immunol. 2002;20:621–67.

225. Iwasaki A, Medzhitov R. Control of adaptive immunity by the innate immune system. Nat Immunol. 2015;16:343–53.

226. Kapsenberg ML. Dendritic-cell control of pathogen-driven T-cell polarization. Nat Rev Immunol. 2003;3:984–93.

227. Blum JS, Wearsch PA, Cresswell P. Pathways of antigen processing. Annu Rev Immunol. 2013;31:443–73.

228. Roche PA, Furuta K. The ins and outs of MHC class II-mediated antigen processing and presentation. Nat Rev Immunol. 2015;15:203–16.

229. Savina A, Amigorena S. Phagocytosis and antigen presentation in dendritic cells. Immunol Rev. 2007;219:143–56.

230. Neefjes J, Jongsma ML, Paul P, Bakke O. Towards a systems understanding of MHC class I and MHC class II antigen presentation. Nat Rev Immunol. 2011;11:823–36.

231. Jensen PE. Recent advances in antigen processing and presentation. Nat Immunol. 2007;8:1041–8.

232. Joffre OP, Segura E, Savina A, Amigorena S. Cross-presentation by dendritic cells. Nat Rev Immunol. 2012;12:557–69.

233. Jutras I, Desjardins M. Phagocytosis: at the crossroads of innate and adaptive immunity. Annu Rev Cell Dev Biol. 2005;21:511–27.

234. Vyas JM, Van der Veen AG, Ploegh HL. The known unknowns of antigen processing and presentation. Nat Rev Immunol. 2008;8:607–18.

235. Lopez-Bravo M, Ardavin C. In vivo induction of immune responses to pathogens by conventional dendritic cells. Immunity. 2008;29:343–51.

236. Alvarez D, Vollmann EH, von Andrian UH. Mechanisms and consequences of dendritic cell migration. Immunity. 2008;29:325–42.

237. Randolph GJ, Angeli V, Swartz MA. Dendritic-cell trafficking to lymph nodes through lymphatic vessels. Nat Rev Immunol. 2005;5:617–28.

238. Chen L, Flies DB. Molecular mechanisms of T cell co-stimulation and co-inhibition. Nat Rev Immunol. 2013;13:227–42.

239. Sims R, van der Lee SJ, Naj AC, Bellenguez C, Badarinarayan N, Jakobsdottir J, et al. Rare coding variants in PLCG2, ABI3, and TREM2 implicate microglial-mediated innate immunity in Alzheimer's disease. Nat Genet. 2017;49:1373–84.

240. Neu KE, Tang Q, Wilson PC, Khan AA. Single-cell genomics: approaches and utility in immunology. Trends Immunol. 2017;38:140–9.

241. Zhou F, Li X, Wang W, Zhu P, Zhou J, He W, et al. Tracing haematopoietic stem cell formation at single-cell resolution. Nature. 2016;533:487–92.

242. Gierahn TM, Wadsworth MH 2nd, Hughes TK, Bryson BD, Butler A, Satija R, et al. Seq-well: portable, low-cost RNA sequencing of single cells at high throughput. Nat Methods. 2017;14:395–8.

T Cell Immunity

Shalu Sharma Kharkwal and Steven A. Porcelli

Abbreviations

AIDS	Acquired immunodeficiency syndrome
APC	Antigen-presenting cell
BCR	B cell receptor
CD	Cluster of differentiation
CTL	Cytotoxic T lymphocyte
CTLA-4	Cytotoxic lymphocyte-associated molecule-4
DC	Dendritic cell
DN	Double negative
GC	Galactosylceramide
HIV	Human immunodeficiency virus
ICOS	Inducible costimulatory signal
IEL	Intraepithelial lymphocytes
IFNγ	Interferon gamma
IL	Interleukin
IPEX	Immune dysregulation, polyendocrinopathy, enteropathy X-linked
MAIT	Mucosa-associated invariant T
MHC	Major histocompatibility complex
NK	Natural killer
NKT	Natural killer T
PD	Programmed death
pMHC	Peptide-MHC complex
Tc	T cytotoxic cell
TCR	T cell receptor
Tfh	Follicular helper T cell
TGFβ	Transforming growth factor β
Th	T helper cell
Treg	T regulatory cell

Introduction

T cells are a remarkably complex and diverse class of lymphocytes that play a central role in many functions of the mammalian immune system. They are at the core of adaptive immunity that is required for effective resistance to many types of pathogens, in particular viruses and many more complex microbes that are able to evade the more primitive mechanisms of innate immunity. Because of their ability to differentiate into long-lived memory cells, T cells are a major component of acquired resistance to infections and a principal target for most types of vaccines [1]. In the absence of T cells, a severe immunodeficiency state occurs with an inability to control infections by common as well as opportunistic microbes. This situation has been strongly emphasized by the consequences of human immunodeficiency virus (HIV) infection, which results in a frequently fatal acquired immunodeficiency syndrome (AIDS) mainly through depletion of T cells. When functioning normally, T cells provide effective control of a wide range of potential infectious agents and also contribute to

S. S. Kharkwal · S. A. Porcelli (✉)
Department of Microbiology and Immunology, Albert Einstein College of Medicine, Bronx, NY, USA
e-mail: shalu.sharma@einstein.yu.edu; steven.porcelli@einstein.yu.edu

© Springer International Publishing AG, part of Springer Nature 2018
B. H. Segal (ed.), *Management of Infections in the Immunocompromised Host*,
https://doi.org/10.1007/978-3-319-77674-3_2

suppression of neoplastic diseases by recognizing and eliminating cancerous cells. A complex process for maintaining self-tolerance of T cells normally prevents recognition of self-antigens, but in rare cases this may fail and result in autoimmunity and a variety of inflammatory diseases. In addition, T cells have a strong tendency to recognize antigens of foreign tissue transplants, even between quite closely related individuals. Thus, they play an important role in many cases of transplant rejection and are a major focus of current efforts to overcome histocompatibility barriers in transplantation.

Origin and Development of T Cells

Like B lymphocytes, T cells also originate from lymphoid progenitors derived from the bone marrow. These progenitor cells migrate to the thymus gland, where they differentiate into mature T cells that populate the peripheral lymphoid tissues and recirculate through the blood and lymph. This process of development is especially active from birth until puberty, after which the production of new T cells is greatly reduced due to involution of the thymus. Like the other major population of lymphocytes, the antibody-producing B cells, T cells express a family of structurally diverse cell surface proteins that serve as receptors for foreign antigens. These T cell receptors (TCRs) are clonally distributed, which means that each T cell generates a unique TCR structure as it develops through a complex process of somatic gene rearrangement. This results in a very large repertoire of specific receptors, each expressed by a different T cell.

The complex process of T cell development in the thymus has been extensively studied, and a sequence of critically important steps has been identified [2]. The process begins with the migration of lymphoid progenitor cells from the fetal liver or the bone marrow into the outer layer or cortex of the thymus. Once in the thymus, these progenitors begin differentiating into thymocytes which are fully committed to progressing along the T cell lineage. Thymocyte development and differentiation is controlled by specific signals

that are unique to the microenvironments of the thymus, initially in the cortex and subsequently in the inner layer or medulla of the organ. Both of these zones of thymic tissue contain a variety of cell types in addition to the thymocytes themselves, including thymic stromal fibroblasts, cortical thymic epithelial cells, medullary thymic epithelial cells, and thymic DCs. A stepwise process has been described by which thymocytes initiate the expression of number of T cell surface markers, most notably the co-receptor molecules CD4 and CD8 and their clonally variable TCRs (Fig. 2.1). This process involves a number of gene rearrangement events as well as both positive and negative selection steps to insure that the TCRs expressed by developing thymocytes are functional but not dangerously autoreactive. Most thymocytes fail to pass the quality control checkpoints of this process, resulting in the vast majority of them undergoing programmed cell death (apoptosis) and being destroyed within the thymus by macrophages. As a result, only a very small fraction, perhaps 0.1% or less, of thymocytes eventually survive to exit the thymic medulla into the circulation as mature, naïve T cells. Encounters with specific antigens that engage the TCRs of these resting, naïve T cells lead to activation and clonal expansion. This is followed by differentiation into effector T cells with a variety of critical functions such as cytokine production or direct cytotoxic activity [3] or conversion into stable memory T cell populations that persist for many years [4]. These stable memory T cells provide improved protection against subsequent exposure to the same or related infections and also form the basis for all vaccine-mediated protection.

Antigen Presentation of Specific T Cell Antigens

The great majority of T cells in humans and most other mammals are specific for peptide fragments of foreign proteins. The complex process of degradation of proteins into small peptides, loading of these peptides onto MHC class I and class II molecules, and their transfer to the surface of

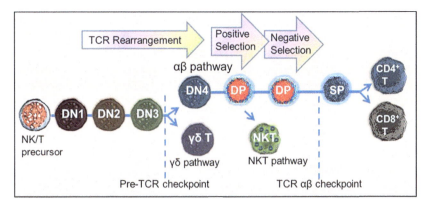

Fig. 2.1 T cell development pathways. The common lymphoid progenitor cell produced in the bone marrow gives rise to the NK/T cell precursor that migrates to the thymus and differentiates into thymocytes. While progressing through a series of "double negative" stages (DN1, DN2, DN3), the developing thymocytes undergo TCRβ gene rearrangements followed by rearrangements of other TCR loci. Thymocytes that successfully assemble a functional TCR progress past the pre-TCR checkpoint. The majority of these cells express TCRαβ and enter into the αβ pathway, whereas a small population expresses TCRγδ and progresses down an alternative γδ pathway. Cells in the αβ pathway then turn on expression of both CD4 and CD8 to become "double positive" (DP) thymocytes. These cells undergo positive and negative selection based on their TCR interactions with molecules expressed on a variety of cells within the thymus. A minor fraction of DP thymocytes enter an alternative selection pathway that generates CD1-restricted T cells including NKT cells. The majority of DP cells downregulate either CD4 or CD8 expression to become "single positive" (SP) thymocytes, a small fraction of which become mature CD4+ or CD8+ T cells that survive and exit the thymus

antigen-presenting cells for probing by T cells is called antigen processing and presentation [5, 6]. Most peptides presented in a healthy individual are of self-origin and pose no danger and elicit no T cell response. However, during infections by viruses or other pathogens, a very large fraction of peptides bound to MHC molecules may be derived from foreign proteins and are recognized by T cells for induction of immune responses [7]. The complexes of peptides bound to MHC molecules (pMHC complexes) are assembled by the exogenous and endogenous antigen processing and presentation pathways [8].

The exogenous pathway for antigen processing and presentation is the principal mechanism by which peptides derived from proteins of extracellular origin become bound to MHC class II molecules for presentation to CD4+ T cells [9]. This pathway is essential for responses of CD4+ T cells against proteins that are internalized by professional antigen-presenting cells (APCs) via phagocytosis or receptor-mediated endocytosis and transferred to the endosomal compartments for degradation. The protease-containing endosomes are highly acidic and degrade the proteins

to yield peptides of varying length. A subset of endosomes, often referred to as MHC class II compartments (MIICs), are enriched for MHC class II molecules as well as other accessory proteins that facilitate the formation of pMHC complexes [10]. The exogenous pathway is most prominently active in professional APCs such as DCs, macrophages, and B cells, which can efficiently take up antigens and express high levels of MHC II molecules. The pMHC II complexes formed in MIICs are packaged into vesicles which are transported to the plasma membrane of the APCs. Fusion of these vesicles with the plasma membrane results in surface expression of pMHC II complexes for surface presentation and recognition by CD4+ T helper cells.

In contrast to the exogenous pathway that is restricted mainly to professional APCs, the endogenous antigen processing pathway, which generates peptides for presentation by MHC class I molecules, is active in all nucleated cells. The endogenous pathway enables the degradation of intracellular proteins by the cytoplasmic proteasome complex into peptides of eight to ten amino acids in length [11]. These are transported into the endoplasmic reticulum (ER) by a specialized transporter complex called TAP. Once in the ER lumen, the peptides associate with newly synthesized MHC class I molecules, which are released into the secretory pathway and transported to the cell surface. Complexes of antigenic peptides and MHC class I molecules formed in this way provide the major targets on the cell surface for recognition by CD8+ T cells.

Notably, it has been shown in some cases that mature DCs are also capable of presenting peptides derived from proteins of extracellular origin on MHC I molecules to induce CD8+ T cell responses. This process is called crosspresentation and is believed to be extremely important for the initial activation and expansion of naïve CD8+ T cells during the initiation of cell-mediated immune responses [12]. This pathway for presentation of exogenously acquired antigens on MHC I molecules has been found to be facilitated by internalization of particulate forms of antigen, particularly apoptotic debris of virally infected cells. The precise intracellular compartments and mechanisms by which endocytosed antigens undergo processing into peptides and loading onto MHC I proteins for cross-presentation to CD8+ T cells remain controversial [13].

In addition to the classical MHC I- and MHC II-dependent antigen-presenting pathways for peptide presentation, it has also been shown that at least three alternative pathways exist for the presentation of nonpeptide antigens (Fig. 2.2) [14]. Among these, the most extensively studied and currently best understood is the CD1-dependent pathway for presentation of lipid and glycolipid antigens. The CD1 molecules that mediate this pathway are structurally related to the classical MHC I molecules but have evolved specialized features to adapt them for the binding and presentation of a variety of highly hydrophobic lipids of microbial or self-origin [15]. Another MHC I-like molecule called MR1 has recently been demonstrated to bind vitamin B metabolites produced by bacteria and present these to a unique population of T cells known as mucosa-associated invariant T (MAIT) cells [16]. In addition, a member of the butyrophilin family of cell surface proteins, BTN3A1, has been shown to serve as the presenting molecule for phosphorylated metabolites of the isoprenoid biosynthesis pathway present in most bacteria and parasites [17]. These alternative antigen presentation pathways, and the unconventional T cell populations that respond through them, are discussed in greater detail in subsequent sections of this chapter.

T Cell Antigen Receptors

The expression of T cell antigen receptors (TCRs) is a phenotypic hallmark of all mature T cells. These are cell surface protein complexes that mediate the specific recognition of antigens. These proteins are induced early in the process of T cell development and mediate both positive and negative selection steps in the thymus [2]. The TCR complex consists of several invariant polypeptide chains comprising the CD3 complex which are noncovalently associated with either TCRαβ or TCRγδ heterodimers [18]. Whereas the invariant CD3 subunits of the complex are principally responsible for signal transduction, the structurally variable TCRαβ or TCRγδ components are responsible for antigen recognition. In humans and most other mammals, the great majority of T cells in the circulation and in lymphoid tissues express TCRαβ, while TCRγδ is often abundant on certain populations of T cells residing in nonlymphoid tissues (e.g., in skin or intestine). In general, both types of TCRs share substantial structural similarities with immunoglobulins and have an analogous domain structure including constant (C) region and variable (V) region domains along with their transmembrane regions and short cytoplasmic tails. However, unlike immunoglobulins which comprise the B cell receptors (BCRs) or secreted antibodies which have two antigen-binding sites, TCRs have only one antigen-binding site and are not secreted. The structural diversity of TCRs is generated through a process of somatic recombination of multiple variable (V) region genes with one of a variety of short diversity (D) and joining (J) gene segments. This process is similar in

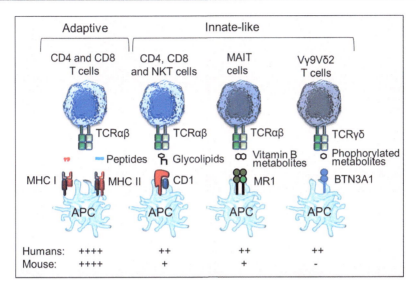

Fig. 2.2 Pathways for antigen presentation to T cells. The four known pathways for antigen presentation are illustrated. In the dominant or "classical" MHC-restricted pathway, peptide antigens derived by processing of larger proteins are presented by MHC class I or class II molecules to the major populations of CD4$^+$ and CD8$^+$ T cells expressing classical TCRαβ antigen receptors. The MHC-dependent peptide presentation pathway is the predominant mode of T cell recognition in both humans and rodent models. The other three known pathways present nonpeptide antigens to T cell subsets that use either TCRαβ receptors with limited diversity or TCRγδ receptors. These alternative pathways are more prominent in humans than in mice, and their roles in host immunity and disease remain largely undefined. While the MHC-restricted peptide presentation pathways generate adaptive immunity with memory T cells that give enhanced responses upon subsequent re-exposure to previously encountered antigens, the alternative pathways appear to function more as "hardwired" innate recognition pathways and have less capacity to generate immunological memory

many respects to the mechanism for generation of diversity in BCRs and antibodies, with the notable difference that TCR genes do not undergo somatic hypermutation. The process of random joining of V, D, and J segments generates a vast repertoire of distinct receptors, enabling T cell recognition of an enormous range of antigens.

The TCRαβ and TCRγδ heterodimers have very short cytoplasmic tails that are not capable of transducing signals upon engagement by antigen and therefore rely on the associated CD3 subunits to carry out this function. Five distinct CD3 polypeptides (CD3γ, CD3δ, CD3ε, CD3ζ, CD3η) are physically associated with the TCRs on the cell surface (Fig. 2.3). After TCRs interact with their cognate antigens, intracellular signaling kinases such as Lck phosphorylate the tyrosine residues in specific cytoplasmic sequences known as immunoreceptor tyrosine-based activation motifs (ITAMs) of several CD3 subunits. This leads to the recruitment of additional kinases

to the CD3 complex to initiate the signaling cascade. Another function of CD3 is to promote the stable assembly and intracellular transport of newly synthesized TCRs to the cell surface. Thus, surface expression of TCR is ablated in mice lacking individual CD3 chains due to the requirement for the TCRαβ or TCRγδ heterodimer to become associated with CD3 in the ER prior to its transport to the Golgi apparatus for glycosylation and transfer to the T cell surface. The extracellular immunoglobulin-like domains of CD3γ, CD3δ, and CD3ε interact with the TCR to keep the entire complex intact during intracellular transport and on the cell surface [19]. Conversely, the CD3ζ chain and its alternatively spliced form known as CD3η are minimally exposed on the cell surface but play a major role in signal transduction through their intracellular domains.

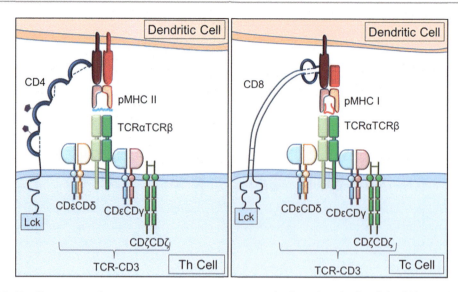

Fig. 2.3 T cell receptor and co-receptor recognition of pMHC complexes. The TCRαβ heterodimer mediates direct recognition of peptides bound to MHC class II in the case of CD4+ T cells (*left*) or MHC class I in the case of CD8+ T cells (*right*). The TCRαβ dimers are bound noncovalently to the subunits of the CD3 complex on the T cell surface. The CD4 and CD8 co-receptors recruit the tyrosine kinase Lck, which contributes to T cell activation by phosphorylating the cytoplasmic domains of the CD3 proteins, particularly the CD3ζ chains

CD4 and CD8 Co-receptors

The CD4 and CD8 molecules are called co-receptors because they assist TCR in establishing interactions with specific pMHC complexes and strengthen the signals resulting from these interactions [20]. Approximately two thirds of mature T cells expressing TCRαβ also express CD4, whereas most of the remaining one third express CD8. Neither CD4 nor CD8 is expressed by the majority of T cells bearing TCRγδ, and these cells are often referred to as double negative (DN). On mature T cells, the expression of CD4 or CD8 is virtually always mutually exclusive and correlates strongly with different functions. Thus, T helper (Th) cells express CD4, which interacts with the MHC II molecule on APCs and stabilizes TCR recognition of pMHC II complexes. Conversely, CD8 is expressed predominantly by cytotoxic T cells (Tc) and assists in TCR recognition of pMHC I complexes (Fig. 2.3). Despite the striking basic similarity in their functions, CD4 and CD8 are structurally very different. CD4 is a single-chain polypeptide with four extracellular immunoglobulin (Ig)-like domains and a cytoplasmic tail. The most membrane distal extracellular domains of CD4 interact with the membrane proximal domains of MHC class II molecules, and the cytosolic tail binds the intracellular signaling kinase Lck to initiate early steps in T cell activation. In contrast, CD8 molecules are most commonly heterodimers composed of similar CD8α and CD8β polypeptides, each having only one Ig-like extracellular domain. The CD8 extracellular domains bind to the membrane proximal domain of MHC class I molecules, and the cytoplasmic tail of the CD8α chain also recruits Lck to the TCR complex. Although the interaction of TCRs with cognate pMHC complexes does not necessarily require CD4 or CD8, the participation of these co-receptors strengthens the interaction and greatly amplifies the signals that result from it.

Costimulatory and Co-inhibitory Receptors

Activation of a resting T cell triggers its proliferation and clonal expansion, followed by its differentiation into effector or memory T cells. The process of T cell activation is tightly controlled and regulated to prevent autoimmunity or excessive inflammation and involves a series of integrated activating signals as well as inhibitory "checkpoints." Although the number of specific molecular interactions or signals involved in T cell activation is large, these can be separated into three types, generally referred to as signals 1, 2, and 3 (Fig. 2.4). Signal 1 is emitted when the TCR makes contact with its specific cognate antigen presented on the surface of an APC. Signal 2 involves interaction of one or more costimulatory receptor molecules on T cells with their membrane-bound ligands on the APC surface. Signal 3 is delivered by cytokines, particularly interleukin-2 (IL-2) which is a major T cell growth factor.

Costimulation (signal 2) is critically important for activation of naïve T cells, especially in the case of naïve CD4+ T cells. The most potent and best studied of the costimulatory receptors on T cells is CD28, a sparsely expressed T cell membrane protein that binds to B7.1 (CD80) and B7.2 (CD86) proteins on APCs during antigen recognition [21]. Delivery of signal 1 by the TCR without engagement of CD28 to provide signal 2 does not result in productive T cell responses but instead leads to a prolonged unresponsive state called anergy. Thus, the requirement for this second signal is likely to represent a mechanism that contributes to the maintenance of self-tolerance [21]. On the other hand, when CD28 engagement by either of its ligands occurs concurrently with signal 1, a cascade of further events is initiated leading to T cell proliferation and expression of effector functions. These include increased expression of CD40L on the T cell, which engages its receptor CD40 on DCs to further amplify their expression of stimulatory surface proteins and cytokines, a process referred to as "licensing" of DCs. CD28 engagement on T cells together with signal 1 also induces the secretion of IL-2 and expression of the high-affinity receptor for this cytokine on the cell surface. The binding of IL-2 to its receptor, along with the binding of other cytokines to their specific receptors, provides signal 3 to further drive proliferation and

differentiation of the antigen-specific T cell clones.

In addition to these central costimulatory pathways, there are multiple secondary mechanisms that further amplify or influence the quality of T cell responses. For example, following initial activation, many T cells express an inducible T cell costimulatory molecule (ICOS, also known as CD278). This receptor is structurally homologous to CD28 and binds to a specific ligand (ICOS-L or B7-H2) to provide further amplification and differentiation of the responding T cells [22]. Other important costimulatory molecules that make significant contributions to T cell activation include members of the TNF receptor superfamily such as the 4-1BB protein (CD137) [23].

After T cell activation has occurred, a series of molecules known as co-inhibitory receptors are upregulated and engaged to control and eventually shut down the T cell response. One of the most important of these is the protein CTLA-4 (CD152), which binds with high affinity to the same ligands that engage the CD28 co-receptor. By competing effectively for these ligands with CD28, the engagement of CTLA-4 delivers a potent inhibitory signal that shuts down T cell responses [24]. Similarly, the co-inhibitory receptor PD-1 (CD279), a related member of the CTLA-4 family, is a major immunoregulatory molecule. This receptor is expressed by T cells as well as B cells and macrophages, implying a broad role in the control of immune responses. The two ligands of PD-1, PD-L1 (CD274) and PD-L2 (CD273), are expressed on leukocytes as well as nonhematopoietic cell types and can be upregulated by inflammatory cytokines such as interferon-γ (IFNγ). Inhibitory signaling by CTLA-4 and PD-1 receptors represents important inhibitory "checkpoints" in the control of normal T cell responses [25], and without them a marked tendency toward autoimmunity or chronic inflammation is observed. However, in some situations these molecules may be associated with unwanted suppression of beneficial immune responses, and favorable clinical effects can be achieved by temporarily blocking these co-inhibitory pathways. Thus, antibodies that

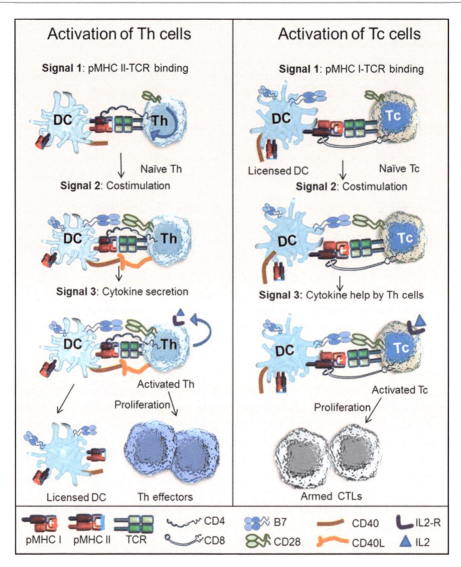

Fig. 2.4 Three distinct signals involved in activation of naïve T cells. Activation of naïve CD4+ T cells (left) is initiated when the TCR interacts with cognate pMHC II complexes on a dendritic cell, thus delivering signal 1 to the T cell. Other factors in the local priming environment, principally signals from innate immune recognition receptors that respond directly to pathogens or inflammation, induce upregulation of B7 molecules on the DC. This engages CD28 on the T cell, providing costimulation as signal 2. Costimulation greatly augments production of IL-2 and other cytokines, which interact with their receptors in an autocrine fashion to deliver signal 3. Together, this sequential signaling cascade induces proliferation and maturation of CD4+ T cells into effector Th cells. In addition, the interaction of CD40L on the T cell with its receptor CD40 on the DCs enhances their antigen processing and presentation functions, converting them from a resting state to a licensed DC. These licensed DCs are highly efficient at initiating a similar cascade of signals for activation of naïve CD8+ T cells (right). They receive signal 1 through engagement of their TCRs by pMHC I complexes on licensed DCs and signal 2 through CD28 engagement. Signal 3 is delivered primarily by paracrine IL-2 or other cytokines provided by Th effector cells. The result is activation and proliferation of Tc resulting in armed CTLs that mediate potent perforin/granzyme or Fas-mediated cytotoxicity

block signaling by CTLA-4 and PD-1 are now well established as effective agents for treatment of multiple types of cancers [24, 26, 27] and also have the ability to restore antiviral activities of T cells [28]. While cancer immunotherapy targeting immune checkpoints has significantly improved patient outcomes, it has also been associated with immune-related adverse effects such as hypophysitis and primary thyroid dysfunction in the case of CTLA4-targeted immunotherapy and with type 1 diabetes and primary thyroid dysfunction with PD1-targeted immunotherapy [27].

Functional Specialization of T Cell Subsets

Although all T cells share certain canonical features, such as the expression of a CD3-TCR complex, many different functionally and phenotypically distinct subsets of T cells have been defined. Early studies of T cell subsets recognized three distinct functional types, designated helper, cytotoxic, and suppressor T cells. More recent work has largely supported and further refined this classification.

Helper T Cells

T cells that express CD4 and recognize peptide antigens presented by MHC class II are generally classified as helper T cells (Th) because of their ability to differentiate into cells that provide help to B cells for augmenting antibody production. This designation is an oversimplification, as naïve CD4+ T cells have the potential to differentiate into a complex variety of different functional subsets with different roles in the immune response (Fig. 2.5) [29]. The significance of the range of effector functions of differentiated and activated CD4+ T cells is evident from diseases that are caused by either loss or perturbation of these functions [30]. Upon initial encounter with antigen and subsequent activation, naïve Th cells initially give rise to IL-2-secreting effectors that are referred to as Th0 cells. These then go on to differentiate into specialized effector cells comprising a number of different specific subsets, depending upon the type of cytokines present in the microenvironment [31]. In general, the presence of the cytokine IL-12, along with the

absence of certain other factors such as IL-4, leads to the generation of Th1 cells that produce IFNγ and mediate critical roles in immune responses against intracellular infections caused by viruses and certain bacteria [31]. In contrast, initial antigen encounter in a milieu rich in IL-4 produced by mast cells, basophils, or other cell types leads to differentiation into Th2 cells. These produce IL-4 and a range of other cytokines associated with humoral and cellular responses primarily to parasitic infections and environmental allergens [32, 33]. The differentiation of naïve Th cells into Th1 and Th2 subsets is controlled to a great extent by the induction of specific transcription factors, T-bet in the case of Th1 cells and Gata-3 for Th2 cells [34].

In addition to the well-established Th1 and Th2 subsets, a number of additional functional subsets of Th cells have been more recently defined, greatly extending the complexity of Th cell differentiation and specialization of function. In general, these subsets are each defined by secretion of one or more specific signature cytokines and by expression of a characteristic master transcriptional regulator. For example, Th17 cells are characterized by their secretion of cytokines of the IL-17 family and by expression of the transcription factor RORγt [35]. These cells localize most prominently to nonlymphoid tissues, such as the skin and gastrointestinal tract. The differentiation of naïve Th cells into Th17 cells is also dependent on the cytokine milieu in which they initially encounter antigen and appears to be driven predominantly by IL-6 and TGF-β. Th17 cells also upregulate the receptor for IL-23, and their proliferation is strongly amplified by that cytokine. Th17 cells are important for recruitment of neutrophils and other effector cells to sites of infection and play a significant part in immunity to many types of extracellular bacteria and fungal pathogens. They are also implicated in the pathogenesis of autoimmune disorders such as multiple sclerosis and rheumatoid arthritis [36, 37]. Another novel subset defined by secretion of IL-9 has been described and classified as Th9 cells [38]. Originally described as a T cell and mast cell growth factor, IL-9 is a multifunctional cytokine secreted by many cell types including T

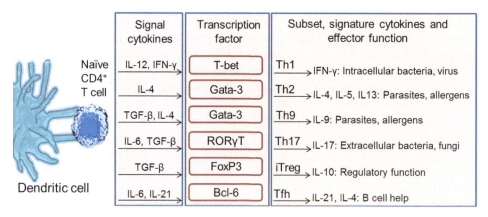

	Signal cytokines	Transcription factor	Subset, signature cytokines and effector function
Naïve CD4+ T cell	IL-12, IFN-γ	T-bet	Th1 → IFN-γ: Intracellular bacteria, virus
	IL-4	Gata-3	Th2 → IL-4, IL-5, IL13: Parasites, allergens
	TGF-β, IL-4	Gata-3	Th9 → IL-9: Parasites, allergens
	IL-6, TGF-β	RORγT	Th17 → IL-17: Extracellular bacteria, fungi
	TGF-β	FoxP3	iTreg → IL-10: Regulatory function
	IL-6, IL-21	Bcl-6	Tfh → IL-21, IL-4: B cell help

Dendritic cell

Fig. 2.5 Differentiation of naïve CD4+ T cells into functional Th subsets. Naïve CD4+ T cells have the capacity to differentiate into at least six well-recognized, distinct functional subsets. This process is driven largely by the cytokines that are most abundant in the environment where the naïve T cell first encounters antigen. The key cytokine signals drive the induction of at least one master transcription factor, which programs the activated Th cell to become one of the functional subsets indicated. These subsets differ with respect to their cytokine secretion signatures and with regard to their principal immunological functions

cells, eosinophils, mast cells, and neutrophils. Th9 cells are believed to have important roles in mediating immunity against helminths and may participate in chronic and acute allergic inflammation. They also have unique requirements for their development that distinguish them from other Th subsets [39–42].

Another distinct subset of differentiated Th cells is designated follicular helper T cells (Tfh). These cells appear to arise from naïve CD4+ T cells during activation by antigens in the paracortical regions of lymph nodes and then migrate to the B cell-rich follicles. Tfh cells express the chemokine receptor CXCR5, which is involved in their attraction to the follicles [43]. They secrete the cytokines IL-21 and B and T lymphocyte attenuator (BTLA) and express the costimulatory molecule ICOS, all of which are important in driving the germinal center reaction that is crucial for triggering B cells to undergo antibody class switching, maturation, and differentiation into antibody-secreting plasma cells and memory B cells [44]. Dysregulation of Tfh cells or genetic defects that affect Tfh cell differentiation are known to cause autoimmunity and primary immune deficiency diseases [44, 45].

Cytotoxic T Cells

Cytotoxic T cells (Tc) as classically defined are CD8+ and recognize peptide antigens presented by MHC class I molecules. Naïve Tc that receive the appropriate combinations of antigenic, costimulatory, and inflammatory cytokine signals differentiate into mature cytolytic T cells (CTLs) that are "armed" with cytolytic granules in their cytoplasm. By recognizing and lysing infected target cells, CTLs play a critically important role in immune defense against intracellular infections such as viruses and certain types of bacteria [46, 47]. In addition to antimicrobial defense, CTLs mediate antitumor immunity. Armed CTLs patrol the body and are attracted to inflamed sites where they independently carry out target killing by forming transient conjugates with infected host cells. Following recognition of an infected cell, CTLs mediate killing of the target cell by several potential mechanisms, the most important of which is probably the exocytosis of granules containing perforin (a pore-forming protein) and proteases (known as granzymes). Other mechanisms for target cell killing involve engagement of the death receptor Fas on the target cell by Fas ligand on the membrane of the armed CTL and production of soluble cytotoxic cytokines such as TNF-α. All of these mechanisms induce programmed cell death (apoptosis) of the target cell, causing it to degenerate into debris that is rapidly scavenged by tissue macrophages.

Regulatory T Cells

Originally described as suppressor T cells (Ts), it has now become standard to refer to T cells that inhibit immune responses as regulatory T cells (Treg). The best described and characterized Treg cells are a subpopulation of $CD4^+$ T cells that maintain tolerance to self-antigens to control autoimmunity, suppress allergic disease, and contribute to feto-maternal tolerance by immune modulation [48]. Current classification divides these into so-called natural Tregs (nTregs), which differentiate from naïve $CD4^+$ T cells before exiting the thymus, and induced Tregs (iTregs) which are derived from mature $CD4^+$ T cells outside of the thymus. The nuclear protein FoxP3 is the major transcriptional regulator that drives differentiation of developing or mature naïve T cells into Tregs [49]. This is associated with expression of a characteristic pattern of several cell surface markers such as CD25, CTLA-4, GITR, and LAG-3. However, these markers are not specific for Tregs as they are also expressed by activated Th cells. Although most Tregs as currently described are $CD4^+$ and recognize antigens presented by MHC class II, a small population of $FoxP3^+$ Tregs has also been found to be MHC class I restricted and $CD8^+$ [50]. In general, Tregs need to be activated by TCR engagement to be able to suppress the activation of other T cells, implying that the suppressive activity is antigen-dependent as well as antigen-specific [50]. However, there is evidence suggesting that Tregs can suppress Th cells that do not share the same antigen specificity but perhaps with less efficiency. Tregs can recognize self- as well as nonself-antigens, as evident from their protective roles in autoimmune diseases such as type I diabetes as well as in chronic inflammation caused by infections [51–53]. It appears that Treg activity is downregulated either directly or indirectly by other immune cells during active immune responses to most infections to allow pathogen

elimination, although some pathogens such as HIV, *Mycobacterium tuberculosis*, and *Leishmania* species are able to manipulate Tregs to suppress host immunity and maintain chronic infection [54, 55]. An increased number of $CD4^+$ Tregs are often associated with malignant tumors and correlate with poor prognosis. Modulating the Treg function in such conditions may restore an effective adaptive immune response and is thus a potential therapeutic strategy for cancer and certain types of persistent infections [56]. A deficiency of Tregs due to mutation in Foxp3 in humans has been identified as the cause of a severe and fatal autoimmune disorder known as the IPEX (immune dysregulation, polyendocrinopathy, enteropathy X-linked) syndrome [57].

Nonconventional T Cells

A number of distinct subsets of T cells have been recognized that do not adhere to the general rules of antigen recognition that apply to the classical Th, Tc, and Treg subsets described above. These nonconventional T cells are characterized by TCR-mediated recognition of nonpeptide antigens, which are presented by molecules distinct from the classical MHC class I or MHC class II molecules (Fig. 2.2). The nonconventional T cell subsets appear to have a more restricted repertoire of antigen receptors and play specialized but possibly important roles in host immunity. The three best characterized groups of nonconventional T cells currently recognized are CD1-restricted T cells, γδ T cells, and mucosa-associated invariant T (MAIT) cells.

CD1-Restricted T Cells

A relatively small subset of T cells in humans recognizes lipid antigens presented by proteins of the CD1 family, which are structurally similar to MHC class I molecules. CD1 exists in five different forms in humans (CD1a, CD1b, CD1c, CD1d, and CD1e), and all are known to function in the binding and presentation of lipid antigens to T cells [15, 58, 59]. The developmental pathways, specificities, and specific immune functions of most CD1-restricted T cells are not currently known. However, it has been established that a subpopulation of these T cells recognizes specific lipid antigens produced by *Mycobacterium tuberculosis* and other related organisms [60, 61]. CD1-restricted T cells possess many of the effector functions associated with conventional T cells, including cytotoxic activity, cytokine secretion, and the ability to provide help to B cells for antibody production. One specific population of T cells recognizing lipids presented by the CD1d molecule (the only form of CD1 that is present in rodents) has been extensively studied in both mice and humans. These are called natural killer T (NKT) cells, and they represent by far the best characterized population of CD1-restricted T cells. Most of these cells express an unusual TCRαβ with an invariant TCRα chain and also express a number of C-type lectin receptors that are more typically found on NK cells [62]. Many features of NKT cells are highly conserved between mice and humans, although the frequency of these cells is much lower in humans suggesting a less prominent role in the overall immune response than in rodents. NKT cells are known to recognize a range of glycolipids, such as various α-glycosylceramides or diacylglycerols produced by bacteria [63], and the availability of synthetic forms of α-galactosylceramide (α-GC) that potently activate NKT cells in vitro and in vivo has greatly facilitated research on this T cell subset [64]. NKT cells have been shown in mouse models to participate in immune responses against many types of pathogens and also contribute to anticancer immunity. Deletion of CD4[+] NKT cells early during HIV infection is associated with subsequent destruction of immune function [65]. Under certain conditions, they also can function as regulatory T cells and have the ability to suppress autoimmune or inflammatory diseases [66, 67].

γδ T Cells

A relatively small subset of T cells expresses TCRs that lack the heterodimer of α and β chains that are found in conventional MHC class I- and II-restricted T cells and instead expresses a related but distinct heterodimer called TCRγδ. These T cells are most abundant in the gut mucosa where they comprise a substantial portion of the intraepithelial lymphocyte (IEL) population [68, 69]. They are also found prominently in the skin in some species (e.g., mice, but not humans) and are present in the circulation and lymphoid organs in low numbers. There are multiple subtypes of γδ T cells which are classified according to the particular variable region genes expressed in their TCRs. The specificities and functions of most of these subtypes remain unknown. However, one population in humans, known as the Vγ9/Vδ2 subset based on its TCR variable region gene usage, has been shown to specifically respond to a class of microbial metabolites which are mainly small phosphorylated molecules [70]. Remarkably, these appear to be presented by a member of the butyrophilin family of cell surface proteins, which are unrelated to MHC class I or II or CD1 molecules [17]. The antigens and antigen-presenting molecules recognized by other subsets of γδ T cells are less well defined, although multiple studies suggest a range of different specificities related to cellular stress and invading pathogens [71]. However, it has also been shown that human Vδ1[+] γδ T cells demonstrate reactivity that is dependent on several members of the CD1 family and most likely recognize lipid ligands presented by these molecules [72]. γδ T cells have been reported to demonstrate a wide range of effector functions and have been frequently characterized as innate-like lymphocytes that may bridge the gap between innate and adaptive components of the immune system [68, 71].

MAIT Cells

Mucosa-associated invariant T (MAIT) cells are another population of innate-like lymphocytes that respond to a limited number of antigens that are mainly pathogen-derived riboflavin metabolites presented by an MHC class I-related molecule called MR1 [73]. MAIT cells reside mainly in the gut lamina propria and are also found at low frequency in other tissues such as the liver and blood. They have unique developmental requirements which depend on the presence of the gut commensal microbiota and B cells [74]. MAIT cells express an unusual αβ TCR with a nearly invariant α chain, similar in principle but distinct from that expressed by NKT cells. A wide variety of bacteria can activate MAIT cells in vitro; however their role in protection against pathogenic bacteria remains largely unclear. The frequency of MAIT cells has been observed to decline significantly during early stages of HIV infection, although residual persisting cells remain functional and may help to control bacterial infections [75]. Activated MAIT cells have cytotoxic activity and may play a role in immunity against intracellular as well as extracellular bacteria [76, 77].

Summary

The paramount importance of T cells in adaptive immunity is a well-established central dogma of immunology, although the variety of ways in which these cells operate remains an area of intensive study. Basic discoveries on the effector functions of T cells and their mechanisms of antigen recognition continue to accumulate and improve our ability to manipulate this crucial arm of the immune system. Ultimately, a thorough understanding of T cell biology will provide a route to rational design of many improved vaccines and immunotherapies.

Acknowledgments The authors acknowledge support from NIH grants AI45889 and AI093649 (both awarded to SAP).

References

1. Seder RA, Darrah PA, Roederer M. T-cell quality in memory and protection: implications for vaccine design. Nat Rev Immunol. 2008;8(4):247–58.
2. Shah DK, Zuniga-Pflucker JC. An overview of the intrathymic intricacies of T cell development. J Immunol. 2014;192(9):4017–23.
3. Broere F, Apasov SG, Sitkovsky MV, Eden WV. In: Nijkamp FP, Parnham MJ, editors. T cell subsets and T cell-mediated immunity. 3rd ed. Basel: Birkhauser; 2011.
4. Farber DL, Yudanin NA, Restifo NP. Human memory T cells: generation, compartmentalization and homeostasis. Nat Rev Immunol. 2014;14(1):24–35.
5. Roche PA, Furuta K. The ins and outs of MHC class II-mediated antigen processing and presentation. Nat Rev Immunol. 2015;15(4):203–16.
6. van Kasteren SI, Overkleeft H, Ovaa H, Neefjes J. Chemical biology of antigen presentation by MHC molecules. Curr Opin Immunol. 2014;26:21–31.
7. Bleek GMV, Nathenson SG. Isolation of an endogenously processed immunodominant viral peptide from the class I H-2Kb molecule. Nature. 1990;348(6298):213–6.
8. Neefjes J, Jongsma ML, Paul P, Bakke O. Towards a systems understanding of MHC class I and MHC class II antigen presentation. Nat Rev Immunol. 2011;11(12):823–36.
9. Watts C. The exogenous pathway for antigen presentation on major histocompatibility complex class II and CD1 molecules. Nat Immunol. 2004;5(7):685–92.
10. Garstka MA, Neefjes J. How to target MHC class II into the MIIC compartment. Mol Immunol. 2013;55(2):162–5.
11. Blum JS, Wearsch PA, Cresswell P. Pathways of antigen processing. Annu Rev Immunol. 2013;31:443–73.
12. Segura E, Amigorena S. Cross-presentation by human dendritic cell subsets. Immunol Lett. 2014;158(1–2):73–8.
13. Basta S, Alatery A. The cross-priming pathway: a portrait of an intricate immune system. Scand J Immunol. 2007;65(4):311–9.
14. Dieli F, Fadda R, Caccamo N. Butyrophilin 3A1 presents phosphoantigens to human gammadelta T cells: the fourth model of antigen presentation in the immune system. Cell Mol Immunol. 2014;11(2):123–5.
15. Adams EJ. Lipid presentation by human CD1 molecules and the diverse T cell populations that respond to them. Curr Opin Immunol. 2014;26:1–6.
16. Birkinshaw RW, Kjer-Nielsen L, Eckle SB, McCluskey J, Rossjohn J. MAITs, MR1 and vitamin B metabolites. Curr Opin Immunol. 2014;26:7–13.
17. Vavassori S, Kumar A, Wan GS, Ramanjaneyulu GS, Cavallari M, El Daker S, et al. Butyrophilin 3A1 binds phosphorylated antigens and stimulates human gammadelta T cells. Nat Immunol. 2013;14(9):908–16.
18. Kuhns MS, Badgandi HB. Piecing together the family portrait of TCR-CD3 complexes. Immunol Rev. 2012;250(1):120–43.
19. Wucherpfennig KW, Gagnon E, Call MJ, Huseby ES, Call ME. Structural biology of the T-cell receptor: insights into receptor assembly, ligand recognition, and initiation of signaling. Cold Spring Harb Perspect Biol. 2010;2(4):a005140.
20. Li Y, Yin Y, Mariuzza RA. Structural and biophysical insights into the role of CD4 and CD8 in T cell activation. Front Immunol. 2013;4:206.

21. Chen L, Flies DB. Molecular mechanisms of T cell co-stimulation and co-inhibition. Nat Rev Immunol. 2013;13(4):227–42.

22. Simpson TR, Quezada SA, Allison JP. Regulation of CD4 T cell activation and effector function by inducible costimulator (ICOS). Curr Opin Immunol. 2010;22(3):326–32.

23. Long AH, Haso WM, Shern JF, Wanhainen KM, Murgai M, Ingaramo M, et al. 4-1BB costimulation ameliorates T cell exhaustion induced by tonic signaling of chimeric antigen receptors. Nat Med 2015; 21(6):581–90.

24. Weber J. Immune checkpoint proteins: a new therapeutic paradigm for cancer – preclinical background: CTLA-4 and PD-1 blockade. Semin Oncol. 2010;37(5):430–9.

25. Engeland CE, Grossardt C, Veinalde R, Bossow S, Lutz D, Kaufmann JK, et al. CTLA-4 and PD-L1 checkpoint blockade enhances oncolytic measles virus therapy. Mol Ther J Am Soc Gene Ther. 2014;22(11):1949–59.

26. Ohigashi Y, Sho M, Yamada Y, Tsurui Y, Hamada K, Ikeda N, et al. Clinical significance of programmed death-1 ligand-1 and programmed death-1 ligand-2 expression in human esophageal cancer. Clin Cancer Res. 2005;11(8):2947–53.

27. Byun DJ, Wolchok JD, Rosenberg LM, Girotra M. Cancer immunotherapy [mdash] immune checkpoint blockade and associated endocrinopathies. Nat Rev Endocrinol. 2017;13(4):195–207.

28. Barber DL, Wherry EJ, Masopust D, Zhu B, Allison JP, Sharpe AH, et al. Restoring function in exhausted CD8 T cells during chronic viral infection. Nature. 2006;439(7077):682–7.

29. Zhu J, Paul WE. CD4 T cells: fates, functions, and faults. Blood. 2008;112(5):1557–69.

30. Al-Herz W, Bousfiha A, Casanova JL, Chapel H, Conley ME, Cunningham-Rundles C, et al. Primary immunodeficiency diseases: an update on the classification from the international union of immunological societies expert committee for primary immunodeficiency. Front Immunol. 2011;2:54.

31. Coquet JM, Rausch L, Borst J. The importance of co-stimulation in the orchestration of T helper cell differentiation. Immunol Cell Biol 2015;93(9):780–8.

32. Gutcher I, Becher B. APC-derived cytokines and T cell polarization in autoimmune inflammation. J Clin Invest. 2007;117(5):1119–27.

33. Moss RB, Moll T, El-Kalay M, Kohne C, Soo Hoo W, Encinas J, et al. Th1/Th2 cells in inflammatory disease states: therapeutic implications. Expert Opin Biol Ther. 2004;4(12):1887–96.

34. Wilson CB, Rowell E, Sekimata M. Epigenetic control of T-helper-cell differentiation. Nat Rev Immunol. 2009;9(2):91–105.

35. Ivanov II, McKenzie BS, Zhou L, Tadokoro CE, Lepelley A, Lafaille JJ, et al. The orphan nuclear receptor RORgammat directs the differentiation program of proinflammatory IL-17+ T helper cells. Cell. 2006;126(6):1121–33.

36. Korn T, Bettelli E, Gao W, Awasthi A, Jager A, Strom TB, et al. IL-21 initiates an alternative pathway to induce proinflammatory T(H)17 cells. Nature. 2007;448(7152):484–7.

37. Fouser LA, Wright JF, Dunussi-Joannopoulos K, Collins M. Th17 cytokines and their emerging roles in inflammation and autoimmunity. Immunol Rev. 2008;226:87–102.

38. Kaplan MH, Hufford MM, Olson MR. The development and in vivo function of T helper 9 cells. Nat Rev Immunol. 2015;15(5):295–307.

39. Stassen M, Schmitt E, Bopp T. From interleukin-9 to T helper 9 cells. Ann N Y Acad Sci. 2012;1247:56–68.

40. Kaplan MH. Th9 cells: differentiation and disease. Immunol Rev. 2013;252(1):104–15.

41. Xie J, Lotoski LC, Chooniedass R, Su RC, Simons FE, Liem J, et al. Elevated antigen-driven IL-9 responses are prominent in peanut allergic humans. PLoS One. 2012;7(10):e45377.

42. Dardalhon V, Awasthi A, Kwon H, Galileos G, Gao W, Sobel RA, et al. IL-4 inhibits TGF-beta-induced Foxp3+ T cells and, together with TGF-beta, generates IL-9+ IL-10+ Foxp3(-) effector T cells. Nat Immunol. 2008;9(12):1347–55.

43. Crotty S. T follicular helper cell differentiation, function, and roles in disease. Immunity. 2014;41(4):529–42.

44. Tangye SG, Ma CS, Brink R, Deenick EK. The good, the bad and the ugly – TFH cells in human health and disease. Nat Rev Immunol. 2013;13(6):412–26.

45. Vinuesa CG, Cook MC, Angelucci C, Athanasopoulos V, Rui L, Hill KM, et al. A RING-type ubiquitin ligase family member required to repress follicular helper T cells and autoimmunity. Nature. 2005;435(7041):452–8.

46. Johnson S, Bergthaler A, Graw F, Flatz L, Bonilla WV, Siegrist CA, et al. Protective efficacy of individual CD8+ T cell specificities in chronic viral infection. J Immunol. 2015;194(4):1755–62.

47. Nizzoli G, Krietsch J, Weick A, Steinfelder S, Facciotti F, Gruarin P, et al. Human CD1c+ dendritic cells secrete high levels of IL-12 and potently prime cytotoxic T-cell responses. Blood. 2013;122(6):932–42.

48. Sakaguchi S, Yamaguchi T, Nomura T, Ono M. Regulatory T cells and immune tolerance. Cell. 2008;133(5):775–87.

49. Fontenot JD, Gavin MA, Rudensky AY. Foxp3 programs the development and function of CD4+CD25+ regulatory T cells. Nat Immunol. 2003;4(4):330–6.

50. Belkaid Y. Regulatory T cells and infection: a dangerous necessity. Nat Rev Immunol. 2007;7(11):875–88.

51. Cobbold SP. Regulatory T cells and transplantation tolerance. J Nephrol. 2008;21(4):485–96.

52. Holaday BJ, Pompeu MM, Jeronimo S, Texeira MJ, Sousa Ade A, Vasconcelos AW, et al. Potential role for interleukin-10 in the immunosuppression associated with kala azar. J Clin Invest. 1993;92(6):2626–32.

53. Muthuswamy R, Urban J, Lee JJ, Reinhart TA, Bartlett D, Kalinski P. Ability of mature dendritic

cells to interact with regulatory T cells is imprinted during maturation. Cancer Res. 2008;68(14):5972–8.

54. Shafiani S, Dinh C, Ertelt JM, Moguche AO, Siddiqui I, Smigiel KS, et al. Pathogen-specific Treg cells expand early during mycobacterium tuberculosis infection but are later eliminated in response to Interleukin-12. Immunity. 2013;38(6):1261–70.

55. Belkaid Y, Piccirillo CA, Mendez S, Shevach EM, Sacks DL. CD4+CD25+ regulatory T cells control Leishmania major persistence and immunity. Nature. 2002;420(6915):502–7.

56. Kitamura T, Qian BZ, Pollard JW. Immune cell promotion of metastasis. Nat Rev Immunol. 2015;15(2):73–86.

57. Le Bras S, Geha RS. IPEX and the role of Foxp3 in the development and function of human Tregs. J Clin Invest. 2006;116(6):1473–5.

58. Vincent MS, Gumperz JE, Brenner MB. Understanding the function of CD1-restricted T cells. Nat Immunol. 2003;4(6):517–23.

59. Barral DC, Brenner MB. CD1 antigen presentation: how it works. Nat Rev Immunol. 2007;7(12):929–41.

60. Van Rhijn I, Ly D, Moody DB. CD1a, CD1b, and CD1c in immunity against mycobacteria. Adv Exp Med Biol. 2013;783:181–97.

61. Van Rhijn I, Moody DB. CD1 and mycobacterial lipids activate human T cells. Immunol Rev. 2015;264(1):138–53.

62. Bendelac A, Savage PB, Teyton L. The biology of NKT cells. Annu Rev Immunol. 2007;25:297–336.

63. Venkataswamy MM, Porcelli SA. Lipid and glycolipid antigens of CD1d-restricted natural killer T cells. Semin Immunol. 2010;22(2):68–78.

64. Carreno LJ, Kharkwal SS, Porcelli SA. Optimizing NKT cell ligands as vaccine adjuvants. Immunotherapy. 2014;6(3):309–20.

65. Fernandez CS, Kelleher AD, Finlayson R, Godfrey DI, Kent SJ. NKT cell depletion in humans during early HIV infection. Immunol Cell Biol. 2014;92(7):578–90.

66. Brigl M, Brenner MB. CD1: antigen presentation and T cell function. Annu Rev Immunol. 2004;22:817–90.

67. Berzins SP, Smyth MJ, Baxter AG. Presumed guilty: natural killer T cell defects and human disease. Nat Rev Immunol. 2011;11(2):131–42.

68. Born WK, Reardon CL, O'Brien RL. The function of gammadelta T cells in innate immunity. Curr Opin Immunol. 2006;18(1):31–8.

69. Kabelitz D, Marischen L, Oberg HH, Holtmeier W, Wesch D. Epithelial defence by gamma delta T cells. Int Arch Allergy Immunol. 2005;137(1):73–81.

70. Morita CT, Jin C, Sarikonda G, Wang H. Nonpeptide antigens, presentation mechanisms, and immunological memory of human Vgamma2Vdelta2 T cells: discriminating friend from foe through the recognition of prenyl pyrophosphate antigens. Immunol Rev. 2007;215:59–76.

71. Chien YH, Meyer C, Bonneville M. Gammadelta T cells: first line of defense and beyond. Annu Rev Immunol. 2014;32:121–55.

72. Uldrich AP, Le Nours J, Pellicci DG, Gherardin NA, McPherson KG, Lim RT, et al. CD1d-lipid antigen recognition by the gammadelta TCR. Nat Immunol. 2013;14(11):1137–45.

73. Kjer-Nielsen L, Patel O, Corbett AJ, Le Nours J, Meehan B, Liu L, et al. MR1 presents microbial vitamin B metabolites to MAIT cells. Nature. 2012;491(7426):717–23.

74. Martin E, Treiner E, Duban L, Guerri L, Laude H, Toly C, et al. Stepwise development of MAIT cells in mouse and human. PLoS Biol. 2009;7(3):e54.

75. Fernandez CS, Amarasena T, Kelleher AD, Rossjohn J, McCluskey J, Godfrey DI, et al. MAIT cells are depleted early but retain functional cytokine expression in HIV infection. Immunol Cell Biol. 2015;93(2):177–88.

76. Bird L. Mucosal immunology: bait for MAIT cells identified. Nat Rev Immunol. 2010;10(8):539.

77. Kurioka A, Ussher JE, Cosgrove C, Clough C, Fergusson JR, Smith K, et al. MAIT cells are licensed through granzyme exchange to kill bacterially sensitized targets. Mucosal Immunol. 2015;8(2):429–40.

B Cell Immunity

3

Lee Ann Garrett-Sinha

General Information on B Cells

B lymphocytes or B cells are immune cells that produce immunoglobulins (antibodies) that are directly involved in countering infection. B cells and the antibodies they secrete comprise the humoral arm of the immune system. However, it has become clear that B cells play other roles in the immune system, beyond their ability to generate antibodies [1–6]. For instance, B cells can internalize antigens and process them for presentation to T cells on MHC class II, thereby inducing T cell activation. B cells also secrete a number of bioactive cytokines that help to modulate the activity of other immune cell subsets. B cells develop from hematopoietic stem cells in the bone marrow via a series of intermediate progenitor stages during which the immunoglobulin light and heavy chains are rearranged by the process of VDJ recombination to yield functional in-frame antibody encoding genes [7–9]. The majority of B cells express only one functional immunoglobulin heavy and light chain and therefore have a defined specificity. Some B cells may recognize more than one antigen if the antibody genes they express are poly-reactive.

L. A. Garrett-Sinha (✉)
Department of Biochemistry, Center of Excellence in Bioinformatics and Life Sciences, State University of New York at Buffalo, Buffalo, NY, USA
e-mail: leesinha@buffalo.edu

The earliest immunoglobulin heavy chain expressed in developing B cells is of the IgM isotype [10, 11]. Later in development when B cells leave the bone marrow, they express both IgM and IgD isotypes, which differ in the C-terminal domain of the heavy chain (the heavy chain constant region) and are derived from the same mRNA transcript by alternate splicing [12]. Upon activation in the peripheral lymphoid organs, B cells can undergo an isotype switch in which they delete DNA sequences encoding the constant regions of IgM and IgD and bring the antigen-binding domain of the gene close to alternate C-terminal exons to generate antibodies of different isotypes – IgG, IgA, or IgE – each of which has specific effector functions [13–16].

B cells can alter the specificity of the antigen-binding region of the antibody heavy and light chain genes by undergoing somatic hypermutation and affinity maturation in germinal centers [17], a process described in more detail below. The ability to change antigen specificity allows B cells that are weakly reactive with an antigen to yield progeny cells that have much higher antigen specificity than the original clone of B cells activated.

Two copies of the immunoglobulin heavy chain protein associate with two copies of the immunoglobulin light chain protein to form a functional antibody. B cells can express both membrane-bound forms of antibodies and secreted forms, which differ based on alternate

© Springer International Publishing AG, part of Springer Nature 2018
B. H. Segal (ed.), *Management of Infections in the Immunocompromised Host*,
https://doi.org/10.1007/978-3-319-77674-3_3

C-terminal exon usage [18]. There appears to be better processing of the secreted form of the heavy chain mRNA leading to more immunoglobulin produced per transcript [19], allowing a high level of antibody secretion. The membrane-bound forms of the antibodies are displayed on the cell surface along with accessory proteins to form the B cell receptor (BCR) [20]. Antigen binding to the BCR triggers an intracellular signaling cascade that results in B cell activation and proliferation. B cells activated appropriately can further differentiate into antibody-secreting cells (ASCs) also known as plasmablasts (if still proliferating) or plasma cells (if nonproliferative). B cells can become ASCs and secrete antibody in either a T cell-dependent or T cell-independent fashion. T cell-dependent responses and germinal center are described in more detail below. T cell-independent responses of B cells can be subdivided into two categories, type I and type II. Type I T cell-independent responses occur when B cells bind an antigen containing a Toll-like receptor (TLR) ligand, such as LPS or DNA containing unmethylated CpG residues, that can act as a polyclonal activator of the cells. Type II T cell-independent responses occur when B cells bind to antigens with highly repetitive carbohydrate structures, similar to the capsules of encapsulated bacteria, which strongly cross-links the BCR. Both of these stimuli can induce B cell activation and the expression of transcription factors that drive an ASC phenotype.

B cell maintenance in the spleen and lymph nodes is dependent on the presence of the cytokine BAFF (B cell-activating factor belonging to the TNF family) [21, 22]. BAFF is a heterotrimeric protein of the TNF family that binds to the BAFF receptor expressed on B cells, triggering survival signals. BAFF is produced mainly by myeloid-derived cells such as neutrophils, macrophages, and dendritic cells (DCs) [23–25]. Limited amounts of BAFF are available in vivo, thus limiting the number of B cells that can be supported. Excess BAFF can lead to increased survival of autoreactive B cells that would normally be eliminated and can therefore promote autoimmune disease [26].

Types of Mature B Cells

Mouse

Once B cells exit the bone marrow, they travel to the spleen and become transitional, immature B cells [27]. They continue maturation to become mature B-2 cells, which can be subdivided into follicular (FO) B cells or marginal zone (MZ) types [28]. FO B cells are found in the B cell follicles of the spleen and lymph nodes but are not static and recirculate through the body via the bloodstream and lymphatic system. FO B cells can be further divided into two subsets, FO-I and FO-II B cells [29]. FO-II B cells, unlike FO-I B cells, do not require antigen binding or the kinase Btk for their development. It remains unclear whether FO-I and FO-II B cells have different functions in vivo.

MZ B cells are localized in the marginal zone of the spleen, a region that surrounds the B cell follicle and is closely adjacent to blood flowing through the marginal sinus [30]. Unlike FO B cells, MZ B cells do not circulate through the body but remain localized in the marginal zone of the spleen. They are specialized to fight blood-borne infections [31]. In addition to FO and MZ B cells, mice possess a separate set of mature B cells known as B-1 cells, which are enriched in the peritoneal and pleural cavities and arise from fetal liver progenitors [32]. They are maintained throughout life by self-renewal [33] and can be further subdivided into B-1a and B-1b B cells, based on expression of CD5 on the B-1a subset. B-1 cells secrete IgM antibody in the absence of overt stimulation and thus generate what is known as "natural" antibodies, which are involved in early antibacterial antibody responses [34, 35]. B-1 cells can contribute to gut IgA responses to pathogens by undergoing isotype switching to IgA [36]. Like MZ B cells, B-1 B cells also do not generally circulate in the body and can respond rapidly to infections [37, 38]. B-1 and MZ B cell subsets are enriched for B cells that harbor self-reactivity and are partially pre-activated, while FO B cells have lower levels of self-reactivity [34].

FO B cells respond most strongly to protein-containing antigens, which are internalized, processed, and presented on MHC class II to T cells. T cell help to FO B cells allows them to generate germinal centers, where they undergo somatic hypermutation, affinity maturation, and class switching. MZ and B-1 B cells on the other hand respond strongly to nonprotein antigens in a T cell-independent fashion to generate early immune responses prior to development of germinal centers. The T cell-independent responses of MZ and B-1 B cells are often dependent on stimulation of Toll-like receptors (TLRs) by bacterial and viral components [39]. Because B-1 and MZ B cells can respond rapidly to pathogens in a T cell-independent fashion, they are referred to as innate-like B lymphocytes.

A more recently described subset of B cells are the regulatory B cells or Breg. Breg cells produce the immunosuppressive cytokines IL-10, IL-35, and/or TGFβ to limit immune responses in the contexts of infection and autoimmunity [40–44]. The subset of these regulatory B cells that produces IL-10 is also known as B10 cells. Several other immunosuppressive mechanisms are proposed for Breg cells including promoting the proliferation, development, and function of regulatory T cells (Treg cells), expression of Fas ligand triggering apoptosis of immune effector populations, and production of extracellular adenosine that regulates activity of various immune cells [45, 46]. Regulatory B cells have been shown to have various cell surface phenotypes, depending on the study. Using in vitro stimulation assays, IL-10-producing B cells have been identified among the transitional or marginal zone precursor subsets in the spleen or in CD5+CD1d^{high} B cells [47, 48]. The surface protein Tim1 has also been reported to be expressed on a large fraction of IL-10-secreting B cells [49]. More recent studies have indicated that the majority of in vivo IL-10-producing B cells in autoimmune disease may actually be CD138$^+$ plasmablasts [40, 50, 51].

Human

Analysis of human B cell subsets is most often done using peripheral blood, because of the ease in obtaining this tissue. B cell phenotypes have also been analyzed fairly extensively in tonsils and less frequently in lymph nodes, spleens, and other organs. B cell subsets in peripheral blood include immature transitional B cells, mature naïve B cells, germinal center B cells, memory B cells, plasmablasts, and plasma cells, and these subsets can be distinguished based on analysis of markers such as CD10, CD20, CD24, CD27, CD38, CD138, and the surface BCR isotype [52, 53]. Most of these human peripheral blood B cells seem to share characteristics of mouse FO B cells. However, there is evidence that humans also have B cell subsets similar to mouse MZ and B-1 cells. Human B cells that express markers similar to those of mouse MZ B cells (IgM^{high}, IgD^{low}, CD21^{high}) are found in peripheral blood, but these cells also typically express markers of memory B cells such as CD27, have mutated immunoglobulin variable regions, and recirculate through the body [54–56]. This has led to some confusion about whether human MZ phenotype B cells are the equivalent of mouse MZ B cells or not. Supporting a close relationship between the MZ subsets in these two species, humans MZ B cells are dependent on Notch2 signaling, a pathway which is also known to be crucial for development of murine MZ B cells [57, 58].

Some evidence also suggests that humans may have an equivalent of mouse B-1 cells. CD5 cannot be used as a B-1 cell marker in humans because it is expressed in immature, transitional B cells of humans [59]. In 2011, a report was published identifying human B-1 cells in umbilical cord blood as CD20+ CD27+ CD43+ CD70- B cells [60], but this study has remained controversial [61–63]. Supporting the possible existence of B-1 cells in humans are observations with nonhuman primates, where cells similar to B-1 B cells have been described [64].

Human B cells producing IL-10 have also been described [65], suggesting that Bregs exist in humans as they do in mice. These cells are capable of limiting the activation of human monocytes in an IL-10-dependent fashion [65]. The numbers of IL-10-secreting B cells are often altered in autoimmune patients as compared to normal controls [66–68].

B Cell Participation in Immune Responses

Naïve B cells are those that have not previously encountered antigen. When antigen binds to the BCR of the naïve B cells, they become activated and divide. The presence of a specific antigen results in activation of only a small number of B cells, whose BCRs specifically recognize that particular antigen. However, antigen binding alone is not typically sufficient to trigger B cells to secrete antibody. Additional signals can coordinate with BCR cross-linking to induce B cells to differentiate into antibody-secreting cells (ASCs), also known as plasma cells. Development of ASCs can be triggered by signals derived from T cells (cytokines and CD40 ligand) or by signals derived from pathogens (Toll-like receptor ligands) [69].

B cells are part of the adaptive immune response and thus contribute to immunological memory, the process whereby immune cells respond more quickly and efficiently to an antigen that they have encountered previously. Immunological memory of B cells depends on the development of memory B cells mostly produced from germinal center B cells that have typically undergone isotype switching and affinity maturation. These memory B cells remain quiescent in the body until they are stimulated by encounter with antigen at which time they rapidly divide and produce antibodies.

Germinal Centers

B cells that receive antigenic stimulation via the BCR and subsequently interact with primed CD4+ T cells can form a germinal center reaction. Germinal center B cells in mice can be detected by their expression of the markers GL7 and Fas and their ability to bind peanut agglutinin (PNA) [70, 71]. In humans, germinal center B cells are usually detected as B cells that are IgD[negative] and express high levels of CD38 [72]. The germinal center can be subdivided into two main zones, the dark zone and light zone whose regions are organized by differential expression of chemokines [73]. B lineage cells known as centroblasts are attracted to the dark zone by local expression of CXCL12. They are rapidly proliferating and are also undergoing a process termed somatic hypermutation in which the variable regions of the antibody genes undergo random mutagenesis dependent on the activity of the enzyme activation-induced cytidine deaminase (AID) [74]. Centroblasts migrate to the light zone of the germinal center in response to a chemokine attraction by CXCL13, where they become centrocytes and cease proliferation and somatic hypermutation [73]. The mutated BCRs on centrocytes can bind to antigen presented on follicular dendritic cells (FDC) [75]. If the mutation results in higher affinity of the BCR for antigen, then that particular B cell will compete efficiently for limited amounts of antigen present on the FDC. If the mutation in the BCR abrogates or lowers the affinity for cognate antigen, the mutated B cell will fail to compete efficiently for antigen presented on FDC.

After binding antigen on the FDC, centrocytes internalize some of the antigen and process it for presentation on MHC II molecules. These centrocytes subsequently interact with a subclass of CD4+ T cells known as T follicular helper cells (T_{FH}) that provide CD40 ligand and cytokine help to the B cells [76]. Interaction of centrocytes with T_{FH} promotes B cell survival and class switching from IgM to IgG or other isotypes. Like somatic hypermutation, class switching also depends on the activity of the AID enzyme [74]. Germinal center B cells with higher-affinity BCRs that have competed more effectively for antigen bound to FDC are able to preferentially form cognate interactions with T_{FH} and receive T cell help [77]. This results in positive selection of those B cells whose BCRs are mutated to the highest affinity for antigen, a process termed affinity maturation. Within 1 week of the initiation of a germinal center reaction, some germinal B cells begin to differentiate into high-affinity class-switched plasma cells and memory B cells.

B Cell Memory

Memory B cells are those that have previously encountered antigen and been activated. They are long-lived cells and characterized by the rapid response to second encounter with antigen [78]. Classically, these cells were thought to be derived from germinal center B cells that had undergone isotype switching and affinity maturation, but evidence indicates that some memory B cells can also be generated outside of germinal centers and can be generated in a T cell-independent fashion [79–84]. Previously, T cell-independent B cell responses were thought not to generate memory B cells, because antigen-specific B cells did not respond more strongly upon second encounter with the same T cell-independent antigen. However, it was later realized that this was due to the formation of antigen-specific IgG in the primary response, which subsequently binds to antigen in secondary exposures and prevents it from interacting with antigen-specific B cells [83].

In humans, memory B cells can be identified because of their expression of the cell surface marker CD27 [55, 85]. Many of these cells are isotype-switched, but non-switched IgM+ memory B cells are also found. As discussed above, these non-switched CD27+ memory B cells in humans may be functionally equivalent to mouse marginal zone B cells [54–56]. Detection of memory B cells in mice is not as easy as it is in humans, because CD27 is not a marker of memory B cells in mice [79, 86]. Mouse memory B cells have been identified as antigen-specific, isotype-switched cells present after germinal center responses have ceased, but some memory

B cells do not switch and therefore this is not an effective way to identify all memory B cells in mice. Using transgenic BCR systems, where antigen specificity is known, it is possible to track memory B cell responses. More recently, CD80, PD-L2, and CD73 have been shown to be enriched in mouse memory B cells, and expression of these proteins at different levels can distinguish multiple subsets of memory B cells, with cells expressing all three markers having increased levels of isotype switching and somatic hypermutation [87, 88]. Memory B cells expressing both CD80 and PDL2 differentiate rapidly to antibody-secreting cells upon encountering antigen, while memory B cells lacking these markers instead gave rise to few early antibody-secreting cells but seeded germinal centers [89]. Other evidence has suggested that IgM+ memory B cells preferentially seed new germinal centers when they encounter an antigen the second time, while IgG+ memory B cells preferentially generate plasma cells [90]. Recent evidence has suggested production of memory B cells peaks during the early and middle stages of germinal center reactions [91].

Antibody-Secreting Cells

Antibody-secreting cells (ASCs) or plasma cells are terminally-differentiated effector cells of the B cell lineage, specialized to secrete large amounts of antigen-specific antibody. ASCs are larger than B cells and have an expanded endoplasmic reticulum allowing them to produce large quantities of antibody [92]. Initially it was thought that the affinity of the BCR for antigen could modulate whether B cells become ASCs or not, with higher-affinity BCRs promoting an ASC fate [93, 94]. However, more recent data have instead shown that early stages of the germinal center reaction give rise to mostly memory B cells, while late stages of the germinal center reaction preferentially give rise to ASCs [91]. ASCs can either be short-lived, surviving for days to weeks, or long-lived, surviving for years to decades. Short-lived ASCs are mainly found in lymphoid tissues (spleen or lymph node) or in sites of inflammation [95]. These cells typically are generated outside of germinal centers and are undergoing proliferation (therefore they are known as plasmablasts). Short-lived ASCs provide early antibody to control initial infection. In contrast, long-lived ASCs are typically derived from germinal centers, although they can also be derived from T cell-independent, non-germinal center responses [96]. They are mainly found in the bone marrow and no longer proliferate [95]. These long-lived ASCs contribute to immunological memory by secreting high-affinity antigen-specific antibodies against pathogens the body has already been exposed to previously.

Most long-lived ASCs home to the bone marrow in response to CXCL12, where they enter specific niches that support their long-term survival [97]. These niches provide the tumor necrosis family ligands APRIL (a proliferation-inducing ligand) and BAFF, which are crucial for ASC survival [98, 99]. APRIL and BAFF bind to the receptor BCMA (B cell maturation antigen) expressed on bone marrow plasma cells. BCMA is also crucial for the survival of long-lived plasma cells [100]. In addition to BAFF and APRIL, the plasma cell niche provides other signals that help ASC survival including cytokines and cell-cell contacts. Several such signals have been shown to play a role, including CXCL12, IL-6, and CD44-mediated adhesion [101]. More recently, it has been appreciated that ASCs express CD28 and that they require signaling via CD28 for their survival in the bone marrow [102, 103]. Non-B cells in the ASC niche provide CD80 and/or CD86 that bind the CD28 receptor on ASCs and promote their survival.

Transcriptional Programs Regulating B Cell Differentiation

B cell development from hematopoietic progenitors, maturation, and functional responses all depend on the expression of certain key transcription factors that control target genes required for these processes. There are several dozen transcription factors known to regulate various aspects of these processes, so they cannot be covered in detail in this space. Here we provide a brief overview of some of the key transcription factors known to regulate peripheral B cell responses.

The transcription factors involved in B cell responses can be subdivided based on their functional roles into several classes: those that maintain naïve B cell phenotype and quiescence, those that are activated upon signaling by cell surface receptors, those that control germinal center kinetics, and those that are important for ASC generation. Among the factors known to be crucial for maintaining mature B cell phenotypes are Pax5, Ets1, Ebf1, and PU.1 [104–107]. Deletion of these factors leads to improper B cell differentiation or to a failure to maintain quiescence. In addition, the transcription factor Notch2 is required for marginal zone B cell development [58]. Among the transcription factors activated by BCR, TLR, or cytokine signaling pathways are NFκB, Stat family members, and IRF proteins [108–114]. Among the transcription factors important for germinal center responses are Bcl6, Bach2, Irf4, E2A, SpiB, c-Rel, and Irf8 [112, 115–119]. The transcription factor Abf1 seems to play an important role in generation of memory B cells [120]. Among those transcription factors needed for ASC generation are RelA, Blimp1, Xbp1, Irf4, and Zbtb20 [112, 121–124]. The above list should not be taken as a complete listing of all transcription factors that control stages of B cell differentiation but rather as a summary of some of the important ones that have been identified.

Immunodeficiency in the Absence of B Cells

Several human diseases are associated with a lack of B cells or with their secreted product, immunoglobulins. Such patients show varying susceptibility to infections, depending on the particular immune responses that are impaired. In severe combined immunodeficiency (SCID), there are genetic defects that impair the functions of both B and T cells. SCID can be caused by a variety of genetic defects, including inactivating mutations in cytokine signaling pathways (IL2RG, IL2RA, JAK3), in T cell receptor signaling (CD3D, CD3E, CD45, CD247), in the VDJ recombination machinery (RAG1, RAG2, DCLRE1C, NHEJ1, LIG4), or in T cell metabolism (ADA) [125]. Various forms of SCID can lead to either a near absence of B cells or impairment in their functions. In either case, antibody levels are very low and SCID patients are extremely susceptible to severe and life-threatening infections. Patients with X-linked agammaglobulinemia (XLA) specifically lack B cells and the antibodies they produce. XLA is caused by genetic defects in the gene encoding the kinase Btk [126]. XLA patients are very susceptible to recurrent and/or severe ear, sinus, or pulmonary infections, particularly those caused by encapsulated bacteria such as *Streptococcus pneumoniae* and *Haemophilus influenzae*.

Other types of immunodeficiencies can have normal numbers of B cells but altered antibody production. For instance, in common variable immunodeficiency (CVID), patients have decreased serum IgG in combination with decreased IgA or IgM [127]. They also show poor antibody responses to vaccines. In selective IgA deficiency or IgG subclass deficiencies (IgG2, IgG3, IgG4), patients lack one class of antibody but produce the other classes normally. Some people with selective IgA deficiency develop recurrent sinus, pulmonary, or gastrointestinal infections, although others are asymptomatic [128]. IgG subclass deficiency can be asymptomatic and clinically insignificant, although some patients may also have recurrent respiratory infections or poor antibody responses to certain vaccines [129].

Additional genetic syndromes can result in aberrations in one or more antibody types. Hyper IgM syndrome (HIGM) has a deficiency in switching antibody isotype from IgM to IgG or other classes. HIGM is most frequently caused by mutations in the CD40 gene or its ligand CD40L [130]. HIGM patients are susceptible to a variety of bacterial and viral infections. Hyper IgE syndrome (HIES or Job's syndrome) is a condition in which the levels of IgE antibodies are much higher than normal. These patients are susceptible to recurrent infections of the skin and lungs caused by bacteria. They also have eczema. Most HIES patients have mutations in the Stat3 gene that impair its activity [131]. Wiskott-Aldrich syndrome (WAS) is a genetic disease caused by mutations in the WAS gene, which leads to immunodeficiency, autoimmunity, and bleeding disorders [132]. It results in reduced antibody production and reduced specific antibody responses to vaccines. The immune system changes in WAS lead to susceptibility to a variety of bacterial and viral pathogens. Ataxia-telangiectasia (AT) is caused by mutations in the ATM gene [133]. ATM is involved in VDJ recombination, so patients with AT have immune system abnormalities including reduced numbers of lymphocytes and reduced antibody production. These defects cause immunodeficiency. WHIM syndrome (warts, hypogammaglobulinemia, infections, and myelokathexis syndrome) is another genetic disease that leads to reduced antibody production. It is caused by mutations in the CXCR4 gene that make it hyperactive [134]. This results in impaired B cell production of antibodies and susceptibility to bacterial infections.

Summary

In the discussion above, we have listed the main phenotypes and functional responses of mouse and human B cells. These functional responses are absolutely crucial in generating protective immunity to certain bacterial pathogens, as loss of B cells or antibodies leads to susceptibility to bacterial infections. Future studies will continue to reveal details of how B cell responses are mechanistically regulated, which will be important in stimulating B cell responses to infection or to vaccines.

References

1. Chan OT, Hannum LG, Haberman AM, Madaio MP, Shlomchik MJ. A novel mouse with B cells but lacking serum antibody reveals an antibody-independent role for B cells in murine lupus. J Exp Med. 1999;189(10):1639–48.

2. Rubtsov AV, Rubtsova K, Kappler JW, Jacobelli J, Friedman RS, Marrack P. CD11c-expressing B cells are located at the T cell/B cell border in spleen and are potent APCs. J Immunol. 2015;195(1):71–9.

3. Molnarfi N, Schulze-Topphoff U, Weber MS, Patarroyo JC, Prod'homme T, Varrin-Doyer M, et al. MHC class II-dependent B cell APC function is required for induction of CNS autoimmunity independent of myelin-specific antibodies. J Exp Med. 2013;210(13):2921–37.

4. Liu Q, Liu Z, Rozo CT, Hamed HA, Alem F, Urban JF Jr, et al. The role of B cells in the development of CD4 effector T cells during a polarized Th2 immune response. J Immunol. 2007;179(6):3821–30.

5. Lino AC, Dorner T, Bar-Or A, Fillatreau S. Cytokine-producing B cells: a translational view on their roles in human and mouse autoimmune diseases. Immunol Rev. 2016;269(1):130–44.

6. Bao Y, Cao X. The immune potential and immunopathology of cytokine-producing B cell subsets: a comprehensive review. J Autoimmun. 2014;55:10–23.

7. Clark MR, Mandal M, Ochiai K, Singh H. Orchestrating B cell lymphopoiesis through interplay of IL-7 receptor and pre-B cell receptor signalling. Nat Rev Immunol. 2014;14(2):69–80.

8. Ichii M, Oritani K, Kanakura Y. Early B lymphocyte development: similarities and differences in human and mouse. World J Stem Cells. 2014;6(4):421–31.

9. Sen R, Oltz E. Genetic and epigenetic regulation of IgH gene assembly. Curr Opin Immunol. 2006;18(3):237–42.

10. Coffman RL, Cohn M. The class of surface immunoglobulin on virgin and memory B lymphocytes. J Immunol. 1977;118(5):1806–15.

11. Abney ER, Cooper MD, Kearney JF, Lawton AR, Parkhouse RM. Sequential expression of immunoglobulin on developing mouse B lymphocytes: a systematic survey that suggests a model for the generation of immunoglobulin isotype diversity. J Immunol. 1978;120(6):2041–9.

12. Blattner FR, Tucker PW. The molecular biology of immunoglobulin D. Nature. 1984;307(5950):417–22.

13. Stavnezer J, Schrader CE. IgH chain class switch recombination: mechanism and regulation. J Immunol. 2014;193(11):5370–8.

14. Vidarsson G, Dekkers G, Rispens T. IgG subclasses and allotypes: from structure to effector functions. Front Immunol. 2014;5:520.

15. Pabst O. New concepts in the generation and functions of IgA. Nat Rev Immunol. 2012;12(12):821–32.

16. Oettgen HC, Burton OT. IgE and mast cells: the endogenous adjuvant. Adv Immunol. 2015;127:203–56.

17. Victora GD, Nussenzweig MC. Germinal centers. Annu Rev Immunol. 2012;30:429–57.

18. Alt FW, Bothwell AL, Knapp M, Siden E, Mather E, Koshland M, et al. Synthesis of secreted and membrane-bound immunoglobulin mu heavy chains is directed by mRNAs that differ at their 3′ ends. Cell. 1980;20(2):293–301.

19. Shell SA, Martincic K, Tran J, Milcarek C. Increased phosphorylation of the carboxyl-terminal domain of RNA polymerase II and loading of polyadenylation and cotranscriptional factors contribute to regulation of the ig heavy chain mRNA in plasma cells. J Immunol. 2007;179(11):7663–73.

20. Hobeika E, Nielsen PJ, Medgyesi D. Signaling mechanisms regulating B-lymphocyte activation and tolerance. J Mol Med (Berl). 2015;93(2):143–58.

21. Batten M, Groom J, Cachero TG, Qian F, Schneider P, Tschopp J, et al. BAFF mediates survival of peripheral immature B lymphocytes. J Exp Med. 2000;192(10):1453–66.

22. Thompson JS, Schneider P, Kalled SL, Wang L, Lefevre EA, Cachero TG, et al. BAFF binds to the tumor necrosis factor receptor-like molecule B cell maturation antigen and is important for maintaining the peripheral B cell population. J Exp Med. 2000;192(1):129–35.

23. Schneider P, MacKay F, Steiner V, Hofmann K, Bodmer JL, Holler N, et al. BAFF, a novel ligand of the tumor necrosis factor family, stimulates B cell growth. J Exp Med. 1999;189(11):1747–56.

24. Shu HB, Hu WH, Johnson H. TALL-1 is a novel member of the TNF family that is down-regulated by mitogens. J Leukoc Biol. 1999;65(5):680–3.

25. Moore PA, Belvedere O, Orr A, Pieri K, LaFleur DW, Feng P, et al. BLyS: member of the tumor necrosis factor family and B lymphocyte stimulator. Science. 1999;285(5425):260–3.

26. Khare SD, Sarosi I, Xia XZ, McCabe S, Miner K, Solovyev I, et al. Severe B cell hyperplasia and autoimmune disease in TALL-1 transgenic mice. Proc Natl Acad Sci U S A. 2000;97(7):3370–5.

27. Vossenkamper A, Spencer J. Transitional B cells: how well are the checkpoints for specificity understood? Arch Immunol Ther Exp. 2011;59(5):379–84.

28. Allman D, Pillai S. Peripheral B cell subsets. Curr Opin Immunol. 2008;20(2):149–57.

29. Cariappa A, Boboila C, Moran ST, Liu H, Shi HN, Pillai S. The recirculating B cell pool contains two functionally distinct, long-lived, posttransitional, follicular B cell populations. J Immunol. 2007;179(4):2270–81.

30. Cerutti A, Cols M, Puga I. Marginal zone B cells: virtues of innate-like antibody-producing lymphocytes. Nat Rev Immunol. 2013;13(2):118–32.

31. Martin F, Kearney JF. Marginal-zone B cells. Nat Rev Immunol. 2002;2(5):323–35.

32. Hayakawa K, Hardy RR, Herzenberg LA, Herzenberg LA. Progenitors for Ly-1 B cells are distinct from progenitors for other B cells. J Exp Med. 1985;161(6):1554–68.

33. Hayakawa K, Hardy RR, Stall AM, Herzenberg LA, Herzenberg LA. Immunoglobulin-bearing B cells reconstitute and maintain the murine Ly-1 B cell lineage. Eur J Immunol. 1986;16(10):1313–6.

34. Hayakawa K, Hardy RR, Honda M, Herzenberg LA, Steinberg AD, Herzenberg LA. Ly-1 B cells: functionally distinct lymphocytes that secrete

IgM autoantibodies. Proc Natl Acad Sci U S A. 1984;81(8):2494–8.

35. Ehrenstein MR, Notley CA. The importance of natural IgM: scavenger, protector and regulator. Nat Rev Immunol. 2010;10(11):778–86.

36. Suzuki K, Maruya M, Kawamoto S, Fagarasan S. Roles of B-1 and B-2 cells in innate and acquired IgA-mediated immunity. Immunol Rev. 2010;237(1):180–90.

37. Martin F, Oliver AM, Kearney JF. Marginal zone and B1 B cells unite in the early response against T-independent blood-borne particulate antigens. Immunity. 2001;14(5):617–29.

38. Lopes-Carvalho T, Foote J, Kearney JF. Marginal zone B cells in lymphocyte activation and regulation. Curr Opin Immunol. 2005;17(3):244–50.

39. Rubtsov AV, Swanson CL, Troy S, Strauch P, Pelanda R, Torres RM. TLR agonists promote marginal zone B cell activation and facilitate T-dependent IgM responses. J Immunol. 2008;180(6):3882–8.

40. Shen P, Roch T, Lampropoulou V, O'Connor RA, Stervbo U, Hilgenberg E, et al. IL-35-producing B cells are critical regulators of immunity during autoimmune and infectious diseases. Nature. 2014;507(7492):366–70.

41. Mizoguchi A, Mizoguchi E, Takedatsu H, Blumberg RS, Bhan AK. Chronic intestinal inflammatory condition generates IL-10-producing regulatory B cell subset characterized by CD1d upregulation. Immunity. 2002;16(2):219–30.

42. Fillatreau S, Sweenie CH, McGeachy MJ, Gray D, Anderton SM. B cells regulate autoimmunity by provision of IL-10. Nat Immunol. 2002;3(10):944–50.

43. Kaku H, Cheng KF, Al-Abed Y, Rothstein TL. A novel mechanism of B cell-mediated immune suppression through CD73 expression and adenosine production. J Immunol. 2014;193(12):5904–13.

44. Zhang HP, Wu Y, Liu J, Jiang J, Geng XR, Yang G, et al. TSP1-producing B cells show immune regulatory property and suppress allergy-related mucosal inflammation. Sci Rep. 2013;3:3345.

45. Ding T, Yan F, Cao S, Ren X. Regulatory B cell: new member of immunosuppressive cell club. Hum Immunol. 2015;76(9):615–21.

46. Ray A, Wang L, Dittel BN. IL-10-independent regulatory B-cell subsets and mechanisms of action. Int Immunol. 2015;27(10):531–6.

47. Yanaba K, Bouaziz JD, Haas KM, Poe JC, Fujimoto M, Tedder TF. A regulatory B cell subset with a unique CD1dhiCD5+ phenotype controls T cell-dependent inflammatory responses. Immunity. 2008;28(5):639–50.

48. Evans JG, Chavez-Rueda KA, Eddaoudi A, Meyer-Bahlburg A, Rawlings DJ, Ehrenstein MR, et al. Novel suppressive function of transitional 2 B cells in experimental arthritis. J Immunol. 2007;178(12):7868–78.

49. Ding Q, Yeung M, Camirand G, Zeng Q, Akiba H, Yagita H, et al. Regulatory B cells are identified by expression of TIM-1 and can be induced through TIM-1 ligation to promote tolerance in mice. J Clin Invest. 2011;121(9):3645–56.

50. Neves P, Lampropoulou V, Calderon-Gomez E, Roch T, Stervbo U, Shen P, et al. Signaling via the MyD88 adaptor protein in B cells suppresses protective immunity during Salmonella typhimurium infection. Immunity. 2010;33(5):777–90.

51. Matsumoto M, Baba A, Yokota T, Nishikawa H, Ohkawa Y, Kayama H, et al. Interleukin-10-producing plasmablasts exert regulatory function in autoimmune inflammation. Immunity. 2014;41(6):1040–51.

52. Kjeldsen MK, Perez-Andres M, Schmitz A, Johansen P, Boegsted M, Nyegaard M, et al. Multiparametric flow cytometry for identification and fluorescence activated cell sorting of five distinct B-cell subpopulations in normal tonsil tissue. Am J Clin Pathol. 2011;136(6):960–9.

53. Kaminski DA, Wei C, Qian Y, Rosenberg AF, Sanz I. Advances in human B cell phenotypic profiling. Front Immunol. 2012;3:302.

54. Dunn-Walters DK, Isaacson PG, Spencer J. Analysis of mutations in immunoglobulin heavy chain variable region genes of microdissected marginal zone (MGZ) B cells suggests that the MGZ of human spleen is a reservoir of memory B cells. J Exp Med. 1995;182(2):559–66.

55. Tangye SG, Liu YJ, Aversa G, Phillips JH, de Vries JE. Identification of functional human splenic memory B cells by expression of CD148 and CD27. J Exp Med. 1998;188(9):1691–703.

56. Weller S, Braun MC, Tan BK, Rosenwald A, Cordier C, Conley ME, et al. Human blood IgM "memory" B cells are circulating splenic marginal zone B cells harboring a prediversified immunoglobulin repertoire. Blood. 2004;104(12):3647–54.

57. Descatoire M, Weller S, Irtan S, Sarnacki S, Feuillard J, Storck S, et al. Identification of a human splenic marginal zone B cell precursor with NOTCH2-dependent differentiation properties. J Exp Med. 2014;211(5):987–1000.

58. Saito T, Chiba S, Ichikawa M, Kunisato A, Asai T, Shimizu K, et al. Notch2 is preferentially expressed in mature B cells and indispensable for marginal zone B lineage development. Immunity. 2003;18(5):675–85.

59. Sims GP, Ettinger R, Shirota Y, Yarboro CH, Illei GG, Lipsky PE. Identification and characterization of circulating human transitional B cells. Blood. 2005;105(11):4390–8.

60. Griffin DO, Holodick NE, Rothstein TL. Human B1 cells in umbilical cord and adult peripheral blood express the novel phenotype CD20+ CD27+ CD43+ CD70. J Exp Med. 2011;208(1):67–80.

61. Perez-Andres M, Grosserichter-Wagener C, Teodosio C, van Dongen JJ, Orfao A, van Zelm MC. The nature of circulating CD27+CD43+ B cells. J Exp Med. 2011;208(13):2565–6.

62. Descatoire M, Weill JC, Reynaud CA, Weller S. A human equivalent of mouse B-1 cells? J Exp Med. 2011;208(13):2563–4.

63. Griffin DO, Holodick NE, Rothstein TL. Human B1 cells are CD3-: a reply to "a human equivalent of mouse B-1 cells?" and "the nature of circulating CD27+CD43+ B cells". J Exp Med. 2011;208(13):2566–9.

64. Yammani RD, Haas KM. Primate B-1 cells generate antigen-specific B cell responses to T cell-independent type 2 antigens. J Immunol. 2013;190(7):3100–8.

65. Iwata Y, Matsushita T, Horikawa M, Dilillo DJ, Yanaba K, Venturi GM, et al. Characterization of a rare IL-10-competent B-cell subset in humans that parallels mouse regulatory B10 cells. Blood. 2011;117(2):530–41.

66. Blair PA, Norena LY, Flores-Borja F, Rawlings DJ, Isenberg DA, Ehrenstein MR, et al. CD19(+) CD24(hi)CD38(hi) B cells exhibit regulatory capacity in healthy individuals but are functionally impaired in systemic Lupus Erythematosus patients. Immunity. 2010;32(1):129–40.

67. Duddy M, Niino M, Adatia F, Hebert S, Freedman M, Atkins H, et al. Distinct effector cytokine profiles of memory and naive human B cell subsets and implication in multiple sclerosis. J Immunol. 2007;178(10):6092–9.

68. Todd SK, Pepper RJ, Draibe J, Tanna A, Pusey CD, Mauri C, et al. Regulatory B cells are numerically but not functionally deficient in anti-neutrophil cytoplasm antibody-associated vasculitis. Rheumatology (Oxford). 2014;53(9):1693–703.

69. Bortnick A, Murre C. Cellular and chromatin dynamics of antibody-secreting plasma cells. Wiley Interdisc Rev Dev Biol. 2015;5(2):136–49.

70. Mandik L, Nguyen KA, Erikson J. Fas receptor expression on B-lineage cells. Eur J Immunol. 1995;25(11):3148–54.

71. Cervenak L, Magyar A, Boja R, Laszlo G. Differential expression of GL7 activation antigen on bone marrow B cell subpopulations and peripheral B cells. Immunol Lett. 2001;78(2):89–96.

72. Pascual V, Liu YJ, Magalski A, de Bouteiller O, Banchereau J, Capra JD. Analysis of somatic mutation in five B cell subsets of human tonsil. J Exp Med. 1994;180(1):329–39.

73. De Silva NS, Klein U. Dynamics of B cells in germinal centres. Nat Rev Immunol. 2015;15(3):137–48.

74. Daniel JA, Nussenzweig A. The AID-induced DNA damage response in chromatin. Mol Cell. 2013;50(3):309–21.

75. Heesters BA, Myers RC, Carroll MC. Follicular dendritic cells: dynamic antigen libraries. Nat Rev Immunol. 2014;14(7):495–504.

76. Craft JE. Follicular helper T cells in immunity and systemic autoimmunity. Nat Rev Rheumatol. 2012;8(6):337–47.

77. Schwickert TA, Victora GD, Fooksman DR, Kamphorst AO, Mugnier MR, Gitlin AD, et al. A dynamic T cell-limited checkpoint regulates affinity-dependent B cell entry into the germinal center. J Exp Med. 2011;208(6):1243–52.

78. Kurosaki T, Kometani K, Ise W. Memory B cells. Nat Rev Immunol. 2015;15(3):149–59.

79. Takemori T, Kaji T, Takahashi Y, Shimoda M, Rajewsky K. Generation of memory B cells inside and outside germinal centers. Eur J Immunol. 2014;44(5):1258–64.

80. Taylor JJ, Pape KA, Jenkins MK. A germinal center-independent pathway generates unswitched memory B cells early in the primary response. J Exp Med. 2012;209(3):597–606.

81. Kaji T, Ishige A, Hikida M, Taka J, Hijikata A, Kubo M, et al. Distinct cellular pathways select germline-encoded and somatically mutated antibodies into immunological memory. J Exp Med. 2012;209(11):2079–97.

82. Alugupalli KR, Leong JM, Woodland RT, Muramatsu M, Honjo T, Gerstein RM. B1b lymphocytes confer T cell-independent long-lasting immunity. Immunity. 2004;21(3):379–90.

83. Obukhanych TV, Nussenzweig MC. T-independent type II immune responses generate memory B cells. J Exp Med. 2006;203(2):305–10.

84. Yang Y, Ghosn EE, Cole LE, Obukhanych TV, Sadate-Ngatchou P, Vogel SN, et al. Antigen-specific memory in B-1a and its relationship to natural immunity. Proc Natl Acad Sci U S A. 2012;109(14):5388–93.

85. Klein U, Rajewsky K, Kuppers R. Human immunoglobulin (Ig)M+IgD+ peripheral blood B cells expressing the CD27 cell surface antigen carry somatically mutated variable region genes: CD27 as a general marker for somatically mutated (memory) B cells. J Exp Med. 1998;188(9):1679–89.

86. Xiao Y, Hendriks J, Langerak P, Jacobs H, Borst J. CD27 is acquired by primed B cells at the centroblast stage and promotes germinal center formation. J Immunol. 2004;172(12):7432–41.

87. Tomayko MM, Steinel NC, Anderson SM, Shlomchik MJ. Cutting edge: hierarchy of maturity of murine memory B cell subsets. J Immunol. 2010;185(12):7146–50.

88. Anderson SM, Tomayko MM, Ahuja A, Haberman AM, Shlomchik MJ. New markers for murine memory B cells that define mutated and unmutated subsets. J Exp Med. 2007;204(9):2103–14.

89. Zuccarino-Catania GV, Sadanand S, Weisel FJ, Tomayko MM, Meng H, Kleinstein SH, et al. CD80 and PD-L2 define functionally distinct memory B cell subsets that are independent of antibody isotype. Nat Immunol. 2014;15(7):631–7.

90. Dogan I, Bertocci B, Vilmont V, Delbos F, Megret J, Storck S, et al. Multiple layers of B cell memory with different effector functions. Nat Immunol. 2009;10(12):1292–9.

91. Weisel FJ, Zuccarino-Catania GV, Chikina M, Shlomchik MJ. A temporal switch in the germinal

center determines differential output of memory B and plasma cells. Immunity. 2016;44(1):116–30.

92. Bayles I, Milcarek C. Plasma cell formation, secretion, and persistence: the short and the long of it. Crit Rev Immunol. 2014;34(6):481–99.

93. Paus D, Phan TG, Chan TD, Gardam S, Basten A, Brink R. Antigen recognition strength regulates the choice between extrafollicular plasma cell and germinal center B cell differentiation. J Exp Med. 2006;203(4):1081–91.

94. O'Connor BP, Vogel LA, Zhang W, Loo W, Shnider D, Lind EF, et al. Imprinting the fate of antigen-reactive B cells through the affinity of the B cell receptor. J Immunol. 2006;177(11):7723–32.

95. Oracki SA, Walker JA, Hibbs ML, Corcoran LM, Tarlinton DM. Plasma cell development and survival. Immunol Rev. 2010;237(1):140–59.

96. Bortnick A, Chernova I, Quinn WJ 3rd, Mugnier M, Cancro MP, Allman D. Long-lived bone marrow plasma cells are induced early in response to T cell-independent or T cell-dependent antigens. J Immunol. 2012;188(11):5389–96.

97. Nutt SL, Hodgkin PD, Tarlinton DM, Corcoran LM. The generation of antibody-secreting plasma cells. Nat Rev Immunol. 2015;15(3):160–71.

98. Benson MJ, Dillon SR, Castigli E, Geha RS, Xu S, Lam KP, et al. Cutting edge: the dependence of plasma cells and independence of memory B cells on BAFF and APRIL. J Immunol. 2008;180(6):3655–9.

99. Belnoue E, Pihlgren M, McGaha TL, Tougne C, Rochat AF, Bossen C, et al. APRIL is critical for plasmablast survival in the bone marrow and poorly expressed by early-life bone marrow stromal cells. Blood. 2008;111(5):2755–64.

100. O'Connor BP, Raman VS, Erickson LD, Cook WJ, Weaver LK, Ahonen C, et al. BCMA is essential for the survival of long-lived bone marrow plasma cells. J Exp Med. 2004;199(1):91–8.

101. Cassese G, Arce S, Hauser AE, Lehnert K, Moewes B, Mostarac M, et al. Plasma cell survival is mediated by synergistic effects of cytokines and adhesion-dependent signals. J Immunol. 2003;171(4):1684–90.

102. Rozanski CH, Utley A, Carlson LM, Farren MR, Murray M, Russell LM, et al. CD28 promotes plasma cell survival, sustained antibody responses, and BLIMP-1 upregulation through its distal PYAP proline motif. J Immunol. 2015;194(10):4717–28.

103. Njau MN, Kim JH, Chappell CP, Ravindran R, Thomas L, Pulendran B, et al. CD28-B7 interaction modulates short- and long-lived plasma cell function. J Immunol. 2012;189(6):2758–67.

104. Medvedovic J, Ebert A, Tagoh H, Busslinger M. Pax5: a master regulator of B cell development and leukemogenesis. Adv Immunol. 2011;111:179–206.

105. Garrett-Sinha LA. Review of Ets1 structure, function, and roles in immunity. Cell Mol life Sci : CMLS. 2013;70:3375–90.

106. Carotta S, Wu L, Nutt SL. Surprising new roles for PU.1 in the adaptive immune response. Immunol Rev. 2010;238(1):63–75.

107. Boller S, Grosschedl R. The regulatory network of B-cell differentiation: a focused view of early B-cell factor 1 function. Immunol Rev. 2014;261(1):102–15.

108. Gardam S, Brink R. Non-canonical NF-kappaB signaling initiated by BAFF influences B cell biology at multiple junctures. Front Immunol. 2014;4:509.

109. Kaileh M, Sen R. NF-kappaB function in B lymphocytes. Immunol Rev. 2012;246(1):254–71.

110. Goenka S, Kaplan MH. Transcriptional regulation by STAT6. Immunol Res. 2011;50(1):87–96.

111. Kane A, Deenick EK, Ma CS, Cook MC, Uzel G, Tangye SG. STAT3 is a central regulator of lymphocyte differentiation and function. Curr Opin Immunol. 2014;28:49–57.

112. De Silva NS, Simonetti G, Heise N, Klein U. The diverse roles of IRF4 in late germinal center B-cell differentiation. Immunol Rev. 2012;247(1):73–92.

113. Lien C, Fang CM, Huso D, Livak F, Lu R, Pitha PM. Critical role of IRF-5 in regulation of B-cell differentiation. Proc Natl Acad Sci U S A. 2010;107(10):4664–8.

114. Wang H, Morse HC 3rd. IRF8 regulates myeloid and B lymphoid lineage diversification. Immunol Res. 2009;43(1–3):109–17.

115. Basso K, Dalla-Favera R. Roles of BCL6 in normal and transformed germinal center B cells. Immunol Rev. 2012;247(1):172–83.

116. Igarashi K, Ochiai K, Itoh-Nakadai A, Muto A. Orchestration of plasma cell differentiation by Bach2 and its gene regulatory network. Immunol Rev. 2014;261(1):116–25.

117. Kwon K, Hutter C, Sun Q, Bilic I, Cobaleda C, Malin S, et al. Instructive role of the transcription factor E2A in early B lymphopoiesis and germinal center B cell development. Immunity. 2008;28(6):751–62.

118. Su GH, Chen HM, Muthusamy N, Garrett-Sinha LA, Baunoch D, Tenen DG, et al. Defective B cell receptor-mediated responses in mice lacking the Ets protein, Spi-B. EMBO J. 1997;16(23):7118–29.

119. Lee CH, Melchers M, Wang H, Torrey TA, Slota R, Qi CF, et al. Regulation of the germinal center gene program by interferon (IFN) regulatory factor 8/IFN consensus sequence-binding protein. J Exp Med. 2006;203(1):63–72.

120. Chiu YK, Lin IY, Su ST, Wang KH, Yang SY, Tsai DY, et al. Transcription factor ABF-1 suppresses plasma cell differentiation but facilitates memory B cell formation. J Immunol. 2014;193(5):2207–17.

121. Heise N, De Silva NS, Silva K, Carette A, Simonetti G, Pasparakis M, et al. Germinal center B cell maintenance and differentiation are controlled by distinct NF-kappaB transcription factor subunits. J Exp Med. 2014;211(10):2103–18.

122. Nutt SL, Taubenheim N, Hasbold J, Corcoran LM, Hodgkin PD. The genetic network controlling plasma cell differentiation. Semin Immunol. 2011;23(5):341–9.

123. Glimcher LH. XBP1: the last two decades. Ann Rheum Dis. 2010;69(Suppl 1):i67–71.

124. Chevrier S, Emslie D, Shi W, Kratina T, Wellard C, Karnowski A, et al. The BTB-ZF transcription factor Zbtb20 is driven by Irf4 to promote plasma cell differentiation and longevity. J Exp Med. 2014;211(5):827–40.

125. Cirillo E, Giardino G, Gallo V, D'Assante R, Grasso F, Romano R, et al. Severe combined immunodeficiency – an update. Ann N Y Acad Sci. 2015;1356:90–106.

126. Vihinen M, Mattsson PT, Smith CI. Bruton tyrosine kinase (BTK) in X-linked agammaglobulinemia (XLA). Front Biosci. 2000;5:D917–28.

127. Jolles S. The variable in common variable immunodeficiency: a disease of complex phenotypes. J Allergy Clin Immunol Pract. 2013;1(6):545–56. quiz 57

128. Yazdani R, Azizi G, Abolhassani H, Aghamohammadi A. Selective IgA deficiency: epidemiology, pathogenesis, clinical phenotype, diagnosis, prognosis and management. Scand J Immunol. 2017;85(1):3–12.

129. Wahn V, von Bernuth H. Short review: IgG subclass deficiencies in children: facts and fiction. Pediatr Allergy Immunol. 2017;28(6):521–4.

130. Qamar N, Fuleihan RL. The hyper IgM syndromes. Clin Rev Allergy Immunol. 2014;46(2):120–30.

131. Mogensen TH. STAT3 and the Hyper-IgE syndrome: clinical presentation, genetic origin, pathogenesis, novel findings and remaining uncertainties. JAKSTAT. 2013;2(2):23435.

132. Buchbinder D, Nugent DJ, Fillipovich AH. Wiskott-Aldrich syndrome: diagnosis, current management, and emerging treatments. Appl Clin Genet. 2014;7:55–66.

133. McKinnon PJ. ATM and ataxia telangiectasia. EMBO Rep. 2004;5(8):772–6.

134. Al Ustwani O, Kurzrock R, Wetzler M. Genetics on a WHIM. Br J Haematol. 2014;164(1):15–23.

Complement

4

Srinjoy Chakraborti and Sanjay Ram

The Complement System

Historical Aspects

The bactericidal activity of normal serum was described as early as the 1880s by von Fodor [1], Nutall [2], and Buchner [3]. Nutall described bactericidal activity of sheep blood against *Bacillus anthracis*, which was lost when blood was heated to 55 °C. Buchner coined the term alexin to describe the heat-labile factor responsible for bacterial killing. Pfeiffer and Issaef [4] demonstrated that whole blood from guinea pigs that survived the challenge with *Vibrio cholerae* could protect naïve animals from developing disease. The following year, Jules Bordet showed that the bactericidal activity of heated immune serum was restored by fresh serum that itself had no intrinsic bactericidal activity [5]. Thus, the bactericidal activity of immune serum was dependent on a heat-stable factor as well as a heat-labile factor (alexin). The combination of heat-stable antibody and alexin was shown to cause hemolysis [6, 7]. Bordet and Gengou described complement fixation and showed the loss of complement activity from serum in the presence of antigen-antibody complexes [8]. Ehrlich, who coined the term "complement," initially believed that each antigen-specific antibody (which he called "amboceptors") had its own complement, while Bordet posited that there was only one type of complement for all antibodies. Bordet was awarded the Nobel Prize in 1919 for his discovery of complement activity.

Ferrata, working in Ehrlich's laboratory, demonstrated that the euglobulin and pseudoglobulin fractions in serum were both required for complement activity, leading to the initial nomenclature of $C'1$ and $C'2$ (the "prime" was omitted following the WHO nomenclature proposed in 1968), and also proved that complement was not a single protein [9]. Loss of a heat-stable component of complement by treatment of serum with cobra venom and absorption of this activity by yeast led to the discovery of the third component (C3). C4 was discovered as the result of loss of complement activity following ammonia extraction of serum; the destroyed component was distinct from C3. Loss of complement activity following methylamine and ammonia treatment predicted the presence of the thioester of C3 and C4. In the 1940s, Manfred Mayer and colleagues developed a standardized method of hemolytic titration. Mayer proposed the "one-hit" theory, whereby only one complete sequence of

This work was supported by grants from the National Institutes of Health/National Institute of Allergy and Infectious Diseases, AI111728, AI118161, AI119327, and AI114790.

S. Chakraborti · S. Ram (✉)
Division of Infectious Diseases and Immunology, Department of Medicine, University of Massachusetts Medical School, Worcester, MA, USA
e-mail: Sanjay.Ram@umassmed.edu

complement proteins was required to lyse an erythrocyte. This method provided a method to titrate the hemolytic activity of sera. However, the "one-hit" theory provided estimates of complement concentrations that were about three orders of magnitude too low (at least for molecules such as C3 and C4). The perception that complement components were trace serum components, coupled with the lack of more advanced protein purification methods, led to stagnation in efforts to characterize complement proteins for almost 20 years. The identification of C3 as a β1c-globulin – a major component of serum that was present at concentration of ~1 mg/ml – by Muller-Eberhard [10] paved the way for further characterization of complement proteins.

Although not appreciated at the time, the existence of the alternative pathway was suggested by experiments where cobra venom factor and zymosan consumed complement activity without affecting the classical heat-labile components [11, 12]. Pillemer and his coworkers first characterized the properdin pathway [13], but his critics ascribed the observations to the presence of small amounts of contaminating antibody [14]. Following Pillemer's untimely suicide in 1957, his work was carried on by Irwin Lepow. Highly competitive work by several groups led to the characterization of the alternative pathway by the early 1970s.

Over the past three decades, the advent of molecular biology, the development of knockout and transgenic animals, and the elucidation of the crystal structures of several complement components have yielded invaluable insights into the intricate functioning of complement. It is now clear that the functions of complement extend well beyond its originally described function, that of combating infections, to include crosstalk with other arms of the immune system (e.g., inflammasome activation) and coagulation system, bridging innate and adaptive immunity, embryogenesis, neural pruning, and modulating tumor growth.

Evolution of the Complement System

The complement system is one of the most ancient arms of innate immunity and developed long before the adaptive arm of immunity. Acquired immunity appears to have arisen early in vertebrate evolution, between the divergence of cyclostomes (lampreys) and cartilaginous fish (sharks). Genes encoding molecules that comprise the acquired immune system, including immunoglobulin (Ig), T-cell receptor (TCR), major histocompatibility complex (MHC) classes I and II, and recombination-activating gene (RAG), have been identified only in sharks and higher vertebrates [15]. The alternative and the lectin pathways are phylogenetically older than the classical pathway. C3, the central molecule of the complement system, C4, and C5 are all derived phylogenetically from a serum protease inhibitor called α2-macroglobulin [16]. Only a single C3/C4/C5 gene that is distinct from the α2-macroglobulin was identified in the lamprey [17], the ascidian [18], and the sea urchin [19], which suggested that the gene duplication that gave rise to distinct C3, C4, and C5 molecules took place later in evolution, around the time of the appearance of jawed vertebrates. It is believed that the classical and terminal complement pathways emerged around the same time as the adaptive immune system, which coincided with the appearance of cartilaginous fish [20].

Insects also possess C3-like molecules. One such protein, called thioester-containing protein 1 (TEP1), possesses ~25% sequence identity with C3 and 31% identity within the thioester domain of C3 (discussed below). Analogous to C3, TEP1 also binds to bacteria covalently through the thioester bond [21].

Synthesis, Distribution, and Catabolism of Complement

Following orthotopic liver transplantation, the "genetic type" (as determined by agarose gel electrophoresis or isoelectric focusing) of complement proteins C3, C6, C8, and factor B (FB) in the serum of the organ recipient was noted to have switched to the phenotype of the liver donor [22]. This observation established the liver as a major site of complement protein synthesis. Several other cell types, such as neutrophils, monocytes, macrophages, adipocytes, microglia, astrocytes, fibroblasts, cervical epithelial cells, and endothelial cells, are also important sites of local complement production [23–25]. Studies in humans using radiolabeled complement components C3, C4, C5, and FB revealed that these molecules have high fractional catabolic rates and are more rapidly metabolized compared to most serum proteins [26]. Several complement components are acute-phase reactants, and their synthesis is modulated by cytokines such as IFN-γ, IL-1, and TNF and by endotoxin [27]. Monocytes and macrophages can synthesize complement in amounts sufficient to opsonize microbes [27]; therefore upregulation of complement production by proinflammatory signals enhances antimicrobial activity locally at sites of infection. Further, the role of locally synthesized complement in several physiologic processes, such as the shaping of adaptive immune responses and neural remodeling, is now apparent.

While most complement is found in plasma, it is also found in almost every mucosal site and body fluid. Complement concentrations at mucosal sites approach 5–10% that seen in serum [28]. An increase in complement concentrations at sites such as the cerebrospinal fluid occurs because of increased vascular permeability and also because of increased production locally as a result of inflammation. Complement levels in the female genital tract are profoundly affected by hormonal regulation [29–31].

Several studies have examined complement levels and activity among neonates and preterm infants. Both preterm and full-term newborns have lower complement function compared to adults [32]. Complement activity and levels of several complement components appear to correlate inversely with the age of gestation [33–39]. Complement activity approaches adult levels at about 6 months of age [40, 41].

Activation of Complement

Complement activation has traditionally been considered as occurring through one of the three pathways – the classical, lectin, or alternative pathways (Fig. 4.1). In most instances, activation of complement often occurs through more than one pathway simultaneously. As an example, C3 deposited through the classical or lectin pathways may recruit the alternative pathway. Here, we will discuss complement activation using a reductionist approach where each pathway is considered separately. Characteristics of each of the components of complement in the fluid phase are listed in Table 4.1. We have used the terminology proposed in 2014 jointly by the International Complement Society (ICS) and the European Complement Network (ECN) [42].

The Classical Pathway

The classical pathway is usually initiated by binding of antibodies to their target antigens. Binding of an antibody to its target exposes a binding site for C1q in the trimolecular C1 complex that comprises a hexameric C1q molecule and two molecules each of C1r and C1s. A single globular head of C1q and Fc interact with very low affinity ($K_d \approx 10^{-4}$ M) [43, 44]. Recently, Diebolder and colleagues showed that binding of antibody molecules to a surface is followed by specific noncovalent interactions between Fc regions of proximate IgG molecules, which results in the formation of ordered hexamers. These hexamers engage each of the six globular heads of C1q, thereby resulting in high-avidity interactions between IgG and C1q [45]. Therefore, to initiate complement activation, it is important for IgG molecules to achieve a critical density on a surface. Certain amino acid point mutations in the Fc portion of IgG – for example, replacing Glu at position 430 with Gly – enhance Fc hexamer formation following binding of antibody to antigen. Such Fc mutations could be employed to enhance the efficacy of therapeutic monoclonal antibodies that rely on complement-dependent cytotoxicity for their activity [45]. C1r and C1s are arranged as a tetramer (C1s-C1r-C1r-C1s) and form a Ca^{2+}-dependent catalytic

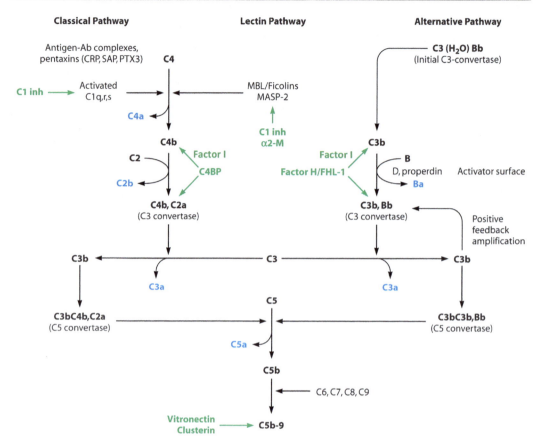

Fig. 4.1 Schematic representing the activation of the complement cascade. The fragments released into solution are indicated in *blue font*. The key fluid-phase regulators are indicated in *green font*. *CRP* C-reactive protein, *SAP* serum amyloid P component, *PTX3* pentraxins 3, *C1 inh* C1 inhibitor, *α2-M* α2-macroglobulin, *C4BP* C4b-binding protein, *FHL-1* factor H-like protein-1 (From Ram et al. [319]. (American Society of Microbiology))

subunit [46, 47]. Binding of C1q generates a conformational signal that results in autoactivation of C1r, which in turn activates C1s. C1r and C1s are both activated through cleavage of an Arg-Ile bond.

Human IgG subclasses differ in their ability to activate complement; in general, IgG1, IgG2, and IgG3 activate complement in the order IgG3>IgG1>IgG2, while IgG4 does not activate complement. In contrast to IgG, where the cooperation between several molecules is required to activate complement, a single IgM molecule can activate complement. This is because IgM is polymer (pentameric or hexameric in the presence or absence of the J chain, respectively) and each target-bound IgM can bind to the C1 complex [48, 49]. Thus, on a molar basis, IgM is the most potent activator of the classical pathway.

The classical pathway can also be activated when members of the pentraxin family (includes C-reactive protein (CRP), serum amyloid P component (SAP), and pentraxin 3 (PTX3)) bind to surfaces and engage C1q [50–52]. A novel mechanism of classical pathway activation described in mice is initiated by the binding of certain pneumococcal polysaccharides to the specific intracellular adhesion molecule (ICAM)-grabbing nonintegrin R1 (SIGN-R1), which was one of five receptors that was discovered during efforts to identify the murine homologue of a human C-type lectin called dendritic cell-specific ICAM-3-grabbing nonintegrin (DC-SIGN) [53].

Table 4.1 Characteristics of soluble proteins of the complement cascade

Component	Approx. serum conc. (µg/ml)	Mol. mass (kD)	Structure	No. of genetic loci	Chromosomal assignment
Proteins that activate complement					
Classical pathway proteins					
C1q	70	459	18 polypeptide chains; 6A, 6B, 6C; A-B and C-C linked by disulfides	3 (A, B, C)	1p34-1p36.3
C1r	34	173	Comprises a CUB (C1r/C1s, uEGF, bone morphogenetic protein) module, an epidermal growth factor (EGF)-like module, a second CUB module, two complement control protein (CCP) modules and a C-terminal chymotrypsin-like serine protease domain; dimer (A and B chains linked by disulfide bond)	1	12p13
C1s	31	80	Dimer (A and B chains linked by disulfide bond); modular structure s described for C1r	1	12p13
C4	600	206	β-α-γ; 1 β-α and 2 α-γ disulfide bonds	2 (C4A, C4B)	6p21.3
C2	11–35	100	1 chain	1	6p21.3
Alternative pathway proteins					
Factor B (FB)	200	90	1 chain	1	6p21.3
Factor D (FD; adipsin)	1–2	25	1 chain	1	19p13.3
Properdin	5–10	55	Cyclic polymers in head-to-tail orientation; dimers/trimers/tetramers in 26:54:20 ratio; each monomer comprises 6 thrombospondin-like repeats (TSRs) and has 14 sites of C-mannosylation	1	Xp11.4-p11.23
Lectin pathway					
Mannan-binding lectin (MBL)	1–5	~25 (subunit monomer)	Subunit – trimers of identical polypeptides; subunits organized into larger oligomers (n ~ 2 for variant (B, C, and D) alleles and 4–6 for wild-type (A) allele)	1	10q11.2-q21
Ficolin-1 (M-ficolin; ficolin/P35-related protein)	0.04–0.1 (monocytes and PMNs main source)	~32 (subunit monomer)	Subunit – trimers of identical polypeptides; subunits organized into larger oligomers	1	9q34
Ficolin-2 (L-ficolin; hucolin; EBP-37; ficolin/P35)	3–4	34 (subunit monomer)	As with ficolin-1	1	9q34

(continued)

Table 4.1 (continued)

Component	Approx. serum conc. (µg/ml)	Mol. mass (kD)	Structure	No. of genetic loci	Chromosomal assignment
Ficolin-3 (H-ficolin; Hakata antigen; thermolabile β-2 macroglycoprotein; thermolabile substance)	18	35 (subunit monomer)	As with ficolin-1	1	Chr 1
MASP-1	6	97	Active form consists of heavy and light chains linked by disulfide bond	1	3q27-28
MASP-2	0.02–0.8	83	Active form consists of A and B chains linked by disulfide bond	1	1p36.3-p36.2
MASP-3	2–12.9	105	Activation splits 105 kD disulfide-linked dimer into A (58 kD) and B (42 kD); B chain is serine protease domain	1	3q27-28
MAp19	?	19	Alternatively spliced version of MASP-2 – contains first 2 domains and 4 additional C-terminal aa's; head-to-tail homodimer	1	1p36.3-p36.2
C3					
C3	1000–1500	190	β-α, linked by disulfide bond. Crystal structure shows organization into 13 domains; 8 macroglobulin domains, and 1 CUB, thioester (TED), anaphylatoxin, linker, and C345c domain	1	19p13.3-p13.2
Terminal complement components					
C5	75	190	β-α, linked by disulfide bond	1	9q34.1
C6	45	100	1 chain	1	5p13
C7	90	95	1 chain	1	5p13
C8	55–80	151	α-γ dimer linked by disulfide, noncovalently associated with β	3	(α,β)1p32; (γ) 9q34.3
C9	60	71	1 chain	1	5p13
Complement inhibitory proteins					
C1 inhibitor (C1-INH)	150	104	1 chain; highly glycosylated	1	11q11-q13.1
C4b-binding protein (C4BP)	150–300	~550	7 disulfide-linked α-chains (8 SCRs) linked to β-chain (3 SCRs) via disulfide (major isoform; α7/β1); minor isoforms α7/β0 and α6/β1. β-chain associated with protein S of the anticoagulation system (C4BP-protein S)	2	(α,β) 1q32

(continued)

Table 4.1 (continued)

Component	Approx. serum conc. (μg/ml)	Mol. mass (kD)	Structure	No. of genetic loci	Chromosomal assignment
Factor H (FH)[a]	500	155	1 chain (20 SCRs)	1	1q32
Factor I (FI)	34	90	1 chain; comprises FI-MAC domain, scavenger receptor cysteine-rich or CD5 domain, two low-density lipoprotein receptor (LDLr) domains and a serine protease domain	1	4q
FHL-1 (factor H-like protein 1)	25	43	1 chain (7 SCRs; identical to 7 N-terminal SCRs of factor H, plus 4 unique C-terminal aa's)	1	1q32
Vitronectin (Vn; S-protein)	500	75 (65 kD proteolytic fragment also seen)	1 chain	1	17q11
Clusterin (Cn; SP-40,40; apolipoprotein J)	100–300	60 (predicted); 80 (observed)	Heterodimer linked by 5-disulfide bond motif	1	8p21-p12

[a]The FH family of proteins includes five FH-related molecules called FHR1, 2, 3, 4, and 5. The function of these proteins remains to be fully elucidated. See text for details

Activated C1s cleaves the 77-amino-acid C4a fragment from the N-terminus of the α-chain of C4 to form the metastable C4b molecule. This exposes the internal thioester bond of C4b [54] that can react readily with nucleophilic (i.e., electron-donating groups) groups such as –OH or $-NH_2$ on surfaces to form covalent ester or amide bonds, respectively [55]. If the nascent carbonyl group in the thioester moiety does not interact with a surface, it reacts with water and remains in solution. There are two isoforms of C4 expressed by most humans, called C4A and C4B [56], which dictate the type of bond formed by C4b (note that C4a and C4b represent activation products of C4 and are distinct from the C4A and C4B isoforms of intact C4). C4B possesses a His residue at position 1106 in the α-chain, which imparts to C4B the ability to form ester linkages, while an Asp residue at position 1106 results in "C4A-like" functionality and preferential amide bond formation [57]. Differences in the binding properties of C4A (amide) and C4B (ester) may have important functional consequences. C4B is believed to possess greater hemolytic activity than C4A [57]. On the other hand, C4A binds to complement receptor 1 (CR1) more efficiently

[58] and may play a key role in clearing immune complexes from the bloodstream, which could explain the association between C4A deficiency and autoimmune diseases [59, 60]. In addition to the fact that C4 exists as distinct isoforms, the number of copies of the C4A and C4B genes varies across individuals. Deletions or duplications of C4 genes occur frequently [61–63] and affect plasma levels of C4. The frequency of C4 gene dosages of 2, 3, 4, 5, and 6 in the Caucasian population is 2%, 25.3%, 52%, 17.3%, and 3.3%, respectively [64]. As a result, complete C4 deficiency is extremely rare [65–67]. Conversely, heterozygous C4 deficiency is very common and occurs in approximately 25% of the general population. A complete deficiency of either of the isoforms of C4, C4A, or C4B is also relatively common and occurs in about 6% of the population [64, 67–69].

In the next step in classical pathway activation, C2 binds to C4b deposited on a surface. C2 is also cleaved by activated C1s into the C2a fragment, which remains attached noncovalently to C4b and C2b, which is released into solution. C4bC2a forms the C3 convertase (C3-cleaving enzyme) of the classical pathway. In this manner, a single C1 complex can cleave several substrate molecules and augment complement activation.

The Lectin Pathway

Activation of complement through the lectin pathway is also important in generating classical pathway C3 convertase, C4b2a. To date, five lectin molecules that can bind to a variety of terminal monosaccharides and initiate complement activation have been described. These include the collectins (collagen-containing C-type [calcium-dependent] lectins), mannan-binding lectin (MBL) [70–73] and collectin 11 [74], and ficolin-1, ficolin-2, and ficolin-3 (also called M-, L-, and H-ficolin, respectively) [75, 76]. Ficolins contain a fibrinogen-like domain combined with a collagen-like domain and thus are not classified as collectins.

The recognition molecules of the lectin pathway are trimers that comprise three identical polypeptide subunits, each terminating in a calcium-dependent carbohydrate recognition domain. These trimers are organized into higher-order oligomers that resemble a bouquet. MBL shares structural and functional homology with C1q [77]. Similar to C1q, MBL is complexed with serine proteases, termed MBL-associated serum proteases (MASPs). Four such molecules – MASP-1, MASP-2, MASP-3, and MBL-associated plasma protein of 19 kD (MAp19) – are the products of two genes arising from a common ancestor shared with C1r and C1s [78]. MASP-1 and MASP-3 are alternatively spliced products of *MASP1*, while MASP-2 and MAp19 are alternatively spliced products of *MASP2*. MASP-2 cleaves C4 and C2 to generate the classical pathway C3 convertase, as described earlier [77, 78]. A role for MASP-1 in complement activation was revealed by a nonfunctional lectin pathway in an individual with a nonsense mutation in *MASP1* (and therefore lacking both MASP-1 and MASP-3) [79]. Reconstitution of the subject's serum with MASP-1 resulted in MASP-2 cleavage and full restoration of lectin pathway activity. Further, MASP-1 and MASP-2 exist as a co-complex with MBL, supporting a model in which MASP-1 trans-activates MASP-2, analogous to C1r and C1s activation.

Levels of MBL are influenced by mutations in the first exon of *MBL2* that encodes the signal peptide and the collagen-like region of the molecule. Three known mutations that result in MBL deficiency are G→D at position 54, G→E at position 57, and R→C at position 57, which are termed the B, C, and D alleles, respectively. These mutant alleles are collectively referred to as the "O" alleles, while the wild-type protein is designated as the "A" allele. Each of these point mutations (O alleles) interferes with oligomerization of the three single chains that form the mature protein and are associated with low levels of MBL. In addition to the mutations in the coding region of the gene, three polymorphic sites are found in the 5′ untranslated promoter region of *mbl2*: H/L, X/Y, and P/Q [80, 81]. The promoter alleles are found in linkage disequilibrium with the exon 1 SNPs, which results in a limited number (seven) of described haplotypes: HYPA, LYPA, LYQA, LXPA, HYPD, LYPB, and LYQC [82]. When the A or wild-type alleles are in cis with promoter −550/−221 haplotypes HY, LY, and LX, the MBL concentrations are high, intermediate, and low, respectively. Studies that use only genotyping to infer MBL levels should be interpreted with caution because individuals with the identical genotype for all MBL variants may have MBL levels that differ by as much as tenfold [83].

MBL binds to a variety of terminal monosaccharides, including mannose, *N*-acetylmannosamine, *N*-acetyl-D-glucosamine, fucose, and glucose [84]. Collectin 11 binds preferentially to L-fucose and D-mannose [85]. The ficolins appear to bind preferentially to acetylated sugars such as N-acetyl-D-glucosamine [75]. In addition, ficolin-1 (M-ficolin) binds to N-acetyl-D-galactosamine and selects sialoglycans, such as those present in the capsule of *Streptococcus agalactiae*. Ligands reported for ficolin-2 (L-ficolin) include β-(1→3)-D-glucan, N-acetylneuraminic acid, lipoteichoic acid, C-reactive protein, fibrinogen, DNA, and certain corticosteroids, while H-ficolin binds to fucose [75, 86]. These sugars frequently decorate microbial surfaces but rarely appear as the terminal unit of oligosaccharides or glycoconjugates on human cells, which enables "self-nonself" discrimination and targets complement activation to foreign surfaces. In these respects, the lectins share several critical features with IgM ("natural antibodies"): both are polyreactive, bind to surface carbohydrates, and require binding of just a single molecule activate complement [77, 87].

Extrinsic proteases such as Hageman factor (factor XII in the clotting cascade) can also activate the classical pathway [88, 89]. Other proteases such as thrombin and kallikrein may activate C5 [90, 91] and FB [92, 93], respectively, although their clinical significance remains to be clarified.

The Alternative Pathway

Similar to the lectin pathway, the alternative pathway does not rely on initiation by antibodies and thus protects the host from pathogens prior to the development of specific immune responses. Activation of the alternative pathway of complement is characterized by a unique positive feedback loop that permits self-amplification of the pathway. The principal component of this feedback loop is C3b, which may be generated by "tickover" of C3, which generates a molecule that is functionally similar to C3b as discussed below, or by alternative or classical pathway C3 convertases. Given its central role in complement activation, the structure of C3 is discussed next.

C3: The Central Component of Complement

All complement pathways converge at the level of C3. C3 is the most abundant complement component (plasma concentrations range from 1.0 to 1.5 mg/ml), and its fragments serve a variety of functions. C3 fragments deposited on surfaces are opsonins for phagocytes, and the anaphylatoxin C3a modulates inflammation, lipid metabolism (C3a-des-Arg, which is generated by cleavage of the C-terminal Arg by carboxypeptidase N, is also called acylation-stimulating protein), and tissue regeneration.

Removal of four Arg residues from the C3 precursor yields a mature C3 molecule, composed of an α- and a β-chain linked by a disulfide bond (Fig. 4.2a). Similar to C4, the α-chain of C3 also possesses an internal thioester moiety that forms covalent bonds with target surfaces. The crystal structure of C3 reveals organization into 13 domains (Fig. 4.2c) [94]. Cleavage of the C3a fragment from C3 results in activation of C3, which is accompanied by marked structural rearrangements among its various domains (Fig. 4.2c). Most notably, the thioester domain that is tucked away in the native molecule moves about 85 Å and becomes completely exposed and capable of reacting with nucleophiles [95]. The thioester forms a highly reactive acyl-imidazole intermediate with an extremely short calculated half-life of ≈ 30 μs [96]. If this reactive group does not bind to a surface –OH (or, in some instances, a –NH$_2$ group) within this short period, it reacts with a water molecule and remain in solution (Fig. 4.2b). The high reactivity and short life of the nascent thioester domain restrict C3 deposition to structures proximate to the site of C3 activation while sparing more distant (and possibly normal) tissue from unwanted damage.

Activation of the Alternative Pathway

Since the discovery of the alternative pathway by Pillemer over 60 years ago [13], "tickover" of C3 (described below) was the traditionally accepted model for the initiation of alternative pathway activation. More recently, properdin binding to select surfaces was proposed as the initiating event for alternative pathway activation.

The "Tickover" Model

As discussed above, the internal thioester bond mediates covalent attachment of C3 to surfaces. Although well concealed in the native C3 molecule, the thioester undergoes spontaneous low-rate hydrolysis at a rate of 0.2–0.4%/h under physiologic conditions [97, 98]. The generated molecule, called C3(H$_2$O), has functional activities and binding properties that are similar to C3b but differs from C3b in that it still possesses the C3a fragment. Similar to C3b, C3(H$_2$O) also can bind to factor B (FB), properdin, and C5, can be further cleaved by the combined action of factor H (FH; cofactor) and factor I (FI; enzyme), and

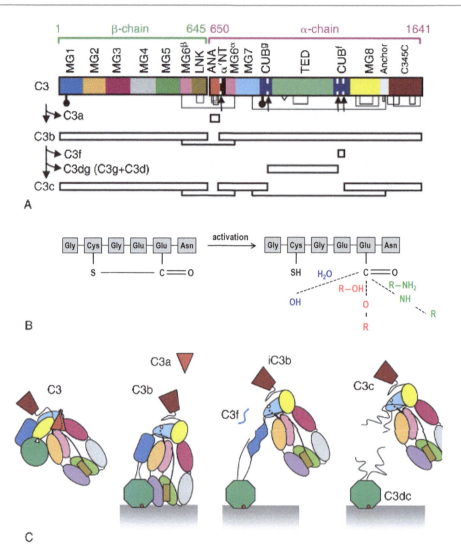

Fig. 4.2 C3 structure and activation. (**a**) The C3 molecule represented as its α and β chains and its degradation products. *Arrows* indicate physiologic cleavage sites. The location of the thioester bond is indicated by the inverted white triangle. Sites of N-linked glycosylation are shown by the "inverted lollipop" symbol. Locations of disulfide bridges are also shown. Colors of the amino acid stretches of the α- and β-chains correspond to domain colors in *C*. (**b**) The internal thioester bond of C3. (**c**) The domain organization of C3 and its degradation products. C3 is organized into 13 domains. During activation, C3a is released from the amino terminus of the ⟨-chain of C3. The exposed internal thioester bond becomes accessible to nucleophilic attack and can react with water or avail-

able hydroxyl or amine groups on cell surfaces (**b**). Analogous reactions occur with C4. Together, these reactions involving C3 and C4 are responsible for covalently linking complement deposition to the cell surface. *Asn* asparagine, *Cys* cysteine, *Glu* glutamic acid, *Gly* glycine, *Met* methionine. Activation of C3 is accompanied by an ~85 Å displacement of the thioester domain, and the resulting C3b molecule can form covalent bonds with targets (**c**). Cleavage of C3b to iC3b also results in conformational changes that contribute to ligand specificity. *MG* macroglobulin, *LNK* linker, *ANA* anaphylatoxin, *CUB* complement C1r/C1s, *uEGF* Bmp1, *TED* thioester-containing domain; α'NT (From Janssen et al. [94], Janssen et al. [95])

can bind to cellular receptors for C3. In the brief period before its degradation by FH and FI, $C3(H_2O)$ can bind to FB to form $C3(H_2O)B$, which in the presence of FD and Mg^{2+} forms $C3(H_2O)Bb$ (the Ba fragment is released from FB). Akin to C3bBb, $C3(H_2O)Bb$ has C3 convertase activity and generates more metastable C3b molecules capable of forming covalent bonds with surfaces. Each C3(H₂O)Bb produces on average three to five metastable C3b molecules before being inactivated by FH [97]. Surface-bound C3b then recruits FB and FD to generate surface-bound C3 convertase (C3bBb) and set into motion the positive feedback loop of the alternative pathway. The sequence of events that generate C3 convertases through the "tickover" of C3 are illustrated in Fig. 4.3a. C3bBb is inherently unstable and dissociates into its components with a $t_{1/2}$ of about 90 s [99]. The binding of properdin – the only known positive regulator of complement – to C3bBb stabilizes the complex and prolongs its half-life five- to tenfold, thereby promoting amplification [99].

The Properdin-Directed Model

The properdin-directed model was put forth by Hourcade et al. [100] and lent support to Pillemer's original proposal of alternative pathway activation made over six decades ago. Properdin is highlypositively charged. Each properin monomer is composed of thrombospondin type 1 repeat (TSR) subunits; subunits oligomerize in a head-to-tail manner to form dimers, trimers, and tetramers at a ratio of 26:54:20, respectively [101]. Phagocytes, in particular neutrophils, are the main site of properdin synthesis and storage [102, 103]. Release of properdin from these cells may increase alternative pathway activation locally at sites of inflammation. Properdin multimers may bind to a select cell surface sulfated glycoconjugates and initiate the alternative pathway [104, 105]. Surface-bound properdin can then recruit C3b or C3(H₂O) that

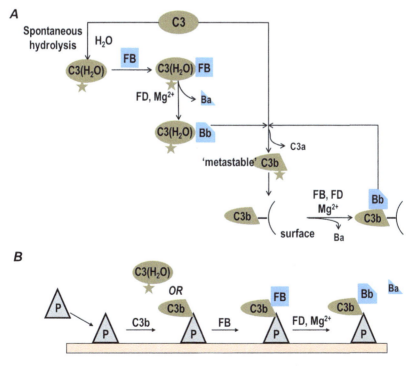

Fig. 4.3 Initiation of alternative pathway activation. (**a**) The "tickover" model. C3 undergoes slow, spontaneous hydrolysis, where the internal thioester bond (indicated by a *star*) that is normally tucked away becomes exposed and reacts with a water molecule to form C3(H₂O). Subsequent Mg²⁺-dependent reactions with FB and FD result in the formation of fluid-phase C3 convertase,

C3(H₂O)Bb, which then activates more native C3 molecules and enables them to bind covalently to surfaces and further activate the alternative pathway. (**b**) The properdin-directed model. Properdin binding to activator surfaces can recruit fluid-phase C3b or C3(H₂O) and serves as a platform for formation of C3 convertases on the surface

then binds FB, to form a platform for further alternative pathway activation (Fig. 4.3b).

Studies using purified properdin should be interpreted with caution because properdin forms higher-order oligomers and aggregates upon freeze-thawing or with prolonged storage [101], which may result in artifactual binding to surfaces. Carefully performed studies by Ferreira and colleagues have shown that freshly isolated properdin in its physiological conformations can initiate alternative pathway activation on *Chlamydia pneumoniae* and activated human platelets [106, 107]. The properdin-directed model provides yet another mechanism whereby complement activation is restricted to sites of tissue injury or on foreign surfaces (i.e., another mechanism of "self-nonself" discrimination).

The Terminal Complement Pathway: Assembly of the Membrane Attack Complex

Binding of an additional C3b molecule to C4b and C3b present in classical and alternative pathway C3 convertases, respectively, generates C5 convertases (C4bC2aC3b and C3bBbC3b) that can cleave C5 and initiate the assembly of membrane attack complex (MAC). C5 bears structural homology with C3 and C4 but lacks a thioester domain. The addition of C3b to C3 convertases alters the K_m for C5 >1000-fold, from far above the physiological concentration of C5 to far below it [108–110]. Therefore, situations that favor complement activation and rapid C3b generation also facilitate the generation of cytolytic MAC. Cleavage of C5 results in the release of the ≈11 kDa C5a fragment, an anaphylatoxin with diverse functions that are discussed below. Removal of the C-terminal Arg residue from C5a by carboxypeptidase N results in formation of C5a-des-Arg, which retains only 1–10% of the inflammatory activity of C5a [111].

Binding of C5b to hydrophobic sites on cell surfaces exposes binding sites for C6 and C7 to form the C5b-7 complex. Incorporation of C7 confers amphiphilic properties to the assembling MAC and permits insertion into cell membranes. C8 then binds to the β-chain of C5b, followed by the addition of one or more C9 molecules. C6, C7, C8, and C9 all belong to the MACPF/CDC (MAC-perforin/cholesterol-dependent cytolysin) superfamily of proteins [112, 113], which contain a common set of four core domains, from the N- to C-terminus, a thrombospondin-1 (TSP1) domain, a low-density lipoprotein receptor-associated (LDLRA) domain, a MACPF domain, and an epidermal growth factor (EGF) domain. In its fully assembled state, MAC comprises one molecule each of C5b, C6, C7, and C8 and up to 18 molecules of C9. The ringlike membrane configuration of MAC is dependent on C9 polymerization. C9 in its free monomeric native state has a globular conformation [114]. Upon polymerization, C9 adopts a tubular structure, where the external aspect of the tubule is hydrophobic and intercalates into membranes, while the inner aspect of the pore is hydrophilic and permits passage of water and ions. While most other pore-forming proteins rely on interactions solely between their MACPF domains, structural studies of poly-C9 revealed unexpected interactions between the TSP1 domain and the MACPF domain of adjacent monomers [115]. The TSP1-MACPF interactions permit recruitment of C9 molecules from solution into the nascent membrane-associated MAC complex. Cryo-electron microscopy analysis of the entire C5b-9 complex revealed a "split-washer" configuration, as opposed to a symmetric closed-ring conformation seen with perforin and other cholesterol-dependent cytolysins [116]. Disruption of the membrane proton-motive force during pore formation and osmotic damage mediated by the channel may both contribute to the cytolytic action of MAC.

The Intracellular Complement System

Complement has long been considered to function mainly in the extracellular milieu. Recent work has shown the presence of intracellular stores of C3 and C5, which can be cleaved by intracellular proteases to release their C3a and C5a fragments, respectively [117]. Activation of the intracellular stores of complement, sometimes referred to as the "complosome" [118], plays an important role in the homeostasis, effector response, and contraction of T cell responses [117, 119]. C3 may be expressed by T cells themselves, or C3(H_2O), the C3b-like hydrolyzed form of C3, may be taken up from the circulation by cells [120] and cleaved to C3a and C3b by the intracellular protease, cathepsin L. Intracellular C3a-C3aR interactions induce low levels of mammalian target of rapamycin (mTOR) activation to facilitate T-cell survival (homoeostasis). The effector phase of T-cell activation is triggered by activation of the T-cell receptor (TCR), which results in translocation of C3a and C3b to the cell surface, where they engage C3aR and CD46, respectively. Activation of CD46 results in increased expression of the CD46 isoform that bears the Cyt-1 intracytoplasmic tail. Cleavage of Cyt-1 by γ-secretase leads to translocation of Cyt-1 to the nucleus which drives the expression of glucose and amino acid transporters, resulting in increased nutrient influx and glycolysis and oxidative phosphorylation [121]. CD46 stimulation also drives expression of NLRP3 and IL-1β to stimulate the NLRP3 inflammasome. Stimulation of CD46 also activates intracellular C5 to generate C5a; C5a-C5aR1 interactions amplify ROS production, which activates the NLRP3 inflammasome [122] and promotes Th1 induction. The contraction phase of the Th1 response is accompanied by dominance of the CD46 isoform with the Cyt-2 tail, which, in conjunction with the IL-2R signaling, produces IL-10. A role for the "complosome" in nonimmune cells was suggested by Satyam et al., who showed that intracellular C3 levels increased during mesenteric ischemia; ischemic damage was limited by treatment with a cathepsin inhibitor or in cathepsin B-deficient mice [123]. These exciting findings have underscored a key role for intracellular complement in diverse cellular processes and merit further study.

Inhibition of Complement Activation

Tight regulation of the cascade is essential to permit complement activation only at sites of tissue injury or on invading microbes and to avoid collateral damage to normal host cells. Targeted activation is achieved by binding of antibody or lectin to specific ligands on microbes. Once complement activation is initiated, amplification occurs through the alternative pathway positive feedback loop, which is facilitated by the positive regulatory action of properdin. However, excessive and uncontrolled activation is limited by the inherently short half-lives of convertases and anaphylatoxins. Several fluid-phase inhibitory proteins that act at various levels of complement activation, including C1, C4b, C3b, and MAC, have been well characterized. It is worth noting that these inhibitory proteins all are present at concentrations far higher than most activators of complement, highlighting their importance in minimizing complement activation during physiological states. Several membrane-associated complement inhibitors also dampen complement activation on cell surfaces. Absence or dysfunction of complement inhibitors is associated with disease entities such as atypical hemolytic uremic syndrome (aHUS), C3 glomerulopathy, and age-related macular degeneration, further underscoring their physiological importance.

Fluid-Phase Complement Inhibitors

In physiological conditions, complement activation in the fluid phase is tightly controlled by C1 inhibitor (C1-INH), C4b-binding protein (C4BP), factor H (FH), FI, vitronectin (Vn), and clusterin (Cn). C1-INH and FI are enzymes, FH and C4BP act as cofactors for FI, while Vn and Cn associate with one or more components of assembling MAC to prevent further pore formation.

C1 Inhibitor (C1-INH)

C1-INH belongs to the family of protease inhibitors called serpins (*ser*ine *p*rotease *in*hibitors) [124]. Protease inactivation by serpins depends on a unique "trapping" mechanism, whereby the enzyme cleaves the inhibitor at its reactive center (between Arg 444 and Thr 445 in C1-INH), which is followed by formation of a covalent complex between the enzyme and the inhibitor. Thus, serpins inhibit enzymes by serving as their "suicide substrates." A unique feature of C1-INH is that N- and O-linked glycans contribute to about a third of its molecular mass, making it one of the most heavily glycosylated serum protein [125]. C1-INH directly inactivates both C1r and C1s [126, 127]. Binding of C1-INH to C1r also dissociates C1r and C1s from the activated C1 macromolecule [128, 129], as well as the entire activated C1 complex (C1q-C1r$_2$-C1s$_2$) from immobilized human IgG [130]. In addition to its well-recognized role as a classical pathway inhibitor, Jiang and colleagues showed that C1-INH also inhibited the alternative pathway by binding to C3b, thereby preventing binding of FB and formation of C3 convertase [131].

Although its name suggests specificity for C1, C1-INH acts on a variety of substrates including the contact system proteases (factor XII, plasma kallikrein), an intrinsic coagulation protease (factor XI), and the fibrinolytic proteases (plasmin, tissue plasminogen activator) [132]. C1-INH deficiency results in hereditary angioneurotic edema, characterized by excessive bradykinin production and increased vascular permeability.

Factor I

Factor I (FI) is a serine protease that controls the classical and alternative pathways of complement. It cleaves the α′ chains of C4b and C3b in the presence of cofactors – C4BP for C4b, FH for C3b and membrane cofactor protein (MCP), and complement receptor 1 (CR1) for both C3b and C4b – to their hemolytically inactive forms. Cleavage of C3b yields iC3b, while cleavage of C4b on either side of the thioester bond yields C4c and C4d. The primary site of FI synthesis is the liver [133] but is also synthesized by other cells including fibroblasts [134], monocytes [135], keratinocytes [136], endothelial cells [137], myoblasts, and primary cervical epithelial cells [23]. FI is an acute-phase protein and is upregulated by LPS and IFN-γ in endothelial cells, hepatocytes, and fibroblasts [134, 138]. The complete absence of FI is rare and is associated with uninhibited complement activation and consumption of complement. Such individuals are functionally deficient in complement and are predisposed to infections, in particular invasive meningococcal disease. Loss of function mutations in FI lead to alternative pathway overactivity and result in aHUS or a form of C3 glomerulopathy characterized by isolated mesangial C3 deposits in the absence of mesangial proliferation [139]. Polymorphisms in FI are associated with an increased risk of AMD [140].

C4b-Binding Protein (C4BP)

C4b-binding protein (C4BP) inhibits the classical pathway by two major mechanisms: (i) acts a cofactor in the factor I (FI)-mediated cleavage of C4b to C4c and C4d and (ii) accelerates dissociation of C2a from the classical pathway C3 convertase (C4bC2a), a property called "decay-accelerating" activity [141–144]. C4BP is composed entirely of short consensus repeat (SCR) domains, also called complement control protein (CCP) domains. Each SCR is comprised of ≈60 amino acids, characterized by four highly invariant cysteine residues and by many conserved amino acids, folded into a compact unit. Several other complement proteins contain SCR domains, including FH, DAF, MCP, CR1, CR2, FB, and C2 [145, 146]. It is worth noting that most SCR-containing complement proteins interact with C3b and/or C4b [145]. A patch of positively charged residues at the interface between the first and second NH$_2$-terminal SCRs plays an important role in the interaction between C4BP and C4b [147].

Factor H (FH) and the FH Family of Proteins

Analogous to inhibition of the classical pathway by C4BP, FH is a cofactor for FI-mediated cleavage of C3b to iC3b and accelerates the decay of C3bBb. FH also prevents binding FB to C3b to prevent formation of the alternative pathway C3 convertase [148–152]. FH contains 20 SCR domains organized as a single chain [153]; only the first four N-terminal SCRs are necessary and sufficient for complement inhibition [154]. In addition to its role as an inhibitor of the alternative pathway in the fluid phase, FH plays a key role in the homeostasis of complement on host cell surfaces. This property stems from the ability of FH to interact simultaneously with C3 fragments deposited on host cells and specific host glycosaminoglycans (including sialic acid in certain configurations) through domains 19 and 20, respectively [155, 156]. The interaction between FH and "self-polyanions" on cells increases the affinity of FH for C3b [157, 158], which simultaneously decreases FB-C3b interactions [151, 152, 157, 158], thus preventing C3 convertase formation. The balance between the affinities of FH and FB for C3b on a surface determines whether the surface is an activator (affinity of FB for C3b greater) or non-activator (affinity of FH for C3b greater) of complement. Similar to complete deficiency of FI, loss of FH is associated with complement consumption and predisposition to meningococcal infections and with renal disease (dense deposit disease). Mutations in FH that impair recognition of cell surfaces and C3d – most of which reside in domains 19 and 20 – result in aHUS. A homozygous polymorphism in domain 7 (His instead of Tyr at position 402) significantly increases the risk of age-related macular degeneration (AMD) [159, 160]. Compared to FH containing Tyr402, FH with His402 shows impaired binding to malondialdehydes that accumulate in "drusen" (the lesions seen in AMD) [161]. Reduced FH bound to drusen permits more alternative pathway activation and consequently increased uptake of malondialdehyde-modified proteins by macrophages, with resulting inflammation and ocular damage.

In addition to FH, there exists an alternatively spliced variant of factor H called factor H-like protein 1 (FHL-1) and five FH-related molecules (FHRs 1 through 5) that are the products of separate genes [162, 163]. All members of the FH family of proteins are arranged in tandem within the regulation of complement activation (*RCA*) gene on human chromosome 1q32. FHL-1 contains the first seven N-terminal SCRs of FH and therefore possesses cofactor and decay-accelerating activity that requires SCRs 1 through 4. The FHRs also are made up entirely of SCR domains, and several of these domains share varying levels of homology with FH. None of the FHRs have cofactor or decay-accelerating activity. FHRs 1, 2, and 5 exist in circulation as homo- or heterodimers. The function of the other FHRs remains to be determined, but they may modulate the function of FH by competing with the binding of FH to C3b or to surfaces. As an example, CFHR3, competes with FH for binding to meningococci and promotes complement activation [164]. The homology and proximity of the FH family of genes result in gene deletions, duplications, and rearrangements that result in the expression of hybrid proteins that are associated with renal disorders, such as atypical hemolytic uremic syndrome, C3 glomerulonephritis, dense deposit disease, and retinal damage in age-related macular degeneration [165]. The role of FH and the FHRs in disease pathogenesis is complex and is the subject of intensive investigation. The reader is referred to several meritorious reviews for a detailed description of their structure, function, and disease associations [165–174].

Vitronectin (Vn)

Vitronectin (Vn; also known as S-protein) can inhibit the terminal complement complex at various stages. The first stage in the formation of the membrane attack complex that can insert into membrane is C5b-7. Vn can occupy the metastable membrane-binding site of the nascent C5b-7 complex [175] to form sC5b-7. Although the sC5b-7 complex can take up further C8 and C9 molecules to form sC5b-8 and sC5b-9, respectively [176], these latter complexes lack hemolytic activity. The wedge-shaped ultrastructure of Vn-containing membrane attack complexes differs from the circular complement lesions that mediate hemolytic activity [177]. In addition, Vn blocks C9 polymerization [178], which limits the number of C9 molecules in the complex to three. Vn also blocks pore formation by perforin, a product of cytotoxic T lymphocytes and natural killer (NK) cells [179]. Vn is a multifunctional protein with several distinct ligands – in addition to complement regulation, it plays roles in coagulation, fibrinolysis, pericellular proteolysis, vascular remodeling, cell attachment, and spreading [180, 181].

Clusterin (Cn)

Clusterin (Cn; also known as apolipoprotein J or serum protein 40,40 (SP40-40)) is a heterodimer linked by five disulfide bonds. The highest levels of Cn occur in semen, which is estimated to contain levels tenfold above the serum concentrations [182]. Although structurally unrelated to Vn, Cn shares functional similarity with Vn by binding to several sites in the membrane attack complex and preventing C9 polymerization [183, 184].

Membrane-Associated Complement Inhibitors

Inhibition of complement activation on host cell surfaces is critical to prevent needless damage to "self" structures. Diseases associated with their absence or dysfunction highlight their physiological importance – as examples, loss of CD46 function is associated with atypical hemolytic uremic syndrome (aHUS) [185] and loss of CD55 and C59 causes paroxysmal nocturnal hemoglobinuria (PNH) [186, 187]. A schematic representation of the five major membrane-associated complement inhibitors discussed in this section is shown in Fig. 4.4.

Complement Receptor 1 (CR1; Also Called CD35 or the Immune Adherence Receptor)

CR1 is an integral membrane glycoprotein composed of a C-terminal transmembrane region and an extracellular region composed of a linear array of 30 SCR units [188, 189]. The N-terminal 28 SCRs are further organized as 4 tandem, long homologous repeats (LHRs) of 7 SCR units each [188, 189]. CR1 is a receptor for C3b, C4b, C1q, and MBL. CR1 possesses cofactor activity and can facilitate FI cleavage of C3b to iC3b and is the only molecule that facilitates further cleavage of iC3b to C3c and C3d. CR1 also mediates decay acceleration of C3 and C5 convertases of the classical and alternative pathways [190].

CR1 is found on erythrocytes, neutrophils, monocytes, glomerular podocytes, and certain T cells. Human erythrocyte CR1 mediates binding of complement-opsonized immune complexes or microorganisms to the cell, and this forms the basis for the phenomenon of immune adherence [191]. These bound complexes or organisms are carried to the spleen or liver where they are removed; in the process CR1 is also lost from the RBC surface [192–196]. CR1 is organized in clusters on the RBC surface, which could explain the multivalent nature of binding of immune

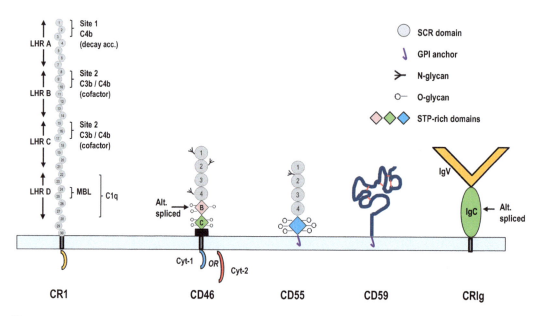

Fig. 4.4 Schematic representation of membrane-bound complement inhibitors. *SCR* short consensus repeat, *LHR* long homologous repeat, *GPI* glycophosphatidylinositol, *STP* serine threonine proline

complexes to RBCs. Furthermore, clustering of CR1 enhances the efficiency of RBCs to bind to opsonized particles despite the relatively low numbers of CR1 molecules per RBC [197–199].

There are four allelic variants of CR1 described in humans [200]. The number of LHRs in these allelic forms varies from three to six and is responsible for the differences in the molecular masses of each allotype [189, 201–205]. Although their frequencies vary across different ethnic groups, CR1*1 (or CR1-A) is the most commonly encountered allotype and occurs in >80% of most populations studied [200]. CR1 copy number on erythrocytes constitutes another polymorphism.

SCR1 of CR1 interacts with the *Plasmodium falciparum* protein PfRh4 [206]. In addition to facilitating the entry of *P. falciparum* into RBCs, CR1 promotes erythrocyte rosetting that is believed to contribute to the pathogenesis of cerebral malaria [207, 208]. Several epidemiologic studies have attempted to correlate CR1 allotypes and expression levels with the severity of malaria, often with conflicting results [208]. Given its importance in clearing immune complexes, CR1 expression levels on erythrocytes may also modulate the severity of systemic lupus erythematosus (SLE) [209–211].

CD46 (Membrane Cofactor Protein or MCP)

CD46 is a cofactor for FI-mediated cleavage of C3b and C4b to iC3b and C4d, respectively [212]. It is expressed on most nucleated cells. Human erythrocytes lack CD46. CD46 comprises 4 SCR domains followed by an O-glycosylated serine/threonine/proline-rich (STP) domain, 12 residues of unknown function, and an intracytoplasmic tail. Alternative splicing of the STP region (encoded by the B and C exons; the A exon is rarely used) to the B exon and the cytoplasmic tail to either Cyt-1 or Cyt-2 gives rise to four major isoforms of CD46 called C1, C2, BC1, and BC2. N-glycans present in SCRs 2 and 4 are required for cofactor activity [213]. The STP region modulates CD46 function. For exam-

ple, the BC isoform binds C4b more efficiently and provides enhanced cytoprotection against the classical pathway than the C isoform [214].

CD55 (Decay-Accelerating Factor [DAF])

CD55 is a single-chain glycoprotein that comprises four SCR domains and a heavily glycosylated STP-rich domain that is anchored to the cell membrane through a glycosylphosphatidylinositol (GPI) residue anchor. As its name suggests, CD55 accelerates the decay of classical and alternative pathway C3 and C5 convertases and protects host cells against autologous complement-mediated injury [186]. DAF is present on all blood cells and most other cell types. It is present at high levels on cells that line extravascular compartments, such as the cornea, conjunctiva, oral and gastrointestinal mucosa, exocrine glands, renal tubules, ureter and bladder, cervical and uterine mucosa, and pleural, pericardial, and synovial membrane [215].

CD59 (Homologous Restriction Factor 20 (HRF-20), Membrane Attack Complex Inhibitory Factor (MACIF), or Protectin)

CD59 is another GPI-anchored membrane-bound complement inhibitor. CD59 binds to C8 in the membrane attack complex (MAC) that is being formed and prevents incorporation of C9 that is necessary for the assembly of the MAC pore [216, 217]. CD59 may also bind to C9 in incompletely assembled MAC complexes. The term "homologous restriction factor" is a misnomer and implies that complement inhibition by CD59 is restricted to the host species. Morgan and colleagues performed a comprehensive analysis of the ability of CD59 derived from various species to inhibit complement from heterologous species and found considerable evidence for protection against "nonhost" complement, albeit to varying degrees. Thus, activity may be host-selective rather than host-restricted [218–220]. Host-selective function also applies to other membrane-bound complement inhibitors such as CD46 and CD55 [218, 221–225]. The ability of nonhuman membrane complement inhibitors to protect against damage by human complement may have implications in xenotransplantation.

Complement Receptor of the Immunoglobulin Superfamily (CRIg)

Human CRIg, previously known as Z39Ig, was cloned from Z39Ig mRNA found in human monocytes that were differentiated with M-CSF and IL-4 [226]. CRIg is a type 1 transmembrane IgG superfamily member and exists as two alternatively spliced forms: the longer form, huCRIg(L), encodes both V and C_2-type terminal Ig domains, while the short form, huCRIg(S), encodes only an IgV domain. CRIg is expressed by Kupffer cells, CD14+ dendritic cells, and non-inflammatory resident macrophages in various tissues, but not on infiltrating macrophages during inflammation or on peripheral blood CD14+ monocytes, suggesting a role for CRIg in maintenance of homeostasis rather that in inflammation processes [227]. CRIg binds to C3b-opsonized particles [228] and accelerates the clearance of *Listeria monocytogenes* and *Staphylococcus aureus* in mice, suggesting a role in host defenses [229]. CRIg also binds to the C3b component of alternative pathway C3 and C5 convertases and prevents their interaction with C3 and C5, thereby inhibiting the alternative pathway [230].

Complement Receptors

Complement receptors may be classified into two categories: (i) receptors that bind to soluble complement fragments (e.g., C3a and C5a) that are released during complement activation and (ii) receptors that engage complement components (e.g., C1q, C3b, iC3b, C3d, and C4b) deposited on surfaces. The characteristics of the membrane-associated complement receptors are summarized in Table 4.2.

Receptors for C5a and C3a

C5aR (CD88; C5aR1) binds to C5a with high affinity (Kd ≈ 1 nM) and C5a-des-Arg with relatively lower affinity (Kd ≈ 660 nM) [231, 232]

Table 4.2 Complement receptors and membrane-bound complement inhibitors

Protein	Characteristics
Membrane-bound complement inhibitors	
CR1	Cofactor for factor I cleavage of C3b to iC3b and further to C3d and C4b to C4d; binds to MBL and C1q; clearance of opsonized pathogens and C3b/C4b associated with immune complexes ("immune adherence")
CD46	Cofactor for factor I cleavage of C3b and C4b. Ligand for Notch family member Jagged1. Roles in T-cell differentiation
CD55	Accelerates the decay of C3 convertase assembled on cells
CD59	Inhibits the assembly of membrane attack complex (C9 polymerization)
CRIg	Ligand for the β-chain of C3b/iC3b; inhibits alternative pathway C3 and C5 convertases by binding to C3b and preventing interaction of the convertases with C3 and C5, respectively; role for pathogen clearance demonstrated in mouse model
Complement receptors	
CR2	Binds primarily to C3d and C3dg; part of the CR2/CD19/CD81 complex that mediates B-cell responses to antigens linked to C3 fragments; receptor for Epstein-Barr virus
CR3	Ligand for iC3b; phagocytosis
CR4	Binds for C3d/C3dg; function not known
C1q receptors (cC1qR and gC1qR)	cC1qR (calreticulin) binds to the collagenous region of C1q; gC1qR binds to the globular domain of C1q; cC1qR – phagocytosis of apoptotic cells, chaperone, Ca^{2+} homeostasis; gC1qR – modulation of complement, kallikrein-kinin, and coagulation systems
SIGN-R1	Complement receptor identified as a murine homologue of DC-SIGN; binds select pneumococcal polysaccharides and C1q and can activate the classical pathway in Ab-independent manner
Receptors for anaphylatoxins	
C3aR	Binds C3a/C3a-des-Arg; vasodilatation
C5aR	Binds C5a/C5a-des-Arg; chemotaxis; modulates inflammation and sepsis, T-cell differentiation

and is expressed on myeloid-derived cells and nonmyeloid cells including vascular smooth muscle, endothelium, epithelium, and glial cells

[233]. C5aR1 is a G protein-coupled receptor [234–237], which interestingly is "pre-coupled" to G proteins even in the absence of its ligand, C5a [236]. Binding of C5a to C5aR1 lies below the level of detection in the absence of the "pre-coupling" of C5aR1 to G proteins. Activation of C5aR1 results in Ca^{2+} fluxes from intracellular stores as well as extracellular sources. Following its activation, β-arrestins 1 and 2 bind to C5aR1 and promote its internalization via clathrin-coated pits [238]. Activation of C5aR1 leads to stimulation of several downstream pathways including PI3K-γ kinase, phospholipase C β2, phospholipase D, and Raf-1/B-Raf-mediated activation of MEK1 [239–241].

A second receptor for C5a, called C5a receptor-like protein (C5L2; C5aR2), is coexpressed with C5aR1 [242]. In addition to its ability to bind to C5a and C5a-des-Arg, C5L2 can also bind to C3a and C3a-des-Arg [243]. Unlike C5aR, C5L2 couples poorly to Gi-like G protein-mediated signaling pathways and does not undergo internalization in response to ligand binding [244]. The role of C5L2 remains controversial. Some studies indicate that C5L2 may serve as a decoy receptor and act as a functional antagonist of C5aR. In support of this hypothesis, neutrophils and macrophages from C5L2$^{-/-}$ mice produce more IL-6 and TNF-α in response to stimulation with C5a and LPS than phagocytes from their wild-type counterparts [245]. C5L2$^{-/-}$ mice also show a greater inflammatory response than wild-type mice in a model of pulmonary immune complex injury [246]. In contrast, Rittirsch et al. showed increased survival of C5L2$^{-/-}$ mice in the cecal ligation and puncture model of "mid-grade" sepsis following ligation of half of the cecum [247]. Chen et al. showed that C5L2 was required for optimal C5a signaling in phagocytes and fibroblasts in vitro and deficiency of C5L2 reduced inflammatory cell infiltration to various stimuli in vivo [248].

Similar to C5aR, C3aR is also a G protein-coupled receptor. Unlike C5aR, stimulation of C3aR initiates Ca^{2+} flux only from the extracellular pool and therefore does not activate PI3K-γ. C3aR activation results in activation of protein kinase C by phospholipase C or mitogen-activated protein (MAP) kinases [249, 250]. C3a-C3aR induces cytokine expression through ERK and Akt phosphorylation [251]. C3aR is present on B lymphocytes, vascular endothelium, adipocytes, and mast cells.

A variety of functions have been ascribed to the anaphylatoxins and their receptors. Their role in sepsis to increase chemotaxis and vascular permeability has been studied extensively. High levels of C3a and C5a have been observed in patients with sepsis, and higher levels often are associated with a poor outcome [252–256]. C3a and C5a may play key roles in guiding T-cell responses [257–263]. Recent work has postulated crosstalk between macrophage FcγRs and C5aR [264, 265]. Treatment of macrophages with C5a upregulates the activating FcγRIII (possess an immunoreceptor tyrosine-based activation motif (ITAM)) and downregulates the inhibiting FcγRIIb (possesses an immunoreceptor tyrosine-based inhibition motif (ITIM)), thereby reducing the threshold for FcγR-mediated stimulation of macrophages [266]. Macrophage activation releases C5, from which C5a is liberated through the activity of proteases, further upregulating activating FcγRs. Engagement of FcγRIIb, on the other hand, inhibits signaling through C5aR [267]. Karsten et al. showed that immune complexes, containing IgG whose Fc contained N-glycans with a high amount of galactose, linked Dectin-1 with FcγRIIb, which eventually blocked C5aR-mediated downstream responses [265].

Receptors for C1q

Two cellular receptors for C1q have been described: cC1qR (calreticulin (CR); cC1q/CR) that binds to the collagen domain of C1q and gC1qR (also known as hyaluronic acid-binding protein 1, or p33) that recognizes the globular domain of C1q. In addition to binding C1q, cC1qR also binds to the collectin surfactant protein A (SP-A) and MBL [268]. cC1qR is expressed in most cell types, except erythrocytes. Calreticulin expressed on the cell surface plays a role in the clearance of C1q-coated apoptotic cells [269]. Calreticulin is predominantly localized in the storage compartments of the endoplasmic reticulum. Intracellular calreticulin, along with calnexin, is a molecular chaperone that regulates glycoprotein folding [270]. By virtue of being a high-affinity Ca^{2+} storage protein, calreticulin regulates Ca^{2+} homeostasis [271].

Ghebrehiwet and colleagues first isolated gC1qR from Raji cells [272]. In addition to binding C1q, gC1qR is part of the receptor complex for high-molecular-weight kininogen (HK) on endothelial cells [273, 274] and may also bind certain microbes [275, 276]. gC1qR modulates the activity of the kallikrein-kinin and coagulation systems [277]. Soluble gC1qR released by endothelial cells acts as an autocrine signal to induce expression of the bradykinin receptor 1 on endothelial cells [278]. Engagement of gC1qR on CD4+ T cell by HIV-1 glycoprotein 41 (gp41) induces expression of a stress molecule called NKp44L, which targets destruction of these CD4+ cells by NK cells and may contribute to CD4+ T-cell depletion in HIV infection [279]. Expressions of gC1qR and cC1qR are both upregulated in almost all types of malignant cells. They appear to have opposing roles in carcinogenesis; cC1qR provides an "eat-me" signal to phagocytes, which targets tumor destruction, while gC1qR promotes tumor growth by enhancing angiogenesis and metastasis [280].

CR2 (CD21)

CR2 (or CD21) is a glycosylated transmembrane protein that is composed of a series 15 or 16 SCRs [281]. C-terminal to the SCRs is a 22–24-amino-acid transmembrane domain followed by a 34-amino-acid intracellular domain [281]. CR2 is found on mature B lymphocytes [282], follicular dendritic cells [283], thymocytes [284], a subpopulation of CD4+ and CD8+ T cells [285], basophils [286], keratinocytes [287], astrocytes [288], and lacrimal and ocular epithelial cells [289]. CR2 is the principal ligand for C3d, but can also bind to iC3b. CR2 is also the receptor for the Epstein-Barr virus glycoprotein 350/220 [290–292]. CR2 plays a key role in coupling the innate recognition of microbial antigens to B-cell activation. Activation of complement results in deposition of C3 fragments on foreign antigens or microbes; the interaction of C3-tagged antigens with CR2 (CD21) results in formation of the CD21/CD19/CD81 complex and B-cell activation, as discussed below.

CR3 (Mac-1, CD11b/CD18, or $\alpha_M\beta_2$-Integrin)

CR3 is one of the four members of the β_2-integrin family that share a common β-subunit (CD18) that is linked noncovalently to one of the four α-subunits forming a glycoprotein heterodimer; the α-subunit of CR3 is CD11b. CR3 mediates binding of neutrophils to endothelial cells and is required for neutrophil recruitment to sites of infection. In addition, CR3 is an important phagocytic receptor for iC3b-coated microbes and plays a key role in extravasation of leukocytes from the circulation to sites of injury or infection and in the homing of lymphocytes to tissues. The three-amino-acid sequence, arginine-glycine-aspartic acid (Arg-Gly-Asp, or the "RGD motif"), which is present in C3 and other CR3 ligands, represents an important binding motif for CR3. The C-terminal domain of CD11b contains a lectin site that recognizes polysaccharides on microbial pathogens such as β-glucan, β-oligomannan, and GlcNAc [293]. Engagement of the lectin site of CD11b plays a critical role in the ability of phagocytes or natural killer (NK) cells to mediate cytotoxicity. When presented with iC3b-coated cells or pathogens that lack ligands for the lectin-binding site on CR3, only adhesion occurs; CR3-dependent cytotoxicity requires engagement of the lectin domain [294]. The lectin site of CR3 also promotes cell surface transmembrane signaling complexes between CR3 and membrane glycoproteins that are attached to cells through GPI anchors and therefore cannot signal, such as CD16b (FcγRIIIB) and CD87 (also called the urokinase plasminogen activator receptor (uPAR)) [295]. Several protein tyrosine kinases (PTKs) [296–298] play important roles in CR3 priming for activation and function of phagocytes, such as cytotoxicity, phagocytosis, respiratory burst, and adhesion. These protein kinases are found in association with CR3 as part of large complexes that include LFA-1 and CD87. CR3 signaling results in activation of phospholipase A2 [299, 300] and phosphatidylinositol 3-kinase [301].

CR4 (CD11c/CD18)

Similar to CR3, CR4 is also an integrin and binds to iC3b. In addition, CR4 binds to fibrinogen, ICAM-1, LPS, and denatured peptides [302–306]. CR4 is expressed on myeloid cells, tissue macrophages, dendritic cells, activated B cells, and lymphoid cells [307–309].

Functions of Complement

Innate Immunity and the Elimination of Pathogens

As discussed above, the complement system is well-adapted to discriminate between self and "nonself" structures such as invading pathogens and target them for elimination. The amplification of C3 and C5 convertases is favored over their decay on "nonself" structures. Complement activation is accompanied by generation of the anaphylatoxins, C3 and C5a, which are proinflammatory and promote vascular dilatation, endothelial permeability, and neutrophil chemotaxis. The deposition of C3 fragments on pathogens is termed opsonization and facilitates their removal by professional phagocytes through the interactions of surface-bound C3b and iC3b with CR1 and CR3, respectively. The majority of opsonophagocytic activity is mediated through iC3b-CR3 interactions in conjunction with IgG Fc engagement of Fc receptors, which trigger microbicidal responses associated with bacterial uptake. Unlike gram-positive bacteria and fungi, whose thick cell walls render them resistant to killing by complement alone (i.e., in the absence of phagocytes), MAC insertion into the membranes of gram-negative bacteria can mediate killing. MAC-mediated killing of gram-negatives occurs before lysis of the organism and may be associated with dissipation of the electrical potential across the inner membrane, although the mechanisms of killing remain to be fully elucidated.

In 1960, Roantree and Rantz showed that gram-negative bacteria isolated from the blood were almost always resistant to killing by complement, whereas most isolates of the same spe-cies isolated from mucosal sites were complement-sensitive [310]. These data point to a central role for complement in host defenses against invading pathogens. Over the years, many mechanisms used by microbes to subvert killing by complement have been elucidated. While a detailed discussion of complement evasion mechanisms of microbes is beyond the scope of this chapter, the reader is referred to several general reviews on the subject [311–316]. Further evidence role for complement in combating infections is supported by the increased incidence of infections in individuals who suffer from defects in complement activation.

The complement system is critical in combating meningococcal infections. The incidence of invasive meningococcal disease in individuals with defects in the alternative (FD and properdin) or terminal complement (C5 through C9) pathways is increased about 1000- to 2000-fold over rates observed in the general population [317–319]. Pharmacologic blockade of C5 by the therapeutic monoclonal antibody eculizumab, which is approved by the FDA for the treatment of paroxysmal nocturnal hemoglobinuria (PNH) and aHUS, is also associated with a rate of meningococcal disease similar to that seen in hereditary terminal pathway defects. Of concern is the observation that vaccination of individuals prior to receiving eculizumab did not fully protect against disease – 16 cases of meningococcal disease, of which 11 were caused by nongroupable (i.e., unencapsulated) strains, were reported in individuals on eculizumab [320], for a rate of ~340/100,000 person years, which is similar to that seen in hereditary complement deficiency. The frequent occurrence of disease caused by rare serogroups and nongroupable strains in patients on eculizumab is consistent with strains isolated from individuals with hereditary terminal complement deficiencies [321–325].

Paradoxically, persons with terminal complement defects and meningococcal infection experience a lower mortality than individuals with an intact complement system. Seminal studies by Brandtzaeg, Mollnes, and colleagues have shown a direct correlation between complement activation, endotoxin levels, and the severity of meningococcal disease [326, 327]. Studies in vitro have shown that an intact terminal pathway is associated with greater lipopolysaccharide release from the surface of *E. coli* strain J5 [328, 329]. This mechanism was illustrated in a C6-deficient woman with meningococcal disease [330]. Shortly receiving fresh frozen plasma (FFP) to correct a coagulopathy, which concomitantly corrected the C6 deficiency, her plasma endotoxin levels increased dramatically and were associated with a transient worsening of hemodynamic parameters. While plasma obtained from the patient prior to FFP treatment did not release endotoxin (LPS) from *E. coli* J5 in vitro, plasma obtained following FFP treatment restored the ability to release *E. coli* LPS. Taken together, these findings suggest that LPS release mediated by membrane attack insertion into gram-negative membranes may contribute to the severity of meningococcal sepsis.

Modulation of the Adaptive Immune Response

B Cells and Humoral Immunity

Complement plays an important role in shaping adaptive immune responses [331, 332]. Evidence suggesting a role of complement in adaptive immunity was provided over 40 years ago, when C3b and C3d were shown to bind to B lymphocytes [333] and follicular dendritic cells (FDCs) [334]. Covalent binding of C3b to an antigen marks the antigen for uptake by phagocytic cells or retention by FDCs for recognition by cognate B cells. CD21, which binds iC3b and C3d, and CD35, which binds to C3b and C4b on B cells, play central roles in enhancing B-cell immunity. Studies of B cells in mice have shown that CD21 (in mice, CD21 and CD35 represent splice products of a single locus called Cr2 [335, 336]) forms a receptor complex with CD19 and CD81. CD19 is a transmembrane protein that serves as a signaling/adaptor molecule. The CD19/CD21/CD81 complex enhances B-cell antigen receptor (BCR) signaling in part by prolonging the association of the BCR with lipid rafts [337], which selectively concentrate activating membrane proteins, including the Src family protein tyrosine kinase Lyn, while excluding negative regulators of BCR signaling, such as CD45 and CD22. When coligated to BCR through the binding of complement-tagged antigens, the CD19/CD21/CD81 complex functions to enhance BCR signaling, thus lowering the threshold for B-cell activation [338, 339]. As an example, hen egg lysozymes bearing two and three copies of C3d were 1000- and 10,000-fold more immunogenic, respectively, than hen egg lysozyme alone [340]. This "adjuvant-like" role for C3d is important to enhance the response to antigens that have a low affinity for the B-cell receptor.

A second mechanism whereby complement enhances B-cell immunity is by localization of antigen to follicular dendritic cells (FDCs) within lymphoid follicles. FDCs are specialized stromal cells that secrete CXCL13, a B-lymphocyte chemoattractant [341], and are important in organizing germinal centers within B-cell follicles [342]. High expression of CD21 and CD35 on FDCs facilitates efficient trapping of immune complexes bound to C3 fragments within the lymphoid compartment. An intact classical pathway, CD21 and CD35 are all necessary for the uptake of immune complexes by FDCs [343].

Studies using C1q-, C4- or C3-, or CD21/CD35-knockout mice have all demonstrated the importance of complement at several stages of B-cell differentiation [344–347]. B cells first express the CD19/CD21/CD81 complex as they migrate from the bone marrow to the periphery [348]. Cross-linking of the BCR at this stage in their development results in cell death or anergy rather than activation and eliminates self-reactive B cells.

B1 cells are the main source of natural antibody and are positively selected during early development. Complement plays a role in the selection or maintenance of B1 cells, because *Cr2* (CD21/CD35)-knockout mice have an altered natural antibody repertoire [349, 350]. Optimum activation of B cells requires an intact classical pathway and ligands for C3 and C4 fragments, evidenced by the observation that mice deficient in C1q, C4, or C3 or mice lacking CD21/CD35 have impaired humoral responses to thymus-dependent and thymus-independent antigens [338, 344, 347].

Regulation of T Cells

C3-deficient mice are highly susceptible to primary infection with influenza virus. C3-knockout mice show delayed viral clearance and increased viral titers in the lung, which is the result of reduced priming of T-helper cells and cytotoxic T lymphocytes (CTLs) in lymph nodes draining the lung and the impaired recruitment into the lung of virus-specific CD4+ and CD8+ effector T cells that produce IFN-γ. Accordingly, T-helper cell-dependent IgG responses are also reduced in C3-knockout mice [351]. Although the mechanism of the role of C3 in T-cell responses to influenza remains unclear, one possibility is that viral particles coated with C3 are taken up by antigen-presenting cells (APCs) through receptors such as CR3 (CD11b/CD18) and CR4 (CD11c/CD18) and results in T-cell priming. Lack of C3 would result in reduced APC function and limited T-cell priming. Separate from a defect in APC function, lack of C3 prevents C3a and C5a generation. Engagement of C3aR and C5aR by these anaphylatoxins may also be important in the pulmonary response to influenza virus.

Cross-linking of CD46 (which is also a receptor for the measles virus) with an anti-CD46 antibody or with C3b (a ligand for CD46) inhibits monocyte IL-12 production, which could contribute to the immunosuppression associated with measles infection [352]. Co-engagement of CD3 and CD46 in the presence of IL-2 induces a T-regulatory 1 (Tr1)-specific cytokine phenotype in CD4+ T cells, which produce IL-10 and thus inhibit the activation of bystander T cells [353]. Recently, CD46 was noted bind to Jagged1, a member of the Notch family of proteins [354]. Loss of CD46-Notch crosstalk resulted in failure to mount appropriate T$_H$1 responses [354].

Local production and activation of complement and signaling through C3aR and C5aR also determine the outcome of T-cell responses [261]. Engagement of Toll-like receptors on dendritic cells (DCs) results in secretion of alternative pathway components, which upregulates the expression of C3aR and C5aR. C3a and C5a act on their cognate receptors on the DCs and induce secretion of IL-6, IL-12, or IL-23. Stimulation of CD28 on T cells induces expression of C3aR and C5aR; engagement of the latter by C3a and C5a generated by DCs induces IL-12R expression and a series of signaling events that result in IFN-γ and IL-2 production. The interleukins secreted by the DCs then determine whether responses are skewed toward T$_H$1 or T$_H$17. In the absence of activation of DCs through pattern recognition receptors, local complement production ceases, and the lack of signaling through C3aR and C5aR is associated with increased production of TGF-β and induction of suppressive Foxp3+ T$_{reg}$ cells [262]. During this process, upregulation of C5L2 sequesters any locally produced C5a ensuring that C5aR is not activated. These events depend on the production of complement locally – not on systemically circulating complement.

Autoimmunity: The Disposal of Immune Complexes and Apoptotic Cells

Complement plays an important role in clearing immune complexes [355]. Immune complex formation is favored under conditions of antibody excess or antigen-antibody equivalence. Fc-Fc interactions that occur under these circumstances lead to precipitation of immune complexes. C1q binding to Fc interferes with Fc-fc interactions and prevents immune complex precipitation. Subsequent C3b deposition, aided by alternative pathway amplification, disrupts forces within the antigen-antibody complex and prevents further lattice formation. Separation of smaller complexes from the lattice results in solubilization of immune complexes [356]. Thus, the classical pathway is important to prevent immune complex precipitation, while C3b deposition facilitates immune complex solubilization. Complement is about ten times more efficient in preventing immune complex precipitation than in solubilizing them. This property of complement may explain the strong association between deficiencies of classical pathway components and lupus [59, 65, 357–366].

Immune complexes bearing C3b are targeted for removal by CR1. Erythrocytes express about 1000 CR1 molecules per cell, while neutrophils express about 60,000 CR1 molecules on their surface [198]. However, because erythrocytes outnumber neutrophils in circulation by a factor of about 1000, over 95% of the CR1 in the circulation is found on erythrocytes. Immune complex removal from the circulation occurs as erythrocytes pass through the liver and spleen, where tissue macrophages lining the sinusoids of these organs remove both CR1 and immune complexes adherent to it [197, 198, 367].

Complement also plays a key role in clearance of apoptotic cells. The surface of apoptotic cells often contains unique phospholipids and proteins that have translocated from the inner to the outer leaflet. Some of these molecules, such as phosphatidylserine [368], annexin 2, and annexin 5 [369], are ligands for C1q, which activates complement. The marked cell is then eliminated through engagement of complement receptors such as C1qR and CR3 on macrophages and dendritic cells. The importance of CR3 in eliminating apoptotic cells is supported by the observation that the R77H variant allele in CD11b (the α-chain of CR3) that results in impaired phagocytosis is a strong risk factor for SLE [370–373]. Complement activation on apoptotic cells is limited because these cells bind to complement inhibitors such as FH and C4BP [374, 375]. Further, elimination through complement receptors such as CR3 may contribute to the minimal inflammation associated with apoptosis [376–378].

Metabolism

Metabolic syndrome is associated with increased systemic inflammation, including activation of complement [379]. Insulin resistance and obesity are associated with increased concentrations of C3. Fat cells are the main source of FD, which is also known as adipsin, as well as FB and C3. Activation of C3 locally results in generation of C3a, which is rapidly converted to C3a-des-Arg

by carboxypeptidase N. C3a-des-Arg is also known as acylation-stimulating protein and promotes triglyceride synthesis in fat cells by increasing the activity of diacylglycerol acyltransferase [380, 381].

Complement and Cancer

Complement may play a role in immune surveillance against malignant cells by promoting antibody-dependent cellular cytotoxicity and also by lysis through the terminal complement complex. However, several reports have elucidated mechanisms whereby various cancer cells have developed mechanisms to limit complement activation on their surfaces. These include expression of high levels of membrane complement inhibitors, such as CD46, CD59, and DAF, and increased recruitment of fluid-phase complement inhibitors such as FH and FHL-1 [382]. The anaphylatoxins C3a and C5a induce the secretion of vascular endothelial growth factor (VEGF), which may promote neovascularization. A similar phenomenon may contribute to retinal neovascularization in the wet form of age-related macular degeneration, where VEGF inhibitors have therapeutic value. Complement can degrade the extracellular matrix, which may facilitate tumor invasion and migration. C5a also attracts myeloid-derived neutrophil- and monocyte-like suppressor cells to tumors, which generate reactive oxygen and nitrogen species that interfere with the ability of T cells to respond to tumor antigens [383]. Signaling through C5aR inhibits apoptosis in neutrophils and T cells [241, 384] and increases proliferation of endothelial and colon cancer cell lines [385, 386]. Activation of C3aR guides cell migration that may promote metastasis [387]. Insertion of sublytic amounts of MAC in cell membranes promotes cell proliferation, inhibits apoptosis, and enhances their resistance to complement-mediated lysis [388–391]. The reader is referred to an excellent review by Afshar-Kharghan for a more detailed discussion of the role of complement in cancer [392].

Tissue Regeneration, Organogenesis, and Synaptic Remodeling

Accumulating experimental evidence suggests a role for complement in tissue growth and regeneration [393]. Certain amphibians such as newts have the capacity to regenerate their limbs and lens, a process that is associated with increased local production of C3 and C5. C3- and C5-knockout mice showed an impaired capacity for liver regeneration [394].

Complement may also be critical in refinement of neural circuits. Studies in mice showed that the classical pathway of complement plays a crucial role in formation of mature neural circuits by eliminating inappropriate or unwanted synapses [395]. A recent study showed an association between higher levels of C4A expression in the brain and the development of schizophrenia [396]. It was postulated that excessive synaptic pruning during adolescence contributes to development of schizophrenia. Consistent with this theory and previous work by Stevens et al. [395], C4-knockout mice also showed defects in synaptic refinement [396].

The C3a-C3aR interaction guides neural crest migration in *Xenopus* embryos [387, 397]. A role for the lectin pathway in development is suggested by the association of collectin 11 (CL-K1) and MASP-1 with the 3MC syndrome [398], a term used to unify four rare autosomal recessive disorders with overlapping clinical features: Mingarelli, Malpuech, Michels, and Carnevale syndromes [399]. The 3MC syndrome is characterized by developmental abnormalities including characteristic facial dysmorphism (high-arched eyebrows, ptosis, cranial synostosis leading to an asymmetric skull, cleft lip, and/or palate and down-turned mouth), learning disability, and genital, limb, and vesicorenal anomalies. Gene-knockdown studies in zebra fish embryos showed that collectin 11 and MASP-1 both played roles in guiding the migration of neural crest cells during development [398].

The context and the extent of complement activation may be important in determining the outcome to the host. Controlled complement activation is important in eliminating apoptotic cells, facilitating adaptive immune responses, aiding tissue regeneration and in organogenesis, while unregulated complement activation may contribute to the pathology of acute myocardial infarction, stroke, hyperacute rejection of organ transplants, and tissue injury in conditions such as hepatic, pulmonary, and renal fibrosis, Alzheimer's disease, Parkinson's disease, and multiple sclerosis.

Concluding Remarks

Complement plays critical roles in protecting hosts from invading pathogens. The past two decades have greatly expanded our understanding of the roles of complement beyond fighting infections. The structure of several proteins has been solved, and structure-function relationships have been elucidated. Several diseases have been associated with complement dysfunction. An understanding of how polymorphisms in complement protein affect their function and how altered function is linked with diseases, coupled with the decreasing costs of gene sequencing, has led to characterizing "complotypes" [400], which may prove useful to define or predict imbalances in complement activity that may contribute to pathology. A deeper appreciation of the various functions of complement proteins in disease states makes them attractive targets for pharmacological intervention. In addition to the C5 inhibitor eculizumab, which has been approved for the treatment of PNH and aHUS, several new candidate molecules that target various arms of the complement system are currently in clinical trials or in various stages of preclinical development. We have only begun to scratch the surface; several more functions for complement will undoubtedly be uncovered, and lead to the development of numerous complement-based therapeutics.

References

1. von Fodor J. Die Faehigkeit des Blutes Bakterien zu vernichten. Deut Med Wschr. 1887;13:745.
2. Nutall G. Experimente uber die bacterienfeindlichen Eiflusse des thierischen. Korpers Z Hyg Infectionskir. 1888;4:353.
3. Buchner H. Uber die nehere Natur der bakterientodtenden Substanz in Blutserum. Zbl Bakt (Naturwiss). 1889;6:561.
4. Pfeiffer F, Issaeff R. Uber die Specifishche der Bedeutung der Choleraimmunitat. Z Hyg Infectionskr. 1894;17:355.
5. Bordet J. Les leukocytes et les proprietes actives du serum chez les vaccines. Ann Inst Pasteur (Paris). 1895;9:462–506.
6. Bordet J. Sur l'agglutination et le dissolution des globules rouges par le sérum d'animaux injectés de sang défibriné. Ann Inst Pasteur (Paris). 1898;12:688.
7. Ehrlich P, Morgenroth J. Zur Theorie der Lysinwirkung. Berlin Klin Wschr. 1899;36:6.
8. Bordet J, Gengou O. Sur l'existence de substances sensibilisatrices dans la plupart des serums antimicrobiens. Ann Inst Pasteur (Paris). 1901;15:289.
9. Ferrata A. Die Unwirksamkeit der Komplexen Hämolysine in salzfreien Lösungen und ihre Ursache. Berlin Klin Wschr. 1907;44:366.
10. Muller-Eberhard HJ, Nilsson U, Aronsson T. Isolation and characterization of two beta1-glycoproteins of human serum. J Exp Med. 1960;111:201–15.
11. Coca AF. A study of the anticomplementary action of yeast of certain bacteria and of cobra venom. Z Immunitaetsforsch. 1914;21:604.
12. Ritz H. Über die Wirkung des Cobragiftes auf die Komplemente. Z Immunitaetsforsch. 1912;13:62.
13. Pillemer L, Blum L, Lepow IH, Ross OA, Todd EW, Wardlaw AC. The properdin system and immunity. I. Demonstration and isolation of a new serum protein, properdin, and its role in immune phenomena. Science. 1954;120:279–85.
14. Nelson RA Jr. An alternative mechanism for the properdin system. J Exp Med. 1958;108:515–35.
15. Fujita T, Matsushita M, Endo Y. The lectin-complement pathway – its role in innate immunity and evolution. Immunol Rev. 2004;198:185–202.
16. Sottrup-Jensen L, Stepanik TM, Kristensen T, Lonblad PB, Jones CM, Wierzbicki DM, Magnusson S, Domdey H, Wetsel RA, Lundwall A, et al. Common evolutionary origin of alpha 2-macroglobulin and complement components C3 and C4. Proc Natl Acad Sci U S A. 1985;82:9–13.
17. Nonaka M, Takahashi M. Complete complementary DNA sequence of the third component of complement of lamprey. Implication for the evolution of thioester containing proteins. J Immunol. 1992;148:3290–5.
18. Nonaka M, Azumi K, Ji X, Namikawa-Yamada C, Sasaki M, Saiga H, Dodds AW, Sekine H, Homma MK, Matsushita M, Endo Y, Fujita T. Opsonic complement component C3 in the solitary ascidian, Halocynthia roretzi. J Immunol. 1999;162:387–91.
19. Al-Sharif WZ, Sunyer JO, Lambris JD, Smith LC. Sea urchin coelomocytes specifically express a homologue of the complement component C3. J Immunol. 1998;160:2983–97.
20. Nonaka M, Miyazawa S. Evolution of the initiating enzymes of the complement system. Genome Biol. 2002;3:REVIEWS1001.
21. Levashina EA, Moita LF, Blandin S, Vriend G, Lagueux M, Kafatos FC. Conserved role of a complement-like protein in phagocytosis revealed by dsRNA knockout in cultured cells of the mosquito, Anopheles gambiae. Cell. 2001;104:709–18.
22. Alper CA, Raum D, Awdeh ZL, Petersen BH, Taylor PD, Starzl TE. Studies of hepatic synthesis in vivo of plasma proteins, including orosomucoid, transferrin, alpha 1-antitrypsin, C8, and factor B. Clin Immunol Immunopathol. 1980;16:84–9.
23. Edwards JL, Apicella MA. The role of lipooligosaccharide in Neisseria gonorrhoeae pathogenesis of cervical epithelia: lipid A serves as a C3 acceptor molecule. Cell Microbiol. 2002;4:585–98.
24. Morgan BP, Gasque P. Extrahepatic complement biosynthesis: where, when and why? Clin Exp Immunol. 1997;107:1–7.
25. Perlmutter DH, Colten HR. Molecular immunobiology of complement biosynthesis: a model of single-cell control of effector-inhibitor balance. Annu Rev Immunol. 1986;4:231–51.
26. Ruddy S, Carpenter CB, Chin KW, Knotsman JN, Soter NA, Gotze O, Muller-Eberhard HJ, Austen KF. Human complement metabolism: an analysis of 144 studies. Medicine. 1975;54:165–78.
27. Mier JW, Dinarello CA, Atkins MB, Punsal PI, Perlmutter DH. Regulation of hepatic acute phase protein synthesis by products of interleukin 2 (IL 2)-stimulated human peripheral blood mononuclear cells. J Immunol. 1987;139:1268–72.
28. Price RJ, Boettcher B. The presence of complement in human cervical mucus and its possible relevance to infertility in women with complement-dependent sperm- immobilizing antibodies. Fertil Steril. 1979;32:61–6.
29. Kaul A, Nagamani M, Nowicki B. Decreased expression of endometrial decay accelerating factor (DAF), a complement regulatory protein, in patients with luteal phase defect. Am J Reprod Immunol. 1995;34:236–40.
30. Nogawa Fonzar-Marana RR, Ferriani RA, Soares SG, Cavalcante-Neto FF, Teixeira JE, Barbosa JE. Expression of complement system regulatory molecules in the endometrium of normal ovulatory and hyperstimulated women correlate with menstrual cycle phase. Fertil Steril. 2006;86:758–61.
31. Palomino WA, Argandona F, Azua R, Kohen P, Devoto L. Complement C3 and decay-accelerating

factor expression levels are modulated by human chorionic gonadotropin in endometrial compartments during the implantation window. Reprod Sci. 2013;20:1103–10.

32. Wolach B, Carmi D, Gilboa S, Satar M, Segal S, Dolfin T, Schlesinger M. Some aspects of the humoral immunity and the phagocytic function in newborn infants. Isr J Med Sci. 1994;30:331–5.

33. Adinolfi M, Beck SE. Human complement C7 and C9 in fetal and newborn sera. Arch Dis Child. 1975;50:562–4.

34. Feinstein PA, Kaplan SR. The alternative pathway of complement activation in the neonate. Pediatr Res. 1975;9:803–6.

35. Hogasen AK, Overlie I, Hansen TW, Abrahamsen TG, Finne PH, Hogasen K. The analysis of the complement activation product SC5 b-9 is applicable in neonates in spite of their profound C9 deficiency. J Perinat Med. 2000;28:39–48.

36. Notarangelo LD, Chirico G, Chiara A, Colombo A, Rondini G, Plebani A, Martini A, Ugazio AG. Activity of classical and alternative pathways of complement in preterm and small for gestational age infants. Pediatr Res. 1984;18:281–5.

37. Prabhakar P, Singhi S, Sharma A, James O. Immunoglobulin and C3 levels in maternal and cord blood in Jamaica. Trop Geogr Med. 1985;37:304–8.

38. Sonntag J, Brandenburg U, Polzehl D, Strauss E, Vogel M, Dudenhausen JW, Obladen M. Complement system in healthy term newborns: reference values in umbilical cord blood. Pediatr Dev Pathol Off J Soc Pediatr Pathol Paediatr Pathol Soc. 1998;1:131–5.

39. Yonemasu K, Kitajima H, Tanabe S, Ochi T, Shinkai H. Effect of age on C1q and C3 levels in human serum and their presence in colostrum. Immunology. 1978;35:523–30.

40. Davis CA, Vallota EH, Forristal J. Serum complement levels in infancy: age related changes. Pediatr Res. 1979;13:1043–6.

41. Drossou V, Kanakoudi F, Diamanti E, Tzimouli V, Konstantinidis T, Germenis A, Kremenopoulos G, Katsougiannopoulos V. Concentrations of main serum opsonins in early infancy. Arch Dis Child Fetal Neonatal Ed. 1995;72:F172–5.

42. Kemper C, Pangburn MK, Fishelson Z. Complement nomenclature 2014. Mol Immunol. 2014;61:56–8.

43. Feinstein A, Richardson N, Taussig MI. Immunoglobulin flexibility in complement activation. Immunol Today. 1986;7:169–74.

44. Hughes-Jones NC, Gardner B. Reaction between the isolated globular sub-units of the complement component C1q and IgG-complexes. Mol Immunol. 1979;16:697–701.

45. Diebolder CA, Beurskens FJ, de Jong RN, Koning RI, Strumane K, Lindorfer MA, Voorhorst M, Ugurlar D, Rosati S, Heck AJ, van de Winkel JG, Wilson IA, Koster AJ, Taylor RP, Saphire EO, Burton DR, Schuurman J, Gros P, Parren PW. Complement is activated by IgG hexamers assembled at the cell surface. Science. 2014;343:1260–3.

46. Arlaud GJ, Gaboriaud C, Thielens NM, Rossi V. Structural biology of C1. Biochem Soc Trans. 2002;30:1001–6.

47. Kishore U, Reid KB. C1q: structure, function, and receptors. Immunopharmacology. 2000;49:159–70.

48. Czajkowsky DM, Shao Z. The human IgM pentamer is a mushroom-shaped molecule with a flexural bias. Proc Natl Acad Sci U S A. 2009;106:14960–5.

49. Muller R, Grawert MA, Kern T, Madl T, Peschek J, Sattler M, Groll M, Buchner J. High-resolution structures of the IgM Fc domains reveal principles of its hexamer formation. Proc Natl Acad Sci U S A. 2013;110:10183–8.

50. Nauta AJ, Bottazzi B, Mantovani A, Salvatori G, Kishore U, Schwaeble WJ, Gingras AR, Tzima S, Vivanco F, Egido J, Tijsma O, Hack EC, Daha MR, Roos A. Biochemical and functional characterization of the interaction between pentraxin 3 and C1q. Eur J Immunol. 2003;33:465–73.

51. Roumenina LT, Ruseva MM, Zlatarova A, Ghai R, Kolev M, Olova N, Gadjeva M, Agrawal A, Bottazzi B, Mantovani A, Reid KB, Kishore U, Kojouharova MS. Interaction of C1q with IgG1, C-reactive protein and pentraxin 3: mutational studies using recombinant globular head modules of human C1q A, B, and C chains. Biochemistry. 2006;45:4093–104.

52. Ying SC, Gewurz AT, Jiang H, Gewurz H. Human serum amyloid P component oligomers bind and activate the classical complement pathway via residues 14–26 and 76–92 of the A chain collagen-like region of C1q. J Immunol. 1993;150:169–76.

53. Kang YS, Yamazaki S, Iyoda T, Pack M, Bruening SA, Kim JY, Takahara K, Inaba K, Steinman RM, Park CG. SIGN-R1, a novel C-type lectin expressed by marginal zone macrophages in spleen, mediates uptake of the polysaccharide dextran. Int Immunol. 2003;15:177–86.

54. Law SK, Lichtenberg NA, Levine RP. Covalent binding and hemolytic activity of complement proteins. Proc Natl Acad Sci U S A. 1980;77:7194–8.

55. Dodds AW, Ren XD, Willis AC, Law SK. The reaction mechanism of the internal thioester in the human complement component C4. Nature. 1996;379:177–9.

56. Awdeh ZL, Alper CA. Inherited structural polymorphism of the fourth component of human complement. Proc Natl Acad Sci U S A. 1980;77:3576–80.

57. Carroll MC, Fathallah DM, Bergamaschini L, Alicot EM, Isenman DE. Substitution of a single amino acid (aspartic acid for histidine) converts the functional activity of human complement C4B to C4A. Proc Natl Acad Sci U S A. 1990;87:6868–72.

58. Reilly BD, Mold C. Quantitative analysis of C4Ab and C4Bb binding to the C3b/C4b receptor (CR1, CD35). Clin Exp Immunol. 1997;110:310–6.

59. Christiansen FT, Dawkins RL, Uko G, McCluskey J, Kay PH, Zilko PJ. Complement allotyping in

SLE: association with C4A null. Aust NZ J Med. 1983;13:483–8.

60. Yang Y, Chung EK, Wu YL, Savelli SL, Nagaraja HN, Zhou B, Hebert M, Jones KN, Shu Y, Kitzmiller K, Blanchong CA, McBride KL, Higgins GC, Rennebohm RM, Rice RR, Hackshaw KV, Roubey RA, Grossman JM, Tsao BP, Birmingham DJ, Rovin BH, Hebert LA, Yu CY. Gene copy-number variation and associated polymorphisms of complement component C4 in human systemic lupus erythematosus (SLE): low copy number is a risk factor for and high copy number is a protective factor against SLE susceptibility in European Americans. Am J Hum Genet. 2007;80:1037–54.

61. Carroll MC, Campbell RD, Bentley DR, Porter RR. A molecular map of the human major histocompatibility complex class III region linking complement genes C4, C2 and factor B. Nature. 1984;307:237–41.

62. Carroll MC, Palsdottir A, Belt KT, Porter RR. Deletion of complement C4 and steroid 21-hydroxylase genes in the HLA class III region. EMBO J. 1985;4:2547–52.

63. Schneider PM, Carroll MC, Alper CA, Rittner C, Whitehead AS, Yunis EJ, Colten HR. Polymorphism of the human complement C4 and steroid 21-hydroxylase genes. Restriction fragment length polymorphisms revealing structural deletions, homoduplications, and size variants. J Clin Invest. 1986;78:650–7.

64. Blanchong CA, Chung EK, Rupert KL, Yang Y, Yang Z, Zhou B, Moulds JM, Yu CY. Genetic, structural and functional diversities of human complement components C4A and C4B and their mouse homologues, Slp and C4. Int Immunopharmacol. 2001;1:365–92.

65. Agnello V. Lupus diseases associated with hereditary and acquired deficiencies of complement. Springer Semin Immunopathol. 1986;9:161–78.

66. Hauptmann G, Goetz J, Uring-Lambert B, Grosshans E. Component deficiencies. 2. The fourth component. Prog Allergy. 1986;39:232–49.

67. Hauptmann G, Tappeiner G, Schifferli JA. Inherited deficiency of the fourth component of human complement. Immunodefic Rev. 1988;1:3–22.

68. Blanchong CA, Zhou B, Rupert KL, Chung EK, Jones KN, Sotos JF, Zipf WB, Rennebohm RM, Yung Yu C. Deficiencies of human complement component C4A and C4B and heterozygosity in length variants of RP-C4-CYP21-TNX (RCCX) modules in Caucasians. The load of RCCX genetic diversity on major histocompatibility complex-associated disease. J Exp Med. 2000;191:2183–96.

69. Simon S, Truedsson L, Marcus-Bagley D, Awdeh Z, Eisenbarth GS, Brink SJ, Yunis EJ, Alper CA. Relationship between protein complotypes and DNA variant haplotypes: complotype-RFLP constellations (CRC). Hum Immunol. 1997;57:27–36.

70. Dommett RM, Klein N, Turner MW. Mannose-binding lectin in innate immunity: past, present and future. Tissue Antigens. 2006;68:193–209.

71. Ikeda K, Sannoh T, Kawasaki N, Kawasaki T, Yamashina I. Serum lectin with known structure activates complement through the classical pathway. J Biol Chem. 1987;262:7451–4.

72. Thiel S. Complement activating soluble pattern recognition molecules with collagen-like regions, mannan-binding lectin, ficolins and associated proteins. Mol Immunol. 2007;44:3875–88.

73. Thiel S, Gadjeva M. Humoral pattern recognition molecules: mannan-binding lectin and ficolins. Adv Exp Med Biol. 2009;653:58–73.

74. Ma YJ, Skjoedt MO, Garred P. Collectin-11/MASP complex formation triggers activation of the lectin complement pathway – the fifth lectin pathway initiation complex. J Innate Immun. 2013;5:242–50.

75. Matsushita M. Ficolins in complement activation. Mol Immunol. 2013;55:22–6.

76. Zhang XL, Ali MA. Ficolins: structure, function and associated diseases. Adv Exp Med Biol. 2008;632:105–15.

77. Jack DL, Klein NJ, Turner MW. Mannose-binding lectin: targeting the microbial world for complement attack and opsonophagocytosis. Immunol Rev. 2001;180:86–99.

78. Schwaeble W, Dahl MR, Thiel S, Stover C, Jensenius JC. The mannan-binding lectin-associated serine proteases (MASPs) and MAp19: four components of the lectin pathway activation complex encoded by two genes. Immunobiology. 2002;205:455–66.

79. Degn SE, Jensen L, Hansen AG, Duman D, Tekin M, Jensenius JC, Thiel S. Mannan-binding lectin-associated serine protease (MASP)-1 is crucial for lectin pathway activation in human serum, whereas neither MASP-1 nor MASP-3 is required for alternative pathway function. J Immunol. 2012;189:3957–69.

80. Madsen HO, Garred P, Kurtzhals JA, Lamm LU, Ryder LP, Thiel S, Svejgaard A. A new frequent allele is the missing link in the structural polymorphism of the human mannan-binding protein. Immunogenetics. 1994;40:37–44.

81. Madsen HO, Garred P, Thiel S, Kurtzhals JA, Lamm LU, Ryder LP, Svejgaard A. Interplay between promoter and structural gene variants control basal serum level of mannan-binding protein. J Immunol. 1995;155:3013–20.

82. Thiel S, Frederiksen PD, Jensenius JC. Clinical manifestations of mannan-binding lectin deficiency. Mol Immunol. 2006;43:86–96.

83. Steffensen R, Thiel S, Varming K, Jersild C, Jensenius JC. Detection of structural gene mutations and promoter polymorphisms in the mannan-binding lectin (MBL) gene by polymerase chain reaction with sequence-specific primers. J Immunol Methods. 2000;241:33–42.

84. Turner MW. The role of mannose-binding lectin in health and disease. Mol Immunol. 2003;40:423–9.

85. Selman L, Hansen S. Structure and function of collectin liver 1 (CL-L1) and collectin 11 (CL-11, CL-K1). Immunobiology. 2012;217:851–63.

86. Laffly E, Lacroix M, Martin L, Vassal-Stermann E, Thielens NM, Gaboriaud C. Human ficolin-2 recognition versatility extended: an update on the binding of ficolin-2 to sulfated/phosphated carbohydrates. FEBS Lett. 2014;588:4694–700.

87. Walport MJ. Complement. First of two parts. N Engl J Med. 2001;344:1058–66.

88. Markiewski MM, Lambris JD. The role of complement in inflammatory diseases from behind the scenes into the spotlight. Am J Pathol. 2007;171:715–27.

89. Schmaier AH. The elusive physiologic role of Factor XII. J Clin Invest. 2008;118:3006–9.

90. Huber-Lang M, Sarma JV, Zetoune FS, Rittirsch D, Neff TA, McGuire SR, Lambris JD, Warner RL, Flierl MA, Hoesel LM, Gebhard F, Younger JG, Drouin SM, Wetsel RA, Ward PA. Generation of C5a in the absence of C3: a new complement activation pathway. Nat Med. 2006;12:682–7.

91. Krisinger MJ, Goebeler V, Lu Z, Meixner SC, Myles T, Pryzdial EL, Conway EM. Thrombin generates previously unidentified C5 products that support the terminal complement activation pathway. Blood. 2012;120:1717–25.

92. DiScipio RG. The activation of the alternative pathway C3 convertase by human plasma kallikrein. Immunology. 1982;45:587–95.

93. Hiemstra PS, Daha MR, Bouma BN. Activation of factor B of the complement system by kallikrein and its light chain. Thromb Res. 1985;38:491–503.

94. Janssen BJ, Huizinga EG, Raaijmakers HC, Roos A, Daha MR, Nilsson-Ekdahl K, Nilsson B, Gros P. Structures of complement component C3 provide insights into the function and evolution of immunity. Nature. 2005;437:505–11.

95. Janssen BJ, Christodoulidou A, McCarthy A, Lambris JD, Gros P. Structure of C3b reveals conformational changes that underlie complement activity. Nature. 2006;444:213–6.

96. Sim RB, Twose TM, Paterson DS, Sim E. The covalent-binding reaction of complement component C3. Biochem J. 1981;193:115–27.

97. Pangburn MK, Muller-Eberhard HJ. Initiation of the alternative complement pathway due to spontaneous hydrolysis of the thioester of C3. Ann N Y Acad Sci. 1983;421:291–8.

98. Pangburn MK, Schreiber RD, Muller-Eberhard HJ. Formation of the initial C3 convertase of the alternative complement pathway. Acquisition of C3b-like activities by spontaneous hydrolysis of the putative thioester in native C3. J Exp Med. 1981;154:856–67.

99. Fearon DT, Austen KF. Properdin: binding to C3b and stabilization of the C3b-dependent C3 convertase. J Exp Med. 1975;142:856–63.

100. Spitzer D, Mitchell LM, Atkinson JP, Hourcade DE. Properdin can initiate complement activation by binding specific target surfaces and providing a plat-

101. Pangburn MK. Analysis of the natural polymeric forms of human properdin and their functions in complement activation. J Immunol. 1989;142:202–7.

102. Schwaeble W, Dippold WG, Schafer MK, Pohla H, Jonas D, Luttig B, Weihe E, Huemer HP, Dierich MP, Reid KB. Properdin, a positive regulator of complement activation, is expressed in human T cell lines and peripheral blood T cells. J Immunol. 1993;151:2521–8.

103. Wirthmueller U, Dewald B, Thelen M, Schafer MK, Stover C, Whaley K, North J, Eggleton P, Reid KB, Schwaeble WJ. Properdin, a positive regulator of complement activation, is released from secondary granules of stimulated peripheral blood neutrophils. J Immunol. 1997;158:4444–51.

104. Holt GD, Pangburn MK, Ginsburg V. Properdin binds to sulfatide [Gal(3-SO4)beta 1-1 Cer] and has a sequence homology with other proteins that bind sulfated glycoconjugates. J Biol Chem. 1990;265:2852–5.

105. Kemper C, Mitchell LM, Zhang L, Hourcade DE. The complement protein properdin binds apoptotic T cells and promotes complement activation and phagocytosis. Proc Natl Acad Sci U S A. 2008;105:9023–8.

106. Cortes C, Ferreira VP, Pangburn MK. Native properdin binds to Chlamydia pneumoniae and promotes complement activation. Infect Immun. 2011;79:724–31.

107. Saggu G, Cortes C, Emch HN, Ramirez G, Worth RG, Ferreira VP. Identification of a novel mode of complement activation on stimulated platelets mediated by properdin and C3(H2O). J Immunol. 2013;190:6457–67.

108. Pangburn MK, Rawal N. Structure and function of complement C5 convertase enzymes. Biochem Soc Trans. 2002;30:1006–10.

109. Rawal N, Pangburn MK. C5 convertase of the alternative pathway of complement. Kinetic analysis of the free and surface-bound forms of the enzyme. J Biol Chem. 1998;273:16828–35.

110. Rawal N, Pangburn MK. Formation of high affinity C5 convertase of the classical pathway of complement. J Biol Chem. 2003;278:38476–83.

111. Matthews KW, Mueller-Ortiz SL, Wetsel RA. Carboxypeptidase N: a pleiotropic regulator of inflammation. Mol Immunol. 2004;40:785–93.

112. Hadders MA, Beringer DX, Gros P. Structure of C8alpha-MACPF reveals mechanism of membrane attack in complement immune defense. Science. 2007;317:1552–4.

113. Rosado CJ, Buckle AM, Law RH, Butcher RE, Kan WT, Bird CH, Ung K, Browne KA, Baran K, Bashtannyk-Puhalovich TA, Faux NG, Wong W, Porter CJ, Pike RN, Ellisdon AM, Pearce MC, Bottomley SP, Emsley J, Smith AI, Rossjohn J, Hartland EL, Voskoboinik I, Trapani JA, Bird PI, Dunstone MA, Whisstock JC. A common fold medi-

form for de novo convertase assembly. J Immunol. 2007;179:2600–8.

ates vertebrate defense and bacterial attack. Science. 2007;317:1548–51.

114. Podack ER, Tschopp J. Polymerization of the ninth component of complement (C9): formation of poly(C9) with a tubular ultrastructure resembling the membrane attack complex of complement. Proc Natl Acad Sci U S A. 1982;79:574–8.

115. Dudkina NV, Spicer BA, Reboul CF, Conroy PJ, Lukoyanova N, Elmlund H, Law RH, Ekkel SM, Kondos SC, Goode RJ, Ramm G, Whisstock JC, Saibil HR, Dunstone MA. Structure of the poly-C9 component of the complement membrane attack complex. Nat Commun. 2016;7:10588.

116. Serna M, Giles JL, Morgan BP, Bubeck D. Structural basis of complement membrane attack complex formation. Nat Commun. 2016;7:10587.

117. Arbore G, West EE, Spolski R, Robertson AAB, Klos A, Rheinheimer C, Dutow P, Woodruff TM, Yu ZX, O'Neill LA, Coll RC, Sher A, Leonard WJ, Kohl J, Monk P, Cooper MA, Arno M, Afzali B, Lachmann HJ, Cope AP, Mayer-Barber KD, Kemper C. T helper 1 immunity requires complement-driven NLRP3 inflammasome activity in CD4(+) T cells. Science. 2016;352:aad1210.

118. Arbore G, Kemper C, Kolev M. Intracellular complement – the complosome – in immune cell regulation. Mol Immunol. 2017;89:2–9.

119. Liszewski MK, Kolev M, Le Friec G, Leung M, Bertram PG, Fara AF, Subias M, Pickering MC, Drouet C, Meri S, Arstila TP, Pekkarinen PT, Ma M, Cope A, Reinheckel T, Rodriguez de Cordoba S, Afzali B, Atkinson JP, Kemper C. Intracellular complement activation sustains T cell homeostasis and mediates effector differentiation. Immunity. 2013;39:1143–57.

120. Elvington M, Liszewski MK, Bertram P, Kulkarni HS, Atkinson JP. A C3(H20) recycling pathway is a component of the intracellular complement system. J Clin Invest. 2017;127:970–81.

121. Kolev M, Dimeloe S, Le Friec G, Navarini A, Arbore G, Povoleri GA, Fischer M, Belle R, Loeliger J, Develioglu L, Bantug GR, Watson J, Couzi L, Afzali B, Lavender P, Hess C, Kemper C. Complement regulates nutrient influx and metabolic reprogramming during Th1 cell responses. Immunity. 2015;42:1033–47.

122. Samstad EO, Niyonzima N, Nymo S, Aune MH, Ryan L, Bakke SS, Lappegard KT, Brekke OL, Lambris JD, Damas JK, Latz E, Mollnes TE, Espevik T. Cholesterol crystals induce complement-dependent inflammasome activation and cytokine release. J Immunol. 2014;192:2837–45.

123. Satyam A, Kannan L, Matsumoto N, Geha M, Lapchak PH, Bosse R, Shi GP, Dalle Lucca JJ, Tsokos MG, Tsokos GC. Intracellular activation of complement 3 is responsible for intestinal tissue damage during mesenteric ischemia. J Immunol. 2017;198:788–97.

124. Patston PA, Gettins P, Beechem J, Schapira M. Mechanism of serpin action: evidence that C1 inhibitor functions as a suicide substrate. Biochemistry. 1991;30:8876–82.

125. Bock SC, Skriver K, Nielsen E, Thogersen HC, Wiman B, Donaldson VH, Eddy RL, Marrinan J, Radziejewska E, Huber R, et al. Human C1 inhibitor: primary structure, cDNA cloning, and chromosomal localization. Biochemistry. 1986;25:4292–301.

126. Sim RB, Reboul A, Arlaud GJ, Villiers CL, Colomb MG. Interaction of 125I-labelled complement subcomponents C-1r and C-1s with protease inhibitors in plasma. FEBS Lett. 1979;97:111–5.

127. Ziccardi RJ. Activation of the early components of the classical complement pathway under physiologic conditions. J Immunol. 1981;126:1769–73.

128. Sim RB, Arlaud GJ, Colomb MG. C1 inhibitor-dependent dissociation of human complement component C1 bound to immune complexes. Biochem J. 1979;179:449–57.

129. Ziccardi RJ, Cooper NR. Active disassembly of the first complement component, C-1, by C-1 inactivator. J Immunol. 1979;123:788–92.

130. Chen CH, Boackle RJ. A newly discovered function for C1 inhibitor, removal of the entire C1qr2s2 complex from immobilized human IgG subclasses. Clin Immunol Immunopathol. 1998;87:68–74.

131. Jiang H, Wagner E, Zhang H, Frank MM. Complement 1 inhibitor is a regulator of the alternative complement pathway. J Exp Med. 2001;194:1609–16.

132. Davis AE 3rd, Lu F, Mejia P. C1 inhibitor, a multi-functional serine protease inhibitor. Thromb Haemost. 2010;104:886–93.

133. Morris KM, Aden DP, Knowles BB, Colten HR. Complement biosynthesis by the human hepatoma-derived cell line HepG2. J Clin Invest. 1982;70:906–13.

134. Vyse TJ, Morley BJ, Bartok I, Theodoridis EL, Davies KA, Webster AD, Walport MJ. The molecular basis of hereditary complement factor I deficiency. J Clin Invest. 1996;97:925–33.

135. Whaley K. Biosynthesis of the complement components and the regulatory proteins of the alternative complement pathway by human peripheral blood monocytes. J Exp Med. 1980;151:501–16.

136. Timar KK, Junnikkala S, Dallos A, Jarva H, Bhuiyan ZA, Meri S, Bos JD, Asghar SS. Human keratinocytes produce the complement inhibitor factor I: synthesis is regulated by interferon-gamma. Mol Immunol. 2007;44:2943–9.

137. Julen N, Dauchel H, Lemercier C, Sim RB, Fontaine M, Ripoche J. In vitro biosynthesis of complement factor I by human endothelial cells. Eur J Immunol. 1992;22:213–7.

138. Dauchel H, Julen N, Lemercier C, Daveau M, Ozanne D, Fontaine M, Ripoche J. Expression of complement alternative pathway proteins by endothelial cells. Differential regulation by interleukin 1 and glucocorticoids. Eur J Immunol. 1990;20:1669–75.

139. Nilsson SC, Sim RB, Lea SM, Fremeaux-Bacchi V, Blom AM. Complement factor I in health and disease. Mol Immunol. 2011;48:1611–20.

140. van Lookeren Campagne M, Strauss EC, Yaspan BL. Age-related macular degeneration: complement in action. Immunobiology. 2016;221:733–9.

141. Fujita T, Gigli I, Nussenzweig V. Human C4-binding protein. II. Role in proteolysis of C4b by C3b- inactivator. J Exp Med. 1978;148:1044–51.

142. Fujita T, Nussenzweig V. The role of C4-binding protein and beta 1H in proteolysis of C4b and C3b. J Exp Med. 1979;150:267–76.

143. Gigli I, Fujita T, Nussenzweig V. Modulation of the classical pathway C3 convertase by plasma proteins C4 binding protein and C3b inactivator. Proc Natl Acad Sci U S A. 1979;76:6596–600.

144. Scharfstein J, Ferreira A, Gigli I, Nussenzweig V. Human C4-binding protein. I. Isolation and characterization. J Exp Med. 1978;148:207–22.

145. Reid KB, Bentley DR, Campbell RD, Chung LP, Sim RB, Kristensen T, Tack BF. Complement system proteins which interact with C3b or C4b A superfamily of structurally related proteins. Immunol Today. 1986;7:230–4.

146. Seya T. Human regulator of complement activation (RCA) gene family proteins and their relationship to microbial infection. Microbiol Immunol. 1995;39:295–305.

147. Villoutreix BO, Hardig Y, Wallqvist A, Covell DG, Garcia de Frutos P, Dahlback B. Structural investigation of C4b-binding protein by molecular modeling: localization of putative binding sites. Proteins. 1998;31:391–405.

148. Fearon DT, Austen KF. Activation of the alternative complement pathway due to resistance of zymosan-bound amplification convertase to endogenous regulatory mechanisms. Proc Natl Acad Sci U S A. 1977;74:1683–7.

149. Pangburn MK, Schreiber RD, Muller-Eberhard HJ. Human complement C3b inactivator: isolation, characterization, and demonstration of an absolute requirement for the serum protein beta1H for cleavage of C3b and C4b in solution. J Exp Med. 1977;146:257–70.

150. Sim E, Wood AB, Hsiung LM, Sim RB. Pattern of degradation of human complement fragment, C3b. FEBS Lett. 1981;132:55–60.

151. Weiler JM, Daha MR, Austen KF, Fearon DT. Control of the amplification convertase of complement by the plasma protein beta1H. Proc Natl Acad Sci U S A. 1976;73:3268–72.

152. Whaley K, Ruddy S. Modulation of the alternative complement pathways by beta 1 H globulin. J Exp Med. 1976;144:1147–63.

153. Ripoche J, Day AJ, Harris TJ, Sim RB. The complete amino acid sequence of human complement factor H. Biochem J. 1988;249:593–602.

154. Sharma AK, Pangburn MK. Identification of three physically and functionally distinct binding sites for C3b in human complement factor H by deletion mutagenesis. Proc Natl Acad Sci U S A. 1996;93:10996–1001.

155. Blaum BS, Hannan JP, Herbert AP, Kavanagh D, Uhrin D, Stehle T. Structural basis for sialic acid-mediated self-recognition by complement factor H. Nat Chem Biol. 2015;11:77–83.

156. Kajander T, Lehtinen MJ, Hyvarinen S, Bhattacharjee A, Leung E, Isenman DE, Meri S, Goldman A, Jokiranta TS. Dual interaction of factor H with C3d and glycosaminoglycans in host-nonhost discrimination by complement. Proc Natl Acad Sci U S A. 2011;108:2897–902.

157. Fearon DT. Regulation by membrane sialic acid of beta1H-dependent decay- dissociation of amplification C3 convertase of the alternative complement pathway. Proc Natl Acad Sci U S A. 1978;75:1971–5.

158. Pangburn MK, Muller-Eberhard HJ. Complement C3 convertase: cell surface restriction of beta1H control and generation of restriction on neuraminidase-treated cells. Proc Natl Acad Sci U S A. 1978;75:2416–20.

159. Haines JL, Hauser MA, Schmidt S, Scott WK, Olson LM, Gallins P, Spencer KL, Kwan SY, Noureddine M, Gilbert JR, Schnetz-Boutaud N, Agarwal A, Postel EA, Pericak-Vance MA. Complement factor H variant increases the risk of age-related macular degeneration. Science. 2005;308:419–21.

160. Klein RJ, Zeiss C, Chew EY, Tsai JY, Sackler RS, Haynes C, Henning AK, SanGiovanni JP, Mane SM, Mayne ST, Bracken MB, Ferris FL, Ott J, Barnstable C, Hoh J. Complement factor H polymorphism in age-related macular degeneration. Science. 2005;308:385–9.

161. Weismann D, Hartvigsen K, Lauer N, Bennett KL, Scholl HP, Charbel Issa P, Cano M, Brandstatter H, Tsimikas S, Skerka C, Superti-Furga G, Handa JT, Zipfel PF, Witztum JL, Binder CJ. Complement factor H binds malondialdehyde epitopes and protects from oxidative stress. Nature. 2011;478:76–81.

162. Pouw RB, Vredevoogd DW, Kuijpers TW, Wouters D. Of mice and men: the factor H protein family and complement regulation. Mol Immunol. 2015;67:12–20.

163. Skerka C, Chen Q, Fremeaux-Bacchi V, Roumenina LT. Complement factor H related proteins (CFHRs). Mol Immunol. 2013;56:170–80.

164. Caesar JJ, Lavender H, Ward PN, Exley RM, Eaton J, Chittock E, Malik TH, Goicoechea De Jorge E, Pickering MC, Tang CM, Lea SM. Competition between antagonistic complement factors for a single protein on N. meningitidis rules disease susceptibility. eLife 2014;3:e04008 DOI: 10.7554/eLife.04008.

165. de Cordoba SR, Tortajada A, Harris CL, Morgan BP. Complement dysregulation and disease: from genes and proteins to diagnostics and drugs. Immunobiology. 2012;217:1034–46.

166. de Cordoba SR, de Jorge EG. Translational mini-review series on complement factor H: genetics and

disease associations of human complement factor H. Clin Exp Immunol. 2008;151:1–13.

167. Fritsche LG, Fariss RN, Stambolian D, Abecasis GR, Curcio CA, Swaroop A. Age-related macular degeneration: genetics and biology coming together. Annu Rev Genomics Hum Genet. 2014;15:151–71.

168. Hofer J, Giner T, Jozsi M. Complement factor H-antibody-associated hemolytic uremic syndrome: pathogenesis, clinical presentation, and treatment. Semin Thromb Hemost. 2014;40:431–43.

169. Kavanagh D, Goodship T. Genetics and complement in atypical HUS. Pediatr Nephrol. 2010;25:2431–42.

170. Liszewski MK, Atkinson JP. Complement regulators in human disease: lessons from modern genetics. J Intern Med. 2015;277:294–305.

171. McHarg S, Clark SJ, Day AJ, Bishop PN. Age-related macular degeneration and the role of the complement system. Mol Immunol. 2015;67:43–50.

172. Pickering MC, Cook HT. Translational mini-review series on complement factor H: renal diseases associated with complement factor H: novel insights from humans and animals. Clin Exp Immunol. 2008;151:210–30.

173. Rodriguez de Cordoba S, Hidalgo MS, Pinto S, Tortajada A. Genetics of atypical hemolytic uremic syndrome (aHUS). Semin Thromb Hemost. 2014;40:422–30.

174. van Lookeren Campagne M, Strauss EC, Yaspan BL. Age-related macular degeneration: complement in action. Immunobiology. 2016;221:733–9.

175. Preissner KT, Wassmuth R, Muller-Berghaus G. Physicochemical characterization of human S-protein and its function in the blood coagulation system. Biochem J. 1985;231:349–55.

176. Bhakdi S, Tranum-Jensen J. Membrane damage by complement. Biochim Biophys Acta. 1983;737:343–72.

177. Preissner KP, Podack ER, Muller-Eberhard HJ. SC5b-7, SC5b-8 and SC5b-9 complexes of complement: ultrastructure and localization of the S-protein (vitronectin) within the macromolecules. Eur J Immunol. 1989;19:69–75.

178. Podack ER, Preissner KT, Muller-Eberhard HJ. Inhibition of C9 polymerization within the SC5b-9 complex of complement by S-protein. Acta Pathol Microbiol Immunol Scand Suppl. 1984;284:89–96.

179. Tschopp J, Masson D, Schafer S, Peitsch M, Preissner KT. The heparin binding domain of S-protein/vitronectin binds to complement components C7, C8, and C9 and perforin from cytolytic T-cells and inhibits their lytic activities. Biochemistry. 1988;27:4103–9.

180. Ekmekci OB, Ekmekci H. Vitronectin in atherosclerotic disease. Clin Chim Acta. 2006;368:77–83.

181. Schvartz I, Seger D, Shaltiel S. Vitronectin. Int J Biochem Cell Biol. 1999;31:539–44.

182. O'Bryan MK, Baker HW, Saunders JR, Kirszbaum L, Walker ID, Hudson P, Liu DY, Glew MD, d'Apice AJ, Murphy BF. Human seminal clusterin (SP-40,40). Isolation and characterization. J Clin Invest. 1990;85:1477–86.

183. Murphy BF, Saunders JR, O'Bryan MK, Kirszbaum L, Walker ID, d'Apice AJ. SP-40,40 is an inhibitor of C5b-6-initiated haemolysis. Int Immunol. 1989;1:551–4.

184. Rosenberg ME, Silkensen J. Clusterin: physiologic and pathophysiologic considerations. Int J Biochem Cell Biol. 1995;27:633–45.

185. Liszewski MK, Atkinson JP. Complement regulator CD46: genetic variants and disease associations. Hum Genomics. 2015;9:7.

186. Nicholson-Weller A, Burge J, Austen KF. Purification from guinea pig erythrocyte stroma of a decay-accelerating factor for the classical c3 convertase, C4b,2a. J Immunol. 1981;127:2035–9.

187. Nicholson-Weller A, Spicer DB, Austen KF. Deficiency of the complement regulatory protein, "decay-accelerating factor," on membranes of granulocytes, monocytes, and platelets in paroxysmal nocturnal hemoglobinuria. N Engl J Med. 1985;312:1091–7.

188. Klickstein LB, Bartow TJ, Miletic V, Rabson LD, Smith JA, Fearon DT. Identification of distinct C3b and C4b recognition sites in the human C3b/C4b receptor (CR1, CD35) by deletion mutagenesis. J Exp Med. 1988;168:1699–717.

189. Klickstein LB, Wong WW, Smith JA, Weis JH, Wilson JG, Fearon DT. Human C3b/C4b receptor (CR1). Demonstration of long homologous repeating domains that are composed of the short consensus repeats characteristics of C3/C4 binding proteins. J Exp Med. 1987;165:1095–112.

190. Krych-Goldberg M, Hauhart RE, Subramanian VB, Yurcisin BM 2nd, Crimmins DL, Hourcade DE, Atkinson JP. Decay accelerating activity of complement receptor type 1 (CD35). Two active sites are required for dissociating C5 convertases. J Biol Chem. 1999;274:31160–8.

191. Nelson RA Jr. The immune-adherence phenomenon; an immunologically specific reaction between microorganisms and erythrocytes leading to enhanced phagocytosis. Science. 1953;118:733–7.

192. Arend WP, Mannik M. Studies on antigen-antibody complexes. II. Quantification of tissue uptake of soluble complexes in normal and complement-depleted rabbits. J Immunol. 1971;107:63–75.

193. Benacerraf B, Sebestyen M, Cooper NS. The clearance of antigen antibody complexes from the blood by the reticuloendothelial system. J Immunol. 1959;82:131–7.

194. Cornacoff JB, Hebert LA, Smead WL, VanAman ME, Birmingham DJ, Waxman FJ. Primate erythrocyte-immune complex-clearing mechanism. J Clin Invest. 1983;71:236–47.

195. Kimberly RP, Edberg JC, Merriam LT, Clarkson SB, Unkeless JC, Taylor RP. In vivo handling of soluble complement fixing Ab/dsDNA immune complexes in chimpanzees. J Clin Invest. 1989;84:962–70.

196. Schifferli JA, Ng YC, Estreicher J, Walport MJ. The clearance of tetanus toxoid/anti-tetanus toxoid immune complexes from the circulation of humans. Complement- and erythrocyte complement receptor 1-dependent mechanisms. J Immunol. 1988;140:899–904.

197. Siegel I, Liu TL, Gleicher N. Red cell immune adherence. Lancet. 1981;2:878–9.

198. Siegel I, Liu TL, Gleicher N. The red-cell immune system. Lancet. 1981;2:556–9.

199. Wilson JG, Murphy EE, Wong WW, Klickstein LB, Weis JH, Fearon DT. Identification of a restriction fragment length polymorphism by a CR1 cDNA that correlates with the number of CR1 on erythrocytes. J Exp Med. 1986;164:50–9.

200. Krych-Goldberg M, Atkinson JP. Structure-function relationships of complement receptor type 1. Immunol Rev. 2001;180:112–22.

201. Dykman TR, Cole JL, Iida K, Atkinson JP. Structural heterogeneity of the C3b/C4b receptor (Cr 1) on human peripheral blood cells. J Exp Med. 1983;157:2160–5.

202. Dykman TR, Hatch JA, Aqua MS, Atkinson JP. Polymorphism of the C3b/C4b receptor (CR1): characterization of a fourth allele. J Immunol. 1985;134:1787–9.

203. Dykman TR, Hatch JA, Atkinson JP. Polymorphism of the human C3b/C4b receptor. Identification of a third allele and analysis of receptor phenotypes in families and patients with systemic lupus erythematosus. J Exp Med. 1984;159:691–703.

204. Hourcade D, Miesner DR, Atkinson JP, Holers VM. Identification of an alternative polyadenylation site in the human C3b/C4b receptor (complement receptor type 1) transcriptional unit and prediction of a secreted form of complement receptor type 1. J Exp Med. 1988;168:1255–70.

205. Wong WW, Wilson JG, Fearon DT. Genetic regulation of a structural polymorphism of human C3b receptor. J Clin Invest. 1983;72:685–93.

206. Park HJ, Guariento M, Maciejewski M, Hauhart R, Tham WH, Cowman AF, Schmidt CQ, Mertens HD, Liszewski MK, Hourcade DE, Barlow PN, Atkinson JP. Using mutagenesis and structural biology to map the binding site for the *Plasmodium falciparum* merozoite protein PfRh4 on the human immune adherence receptor. J Biol Chem. 2014;289:450–63.

207. Rowe JA, Moulds JM, Newbold CI, Miller LH. *P. falciparum* rosetting mediated by a parasite-variant erythrocyte membrane protein and complement-receptor 1. Nature. 1997;388:292–5.

208. Stoute JA. Complement receptor 1 and malaria. Cell Microbiol. 2011;13:1441–50.

209. Arora V, Grover R, Kumar A, Anand D, Das N. Relationship of leukocyte CR1 transcript and protein with the pathophysiology and prognosis of systemic lupus erythematosus: a follow-up study. Lupus. 2011;20:1010–8.

210. Birmingham DJ, Gavit KF, McCarty SM, Yu CY, Rovin BH, Nagaraja HN, Hebert LA. Consumption of erythrocyte CR1 (CD35) is associated with protection against systemic lupus erythematosus renal flare. Clin Exp Immunol. 2006;143:274–80.

211. Marzocchi-Machado CM, Alves CM, Azzolini AE, Polizello AC, Carvalho IF, Lucisano-Valim YM. CR1 on erythrocytes of Brazilian systemic lupus erythematosus patients: the influence of disease activity on expression and ability of this receptor to bind immune complexes opsonized with complement from normal human serum. J Autoimmun. 2005;25:289–97.

212. Liszewski MK, Post TW, Atkinson JP. Membrane cofactor protein (MCP or CD46): newest member of the regulators of complement activation gene cluster. Annu Rev Immunol. 1991;9:431–55.

213. Liszewski MK, Leung MK, Atkinson JP. Membrane cofactor protein: importance of N- and O-glycosylation for complement regulatory function. J Immunol. 1998;161:3711–8.

214. Liszewski MK, Farries TC, Lublin DM, Rooney IA, Atkinson JP. Control of the complement system. Adv Immunol. 1996;61:201–83.

215. Medof ME, Walter EI, Rutgers JL, Knowles DM, Nussenzweig V. Identification of the complement decay-accelerating factor (DAF) on epithelium and glandular cells and in body fluids. J Exp Med. 1987;165:848–64.

216. Meri S, Morgan BP, Davies A, Daniels RH, Olavesen MG, Waldmann H, Lachmann PJ. Human protectin (CD59), an 18,000–20,000 MW complement lysis restricting factor, inhibits C5b-8 catalysed insertion of C9 into lipid bilayers. Immunology. 1990;71:1–9.

217. Rollins SA, Sims PJ. The complement-inhibitory activity of CD59 resides in its capacity to block incorporation of C9 into membrane C5b-9. J Immunol. 1990;144:3478–83.

218. Morgan BP, Berg CW, Harris CL. "Homologous restriction" in complement lysis: roles of membrane complement regulators. Xenotransplantation. 2005;12:258–65.

219. Powell MB, Marchbank KJ, Rushmere NK, van den Berg CW, Morgan BP. Molecular cloning, chromosomal localization, expression, and functional characterization of the mouse analogue of human CD59. J Immunol. 1997;158:1692–702.

220. van den Berg CW, Morgan BP. Complement-inhibiting activities of human CD59 and analogues from rat, sheep, and pig are not homologously restricted. J Immunol. 1994;152:4095–101.

221. Harris CL, Spiller OB, Morgan BP. Human and rodent decay-accelerating factors (CD55) are not species restricted in their complement-inhibiting activities. Immunology. 2000;100:462–70.

222. Mead R, Hinchliffe SJ, Morgan BP. Molecular cloning, expression and characterization of the rat analogue of human membrane cofactor protein (MCP/CD46). Immunology. 1999;98:137–43.

223. Perez de la Lastra JM, Harris CL, Hinchliffe SJ, Holt DS, Rushmere NK, Morgan BP. Pigs express multiple forms of decay-accelerating factor (CD55), all

of which contain only three short consensus repeats. J Immunol. 2000;165:2563–73.

224. Tsujimura A, Shida K, Kitamura M, Nomura M, Takeda J, Tanaka H, Matsumoto M, Matsumiya K, Okuyama A, Nishimune Y, Okabe M, Seya T. Molecular cloning of a murine homologue of membrane cofactor protein (CD46): preferential expression in testicular germ cells. Biochem J. 1998;330(Pt 1):163–8.

225. van den Berg CW, Perez de la Lastra JM, Llanes D, Morgan BP. Purification and characterization of the pig analogue of human membrane cofactor protein (CD46/MCP). J Immunol. 1997;158:1703–9.

226. Langnaese K, Colleaux L, Kloos DU, Fontes M, Wieacker P. Cloning of Z39Ig, a novel gene with immunoglobulin-like domains located on human chromosome X. Biochim Biophys Acta. 2000;1492:522–5.

227. He JQ, Wiesmann C, van Lookeren Campagne M. A role of macrophage complement receptor CRIg in immune clearance and inflammation. Mol Immunol. 2008;45:4041–7.

228. Gorgani NN, He JQ, Katschke KJ Jr, Helmy KY, Xi H, Steffek M, Hass PE, van Lookeren Campagne M. Complement receptor of the Ig superfamily enhances complement-mediated phagocytosis in a subpopulation of tissue resident macrophages. J Immunol. 2008;181:7902–8.

229. Helmy KY, Katschke KJ Jr, Gorgani NN, Kljavin NM, Elliott JM, Diehl L, Scales SJ, Ghilardi N, van Lookeren Campagne M. CRIg: a macrophage complement receptor required for phagocytosis of circulating pathogens. Cell. 2006;124:915–27.

230. Katschke KJ Jr, Helmy KY, Steffek M, Xi H, Yin J, Lee WP, Gribling P, Barck KH, Carano RA, Taylor RE, Rangell L, Diehl L, Hass PE, Wiesmann C, van Lookeren Campagne M. A novel inhibitor of the alternative pathway of complement reverses inflammation and bone destruction in experimental arthritis. J Exp Med. 2007;204:1319–25.

231. Gerard NP, Gerard C. The chemotactic receptor for human C5a anaphylatoxin. Nature. 1991;349:614–7.

232. Gerard NP, Hodges MK, Drazen JM, Weller PF, Gerard C. Characterization of a receptor for C5a anaphylatoxin on human eosinophils. J Biol Chem. 1989;264:1760–6.

233. Zwirner J, Fayyazi A, Gotze O. Expression of the anaphylatoxin C5a receptor in non-myeloid cells. Mol Immunol. 1999;36:877–84.

234. Amatruda TT 3rd, Gerard NP, Gerard C, Simon MI. Specific interactions of chemoattractant factor receptors with G-proteins. J Biol Chem. 1993;268:10139–44.

235. Monk PN, Partridge LJ. Characterization of a complement-fragment-C5a-stimulated calcium-influx mechanism in U937 monocytic cells. Biochem J. 1993;295(Pt 3):679–84.

236. Siciliano SJ, Rollins TE, Springer MS. Interaction between the C5a receptor and Gi in both the membrane-bound and detergent-solubilized states. J Biol Chem. 1990;265:19568–74.

237. Skokowa J, Ali SR, Felda O, Kumar V, Konrad S, Shushakova N, Schmidt RE, Piekorz RP, Nurnberg B, Spicher K, Birnbaumer L, Zwirner J, Claassens JW, Verbeek JS, van Rooijen N, Kohl J, Gessner JE. Macrophages induce the inflammatory response in the pulmonary Arthus reaction through G alpha i2 activation that controls C5aR and Fc receptor cooperation. J Immunol. 2005;174:3041–50.

238. Braun L, Christophe T, Boulay F. Phosphorylation of key serine residues is required for internalization of the complement 5a (C5a) anaphylatoxin receptor via a beta-arrestin, dynamin, and clathrin-dependent pathway. J Biol Chem. 2003;278:4277–85.

239. Buhl AM, Avdi N, Worthen GS, Johnson GL. Mapping of the C5a receptor signal transduction network in human neutrophils. Proc Natl Acad Sci U S A. 1994;91:9190–4.

240. Mullmann TJ, Siegel MI, Egan RW, Billah MM. Complement C5a activation of phospholipase D in human neutrophils. A major route to the production of phosphatidates and diglycerides. J Immunol. 1990;144:1901–8.

241. Perianayagam MC, Balakrishnan VS, King AJ, Pereira BJ, Jaber BL. C5a delays apoptosis of human neutrophils by a phosphatidylinositol 3-kinase-signaling pathway. Kidney Int. 2002;61:456–63.

242. Lee H, Whitfeld PL, Mackay CR. Receptors for complement C5a. The importance of C5aR and the enigmatic role of C5L2. Immunol Cell Biol. 2008;86:153–60.

243. Kalant D, Cain SA, Maslowska M, Sniderman AD, Cianflone K, Monk PN. The chemoattractant receptor-like protein C5L2 binds the C3a des-Arg77/acylation-stimulating protein. J Biol Chem. 2003;278:11123–9.

244. Cain SA, Monk PN. The orphan receptor C5L2 has high affinity binding sites for complement fragments C5a and C5a des-Arg(74). J Biol Chem. 2002;277:7165–9.

245. Gao H, Neff TA, Guo RF, Speyer CL, Sarma JV, Tomlins S, Man Y, Riedemann NC, Hoesel LM, Younkin E, Zetoune FS, Ward PA. Evidence for a functional role of the second C5a receptor C5L2. FASEB J. 2005;19:1003–5.

246. Gerard NP, Lu B, Liu P, Craig S, Fujiwara Y, Okinaga S, Gerard C. An anti-inflammatory function for the complement anaphylatoxin C5a-binding protein, C5L2. J Biol Chem. 2005;280:39677–80.

247. Rittirsch D, Flierl MA, Nadeau BA, Day DE, Huber-Lang M, Mackay CR, Zetoune FS, Gerard NP, Cianflone K, Kohl J, Gerard C, Sarma JV, Ward PA. Functional roles for C5a receptors in sepsis. Nat Med. 2008;14:551–7.

248. Chen NJ, Mirtsos C, Suh D, Lu YC, Lin WJ, McKerlie C, Lee T, Baribault H, Tian H, Yeh WC. C5L2 is critical for the biological activities of the anaphylatoxins C5a and C3a. Nature. 2007;446:203–7.

249. Langkabel P, Zwirner J, Oppermann M. Ligand-induced phosphorylation of anaphylatoxin receptors C3aR and C5aR is mediated by "G protein-coupled receptor kinases". Eur J Immunol. 1999;29:3035–46.

250. Sayah S, Jauneau AC, Patte C, Tonon MC, Vaudry H, Fontaine M. Two different transduction pathways are activated by C3a and C5a anaphylatoxins on astrocytes. Brain Res Mol Brain Res. 2003;112:53–60.

251. Venkatesha RT, Berla Thangam E, Zaidi AK, Ali H. Distinct regulation of C3a-induced MCP-1/CCL2 and RANTES/CCL5 production in human mast cells by extracellular signal regulated kinase and PI3 kinase. Mol Immunol. 2005;42:581–7.

252. Hack CE, Nuijens JH, Felt-Bersma RJ, Schreuder WO, Eerenberg-Belmer AJ, Paardekooper J, Bronsveld W, Thijs LG. Elevated plasma levels of the anaphylatoxins C3a and C4a are associated with a fatal outcome in sepsis. Am J Med. 1989;86:20–6.

253. Heideman M, Norder-Hansson B, Bengtson A, Mollnes TE. Terminal complement complexes and anaphylatoxins in septic and ischemic patients. Arch Surg. 1988;123:188–92.

254. Selberg O, Hecker H, Martin M, Klos A, Bautsch W, Kohl J. Discrimination of sepsis and systemic inflammatory response syndrome by determination of circulating plasma concentrations of procalcitonin, protein complement 3a, and interleukin-6. Crit Care Med. 2000;28:2793–8.

255. Stove S, Welte T, Wagner TO, Kola A, Klos A, Bautsch W, Kohl J. Circulating complement proteins in patients with sepsis or systemic inflammatory response syndrome. Clin Diagn Lab Immunol. 1996;3:175–83.

256. Weinberg PF, Matthay MA, Webster RO, Roskos KV, Goldstein IM, Murray JF. Biologically active products of complement and acute lung injury in patients with the sepsis syndrome. Am Rev Respir Dis. 1984;130:791–6.

257. Cravedi P, Leventhal J, Lakhani P, Ward SC, Donovan MJ, Heeger PS. Immune cell-derived C3a and C5a costimulate human T cell alloimmunity. Am J Transplant. 2013;13:2530–9.

258. Kemper C, Atkinson JP. T-cell regulation: with complements from innate immunity. Nat Rev Immunol. 2007;7:9–18.

259. Kwan WH, van der Touw W, Paz-Artal E, Li MO, Heeger PS. Signaling through C5a receptor and C3a receptor diminishes function of murine natural regulatory T cells. J Exp Med. 2013;210:257–68.

260. Lim H, Kim YU, Drouin SM, Mueller-Ortiz S, Yun K, Morschl E, Wetsel RA, Chung Y. Negative regulation of pulmonary Th17 responses by C3a anaphylatoxin during allergic inflammation in mice. PLoS One. 2012;7:e52666.

261. Strainic MG, Liu J, Huang D, An F, Lalli PN, Muqim N, Shapiro VS, Dubyak GR, Heeger PS, Medof ME. Locally produced complement fragments C5a and C3a provide both costimulatory and survival signals to naive CD4+ T cells. Immunity. 2008;28:425–35.

262. Strainic MG, Shevach EM, An F, Lin F, Medof ME. Absence of signaling into CD4(+) cells via C3aR and C5aR enables autoinductive TGF-beta1 signaling and induction of Foxp3(+) regulatory T cells. Nat Immunol. 2013;14:162–71.

263. van der Touw W, Cravedi P, Kwan WH, Paz-Artal E, Merad M, Heeger PS. Cutting edge: receptors for C3a and C5a modulate stability of alloantigen-reactive induced regulatory T cells. J Immunol. 2013;190:5921–5.

264. Karsten CM, Kohl J. The immunoglobulin, IgG Fc receptor and complement triangle in autoimmune diseases. Immunobiology. 2012;217:1067–79.

265. Karsten CM, Pandey MK, Figge J, Kilchenstein R, Taylor PR, Rosas M, McDonald JU, Orr SJ, Berger M, Petzold D, Blanchard V, Winkler A, Hess C, Reid DM, Majoul IV, Strait RT, Harris NL, Kohl G, Wex E, Ludwig R, Zillikens D, Nimmerjahn F, Finkelman FD, Brown GD, Ehlers M, Kohl J. Anti-inflammatory activity of IgG1 mediated by Fc galactosylation and association of FcgammaRIIB and dectin-1. Nat Med. 2012;18:1401–6.

266. Shushakova N, Skokowa J, Schulman J, Baumann U, Zwirner J, Schmidt RE, Gessner JE. C5a anaphylatoxin is a major regulator of activating versus inhibitory Fc gamma Rs in immune complex-induced lung disease. J Clin Invest. 2002;110:1823–30.

267. Nimmerjahn F, Ravetch JV. Fc gamma receptors as regulators of immune responses. Nat Rev Immunol. 2008;8:34–47.

268. Malhotra R, Sim RB, Reid KB. Interaction of C1q, and other proteins containing collagen-like domains, with the C1q receptor. Biochem Soc Trans. 1990;18:1145–8.

269. Henson PM. A role for calreticulin in the clearance of apoptotic cells in the innate immune system. In: Eggleton P, Michalek M, editors. Calreticulin. 2nd ed. New York: Kluwer Academic/Plenum Publishers; 2003. p. 151–61.

270. Lamriben L, Graham JB, Adams BM, Hebert DN. N-glycan based ER molecular chaperone and protein quality control system: the calnexin binding cycle. Traffic. 2016;17:308–26.

271. Michalak M, Groenendyk J, Szabo E, Gold LI, Opas M. Calreticulin, a multi-process calcium-buffering chaperone of the endoplasmic reticulum. Biochem J. 2009;417:651–66.

272. Ghebrehiwet B, Lim BL, Peerschke EI, Willis AC, Reid KB. Isolation, cDNA cloning, and overexpression of a 33-kD cell surface glycoprotein that binds to the globular "heads" of C1q. J Exp Med. 1994;179:1809–21.

273. Joseph K, Ghebrehiwet B, Peerschke EI, Reid KB, Kaplan AP. Identification of the zinc-dependent endothelial cell binding protein for high molecular weight kininogen and factor XII: identity with the receptor that binds to the globular "heads" of C1q (gC1q-R). Proc Natl Acad Sci U S A. 1996;93:8552–7.

274. Joseph K, Tholanikunnel BG, Ghebrehiwet B, Kaplan AP. Interaction of high molecular weight kininogen binding proteins on endothelial cells. Thromb Haemost. 2004;91:61–70.

275. Braun L, Ghebrehiwet B, Cossart P. gC1q-R/p32, a C1q-binding protein, is a receptor for the InlB invasion protein of *Listeria monocytogenes*. EMBO J. 2000;19:1458–66.

276. Kittlesen DJ, Chianese-Bullock KA, Yao ZQ, Braciale TJ, Hahn YS. Interaction between complement receptor gC1qR and hepatitis C virus core protein inhibits T-lymphocyte proliferation. J Clin Invest. 2000;106:1239–49.

277. Bossi F, Peerschke EI, Ghebrehiwet B, Tedesco F. Cross-talk between the complement and the kinin system in vascular permeability. Immunol Lett. 2011;140:7–13.

278. Ghebrehiwet B, Ji Y, Valentino A, Pednekar L, Ramadass M, Habiel D, Kew RR, Hosszu KH, Galanakis DK, Kishore U, Peerschke EI. Soluble gC1qR is an autocrine signal that induces B1R expression on endothelial cells. J Immunol. 2014;192:377–84.

279. Fausther-Bovendo H, Vieillard V, Sagan S, Bismuth G, Debre P. HIV gp41 engages gC1qR on CD4+ T cells to induce the expression of an NK ligand through the PIP3/H2O2 pathway. PLoS Pathog. 2010;6:e1000975.

280. Peerschke EI, Ghebrehiwet B. cC1qR/CR and gC1qR/p33: observations in cancer. Mol Immunol. 2014;61:100–9.

281. Weis JJ, Toothaker LE, Smith JA, Weis JH, Fearon DT. Structure of the human B lymphocyte receptor for C3d and the Epstein-Barr virus and relatedness to other members of the family of C3/C4 binding proteins. J Exp Med. 1988;167:1047–66.

282. Tedder TF, Clement LT, Cooper MD. Expression of C3d receptors during human B cell differentiation: immunofluorescence analysis with the HB-5 monoclonal antibody. J Immunol. 1984;133:678–83.

283. Reynes M, Aubert JP, Cohen JH, Audouin J, Tricottet V, Diebold J, Kazatchkine MD. Human follicular dendritic cells express CR1, CR2, and CR3 complement receptor antigens. J Immunol. 1985;135:2687–94.

284. Watry D, Hedrick JA, Siervo S, Rhodes G, Lamberti JJ, Lambris JD, Tsoukas CD. Infection of human thymocytes by Epstein-Barr virus. J Exp Med. 1991;173:971–80.

285. Fischer E, Delibrias C, Kazatchkine MD. Expression of CR2 (the C3dg/EBV receptor, CD21) on normal human peripheral blood T lymphocytes. J Immunol. 1991;146:865–9.

286. Bacon K, Gauchat JF, Aubry JP, Pochon S, Graber P, Henchoz S, Bonnefoy JY. CD21 expressed on basophilic cells is involved in histamine release triggered by CD23 and anti-CD21 antibodies. Eur J Immunol. 1993;23:2721–4.

287. Hunyadi J, Simon M Jr, Kenderessy AS, Dobozy A. Expression of complement receptor CR2 (CD21) on human subcorneal keratinocytes in normal and diseased skin. Dermatologica. 1991;183:184–6.

288. Gasque P, Fontaine M, Morgan BP. Complement expression in human brain. Biosynthesis of terminal pathway components and regulators in human glial cells and cell lines. J Immunol. 1995;154:4726–33.

289. Levine J, Pflugfelder SC, Yen M, Crouse CA, Atherton SS. Detection of the complement (CD21)/Epstein-Barr virus receptor in human lacrimal gland and ocular surface epithelia. Reg Immunol. 1990;3:164–70.

290. Fingeroth JD, Weis JJ, Tedder TF, Strominger JL, Biro PA, Fearon DT. Epstein-Barr virus receptor of human B lymphocytes is the C3d receptor CR2. Proc Natl Acad Sci U S A. 1984;81:4510–4.

291. Nemerow GR, Mold C, Schwend VK, Tollefson V, Cooper NR. Identification of gp350 as the viral glycoprotein mediating attachment of Epstein-Barr virus (EBV) to the EBV/C3d receptor of B cells: sequence homology of gp350 and C3 complement fragment C3d. J Virol. 1987;61:1416–20.

292. Nemerow GR, Wolfert R, McNaughton ME, Cooper NR. Identification and characterization of the Epstein-Barr virus receptor on human B lymphocytes and its relationship to the C3d complement receptor (CR2). J Virol. 1985;55:347–51.

293. Thornton BP, Vetvicka V, Pitman M, Goldman RC, Ross GD. Analysis of the sugar specificity and molecular location of the beta-glucan-binding lectin site of complement receptor type 3 (CD11b/CD18). J Immunol. 1996;156:1235–46.

294. Vetvicka V, Thornton BP, Ross GD. Soluble beta-glucan polysaccharide binding to the lectin site of neutrophil or natural killer cell complement receptor type 3 (CD11b/CD18) generates a primed state of the receptor capable of mediating cytotoxicity of iC3b-opsonized target cells. J Clin Invest. 1996;98:50–61.

295. Petty HR, Todd RF 3rd. Integrins as promiscuous signal transduction devices. Immunol Today. 1996;17:209–12.

296. Berton G, Fumagalli L, Laudanna C, Sorio C. Beta 2 integrin-dependent protein tyrosine phosphorylation and activation of the FGR protein tyrosine kinase in human neutrophils. J Cell Biol. 1994;126:1111–21.

297. Lowell CA, Fumagalli L, Berton G. Deficiency of Src family kinases p59/61hck and p58c-fgr results in defective adhesion-dependent neutrophil functions. J Cell Biol. 1996;133:895–910.

298. Zaffran Y, Escallier JC, Ruta S, Capo C, Mege JL. Zymosan-triggered association of tyrosine phosphoproteins and lyn kinase with cytoskeleton in human monocytes. J Immunol. 1995;154:3488–97.

299. Goldman R, Ferber E, Meller R, Zor U. A role for reactive oxygen species in zymosan and beta-glucan induced protein tyrosine phosphorylation and phospholipase A2 activation in murine macrophages. Biochim Biophys Acta. 1994;1222:265–76.

300. Hazan I, Dana R, Granot Y, Levy R. Cytosolic phospholipase A2 and its mode of activation in human neutrophils by opsonized zymosan. Correlation

between 42/44 kDa mitogen-activated protein kinase, cytosolic phospholipase A2 and NADPH oxidase. Biochem J. 1997;326(Pt 3):867–76.

301. Jones SL, Knaus UG, Bokoch GM, Brown EJ. Two signaling mechanisms for activation of alphaM beta2 avidity in polymorphonuclear neutrophils. J Biol Chem. 1998;273:10556–66.

302. Davis GE. The Mac-1 and p150,95 beta 2 integrins bind denatured proteins to mediate leukocyte cell-substrate adhesion. Exp Cell Res. 1992;200:242–52.

303. de Fougerolles AR, Diamond MS, Springer TA. Heterogenous glycosylation of ICAM-3 and lack of interaction with Mac-1 and p150,95. Eur J Immunol. 1995;25:1008–12.

304. Ingalls RR, Golenbock DT. CD11c/CD18, a transmembrane signaling receptor for lipopolysaccharide. J Exp Med. 1995;181:1473–9.

305. Loike JD, Sodeik B, Cao L, Leucona S, Weitz JI, Detmers PA, Wright SD, Silverstein SC. CD11c/CD18 on neutrophils recognizes a domain at the N terminus of the A alpha chain of fibrinogen. Proc Natl Acad Sci U S A. 1991;88:1044–8.

306. Postigo AA, Corbi AL, Sanchez-Madrid F, de Landazuri MO. Regulated expression and function of CD11c/CD18 integrin on human B lymphocytes. Relation between attachment to fibrinogen and triggering of proliferation through CD11c/CD18. J Exp Med. 1991;174:1313–22.

307. Freudenthal PS, Steinman RM. The distinct surface of human blood dendritic cells, as observed after an improved isolation method. Proc Natl Acad Sci U S A. 1990;87:7698–702.

308. Hogg N, Takacs L, Palmer DG, Selvendran Y, Allen C. The p150,95 molecule is a marker of human mononuclear phagocytes: comparison with expression of class II molecules. Eur J Immunol. 1986;16:240–8.

309. Keizer GD, Borst J, Visser W, Schwarting R, de Vries JE, Figdor CG. Membrane glycoprotein p150,95 of human cytotoxic T cell clone is involved in conjugate formation with target cells. J Immunol. 1987;138:3130–6.

310. Roantree RJ, Rantz LA. A study of the relationship of the normal bactericidal activity of human serum to bacterial infection. J Clin Invest. 1960;39:72–81.

311. Berends ET, Kuipers A, Ravesloot MM, Urbanus RT, Rooijakkers SH. Bacteria under stress by complement and coagulation. FEMS Microbiol Rev. 2014;38:1146–71.

312. Blom AM, Hallstrom T, Riesbeck K. Complement evasion strategies of pathogens-acquisition of inhibitors and beyond. Mol Immunol. 2009;46:2808–17.

313. Jongerius I, Ram S, Rooijakkers S. Bacterial complement escape. Adv Exp Med Biol. 2009;666:32–48.

314. Kraiczy P, Wurzner R. Complement escape of human pathogenic bacteria by acquisition of complement regulators. Mol Immunol. 2006;43:31–44.

315. Wurzner R. Evasion of pathogens by avoiding recognition or eradication by complement, in part via molecular mimicry. Mol Immunol. 1999;36:249–60.

316. Zipfel PF, Hallstrom T, Riesbeck K. Human complement control and complement evasion by pathogenic microbes – tipping the balance. Mol Immunol. 2013;56:152–60.

317. Figueroa J, Andreoni J, Densen P. Complement deficiency states and meningococcal disease. Immunol Res. 1993;12:295–311.

318. Figueroa JE, Densen P. Infectious diseases associated with complement deficiencies. Clin Microbiol Rev. 1991;4:359–95.

319. Ram S, Lewis LA, Rice PA. Infections of people with complement deficiencies and patients who have undergone splenectomy. Clin Microbiol Rev. 2010;23:740–80.

320. McNamara LA, Topaz N, Wang X, Hariri S, Fox L, MacNeil JR. High risk for invasive meningococcal disease among patients receiving Eculizumab (Soliris) despite receipt of meningococcal vaccine. MMWR Morb Mortal Wkly Rep. 2017;66:734–7.

321. Fijen CA, Kuijper EJ, Dankert J, Daha MR, Caugant DA. Characterization of Neisseria meningitidis strains causing disease in complement-deficient and complement-sufficient patients. J Clin Microbiol. 1998;36:2342–5.

322. Fijen CA, Kuijper EJ, Hannema AJ, Sjoholm AG, van Putten JP. Complement deficiencies in patients over ten years old with meningococcal disease due to uncommon serogroups [see comments]. Lancet. 1989;2:585–8.

323. Fijen CA, Kuijper EJ, te Bulte MT, Daha MR, Dankert J. Assessment of complement deficiency in patients with meningococcal disease in The Netherlands. Clin Infect Dis. 1999;28:98–105.

324. Fijen CA, Kuijper EJ, Tjia HG, Daha MR, Dankert J. Complement deficiency predisposes for meningitis due to nongroupable meningococci and Neisseria-related bacteria. Clin Infect Dis. 1994;18:780–4.

325. Orren A, Caugant DA, Fijen CA, Dankert J, van Schalkwyk EJ, Poolman JT, Coetzee GJ. Characterization of strains of Neisseria meningitidis recovered from complement-sufficient and complement-deficient patients in the Western Cape Province, South Africa. J Clin Microbiol. 1994;32:2185–91.

326. Brandtzaeg P, Hogasen K, Kierulf P, Mollnes TE. The excessive complement activation in fulminant meningococcal septicemia is predominantly caused by alternative pathway activation. J Infect Dis. 1996;173:647–55.

327. Brandtzaeg P, Mollnes TE, Kierulf P. Complement activation and endotoxin levels in systemic meningococcal disease. J Infect Dis. 1989;160:58–65.

328. O'Hara AM, Moran AP, Wurzner R, Orren A. Complement-mediated lipopolysaccharide release and outer membrane damage in Escherichia coli J5: requirement for C9. Immunology. 2001;102:365–72.

329. Tesh VL, Duncan RL Jr, Morrison DC. The interaction of Escherichia coli with normal human serum: the kinetics of serum-mediated lipopolysaccharide

release and its dissociation from bacterial killing. J Immunol. 1986;137:1329–35.

330. Lehner PJ, Davies KA, Walport MJ, Cope AP, Wurzner R, Orren A, Morgan BP, Cohen J. Meningococcal septicaemia in a C6-deficient patient and effects of plasma transfusion on lipopolysaccharide release. Lancet. 1992;340:1379–81.

331. Carroll MC. Complement and humoral immunity. Vaccine. 2008;26(Suppl 8):I28–33.

332. Carroll MC, Isenman DE. Regulation of humoral immunity by complement. Immunity. 2012;37:199–207.

333. Eden A, Miller GW, Nussenzweig V. Human lymphocytes bear membrane receptors for C3b and C3d. J Clin Invest. 1973;52:3239–42.

334. Papamichail M, Gutierrez C, Embling P, Johnson P, Holborow EJ, Pepys MB. Complement dependence of localisation of aggregated IgG in germinal centres. Scand J Immunol. 1975;4:343–7.

335. Kurtz CB, O'Toole E, Christensen SM, Weis JH. The murine complement receptor gene family. IV. Alternative splicing of Cr2 gene transcripts predicts two distinct gene products that share homologous domains with both human CR2 and CR1. J Immunol. 1990;144:3581–91.

336. Molina H, Kinoshita T, Inoue K, Carel JC, Holers VM. A molecular and immunochemical characterization of mouse CR2. Evidence for a single gene model of mouse complement receptors 1 and 2. J Immunol. 1990;145:2974–83.

337. Cherukuri A, Cheng PC, Sohn HW, Pierce SK. The CD19/CD21 complex functions to prolong B cell antigen receptor signaling from lipid rafts. Immunity. 2001;14:169–79.

338. Fearon DT, Carroll MC. Regulation of B lymphocyte responses to foreign and self-antigens by the CD19/CD21 complex. Annu Rev Immunol. 2000;18:393–422.

339. Tedder TF, Inaoki M, Sato S. The CD19-CD21 complex regulates signal transduction thresholds governing humoral immunity and autoimmunity. Immunity. 1997;6:107–18.

340. Dempsey PW, Allison ME, Akkaraju S, Goodnow CC, Fearon DT. C3d of complement as a molecular adjuvant: bridging innate and acquired immunity. Science. 1996;271:348–50.

341. Gunn MD, Ngo VN, Ansel KM, Ekland EH, Cyster JG, Williams LT. A B-cell-homing chemokine made in lymphoid follicles activates Burkitt's lymphoma receptor-1. Nature. 1998;391:799–803.

342. Liu YJ, Grouard G, de Bouteiller O, Banchereau J. Follicular dendritic cells and germinal centers. Int Rev Cytol. 1996;166:139–79.

343. Barrington RA, Pozdnyakova O, Zafari MR, Benjamin CD, Carroll MC. B lymphocyte memory: role of stromal cell complement and FcgammaRIIB receptors. J Exp Med. 2002;196:1189–99.

344. Ahearn JM, Fischer MB, Croix D, Goerg S, Ma M, Xia J, Zhou X, Howard RG, Rothstein TL, Carroll MC. Disruption of the Cr2 locus results in a reduc-

tion in B-1a cells and in an impaired B cell response to T-dependent antigen. Immunity. 1996;4:251–62.

345. Cutler AJ, Botto M, van Essen D, Rivi R, Davies KA, Gray D, Walport MJ. T cell-dependent immune response in C1q-deficient mice: defective interferon gamma production by antigen-specific T cells. J Exp Med. 1998;187:1789–97.

346. Fischer MB, Ma M, Goerg S, Zhou X, Xia J, Finco O, Han S, Kelsoe G, Howard RG, Rothstein TL, Kremmer E, Rosen FS, Carroll MC. Regulation of the B cell response to T-dependent antigens by classical pathway complement. J Immunol. 1996;157:549–56.

347. Molina H, Holers VM, Li B, Fung Y, Mariathasan S, Goellner J, Strauss-Schoenberger J, Karr RW, Chaplin DD. Markedly impaired humoral immune response in mice deficient in complement receptors 1 and 2. Proc Natl Acad Sci U S A. 1996;93:3357–61.

348. Carsetti R, Kohler G, Lamers MC. Transitional B cells are the target of negative selection in the B cell compartment. J Exp Med. 1995;181:2129–40.

349. Fleming SD, Shea-Donohue T, Guthridge JM, Kulik L, Waldschmidt TJ, Gipson MG, Tsokos GC, Holers VM. Mice deficient in complement receptors 1 and 2 lack a tissue injury-inducing subset of the natural antibody repertoire. J Immunol. 2002;169:2126–33.

350. Reid RR, Woodcock S, Shimabukuro-Vornhagen A, Austen WG Jr, Kobzik L, Zhang M, Hechtman HB, Moore FD Jr, Carroll MC. Functional activity of natural antibody is altered in Cr2-deficient mice. J Immunol. 2002;169:5433–40.

351. Kopf M, Abel B, Gallimore A, Carroll M, Bachmann MF. Complement component C3 promotes T-cell priming and lung migration to control acute influenza virus infection. Nat Med. 2002;8:373–8.

352. Karp CL, Wysocka M, Wahl LM, Ahearn JM, Cuomo PJ, Sherry B, Trinchieri G, Griffin DE. Mechanism of suppression of cell-mediated immunity by measles virus. Science. 1996;273:228–31.

353. Kemper C, Chan AC, Green JM, Brett KA, Murphy KM, Atkinson JP. Activation of human CD4+ cells with CD3 and CD46 induces a T-regulatory cell 1 phenotype. Nature. 2003;421:388–92.

354. Le Friec G, Sheppard D, Whiteman P, Karsten CM, Shamoun SA, Laing A, Bugeon L, Dallman MJ, Melchionna T, Chillakuri C, Smith RA, Drouet C, Couzi L, Fremeaux-Bacchi V, Kohl J, Waddington SN, McDonnell JM, Baker A, Handford PA, Lea SM, Kemper C. The CD46-Jagged1 interaction is critical for human T(H)1 immunity. Nat Immunol. 2012;13:1213–21.

355. Schifferli JA, Ng YC, Peters DK. The role of complement and its receptor in the elimination of immune complexes. N Engl J Med. 1986;315:488–95.

356. Miller GW, Nussenzweig V. A new complement function: solubilization of antigen-antibody aggregates. Proc Natl Acad Sci U S A. 1975;72:418–22.

357. Atkinson JP. Complement deficiency. Predisposing factor to autoimmune syndromes. Am J Med. 1988;85:45–7.

358. Atkinson JP. Complement deficiency: predisposing factor to autoimmune syndromes. Clin Exp Rheumatol. 1989;7(Suppl 3):S95–101.

359. Ehrenfeld M, Urowitz MB, Platts ME. Selective C4 deficiency, systemic lupus erythematosus, and Whipple's disease. Ann Rheum Dis. 1984;43:91–4.

360. Gewurz A, Lint TF, Roberts JL, Zeitz H, Gewurz H. Homozygous C2 deficiency with fulminant lupus erythematosus: severe nephritis via the alternative complement pathway. Arthritis Rheum. 1978;21:28–36.

361. Hannema AJ, Kluin-Nelemans JC, Hack CE, Eerenberg-Belmer AJ, Mallee C, van Helden HP. SLE like syndrome and functional deficiency of C1q in members of a large family. Clin Exp Immunol. 1984;55:106–14.

362. Meyer O, Hauptmann G, Tappeiner G, Ochs HD, Mascart-Lemone F. Genetic deficiency of C4, C2 or C1q and lupus syndromes. Association with anti-Ro (SS-A) antibodies. Clin Exp Immunol. 1985;62:678–84.

363. Pickering MC, Walport MJ. Links between complement abnormalities and systemic lupus erythematosus. Rheumatology (Oxford). 2000;39:133–41.

364. Truedsson L, Bengtsson AA, Sturfelt G. Complement deficiencies and systemic lupus erythematosus. Autoimmunity. 2007;40:560–6.

365. Walport MJ. Complement and systemic lupus erythematosus. Arthritis Res. 2002;4(Suppl 3):S279–93.

366. Walport MJ, Davies KA, Botto M. C1q and systemic lupus erythematosus. Immunobiology. 1998;199:265–85.

367. Melhorn MI, Brodsky AS, Estanislau J, Khoory JA, Illigens B, Hamachi I, Kurishita Y, Fraser AD, Nicholson-Weller A, Dolmatova E, Duffy HS, Ghiran IC. CR1-mediated ATP release by human red blood cells promotes CR1 clustering and modulates the immune transfer process. J Biol Chem. 2013;288:31139–53.

368. Paidassi H, Tacnet-Delorme P, Verneret M, Gaboriaud C, Houen G, Duus K, Ling WL, Arlaud GJ, Frachet P. Investigations on the C1q-calreticulin-phosphatidylserine interactions yield new insights into apoptotic cell recognition. J Mol Biol. 2011;408:277–90.

369. Martin M, Leffler J, Blom AM. Annexin A2 and A5 serve as new ligands for C1q on apoptotic cells. J Biol Chem. 2012;287:33733–44.

370. Harley JB, Alarcon-Riquelme ME, Criswell LA, Jacob CO, Kimberly RP, Moser KL, Tsao BP, Vyse TJ, Langefeld CD, Nath SK, Guthridge JM, Cobb BL, Mirel DB, Marion MC, Williams AH, Divers J, Wang W, Frank SG, Namjou B, Gabriel SB, Lee AT, Gregersen PK, Behrens TW, Taylor KE, Fernando M, Zidovetzki R, Gaffney PM, Edberg JC, Rioux JD, Ojwang JO, James JA, Merrill JT, Gilkeson GS, Seldin MF, Yin H, Baechler EC, Li QZ, Wakeland EK, Bruner GR, Kaufman KM, Kelly JA. Genome-wide association scan in women with systemic lupus erythematosus identifies susceptibility variants in ITGAM, PXK, KIAA1542 and other loci. Nat Genet. 2008;40:204–10.

371. Hom G, Graham RR, Modrek B, Taylor KE, Ortmann W, Garnier S, Lee AT, Chung SA, Ferreira RC, Pant PV, Ballinger DG, Kosoy R, Demirci FY, Kamboh MI, Kao AH, Tian C, Gunnarsson I, Bengtsson AA, Rantapaa-Dahlqvist S, Petri M, Manzi S, Seldin MF, Ronnblom L, Syvanen AC, Criswell LA, Gregersen PK, Behrens TW. Association of systemic lupus erythematosus with C8orf13-BLK and ITGAM-ITGAX. N Engl J Med. 2008;358:900–9.

372. Nath SK, Han S, Kim-Howard X, Kelly JA, Viswanathan P, Gilkeson GS, Chen W, Zhu C, McEver RP, Kimberly RP, Alarcon-Riquelme ME, Vyse TJ, Li QZ, Wakeland EK, Merrill JT, James JA, Kaufman KM, Guthridge JM, Harley JB. A nonsynonymous functional variant in integrin-alpha(M) (encoded by ITGAM) is associated with systemic lupus erythematosus. Nat Genet. 2008;40:152–4.

373. Rhodes B, Furnrohr BG, Roberts AL, Tzircotis G, Schett G, Spector TD, Vyse TJ. The rs1143679 (R77H) lupus associated variant of ITGAM (CD11b) impairs complement receptor 3 mediated functions in human monocytes. Ann Rheum Dis. 2012;71:2028–34.

374. Leffler J, Herbert AP, Norstrom E, Schmidt CQ, Barlow PN, Blom AM, Martin M. Annexin-II, DNA, and histones serve as factor H ligands on the surface of apoptotic cells. J Biol Chem. 2010;285:3766–76.

375. Trouw LA, Bengtsson AA, Gelderman KA, Dahlback B, Sturfelt G, Blom AM. C4b-binding protein and factor H compensate for the loss of membrane-bound complement inhibitors to protect apoptotic cells against excessive complement attack. J Biol Chem. 2007;282:28540–8.

376. Mevorach D, Mascarenhas JO, Gershov D, Elkon KB. Complement-dependent clearance of apoptotic cells by human macrophages. J Exp Med. 1998;188:2313–20.

377. Taylor PR, Carugati A, Fadok VA, Cook HT, Andrews M, Carroll MC, Savill JS, Henson PM, Botto M, Walport MJ. A hierarchical role for classical pathway complement proteins in the clearance of apoptotic cells in vivo. J Exp Med. 2000;192:359–66.

378. Verbovetski I, Bychkov H, Trahtemberg U, Shapira I, Hareuveni M, Ben-Tal O, Kutikov I, Gill O, Mevorach D. Opsonization of apoptotic cells by autologous iC3b facilitates clearance by immature dendritic cells, down-regulates DR and CD86, and up-regulates CC chemokine receptor 7. J Exp Med. 2002;196:1553–61.

379. Onat A, Can G, Rezvani R, Cianflone K. Complement C3 and cleavage products in cardio-metabolic risk. Clin Chim Acta. 2011;412:1171–9.

380. Barbu A, Hamad OA, Lind L, Ekdahl KN, Nilsson B. The role of complement factor C3 in lipid metabolism. Mol Immunol. 2015;67:101–7.

381. Cianflone K, Xia Z, Chen LY. Critical review of acylation-stimulating protein physiology in humans and rodents. Biochim Biophys Acta. 2003;1609:127–43.

382. Markiewski MM, Lambris JD. Is complement good or bad for cancer patients? A new perspective on an old dilemma. Trends Immunol. 2009;30:286–92.

383. Rutkowski MJ, Sughrue ME, Kane AJ, Mills SA, Parsa AT. Cancer and the complement cascade. Mol Cancer Res. 2010;8:1453–65.

384. Lalli PN, Strainic MG, Yang M, Lin F, Medof ME, Heeger PS. Locally produced C5a binds to T cell-expressed C5aR to enhance effector T-cell expansion by limiting antigen-induced apoptosis. Blood. 2008;112:1759–66.

385. Cao Q, McIsaac SM, Stadnyk AW. Human colonic epithelial cells detect and respond to C5a via apically expressed C5aR through the ERK pathway. Am J Phys Cell Phys. 2012;302:C1731–40.

386. Kurihara R, Yamaoka K, Sawamukai N, Shimajiri S, Oshita K, Yukawa S, Tokunaga M, Iwata S, Saito K, Chiba K, Tanaka Y. C5a promotes migration, proliferation, and vessel formation in endothelial cells. Inflamm Res. 2010;59:659–66.

387. Carmona-Fontaine C, Theveneau E, Tzekou A, Tada M, Woods M, Page KM, Parsons M, Lambris JD, Mayor R. Complement fragment C3a controls mutual cell attraction during collective cell migration. Dev Cell. 2011;21:1026–37.

388. Kraus S, Seger R, Fishelson Z. Involvement of the ERK mitogen-activated protein kinase in cell resistance to complement-mediated lysis. Clin Exp Immunol. 2001;123:366–74.

389. Niculescu F, Badea T, Rus H. Sublytic C5b-9 induces proliferation of human aortic smooth muscle cells: role of mitogen activated protein kinase and phosphatidylinositol 3-kinase. Atherosclerosis. 1999;142:47–56.

390. Soane L, Cho HJ, Niculescu F, Rus H, Shin ML. C5b-9 terminal complement complex protects oligodendrocytes from death by regulating bad through phosphatidylinositol 3-kinase/Akt pathway. J Immunol. 2001;167:2305–11.

391. Tegla CA, Cudrici C, Patel S, Trippe R 3rd, Rus V, Niculescu F, Rus H. Membrane attack by complement: the assembly and biology of terminal complement complexes. Immunol Res. 2011;51:45–60.

392. Afshar-Kharghan V. The role of the complement system in cancer. J Clin Invest. 2017;127:780–9.

393. Rutkowski MJ, Sughrue ME, Kane AJ, Ahn BJ, Fang S, Parsa AT. The complement cascade as a mediator of tissue growth and regeneration. Inflamm Res. 2010;59:897–905.

394. Kimura Y, Madhavan M, Call MK, Santiago W, Tsonis PA, Lambris JD, Del Rio-Tsonis K. Expression of complement 3 and complement 5 in newt limb and lens regeneration. J Immunol. 2003;170:2331–9.

395. Stevens B, Allen NJ, Vazquez LE, Howell GR, Christopherson KS, Nouri N, Micheva KD, Mehalow AK, Huberman AD, Stafford B, Sher A, Litke AM, Lambris JD, Smith SJ, John SW, Barres BA. The classical complement cascade mediates CNS synapse elimination. Cell. 2007;131:1164–78.

396. Sekar A, Bialas AR, de Rivera H, Davis A, Hammond TR, Kamitaki N, Tooley K, Presumey J, Baum M, Van Doren V, Genovese G, Rose SA, Handsaker RE, Daly MJ, Carroll MC, Stevens B, McCarroll SA. Schizophrenia risk from complex variation of complement component 4. Nature. 2016;530:177–83.

397. McLin VA, Hu CH, Shah R, Jamrich M. Expression of complement components coincides with early patterning and organogenesis in *Xenopus laevis*. Int J Dev Biol. 2008;52:1123–33.

398. Rooryck C, Diaz-Font A, Osborn DP, Chabchoub E, Hernandez-Hernandez V, Shamseldin H, Kenny J, Waters A, Jenkins D, Kaissi AA, Leal GF, Dallapiccola B, Carnevale F, Bitner-Glindzicz M, Lees M, Hennekam R, Stanier P, Burns AJ, Peeters H, Alkuraya FS, Beales PL. Mutations in lectin complement pathway genes COLEC11 and MASP1 cause 3MC syndrome. Nat Genet. 2011;43:197–203.

399. Titomanlio L, Bennaceur S, Bremond-Gignac D, Baumann C, Dupuy O, Verloes A. Michels syndrome, Carnevale syndrome, OSA syndrome, and Malpuech syndrome: variable expression of a single disorder (3MC syndrome)? Am J Med Genet A. 2005;137A:332–5.

400. Harris CL, Heurich M, Rodriguez de Cordoba S, Morgan BP. The complotype: dictating risk for inflammation and infection. Trends Immunol. 2012;33:513–21.

Srinjoy Chakraborti and Sanjay Ram

Introduction

In 1922, Alexander Fleming isolated lysozyme, the first identified antimicrobial peptide from nasal mucus. Subsequently, several antimicrobial proteins and peptides have been identified in organisms from each of the six kingdoms of life. Interest in antimicrobial proteins and peptides surged in the 1960s when antibiotic-resistant bacteria began to emerge. These antimicrobial molecules vary greatly in size and structure. In some instances, antimicrobial functions have been discovered for molecules that have traditionally been associated with other physiological functions – examples include laminin and histones. A comprehensive catalog of over 2600 naturally occurring antimicrobial molecules, including 112 human host defense peptides, can be found on the antimicrobial peptide database (http://aps.unmc.edu/AP/main.php; [1]).

This review focuses mainly on antimicrobial peptides (AMPs), which are small (in most instances, fewer than 50 amino acids) soluble peptides with effector functions similar to the complement proteins. Like complement proteins, most AMPs are activated posttranslationally from precursor peptides on specific surfaces (most commonly of microbial origin), and neutralize their targets. Similar to membrane attack complex, the terminal pore-forming step of the complement cascade, some AMPs form barrel-stave pores on their target membranes. Other functions shared by complement and antimicrobial peptides include phagocyte chemotaxis, induction of chemokines and cytokines, and regulation of inflammation [2].

In addition to protecting the host against a broad spectrum of microbial pathogens, AMPs maintain the normal microbiome, modulate innate and adaptive immune responses, and may participate in tissue remodeling. Most AMPs are amphipathic or cationic, although anionic peptides have also been described. AMPs are usually synthesized as precursor peptides, which include a signal sequence, and subsequently undergo post-translational modifications such as proteolytic cleavage, glycosylation, C-terminal amidation, amino acid isomerization, or cyclization [3–6].

It is believed that AMPs have evolved separately on multiple occasions. Thus, it has been difficult to study their evolution even within the same gene families. For example, in humans a cluster of three β-defensin genes can exist in copy numbers of 2–12 per haploid genome

This work was supported by grants from the National Institutes of Health/National Institutes of Allergy and Infectious Diseases, AI111728, AI118161, AI119327, and AI114790.

S. Chakraborti · S. Ram (✉)
Division of Infectious Diseases and Immunology, Department of Medicine, University of Massachusetts Medical School, Worcester, MA, USA
e-mail: Sanjay.Ram@umassmed.edu

because of duplication events [7]. It is believed that gene duplication followed by adaptive evolution could yield peptides with enhanced antimicrobial properties, or in some instances novel functions, while still retaining the function of the original peptide [5].

Synthesis of Human AMPs

Most canonical AMPs are synthesized by leukocytes, which transport them to sites of infection, or by epithelial cells and then released into the interstitial milieu [3]. For instance, cathelicidin, the precursor form of LL-37, is expressed in the epithelial cells of the eye, skin, and gastrointestinal, genitourinary, and respiratory tracts and also by neutrophils, natural killer, and mast cells [8]. Histatin (Hst) 1 is synthesized by the ocular epithelium, while Hst5 is produced by epithelial surfaces in the oral cavity. Human α-defensins like human neutrophil peptides (HNPs) 1, 3, 4 and human defensin (HD) 6 were originally described in neutrophils but are also found in Paneth cells, tracheal epithelium, oral mucosa, and salivary glands. HD5 is found at female reproductive mucosal surfaces and airway and digestive epithelium and in neutrophils. Human β-defensins (HBDs) 1, 2, 3, and 4 are secreted at gastrointestinal surfaces (small intestine, colon), pancreas, parotid glands, mammary glands, thymus, both male and female reproductive tracts (prostate, vagina, cervix, uterus, oviduct, and placenta), tracheobronchial epithelium, keratinocytes, skin, as well as by leukocytes such as macrophages and neutrophils [3]. Bactericidal/permeability-increasing protein (BPI), which bears structural homology with lipopolysaccharide (LPS)-binding protein (LBP), is expressed in neutrophils and eosinophils and by some epithelial cells. Certain proteins with physiological "noninfective" functions, which upon processing may assume AMP-like properties, are more widely distributed. For example, the matrix protein laminin is widely distributed in the musculoskeletal, vascular, nervous, endocrine, respiratory, and reproductive systems [9]. Histone H2A is synthesized in excess of what is required for DNA pack-

aging at the gastric mucosa and is stored in the secretory vesicles of cells at the site [3].

Functions of AMPs

Although AMPs have traditionally been construed as antimicrobial defense effectors, it is now evident that they participate in diverse processes, such as wound healing, distinguishing self from nonself, and maintenance of a healthy and normal microbiome. HBDs and the cathelicidin LL-37 facilitate tissue remodeling and wound healing through EGFR-mediated chemotaxis of epithelial cells and production of metalloproteinases [10]. TGF-β and insulin-like growth factor 1 (IGF-1) in wounds lead to LL-37 production, which stimulates angiogenesis and granulation tissue formation by activating fibroblasts. HNP1 upregulates procollagen mRNA transcripts and protein from fibroblasts, while HBD-1, 2, and 3 cause keratinocyte proliferation [11]. LL-37 also regulates genes responsible for autophagy, apoptosis, and pyroptosis in neutrophils and macrophages, thereby controlling inflammation [10].

Dysregulation of AMP homeostasis has been associated with autoimmune disorders. AMPs may also contribute to inflammation and the pathogenesis of autoimmune diseases [12]. For example, LL-37 can bind to self-DNA and self-RNA, facilitating their recognition by Toll-like receptors (TLR) 9 and 7 or 8, respectively. Enhanced stimulation of TLR9 on plasmacytoid dendritic cells leading to upregulation of IFN-α (type I IFN) may lead to autoimmune T-cell activation and exacerbation of the skin lesions of psoriasis [13]. LL-37 may also modulate activation of TLR4 by LPS [14, 15]. Downregulation of LL-37 and HBDs 2 and 3 that is observed in atopic dermatitis can predispose such individuals to infections with *Staphylococcus aureus* [6]. Enhanced proteolysis of cathelicidin to LL-37 by cutaneous serine proteases is thought to contribute to the pathology of rosacea [16]; direct inhibition of serine proteases by topical azelaic acid reduced cathelicidin levels and alleviated symptoms [8]. Dysregulation of AMPs has also been associated with inflammatory bowel disease.

Significantly diminished mRNA levels of α-defensins (HDs 5 and 6) were seen in Paneth cells of patients with ileal Crohn's disease [17]. On the other hand, these patients had elevated levels of β-defensins (HBDs 2 and 3) in their serum and terminal ileum, respectively [12]. Therefore, while AMP-mediated innate immune signaling cascades can on the one hand control infection and inflammation, on the other hand they can also precipitate immune dysregulation [6].

Thus, given their diverse mechanisms of action, and increasing repertoire of functions, AMPs are now being evaluated for potential therapeutic applications not only in control of infections but also in wound healing and immune regulation and for treatment of cancer.

Classification of AMPs

AMPs are diverse in structure, function, and origin, and thus there is no clear consensus on their classification scheme. They may be classified based on their biological source (e.g., bacterial, plant, animal), function (e.g., antibacterial, antiviral, insecticidal, chemotactic), peptide properties (charge or hydrophobicity), molecular targets (cell surface targeting properties or intracellular targeting peptides), and covalent bonding pattern (also called the universal classification (UC) scheme, proposed by Wang) [18]. Some authors have proposed the classification of AMPs based on their structure (Fig. 5.1), which is discussed below.

α-Helical AMPs

Linear α-helical peptides are the most widely studied class of AMPs. Notable examples of this class of AMPs include the cathelicidin LL-37 and magainin-2 (pexiganan). Cathelicidins share a highly conserved N-terminal "cathelin" domain, but highly variable antimicrobial sequences, ranging from proline- and arginine-rich peptides to helical peptides to disulfide-linked peptides [19]. LL-37 is released following cleavage of the cathelin domain from the only known human cathelicidin, hCAP-18 (human cationic peptide of 18 kDa). The term cathelicidin was originally used to refer to the entire precursor protein but now is often used interchangeably to refer to the antimicrobial peptide. α-Helical AMPs are amphipathic and often 30–40 amino acids in length, and some are rich in lysine and arginine residues. A few peptides in this class have a kink or a bend at the center, which is essential for their ability to disrupt membranes. While some of these peptides might be disordered in solution, all of them undergo an α-helical conformation when inserted into biological membranes [20, 21].

β-Sheet AMPs

A second class of AMPs comprise β-sheets. Gramicidins, hepcidins, and α- and β-defensins belong to this class of peptides. Some of these AMPs have two or more antiparallel β-sheets stabilized by disulfide bridges, while others such as the human hepcidins contain β-sheets with smaller intervening α-helices [4, 6, 20, 22].

All defensins are cationic and have six conserved cysteine residues linked by three intramolecular disulfide bridges; coupling of the Cys residues defines the three subfamilies, α, β, and θ (Fig. 5.1) [23, 24]. θ-Defensins are macrocyclic peptides with 18 amino acid residues formed by head-to-tail splicing of two separate 9-mer precursors linked by three intramolecular disulfide bridges. These are not found in humans because of a premature stop codon in sequence of one of the precursors. They are however abundant in rhesus macaques and one of them called retrocyclin-1 inhibits cellular entry of HIV-1, HSV, and influenza A virus and protects against *Bacillus anthracis* spores. Their unique characteristics make them attractive therapeutic candidates [24].

Extended AMPs

These peptides contain an abundance of amino acids such as proline, glycine, histidine, arginine, and tryptophan, which prevent formation of

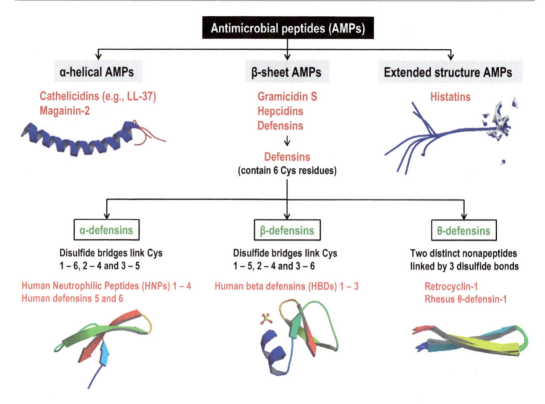

Fig. 5.1 Classification of antimicrobial peptides based on their structure. Structures of representative molecules are shown: α-helical peptides, LL-37 (https://doi.org/10.2210/pdb2k6o/pdb); β-sheet peptides, human neutrophil peptide (HNP) 1 (https://doi.org/10.2210/pdb3hjd/pdb), human beta-defensin (HBD) 1 (https://doi.org/10.2210/pdb1iju/pdb), and rhesus theta defensin-1 (https://doi.org/10.2210/pdb2lyf/pdb); extended structure AMPs, indolicidin (https://doi.org/10.2210/pdb1g8c/pdb)

specific structural motifs. Unlike other AMPs, the structures they assume do not result from inter-residue hydrogen bonds but occur through hydrogen bonds and van der Waals interactions with membrane lipids. Human histatins are representative of this class of AMPs [4, 6].

Mechanisms of Action

While some AMPs exert direct bactericidal effects, others may kill microorganisms and cause damage to eukaryotic cells through modulation of the immune system. In this light, it is reasonable to conclude that their functions cannot be generalized, but are contextual and specific to the infection or the inflammatory process in question. AMPs may target extracellular membranes or intracellular processes to mediate

microbial or cellular damage. Table 5.1 summarizes their mechanisms of action.

Extracellular Targets of AMPs

Membrane Damage by Pore Formation

The initial interaction between the negatively charged microbial membrane and AMPs is driven by electrostatic forces. Thus membrane-active AMPs are often cationic or complexed to a metal cation, such as zinc. Subsequent to initial membrane targeting, α-helical peptides, which are relatively disordered in solution, undergo a phase transition. Upon interaction with phospholipid bilayers and LPS or lipid A, they quickly assume an amphipathic α-helical structure. β-Sheets

Table 5.1 Mechanisms of action of AMPs

Mechanism	Examples	Target
Formation of membrane pores	Dermacidins, BPI	*S. epidermidis, E. faecalis, S. typhimurium, E. coli, Candida* spp.
Inhibition of peptidoglycan synthesis	HBD-3, HNP1	*S. aureus*
Membrane splitting and blebbing	hRNAse7	*P. aeruginosa, P. mirabilis, S. saprophyticus, E. faecalis*
Neutralization of virulence factors		
Inhibition of PAMP recognition	H2A, H2B	Gram-negatives
Inhibition of cellular entry	HNPs1–3, HD5, HBD-3, and HBD-5	HSV
Inhibition of protein function		
Disruption of cellular energetics	Hst5, BPI	*Candida, Leishmania* and *Salmonella* spp., *E. coli*
Inhibition of translation	HNP1, tPMP-1	*Staphylococci*
Inhibition of nucleic acid functions	L4-L5 peptide fragment of laminin	*E. coli, S. aureus*
Chemotaxis	HNPs1 and 2, LL-37, α- and β-defensins	Neutrophils, macrophages, dendritic cells, T cells
Chemokine and cytokine induction	HNPs 1, 2, 3, and 4	Mast cells, epithelial cells, monocytes, T cells, B cells, NK cells
Modulation of complement	HNPs 1–3	Complement C1q

which are more structured in solution may undergo multimer disassembly and form quaternary structures. Once the concentration of AMPs on the membrane reaches a critical threshold, the peptides undergo an amphipathicity-dependent second structural reorganization that leads to formation of pores in membranes. Their hydrophobicity enables these peptides to partition into the membrane lipid bilayer. Additionally, membrane damage is often brought about either by cationic AMPs or anionic AMPs complexed with a metal cation like zinc, which enables them to target anionic microbial membranes. Upon formation of pores, critical cellular functions such as maintenance of electrochemical gradients, selective permeability, respiration, and scaffolding of essential microbial proteins are perturbed, leading to rapid cell death [21, 25]. Multiple models of pore formation have been proposed (Fig. 5.2) and are discussed below.

A. *Barrel-Stave Model*

Alamethicin and gramicidin S are examples of AMPs that form barrel-stave pores in microbial membranes [26]. Upon reaching a critical lipid/peptide ratio, the AMPs oligomerize and insert perpendicularly into the microbial membrane, forming a transmembrane pore (internal and external diameters of 1.8 nm and 4 nm, respectively), akin to the staves that form a barrel. The hydrophobic regions of the peptide associate with lipid head groups, while the hydrophilic regions form the lumen. About 3–11 peptides are usually required to form barrel-stave pores [4, 21].

B. *Toroidal/Disordered Toroidal Pore Model*

Peptides such as magainin and protegrin form toroidal pores. Toroidal pores are distinctive from barrel-stave pores in that the lumen of the pore facing the water core is lined by polar lipid head groups even when peptides are perpendicularly inserted into the membrane. Peptides bind to the membrane, causing strain such that it leads to progressive membrane thinning until the lamellar normal finally gives way and peptides get inserted perpendicularly and on the inner aspect of the membrane, such that a continuous peptide lined hole is formed. Such pores are usually larger than barrel-stave pores, with an internal diameter of 3–5 nm and an external diameter of 7–8.4 nm. These pores comprise 4–7 peptide monomers and about 90 lipid head groups. In this model, while most of the peptides line the external opening and a few line the internal leaflet, all are parallel to the membrane normal. Only a single peptide tilting inward is usually observed in the water core [21, 27, 28].

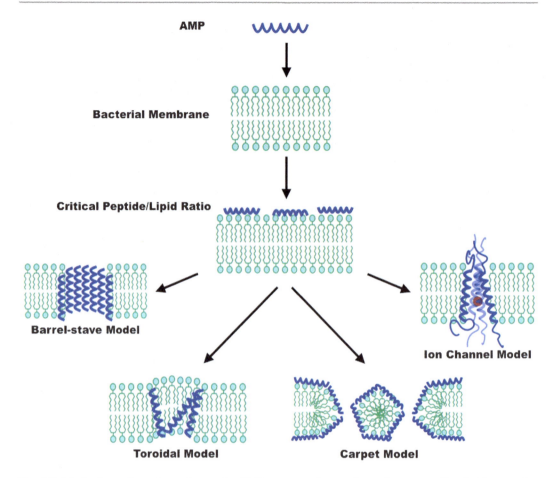

Fig. 5.2 Mechanisms of membrane damage by AMPs. AMPs are attracted to biological membranes by electrostatic interactions. When a critical peptide to lipid ratio is reached, peptides are inserted and oriented along membranes to form pores. Barrel-stave model: peptides are inserted into membrane parallel to each other to form a pore lined only with peptides. Toroidal model: peptides create a strain on the membrane causing it to thin progressively until the strain creates a water pore lined by both peptide as well as lipid head groups. Carpet model: AMPs cover the membrane in a carpet like fashion, causing strain. The membrane bends over and peptides line the cytoplasmic leaflet as well. Micelles are formed from intervening lipid bilayers. Ion channel: formed by AMPs which have no distinct structure in solution, but when they come in contact with bacterial membrane they form an α-helical structure and multiple peptides are stabilized by cations such as Zn^{2+} to form ion channels that cause membrane depolarization

C. *Carpet Model*

At very high concentrations, cationic peptides lie *in-plane* with the anionic microbial membranes covering it like a carpet and finally forming micelles in a detergent-like fashion. This leads to increases in membrane permeability without actually forming pores and is considered an extreme form of the toroidal pore. Cercopin derivatives, such as HB-50, HP-107, and LL-37, are thought to function via this model [4, 21, 25, 27].

D. *Formation of Ion Channels and Membrane Depolarization*

The anionic antimicrobial peptide found in human sweat, dermacidin, is a broad-spectrum antimicrobial that is active against gram-positives such as *Staphylococcus aureus*, *S. epidermidis*, *Enterococcus faecalis*, and *Listeria monocytogenes*; gram-negatives such as *Pseudomonas putida*, *Salmonella typhimurium*, and *Escherichia coli*; and fungi such as *Candida albicans*. The protein is a random coil stabilized by the low pH and Zn^{2+} ions. However, when in proximity to an anionic microbial membrane, the cationic N-terminus of the protein interacts electrostatically with the membrane, assumes an α-helical secondary structure, and oligomerizes and inserts into the membrane via its C-terminus, forming an ion channel stabilized by the Zn^{2+} ions at its N-terminus. Loss of ions through this channel ultimately leads to disruption of membrane potential and cell death [29].

Inhibition of Peptidoglycan Cell Wall Synthesis

HBD-3 secreted by epithelial cells and neutrophils inhibits penicillin-binding protein 2-mediated transglycosylation of the monomeric lipid II pentapeptide molecules into the polymeric murein sacculus of *S. aureus* [30]. Human neutrophil defensin (HNP) 1 also interacts with lipid II of *S. aureus* to inhibit peptidoglycan synthesis [31].

Disruption of Membrane Integrity

Human ribonuclease 7 (hRNAse 7) is a 128 amino acid cationic protein which is abundant in epithelial tissues, skin, and respiratory and urogenital tracts. It is active against gram-positive as well as gram-negative bacteria such as *Proteus mirabilis, P. aeruginosa, E. coli, Klebsiella pneumoniae, S. saprophyticus,* and *E. faecalis.* Bacteria exposed to this CAMP showed extensive membrane splitting and blebbing ultimately leading to cell death [32]. Although the exact mechanism of action of this AMP has not been elucidated, evidence suggests that this AMP probably interacts with proteins tethering the bacterial cell membrane to underlying structures, thereby causing membrane release. For example, it disrupts the outer membrane protein (Opr) I (a homolog of Braun's lipoprotein found in other gram-negatives such as *E. coli* and *Klebsiella* spp.) in *Pseudomonas* which tethers the outer membrane to the murein sacculus [33].

Neutralization of Extracellular Virulence Factors

Recent work demonstrated that cationic histone proteins H2A and H2B are expressed in cytosolic compartments, at cell surfaces, as well as in the extracellular milieu in the human placenta. In fact, the bactericidal effects of the amniotic fluid stems from the ability of H2A and H2B to bind strongly to the anionic lipid A and core oligosaccharides of gram-negative pathogens. Although not directly microbicidal, binding of these histone proteins to lipid A prevents lipid A signaling through TLR4, thereby limiting production of IL-1, IL-6, and TNF-α, all of which contribute to septic shock [34].

Human α- and β-defensins protect against herpes simplex virus (HSV) infections by inhibiting the virus from attaching to its cell receptor and entering cells. Several HNPs and HDs bind to various viral glycoproteins as well as to heparan sulfate (the cell surface receptor for HSV), thereby preventing viral penetration into host cells [35].

Intracellular Targets of AMPs

Disruption of Protein Synthesis and Function

Hst-5 is a strongly basic α-helical peptide which has been demonstrated to be effective against fungi such as *Candida* as well as parasites such as *Leishmania.* This AMP disrupts mitochondrial membrane integrity, resulting in malformation of cristae and dissipation of membrane potential, thereby abrogating ATP synthesis and cellular energetics [36, 37]. While this AMP undergoes receptor-mediated endocytosis to gain entry into *Candida,* the mechanism of its entry into *Leishmania* remains unclear [38]. Although not as conclusively documented as with Hst-5, there is some evidence that human bactericidal/

permeability-increasing protein (BPI) also interferes with the bacterial NADH, ubiquinone oxidoreductase system in *E. coli* and *Salmonella*, thereby interfering with bacterial respiration and energy production [39]. HNP1 and thrombin-induced platelet microbicidal protein-1 (tPMP-1) are believed to inhibit translation by binding to staphylococcal 30s and 50s ribosomal subunits [40].

Inhibition of DNA Function

Laminins are a group of matrix proteins found throughout the human body that comprise three chains (α, β, and γ) linked by disulfide bridges. The globular C-terminus of the α-chain has 5 laminin G (LG) domain-like modules, two of which (LG4 and LG5) are secreted into the fluid phase following proteolytic cleavage, and can then bind to the DNA of *S. aureus* and *E. coli* and inhibit bacterial growth [9].

Immunological Functions of AMP

Chemotactic Function

AMPs are among the multiple chemotactic signals responsible for the influx of immune effector cells to the site of inflammation following tissue injury or infection. Defensins such as HNP1 and HNP2 that are released from neutrophil azurophilic granules cause the influx of monocytes and macrophages [41]. Human α- and β- defensins serve as chemoattractants for T cells and immature dendritic cells [42]; α-defensins attract CD45RA$^+$ naïve T cells, while β-defensins attract CD45RO$^+$ memory T cells and immature dendritic cells. The human cathelicidin LL-37 induces Ca^{2+} mobilization that is required for vesicle fusion and other cellular functions and also attracts neutrophils, monocytes, and T cells through the formyl peptide receptor-like 1 (FPRL1) [43].

Cytokine and Chemokine Induction

AMPs have also been implicated in chemokine and cytokine induction which lead to cellular influx and pro-inflammatory processes. For example, HNP1 and HNP4 cause mast cell degranulation and histamine release [44]. HNPs 1, 2, and 3 stimulate production of IL-8 by the bronchial epithelium and release of TNF-α, and IL-1 by monocytes, while simultaneously suppressing anti-inflammatory cytokines such as IL-10 [45]. HBD-3 can upregulate expression of co-stimulatory molecules such as CD80, CD86, and CD40 on monocytes and myeloid dendritic cells in a TLR 1- and TLR 2-dependent fashion that also involves downstream MyD88 and signaling IRAK-1 phosphorylation [46]. HBDs 2, 3, and 4 and LL-37 also induce the production of IL-18, IL-20, and IL-8 from human keratinocytes; these pro-inflammatory cytokines have been implicated in the pathogenesis of skin diseases such as psoriasis. HNPs 1, 2, and 3 stimulate IL-1, IL-4, IL-6, TNF-α, and IFN-γ from monocytes, and chemokines such as MCP-1 and MIP-2 from pulmonary epithelial cells, while the cathelicidin LL-37 induces IL-8, MCP-1, and MCP-3 production from monocytes and airway epithelium [47]. Such cytokine induction may subsequently trigger cascades where other immune cells like T, B, and NK cells are also activated to produce chemokines [42].

Defensins may also modulate activity of the complement system, although their role remains controversial. HNPs 1–3 immobilized to microtiter wells bind C1q and activate the classical pathway [48]. Although the C1q binding motif on defensins has not been localized, they possess structural and sequence homology with HIV gp41, which also binds C1q. Both gp41 and defensins contain charged amino acids arranged in a loop-like structure similar to the C1q binding motif in IgG (ExKxK) [48]. By contrast, Groeneveld and colleagues showed that HNP-1 binds to the collagen stalk regions of C1q and MBL in a Ca^{2+}-independent manner and blocked

Table 5.2 Mechanisms of AMP resistance

Mechanism	Examples
Reducing cell surface electronegativity[a]	Addition of positively charged residues
	Aminoarabinose to lipid A – *Burkholderia, Salmonella enterica, P. mirabilis*
	Phosphoethanolamine (PEtn) to lipid A – *Neisseriae*
	Glycine and diglycine to lipid A – *Vibrio cholerae* El Tor
	D-alanine to polyteichoic acid – *S. aureus*, group B streptococci, *Listeria monocytogenes*
	L-lysine to phosphatidylglycerol – *S. aureus*
	Removal of negatively charged resides
	Dephosphorylation of the LPS – *Helicobacter pylori, Francisella novicida*
Decoy targets and trapping of AMPs	Alginate capsule – *Pseudomonas aeruginosa* traps CAMPs
	Polyanionic capsules –several, including *Neisseria meningitidis, Haemophilus influenzae, Legionella pneumophila, Streptococcus pneumoniae, Bacillus anthracis*
	Staphylokinase – *S. aureus* (binds HNPs 1, 2)
	Streptococcal inhibitor of complement (SIC) – *Streptococcus pyogenes* (binds HNP1, LL-37)
Expression of drug efflux pumps	MtrCDE – *Neisseria gonorrhoeae*
	AcrAB – *Klebsiella pneumoniae*
	RosA/B – *Yersinia* spp.
	QacA – *S. aureus*, coagulase-negative staphylococci
	YejA-F – *S. typhimurium*
Proteolytic degradation of AMPs	OmpT – *E. coli* (C18G)
	PgtE – *Salmonella enterica* (C18G)
	Gingipains – *P. gingivalis* (HBD-3)
	Aureolysin – *S. aureus* (LL-37)
	ZmpA, ZmpB – *Burkholderia cepacia* (LL-37, protamine, HBD-1)
Regulation of host AMP production and activity	*Shigella* spp., cholera toxin, labile toxin of *E. coli* – transcriptionally represses LL-37 and HBD-1 production
	P aeruginosa - upregulates host cathepsins, which degrade AMP HBDs 2 and 3
	S. pyogenes – represses HBD-2 production by keratinocytes
	N. gonorrhoeae – represses LL-37 production

[a]See text for genetic control of charge modulation

activation of the classical and lectin pathways, respectively [49]. The authors posited that defensins may limit excessive complement activation at sites of tissue injury.

Resistance to Antimicrobial Peptides

Successful establishment of infection requires the pathogen to evade host defenses. While widespread resistance to currently available antibiot-ics has generated considerable interest in AMPs as possible alternatives in the management of infectious diseases, it is not surprising that resistance to these agents have been documented in several pathogens (summarized in Table 5.2).

Alteration of Cell Surface Properties

Cationic AMPs attack the negatively charged bacterial outer membrane. Bacteria have evolved mechanisms to decrease the affinity of their interaction with AMPs by making their cell surfaces less electronegative, either by adding positively charged residues or by removing negatively charged moieties. For instance, members of the *Burkholderia cepacia* complex, *S. enterica* serovar *typhimurium*, and *Proteus mirabilis* add a 4-amino-4-deoxy-T-arabinose group to the lipid A moiety of LPS that imparts a positive charge that neutralizes the negative charge of the phosphate group, thereby conferring resistance to polymyxin B. Similarly, the addition of phosphoethanolamine (PEtn) residues to the lipid A of *Neisserial* lipooligosaccharides renders them resistant to polymyxin, LL-37, and protegrin [50, 51]. While the classical biotype of *Vibrio cholerae* is susceptible to polymyxin, the O1 El Tor biotype is resistant to this AMP because it possesses glycine and diglycine residues in its lipid A [50]. Gram-positive bacteria like *S. aureus*, group B streptococci, and *Listeria monocytogenes* all possess a four-gene operon *dltABCD*, the products of which add D-alanine to the negatively charged polyanionic teichoic acid backbone. However, some authors suggest that D-alanylation-mediated AMP resistance is not because of decreased negative charge of the surface, but the result of enhanced cell wall density, which inhibits the interaction with AMPs. The addition of L-lysine to the anionic phosphatidylglycerol by the product of *mprF* of *S. aureus* renders it resistant to neutrophil defensins [50]. *Francisella novicida* and *Helicobacter pylori* resist polymyxin B by reducing the negative charge of their lipid A through lipid A phosphatase-mediated elimination of the 4′ phosphate [51].

Decoy Targets and Trapping of AMPs

Several bacteria and fungi elaborate capsules or glycocalyces or other exopolysaccharides that act as decoy targets or matrices for AMPs and sequester them such that they cannot reach their target membranes. A notable example is the anionic alginic acid capsule of *Pseudomonas aeruginosa*, which traps cationic AMPs before they can traverse to the membrane, thereby rendering the organism resistant to their bactericidal activity. Capsules and slime layers of most pathogens bear a negative charge and can be hypothesized to confer resistance against AMPs in a similar fashion [52]. Resistance of serogroup B *Neisseria meningitidis* to polymyxin B, α- and β-defensins, cathelicidin, and mCRAMP has been attributed to its capsular polysaccharide [51]. Other pathogens such as *Klebsiella pneumoniae*, *Haemophilus influenzae*, *Legionella pneumophila*, *Streptococcus pneumoniae*, and *Bacillus anthracis* may also employ similar AMP defense mechanisms [52]. Staphylokinase released by *S. aureus* forms complexes with α-defensins such as HNP1 and HNP2 and protects bacteria from their bactericidal effects [53]. Another protein, streptococcal inhibitor of complement (SIC), that is produced in copious amounts by *Streptococcus pyogenes* binds to and neutralizes the activities of HNP1 and LL-37 [54].

Active Efflux

Efflux pumps are energy-dependent protein complexes that extrude a variety of toxic molecules that may traverse the outer membrane, including AMPs. The resistance-nodulation-cell division (RND) pumps are driven by proton-motive force and anti-port H+ ions into the cell while expelling AMPs from the intracellular compartment [55]. For example, the MtrCDE pump (encoded by multiple transferable resistance genes *mtrC*, *D*, and *E*) in *Neisseria gonorrhoeae* confers resistance to LL-37 and protegrin-1. Similarly, deleting *mtrC* in *Haemophilus ducreyi* enhances sensitivity to LL-37 and β-defensins [51]. The plasmid-encoded quaternary ammonium compounds A (QacA) multidrug efflux pump, a member of the major facilitator superfamily (MFS) of pumps, found in *S. aureus* as well as coagulase-negative *Staphylococci* anti-ports an AMP called thrombin-induced platelet microbicidal protein (tPMP-1) in exchange for H+ ions [56]. Others suggest that QacA-dependent alterations in the cytoplasmic membrane confer AMP resistance [57]. RosA/B, a potassium anti-porter efflux pump of the MFS family driven by proton-motive force in *Yersinia* spp. confers resistance to CAMPs such as polymyxin B [58]. Similarly, genetic deletion of the AcrAB efflux pump in *Klebsiella pneumoniae* significantly decreased bacterial survival in the presence of AMPs including polymyxin B, HNP1, HBD-1, and HBD-2 when compared to the wild-type strains [59]. The ATP-binding cassette (ABC) transporters utilize energy from ATP hydrolysis to scavenge and extrude AMPs from the periplasmic space [60]. Mutations of the ATP-binding domains of the ABC transporter encoded by *yejABCDEF* in *S. typhimurium* render it more sensitive to protamine, polymyxin B, melittin, HBD-1, and HBD-2 [61]. The action of efflux pumps appears to be AMP and bacteria specific because ectopic expression of such pumps in other bacteria does not confer resistance to AMPs. Further, overexpression of pumps that are responsible for resistance against particular AMPs in one genus may not confer resistance against the same AMPs in other genera [57].

Proteolytic Degradation

A number of pathogenic bacteria proteolytically degrade and inactivate AMPs. For instance, *P. aeruginosa* isolated from cutaneous ulcers expresses an elastase that proteolytically degrades LL-37, which allows the pathogen to survive in the presence of high concentrations of the AMP [62]. *Burkholderia cepacia* produces two zinc metalloproteases ZmpA and ZmpB, which degrade LL-37 and protamine, and HBD-1, respectively [63]. Aureolysin, a metalloproteinase expressed by *S. aureus*, cleaves LL-37 at multiple sites within its antibacterial C-terminal region. Bacterial survival in the presence of LL-37 correlated inversely with the amount of aureolysin expressed [64].The periodontal pathogen, *Porphyromonas gingivalis* elaborates proteases called gingipains, which degrade AMPs such as HBD-3 [65]. Omptins, a class of β-barrel membrane spanning aspartate proteases that

hydrolyze proteins, are conserved across multiple genera within the Enterobacteriaceae family. They have five extracellular loops that determine substrate specificity. Both enterohemorrhagic and enteropathogenic *E. coli* (EHEC and EPEC, respectively) have an outer membrane omptin family protease, OmpT that cleaves α-helical AMPs such as LL-37 and C18G. The rate of cleavage is more rapid with EHEC OmpT than with EPEC OmpT [66]. PgtE which is a functional homolog of OmpT in *Salmonella enterica* cleaves the AMP C18G [67, 68].

Regulation of Host AMP Production and Activity

Stimulation of pattern recognition receptors (PRRs) such as TLRs by pathogen-associated molecular patterns (PAMPs) including LPS and teichoic acids results in activation of NF-κB, which upregulates host AMP production. The process is further amplified by chemokines and cytokines such as IL-1, IL-6, and TNF-α [50]. However, many pathogens have evolved to limit AMP production. For example, *Streptococcus pyogenes* is a poor inducer of HBD-2 production in terminally differentiated human epidermal keratinocytes [69]. RNA analysis from tissue biopsies from infected individuals and from epithelial and monocyte cell lines infected in vitro revealed that *Shigella dysenteriae* type I and *S. flexneri* actively suppress LL-37 and HBD-1 production during early phases of infection through a plasmid DNA-mediated process [70]. Cholera toxin from the *Vibrio cholera* O139 Bengal strain and labile toxin from enterotoxigenic *E. coli* (ETEC) transcriptionally repress the production of LL-37 and HBD-1 by activating several intracellular signaling pathways [71]. *N. gonorrhoeae* actively represses the production of LL-37 by epithelial cells [72]. *P. aeruginosa* that often colonizes the airways of individuals with cystic fibrosis upregulates the production of host cysteine proteases including cathepsins B, L, and S, which in turn degrade AMPs such as HBD-2 and HBD-3 [73].

Genetic Regulation of AMP Resistance

Bacterial genes that mediate AMP resistance are often transcribed only when the bacterium senses AMPs using two-component signaling systems (TCSSs). TCSSs comprise a homodimeric membrane-bound periplasmic sensory protein that contains a histidine kinase (HK) domain and a cytoplasmic transcriptional response regulator (RR) protein, also organized as a homodimer. Upon stimulation, the HK domain catalyzes the ATP-dependent autophosphorylation of a conserved His residue within the HK dimerization region. The RR domain then catalyzes a phosphorelay whereby phosphate from the phospho-His in the HK domain is transferred to a conserved Asp residue in the RR. This event is followed by downstream activation of transcriptional regulators [74, 75].

In the PhoP/Q TCSS of *Salmonella*, PhoQ (the HK) senses low concentrations of divalent cations such as Mg^{2+} and Ca^{2+}, or acidic pH within phagolysosomes, and phosphorylates PhoP (the RR), which in turn upregulates expression of *pagP* that palmitoylates lipid A. The resulting hepta-acylated lipid A alters membrane fluidity by enhancing hydrophobic interactions and renders it impermeable to α-helical AMPs [76, 77]. Phosphorylation of PhoP also upregulates PgtE, a membrane protease in *Salmonella* that cleaves α-helical AMPs such as C18G [77]. The HK of another *Salmonella* TCSS, PmrB, senses acidic pH and phosphorylates PmrA (the RR), which in turn regulates the *pmrE/pmrF* operon that adds positively charged moieties such as PEtn and aminoarabinose to LPS, thereby decreasing its negative charge and conferring resistance to polymyxin B as discussed above [77]. A TCSS homologous to the PmrA/PmrB is also present in *P. aeruginosa*, which upon stimulation adds aminoarabinose to the LPS and makes the organism polymyxin B resistant [78]. Additionally, *P. aeruginosa* has two TCSSs called CprRS and ParRS that directly sense CAMPs such as CP28, indolicidin, and polymyxin B and activate the *arn-BCADTEF* operon, which adds positively charged aminoarabinose to LPS, rendering the organism AMP resistant [79].

Clinical Use of Host Antimicrobial Peptides

Because of the widespread emergence of resistance to conventional antibiotics, AMPs may constitute an attractive alternative for the treatment of infectious diseases. They are effective against a broad spectrum of microorganisms, have a rapid onset of activity, and are relatively protected against development of resistance. Currently, only few AMPs, including polymyxin B, bacitracin, gramicidin, and glycopeptides such as vancomycin and teicoplanin, are licensed for clinical use. Some of the AMPs that have undergone or are currently undergoing clinical trials are discussed below.

Neuprex

Neuprex or $rBPI_{21}$ is a 21 kDa recombinant form of the first 193 amino acid residues of N-terminal region of the 55 kDa bactericidal/permeability-increasing protein (BPI), where the cysteine at position 132 is replaced by alanine. BPI binds to LPS with high affinity, which forms the basis for its activity against gram-negative bacteria. Upon interaction with negatively charged membranes, $rBPI_{21}$ induces aggregation and causes leakage through pores through hemifusion of inner and outer membranes enriched in phosphatidylglycerol [80, 81]. A phase 3 clinical trial assessed the efficacy of $rBPI_{21}$ as adjunctive treatment of children with meningococcemia. The 60-day mortality among the 190 children who received $rBPI_{21}$ and the 203 children who received placebo was 7.4% and 9.9%, respectively [82]. The lower than expected mortality in the placebo group led to the study being underpowered to obtain the desired improvement in survival with $rBPI_{21}$. Among subjects who survived to receive the complete infusion of the study drug, mortality was 6.2% in the placebo group versus 2.2% in the rBPI$_{21}$ group ($P = 0.07$). There were trends toward reduced requirement for renal replacement therapy, decreased need for blood products, and shorter time on ventilators in children who received rBPI$_{21}$. Administration of rBPI$_{21}$ was not associated with any major adverse effects. rBPI$_{21}$ was also used in conjunction with conventional antibiotics in intra-abdominal infections and lung infection in persons with cystic fibrosis because this peptide may render otherwise drug-resistant organisms more sensitive to antibiotics. In a phase 2 trial in patients with hemorrhagic trauma, patients on Neuprex showed significantly better outcomes versus those on placebo [83].

Omiganan

Omiganan is a 12-amino acid peptide analog of indolicidin, an AMP found naturally in bovine neutrophil granules, with microbicidal activity against gram-positive and gram-negative bacteria, as well as fungi. Although its mechanism of action remains unclear, omiganan is hypothesized to cause cell death primarily by membrane depolarization and disintegration. It may also interact with DNA, thereby inhibiting the activity of DNA-binding enzymes and cause filamentation of genetic material [27]. Clinical trials suggest that topical omiganan gel may be effective for the prevention of intravascular catheter-related infections and the treatment of papulo-pustular rosacea. A study of topical omiganan for treatment of acne vulgaris is underway.

Pexiganan/MSI-78

Pexiganan is a synthetic derivative of the magainin-2, a naturally occurring AMP in the frog *Xenopus laevis* that has broad-spectrum (including anaerobes) bactericidal properties by forming toroidal pores in membranes [84]. Topical pexiganan is being evaluated for treatment of diabetic foot ulcers.

Iseganan/IB-367

Iseganan is derived from porcine protegrin-1 and also functions by forming pores in bacterial and fungal membranes [85]. Although topical iseganan reduced microbial colonization of the oropharynx, it failed to decrease the incidence of ventilator-associated pneumonia [86]. The drug is being evaluated to reduce the severity of oral mucositis in patients undergoing radiotherapy for head and neck cancer.

hLF1-11

Human lactoferrin-derived peptide, hLF1-11, is a synthetic peptide comprising the first 11 N-terminal residues of the native protein. It has activity against methicillin-resistant *S. aureus*, *K. pneumoniae*, *L. monocytogenes*, *A. baumannii*, and fluconazole-resistant *C. albicans* [87]. This peptide has direct microbicidal as well as immunomodulatory modes of action. It associates with anionic membranes through its positively charged N-terminal region and enhances membrane permeability [88, 89]. Upon stimulation with hLF1-11, monocyte differentiation was directed toward a subset of macrophages with a TLR 4-, 5-, and 7-mediated pro-inflammatory cytokine profile and enhanced effector functions against *S. aureus* and *C. albicans* [90, 91]. The peptide is currently being evaluated in hematopoietic stem cell transplant recipients to treat bacterial and fungal infections [92].

CZEN-002/8-mer α-Melanocyte-Stimulating Hormone (α-MSH) Derivative

This α-MSH derivative causes cAMP accumulation in *C. albicans*, thereby disrupting signaling pathways. CZEN-002 is also anti-inflammatory and suppresses TNF-α production [87]. CZEN-002 is currently in phase 2 trials for treatment of vulvovaginal candidiasis [92]. The peptide is also effective against *C. krusei* and *C. glabrata*, which are becoming increasingly drug-resistant.

PAC-113/Histatin 5 Derivative

PAC-113 is a derivative of the human salivary α-helical peptide histatin 5 (Hst-5) and has been granted an Investigational New Drug (IND) status by the FDA for treatment of oral candidiasis [87, 92]. It is active against several species of *Candida* such as *C. albicans*, *C. glabrata*, *C. parapsilosis*, and *C. tropicalis*, including drug-resistant isolates [87]. The mechanism of action of Hst-5 is dichotomous. On the one hand, Hst-5 can bind to the candidial membrane-bound heat shock protein (Ssa1/2), undergo receptor-mediated endocytosis, and subsequently target the mitochondria and intracellular plasma membranes. Alternatively, it can also function as a classical α-helical cationic AMP and interact with anionic membranes, causing membrane damage and cell death [38].

Several other antibacterial peptides are either in clinical development or in early stage clinical trials. The reader is referred to more detailed reviews on this subject [92–94].

Despite their broad spectrum of antimicrobial activity, often greater microbicidal efficacy on a molar basis when compared with conventional antibiotics, and limited evidence of development of acquired resistance, there are several considerations which have slowed development of these peptides as anti-infectives. Most AMPs are labile and susceptible to pH changes and proteolytic degradation within the host [87, 92]. This necessitates their use at high concentrations at which point they lose specificity for microbial membranes and often damage host cell membranes [95]. Toxicity following systemic administration often restricts their use to topical formulations. Moreover, effective drug delivery to locations where drug penetration is characteristically poor, or to intracellular sites, is another practical hurdle that hinders widespread use of these compounds. Finally, the costs of production of AMPs are often prohibitive, although engineering shorter peptides may help alleviate this problem [87, 92]. To overcome some of these obstacles, synthetic compounds called "peptidomimetics" are being developed. These molecules retain the function of AMPs but lack some of the drawbacks of AMPs listed above [94, 96].

Dysregulation of AMPs in Human Disease

The role of AMPs in human physiology is becoming increasingly appreciated. While causality between dysregulated AMP production and disease mechanisms is yet to be firmly established, associations between certain infections and diseases with presumed immunological origins and altered AMP levels have been documented. For instance, patients with atopic dermatitis (AD) have lower levels of dermicidin (DCD)-derived peptides in their sweat compared to healthy volunteers. Moreover, AD patients with histories of recurrent bacterial and viral skin infections had less DCD and DCD-1L in their sweat in comparison to AD patients with no prior history of infectious complications [97]. Skin biopsies of AD patients also revealed lower amounts of the cathelicidin LL-37 and human β-defensin 2 (HBD-2) compared to patients with psoriasis. These observations may account for the predisposition of AD patients to *S. aureus* infections [98]. On the other hand, enhanced inflammation as suggested by increased levels of LL-37 and HBD-2 may play a role in the pathogenesis of psoriasis [98] and rosacea [16]. Low levels of HBD-2, HBD-3, and LL-37 are also associated with atopic eczema [99]. The amount of HBD-2 in the intestinal mucosa correlates with copy number of the HBD-2. While normal hosts and individuals with ulcerative colitis or ileal Crohn's disease (CD) possess four copies of the HBD-2 gene, the median copy number of the HBD-2 gene in patients with colonic CD is three (the difference was statistically significant), which led the authors to conclude that low HBD-2 production might be a predisposing factor for colonic CD [100].

Single-nucleotide polymorphisms (SNPs) in the DEFB1 gene that encodes for HBD-1 are associated with higher levels of oral carriage of *Candida albicans* [101]. Two independent studies have also associated SNPs in the DEFB1 gene with enhanced risk of perinatal acquisition of HIV-1 infections [102, 103].

Recurrent oral bacterial infections, especially periodontal infections associated with overgrowth of *Actinobacillus actinomycetemcomitans*, are a common feature of patients with Kostmann syndrome (severe congenital neutropenia). The neutrophils of these patients lack LL-37 and have diminished levels of HNPs 1–3. These individuals also lack LL-37 in their saliva and plasma. A patient in this cohort who underwent bone marrow transplantation, which restored normal plasma levels of LL-37, did not suffer from periodontal infections. These data suggest that LL-37 and HNPs 1–3 protect against periodontal infections [104]. Inadequate LL-37 activity may exacerbate the pathology of cystic fibrosis (CF). Under high salt concentrations seen in the alveolar surface fluid of persons with CF, LL-37 that is present at subinhibitory concentrations crosses the cell walls of *P. aeruginosa*, forms complexes with its DNA, and promotes mutations in the *mucA* gene, which controls alginate capsule production. These events culminate in the conversion of *P. aeruginosa* to a mucoid phenotype that produces high amounts of alginate, which promotes resistance to killing by LL-37 and correlates with a poor prognosis [105]. Other conditions associated with dysregulation of neutrophil AMP contents that lead to frequent severe bacterial infections are specific granule deficiency (SGD) and Chediak-Higashi syndrome (CHS). SGD patients have normal levels of cathepsins and elastase, but lack defensins, while the converse occurs in CHS [106]. In a study conducted in Zambia, intestinal biopsy specimens from adults who had recently suffered from diarrhea but were disease-free for a month had tenfold lower mRNA transcripts of α-defensins (HD5 and HD6) compared to patients with no history of diarrhea. While the authors suggested that decreased α-defensins may predispose to diarrhea, it should be noted that the intestinal microbiome itself regulates AMP production, which could confound interpretation of the results [107]. The examples listed above only associate dysregulation of AMPs and disease; further research is required to establish causality.

Concluding Remarks

The widespread emergence of antibiotic resistance has led the scientific community to look for newer therapies, which has led to renewed interest in AMPs. The role of AMPs in physiology is becoming more clearly elucidated. While the prevailing view is that AMPs have an important role in antimicrobial defenses, some argue that this hypothesis is supported mostly by in vitro experiments that have used supraphysiologic concentrations of AMPs. They suggest that physiologic concentrations AMPs may play important roles in immunomodulation and processes such as wound healing. Studies have associated dysregulation of AMPs with immune-mediated disorders, normal physiology, and infections. While further research is needed to establish firm causality between defects in AMPs and diseases, the information harnessed so far has provided the foundation for development of AMP-based therapies. Although AMP-based therapies have not yet met with much clinical success, increasing knowledge in the field, coupled with advances in protein engineering, could witness successful AMP-based therapies in the near future.

References

1. Wang G, Li X, Wang Z. APD3: the antimicrobial peptide database as a tool for research and education. Nucleic Acids Res. 2016;44(D1):D1087–93.
2. Zimmer J, Hobkirk J, Mohamed F, Browning M, Stover CM. On the functional overlap between complement and antimicrobial peptides. Front Immunol. 2015;5
3. Zasloff M. Antimicrobial peptides of multicellular organisms. Nature. 2002;415(6870):389–95.
4. Park Y, Hahm KS. Antimicrobial peptides (AMPs): peptide structure and mode of action. J Biochem Mol Biol. 2005;38(5):507–16.
5. Tennessen JA. Molecular evolution of animal antimicrobial peptides: widespread moderate positive selection. J Evol Biol. 2005;18(6):1387–94.
6. Zhang LJ, Gallo RL. Antimicrobial peptides. Curr Biol. 2016;26(1):R14–9.
7. Hollox EJ, Armour JA, Barber JC. Extensive normal copy number variation of a beta-defensin antimicrobial-gene cluster. Am J Hum Genet. 2003;73(3):591–600.

8. Coda AB, et al. Cathelicidin, kallikrein 5, and serine protease activity is inhibited during treatment of rosacea with azelaic acid 15% gel. J Am Acad Dermatol. 2013;69(4):570–7.

9. Senyurek I, Klein G, Kalbacher H, Deeg M, Schittek B. Peptides derived from the human laminin alpha 4 and alpha 5 chains exhibit antimicrobial activity. Peptides. 2010;31(8):1468–72.

10. Mansour SC, Pena OM, Hancock REW. Host defense peptides: front-line immunomodulators. Trends Immunol. 2014;35(9):443–50.

11. Steinstraesser L, Kraneburg U, Jacobsen F, Al-Benna S. Host defense peptides and their antimicrobial-immunomodulatory duality. Immunobiology. 2011;216(3):322–33.

12. Meisch JP, et al. Human beta-defensin 3 peptide is increased and redistributed in Crohn's ileitis. Inflamm Bowel Dis. 2013;19(5):942–53.

13. Lande R, et al. Plasmacytoid dendritic cells sense self-DNA coupled with antimicrobial peptide. Nature. 2007;449(7162):564–9.

14. Scott MG, Davidson DJ, Gold MR, Bowdish D, Hancock RE. The human antimicrobial peptide LL-37 is a multifunctional modulator of innate immune responses. J Immunol. 2002;169(7):3883–91.

15. Rosenfeld Y, Papo N, Shai Y. Endotoxin (lipopolysaccharide) neutralization by innate immunity host-defense peptides. Peptide properties and plausible modes of action. J Biol Chem. 2006;281(3):1636–43.

16. Yamasaki K, et al. Increased serine protease activity and cathelicidin promotes skin inflammation in rosacea. Nat Med. 2007;13(8):975–80.

17. Courth LF, et al. Crohn's disease-derived monocytes fail to induce Paneth cell defensins. Proc Natl Acad Sci U S A. 2015;112(45):14000–5.

18. Wang G. Improved methods for classification, prediction, and design of antimicrobial peptides. Methods Mol Biol. 2015;1268:43–66.

19. Zanetti M. Cathelicidins, multifunctional peptides of the innate immunity. J Leukoc Biol. 2004;75(1):39–48.

20. Bulet P, Stocklin R, Menin L. Anti-microbial peptides: from invertebrates to vertebrates. Immunol Rev. 2004;198:169–84.

21. Brogden KA. Antimicrobial peptides: pore formers or metabolic inhibitors in bacteria? Nat Rev Microbiol. 2005;3(3):238–50.

22. Ahmad A, et al. Identification and design of antimicrobial peptides for therapeutic applications. Curr Protein Pept Sci. 2012;13(3):211–23.

23. White SH, Wimley WC, Selsted ME. Structure, function, and membrane integration of defensins. Curr Opin Struct Biol. 1995;5(4):521–7.

24. Lehrer RI, Cole AM, Selsted ME. θ-Defensins: cyclic peptides with endless potential. J Biol Chem. 2012;287(32):27014–9.

25. Yount NY, Yeaman MR. Immunocontinuum: perspectives in antimicrobial peptide mecha-nisms of action and resistance. Protein Pept Lett. 2005;12(1):49–67.

26. Shah P, Hsiao FS, Ho YH, Chen CS. The proteome targets of intracellular targeting antimicrobial peptides. Proteomics. 2015.

27. Nguyen LT, Haney EF, Vogel HJ. The expanding scope of antimicrobial peptide structures and their modes of action. Trends Biotechnol. 2011;29(9):464–72.

28. Cho J, et al. The novel biological action of antimicrobial peptides via apoptosis induction. J Microbiol Biotechnol. 2012;22(11):1457–66.

29. Burian M, Schittek B. The secrets of dermcidin action. Int J Med Microbiol. 2015;305(2):283–6.

30. Sass V, et al. Human beta-defensin 3 inhibits cell wall biosynthesis in Staphylococci. Infect Immun. 2010;78(6):2793–800.

31. de Leeuw E, et al. Functional interaction of human neutrophil peptide-1 with the cell wall precursor lipid II. FEBS Lett. 2010;584(8):1543–8.

32. Spencer JD, et al. Ribonuclease 7, an antimicrobial peptide upregulated during infection, contributes to microbial defense of the human urinary tract. Kidney Int. 2013;83(4):615–25.

33. Lin YM, et al. Outer membrane protein I of Pseudomonas aeruginosa is a target of cationic antimicrobial peptide/protein. J Biol Chem. 2010;285(12):8985–94.

34. Kim HS, et al. Endotoxin-neutralizing antimicrobial proteins of the human placenta. J Immunol. 2002;168(5):2356–64.

35. Hazrati E, et al. Human α- and β-Defensins block multiple steps in herpes simplex virus infection. J Immunol. 2006;177(12):8658–66.

36. Helmerhorst EJ, et al. The cellular target of histatin 5 on Candida albicans is the energized mitochondrion. J Biol Chem. 1999;274(11):7286–91.

37. Luque-Ortega JR, van't Hof W, Veerman EC, Saugar JM, Rivas L. Human antimicrobial peptide histatin 5 is a cell-penetrating peptide targeting mitochondrial ATP synthesis in Leishmania. FASEB J. 2008;22(6):1817–28.

38. Mochon AB, Liu H. The antimicrobial peptide histatin-5 causes a spatially restricted disruption on the Candida albicans surface, allowing rapid entry of the peptide into the cytoplasm. PLoS Pathog. 2008;4(10):e1000190.

39. Barker HC, Kinsella N, Jaspe A, Friedrich T, O'Connor CD. Formate protects stationary-phase Escherichia coli and Salmonella cells from killing by a cationic antimicrobial peptide. Mol Microbiol. 2000;35(6):1518–29.

40. Backo M, Gaenger E, Burkart A, Chai YL, Bayer AS. Treatment of experimental staphylococcal endocarditis due to a strain with reduced susceptibility in vitro to vancomycin: efficacy of ampicillin-sulbactam. Antimicrob Agents Chemother. 1999;43(10):2565–8.

41. Territo MC, Ganz T, Selsted ME, Lehrer R. Monocyte-chemotactic activity of defensins from human neutrophils. J Clin Invest. 1989;84(6):2017–20.

42. Lai Y, Gallo RL. AMPed up immunity: how antimicrobial peptides have multiple roles in immune defense. Trends Immunol. 2009;30(3):131–41.

43. De Y, et al. LL-37, the neutrophil granule- and epithelial cell-derived cathelicidin, utilizes formyl peptide receptor-like 1 (FPRL1) as a receptor to chemoattract human peripheral blood neutrophils, monocytes, and T cells. J Exp Med. 2000;192(7):1069–74.

44. Befus AD, et al. Neutrophil defensins induce histamine secretion from mast cells: mechanisms of action. J Immunol. 1999;163(2):947–53.

45. Yang D, Biragyn A, Kwak LW, Oppenheim JJ. Mammalian defensins in immunity: more than just microbicidal. Trends Immunol. 2002;23(6):291–6.

46. Funderburg N, et al. Human -defensin-3 activates professional antigen-presenting cells via Toll-like receptors 1 and 2. Proc Natl Acad Sci U S A. 2007;104(47):18631–5.

47. Niyonsaba F, Ushio H, Nagaoka I, Okumura K, Ogawa H. The human beta-defensins (-1, -2, -3, -4) and cathelicidin LL-37 induce IL-18 secretion through p38 and ERK MAPK activation in primary human keratinocytes. J Immunol. 2005;175(3):1776–84.

48. Prohaszka Z, et al. Defensins purified from human granulocytes bind C1q and activate the classical complement pathway like the transmembrane glycoprotein gp41 of HIV-1. Mol Immunol. 1997;34(11):809–16.

49. Groeneveld TW, et al. Human neutrophil peptide-1 inhibits both the classical and the lectin pathway of complement activation. Mol Immunol. 2007;44(14):3608–14.

50. Nizet V. Antimicrobial peptide resistance mechanisms of human bacterial pathogens. Curr Issues Mol Biol. 2006;8:11–26.

51. Gruenheid S, Le Moual H. Resistance to antimicrobial peptides in Gram-negative bacteria. FEMS Microbiol Lett. 2012;330(2):81–9.

52. Yeaman MR, Yount NY. Mechanisms of antimicrobial peptide action and resistance. Pharmacol Rev. 2003;55(1):27–55.

53. Jin T, et al. Staphylococcus aureus resists human defensins by production of staphylokinase, a novel bacterial evasion mechanism. J Immunol. 2004;172(2):1169–76.

54. Frick IM, Akesson P, Rasmussen M, Schmidtchen A, Bjorck L. SIC, a secreted protein of Streptococcus pyogenes that inactivates antibacterial peptides. J Biol Chem. 2003;278(19):16561–6.

55. Paulsen IT, Brown MH, Skurray RA. Proton-dependent multidrug efflux systems. Microbiol Rev. 1996;60(4):575–608.

56. Xu Z, O'Rourke BA, Skurray RA, Brown MH. Role of transmembrane segment 10 in efflux mediated by the staphylococcal multidrug transport protein QacA. J Biol Chem. 2006;281(2):792–9.

57. Guilhelmelli F, et al. Antibiotic development challenges: the various mechanisms of action of antimicrobial peptides and of bacterial resistance. Front Microbiol. 2013;4:353.

58. Bengoechea JA, Skurnik M. Temperature-regulated efflux pump/potassium antiporter system mediates resistance to cationic antimicrobial peptides in Yersinia. Mol Microbiol. 2000;37(1):67–80.

59. Padilla E, et al. Klebsiella pneumoniae AcrAB efflux pump contributes to antimicrobial resistance and virulence. Antimicrob Agents Chemother. 2010;54(1):177–83.

60. Nikaido H, Hall JA. Overview of bacterial ABC transporters. Methods Enzymol. 1998;292:3–20.

61. Eswarappa SM, Panguluri KK, Hensel M, Chakravortty D. The yejABEF operon of Salmonella confers resistance to antimicrobial peptides and contributes to its virulence. Microbiology. 2008;154(Pt 2):666–78.

62. Schmidtchen A, Frick IM, Andersson E, Tapper H, Bjorck L. Proteinases of common pathogenic bacteria degrade and inactivate the antibacterial peptide LL-37. Mol Microbiol. 2002;46(1):157–68.

63. Kooi C, Sokol PA. Burkholderia cenocepacia zinc metalloproteases influence resistance to antimicrobial peptides. Microbiology. 2009;155(Pt 9):2818–25.

64. Sieprawska-Lupa M, et al. Degradation of human antimicrobial peptide LL-37 by Staphylococcus aureus-derived proteinases. Antimicrob Agents Chemother. 2004;48(12):4673–9.

65. Maisetta G, Brancatisano FL, Esin S, Campa M, Batoni G. Gingipains produced by Porphyromonas gingivalis ATCC49417 degrade human-beta-defensin 3 and affect peptide's antibacterial activity in vitro. Peptides. 2011;32(5):1073–7.

66. Thomassin JL, Brannon JR, Gibbs BF, Gruenheid S, Le Moual H. OmpT outer membrane proteases of enterohemorrhagic and enteropathogenic Escherichia coli contribute differently to the degradation of human LL-37. Infect Immun. 2012;80(2):483–92.

67. Grodberg J, Dunn JJ. Comparison of Escherichia coli K-12 outer membrane protease OmpT and Salmonella typhimurium E protein. J Bacteriol. 1989;171(5):2903–5.

68. Guina T, Yi EC, Wang H, Hackett M, Miller SI. A PhoP-regulated outer membrane protease of Salmonella enterica serovar typhimurium promotes resistance to alpha-helical antimicrobial peptides. J Bacteriol. 2000;182(14):4077–86.

69. Dinulos JG, Mentele L, Fredericks LP, Dale BA, Darmstadt GL. Keratinocyte expression of human beta defensin 2 following bacterial infection: role in cutaneous host defense. Clin Diagn Lab Immunol. 2003;10(1):161–6.

70. Islam D, et al. Downregulation of bactericidal peptides in enteric infections: a novel immune escape mechanism with bacterial DNA as a potential regulator. Nat Med. 2001;7(2):180–5.

71. Chakraborty K, et al. Bacterial exotoxins down-regulate cathelicidin (hCAP-18/LL-37) and human beta-defensin 1 (HBD-1) expression in the intestinal epithelial cells. Cell Microbiol. 2008;10(12):2520–37.

72. Bergman P, et al. Neisseria gonorrhoeae downregulates expression of the human antimicrobial peptide LL-37. Cell Microbiol. 2005;7(7):1009–17.

73. Taggart CC, et al. Inactivation of human beta-defensins 2 and 3 by elastolytic cathepsins. J Immunol. 2003;171(2):931–7.

74. West AH, Stock AM. Histidine kinases and response regulator proteins in two-component signaling systems. Trends Biochem Sci. 2001;26(6):369–76.

75. Beier D, Gross R. Regulation of bacterial virulence by two-component systems. Curr Opin Microbiol. 2006;9(2):143–52.

76. Guo L, et al. Lipid A acylation and bacterial resistance against vertebrate antimicrobial peptides. Cell. 1998;95(2):189–98.

77. Ernst RK, Guina T, Miller SI. Salmonella typhimurium outer membrane remodeling: role in resistance to host innate immunity. Microbes Infect. 2001;3(14–15):1327–34.

78. Moskowitz SM, Ernst RK, Miller SI. PmrAB, a two-component regulatory system of Pseudomonas aeruginosa that modulates resistance to cationic antimicrobial peptides and addition of aminoarabinose to lipid A. J Bacteriol. 2004;186(2):575–9.

79. Fernandez L, et al. The two-component system CprRS senses cationic peptides and triggers adaptive resistance in Pseudomonas aeruginosa independently of ParRS. Antimicrob Agents Chemother. 2012;56(12):6212–22.

80. Domingues MM, Castanho MA, Santos NC. rBPI(21) promotes lipopolysaccharide aggregation and exerts its antimicrobial effects by (hemi)fusion of PG-containing membranes. PLoS One. 2009;4(12):e8385.

81. Domingues MM, Lopes SC, Santos NC, Quintas A, Castanho MA. Fold-unfold transitions in the selectivity and mechanism of action of the N-terminal fragment of the bactericidal/permeability-increasing protein (rBPI(21)). Biophys J. 2009;96(3):987–96.

82. Levin M, et al. Recombinant bactericidal/permeability-increasing protein (rBPI21) as adjunctive treatment for children with severe meningococcal sepsis: a randomised trial. rBPI21 Meningococcal Sepsis Study Group. Lancet. 2000;356(9234):961–7.

83. Mackin WM. Neuprex XOMA Corp. IDrugs. 1998;1(6):715–23.

84. Gottler LM, Ramamoorthy A. Structure, membrane orientation, mechanism, and function of pexiganan – a highly potent antimicrobial peptide designed from magainin. Biochim Biophys Acta. 2009;1788(8):1680–6.

85. Bolintineanu DS, Vivcharuk V, Kaznessis YN. Multiscale models of the antimicrobial peptide protegrin-1 on Gram-negative bacteria membranes. Int J Mol Sci. 2012;13(9):11000–11.

86. Jerse AE, et al. Multiple gonococcal opacity proteins are expressed during experimental urethral infection in the male. J Exp Med. 1994;179(3):911–20.

87. Seo MD, Won HS, Kim JH, Mishig-Ochir T, Lee BJ. Antimicrobial peptides for therapeutic applications: a review. Molecules. 2012;17(10):12276–86.

88. Nibbering PH, et al. Human lactoferrin and peptides derived from its N terminus are highly effective against infections with antibiotic-resistant bacteria. Infect Immun. 2001;69(3):1469–76.

89. Lupetti A, et al. Human lactoferrin-derived peptide's antifungal activities against disseminated Candida albicans infection. J Infect Dis. 2007;196(9):1416–24.

90. van der Does AM, et al. The human lactoferrin-derived peptide hLF1-11 primes monocytes for an enhanced TLR-mediated immune response. Biometals. 2010;23(3):493–505.

91. van der Does AM, et al. Antimicrobial peptide hLF1-11 directs granulocyte-macrophage colony-stimulating factor-driven monocyte differentiation toward macrophages with enhanced recognition and clearance of pathogens. Antimicrob Agents Chemother. 2010;54(2):811–6.

92. Hancock RE, Sahl HG. Antimicrobial and host-defense peptides as new anti-infective therapeutic strategies. Nat Biotechnol. 2006;24(12):1551–7.

93. Fjell CD, Hiss JA, Hancock RE, Schneider G. Designing antimicrobial peptides: form follows function. Nat Rev Drug Discov. 2012;11(1):37–51.

94. Mendez-Samperio P. Peptidomimetics as a new generation of antimicrobial agents: current progress. Infect Drug Resist. 2014;7:229–37.

95. Aoki W, Kuroda K, Ueda M. Next generation of antimicrobial peptides as molecular targeted medicines. J Biosci Bioeng. 2012;114(4):365–70.

96. Mojsoska B, Jenssen H. Peptides and Peptidomimetics for antimicrobial drug design. Pharmaceuticals (Basel). 2015;8(3):366–415.

97. Rieg S, et al. Deficiency of dermcidin-derived antimicrobial peptides in sweat of patients with atopic dermatitis correlates with an impaired innate defense of human skin in vivo. J Immunol. 2005;174(12):8003–10.

98. Ong PY, et al. Endogenous antimicrobial peptides and skin infections in atopic dermatitis. N Engl J Med. 2002;347(15):1151–60.

99. Rivas-Santiago B, Serrano CJ, Enciso-Moreno JA. Susceptibility to infectious diseases based on antimicrobial peptide production. Infect Immun. 2009;77(11):4690–5.

100. Fellermann K, et al. A chromosome 8 gene-cluster polymorphism with low human beta-defensin 2 gene copy number predisposes to Crohn disease of the colon. Am J Hum Genet. 2006;79(3):439–48.

101. Jurevic RJ, Bai M, Chadwick RB, White TC, Dale BA. Single-nucleotide polymorphisms (SNPs) in human beta-defensin 1: high-throughput SNP assays and association with Candida carriage in type I diabetics and nondiabetic controls. J Clin Microbiol. 2003;41(1):90–6.

102. Segat L, et al. DEFB-1 genetic polymorphism screening in HIV-1 positive pregnant women and their children. J Matern Fetal Neonatal Med. 2006;19(1):13–6.

103. Milanese M, et al. DEFB1 gene polymorphisms and increased risk of HIV-1 infection in Brazilian children. AIDS. 2006;20(12):1673–5.

104. Pütsep K, Carlsson G, Boman HG, Andersson M. Deficiency of antibacterial peptides in patients with morbus Kostmann: an observation study. Lancet. 2002;360(9340):1144–9.

105. Limoli DH, et al. Cationic antimicrobial peptides promote microbial mutagenesis and patho-adaptation in chronic infections. PLoS Pathog. 2014;10(4):e1004083.

106. Ganz T, Metcalf JA, Gallin JI, Boxer LA, Lehrer RI. Microbicidal/cytotoxic proteins of neutrophils are deficient in two disorders: Chediak-Higashi syndrome and "specific" granule deficiency. J Clin Invest. 1988;82(2):552–6.

107. Kelly P, et al. Reduced gene expression of intestinal alpha-defensins predicts diarrhea in a cohort of African adults. J Infect Dis. 2006;193(10):1464–70.

Role of Deficits in Pathogen Recognition Receptors in Infection Susceptibility

Cristina Cunha, Samuel M. Gonçalves,
and Agostinho Carvalho

Introduction: A Genetic Perspective of the Host-Pathogen Interaction

The determinism of human infectious diseases is still vastly misconstrued. Because exposure to a pathogen is requisite for infection and disease to occur, infectious diseases are often regarded as textbook examples of purely environmental diseases. However, a characteristic feature of many human infectious diseases is the interindividual variability in the development and progression of clinical disease. While a significant contribution might be credited to virulence traits of the infectious agent, recent evidence has highlighted the dominant role of heritable factors in defining susceptibility to infection [1–6]. Twin studies have played a significant part in unraveling host genetic factors involved in susceptibility to infectious diseases, although the relative contribution of heredity and environment to infection in twins remains disputed [7]. Nonetheless, a groundbreaking study from the late 1980s reported that adopted children had a prominently increased risk of death from infectious diseases if at least one of their biological parents had died prematurely from the same infection [8]. Mouse studies have also widely illustrated the importance of host genetic-driven effects, by showing disparities between inbred strains concerning pathogen loads, cytokine responses, and outcomes following infection [9]. Thus, there is considerable evidence supporting the contribution of host genetics to infectious disease; a well-known example is the protective role of the sickle cell trait against the severe forms of malaria caused by *Plasmodium falciparum* [10].

Our current understanding of the genetic susceptibility to human infectious diseases is derived from the study of individuals with rare monogenic defects underlying susceptibility to a narrow range of pathogens and from population-based studies to identify common polymorphisms associated with disease. Such landmark discoveries have established that predisposition to infection segregates in either a Mendelian (monogenic) or a polygenic pattern of inheritance. By implicating these genetic variants in the immune response to selected pathogens, these reports have provided crucial insights into the genetic control of antimicrobial host defenses in humans. Extension of these genetic approaches to the dissection of the associated molecular and cellular mechanisms may further unravel the genetic architecture of susceptibility to infectious diseases and support future studies evaluating host-pathogen genetic interactions and potentially driving clinical translation. In particular, the analysis of the

C. Cunha · S. M. Gonçalves · A. Carvalho (✉)
Life and Health Sciences Research Institute (ICVS),
School of Medicine, University of Minho,
Braga, Portugal

ICVS/3B's – PT Government Associate Laboratory,
Braga/Guimarães, Portugal
e-mail: agostinhocarvalho@med.uminho.pt

transcriptional landscape of the host-pathogen interaction under conditions of specific immune deficiency may contribute to the disclosure of the permissive conditions underlying the emergence of different infectious diseases. In this chapter, we focus on genetic variation in pattern recognition receptors (PRRs) and its role in susceptibility to infectious diseases in patients with primary and acquired immunodeficiencies. Also discussed is the impact of genetic variation in these receptors on the activation of antimicrobial immune responses and how these processes can be exploited in personalized medical interventions based on individual host genetic profiles.

Genetic Principles and Approaches for Identifying Susceptibility Genes

Perhaps the most compelling evidence that host genetics indeed determines the development of infectious disease arises from primary immunodeficiencies, first described in the late 1940s and early 1950s [1]. Primary immunodeficiencies usually present with infections due to common or opportunistic pathogens, resulting from a clear-cut deficit in a single gene. Such immune dysfunction is usually limited to a very small number of individuals or families, but the identification of the underlying genetic defects is very informative on immune defense mechanisms. On the other hand, susceptibility to infections in the general population can be influenced by polymorphisms across multiple genes, with the specific contribution to the phenotype being typically more difficult to establish.

The current interest in the role of rare, large-effect variants as predisposing factors to infectious diseases has prompted the description of an increasing number of single-gene defects underlying phenotypes associated with a certain pathogen selectivity. The identification of mutations in individual immune-related genes influencing susceptibility to a narrow range of different pathogens has led to the evolving concept of pathogen-selective immunodeficiency [11]. It should be stressed that although these immunodeficiency states are widely considered

to be discriminating, the specificity of pathogen susceptibility is not always absolute. Nevertheless, the range of pathogen diversity is typically much narrower in humans than that observed in the corresponding mouse knockout models. One difference is that human studies involve naturally acquired infection while mouse models generally involve administration of pathogens, often at high inocula to induce disease.

Early studies of genetic susceptibility to infectious diseases resorted to genome-wide linkage analyses and candidate gene approaches and identified only a restricted number of strongly associated loci that have been independently validated. Linkage approaches have been employed successfully in the study of monogenic diseases and were successively applied in attempts to define the susceptibility loci underlying common diseases. The most commonly used design involved the study of affected sibling pairs and had some degree of success in identifying loci linked to some infectious diseases, in particular leprosy [12]. However, a major drawback of linkage analyses lies in the difficulty in recruiting numerous multicase families in which two siblings are affected and by the lack of adequate study power [3].

Candidate gene studies comprise the genotyping of common polymorphisms in biologically plausible genes and pathways, typically in unrelated case and control individuals. The degree of replication between candidate gene studies is often poor, most likely due to small sample sizes limiting the study power, unrecognized population stratification, failure to correct for multiple testing during statistical analysis, and missing or inaccurate clinical information. Additional causes for lack of replication may include differences across studies in the phenotypic definition of cases (e.g., a significant bias might be introduced by the use of different diagnostic procedures) and controls, unidentified variation in gene-environment interactions, and actual genetic heterogeneity between populations [13]. The candidate gene approach is further hampered by its reliance on existing and possibly inaccurate biological hypotheses to select genes for study. Despite these limitations, candidate gene studies have disclosed a number of robust, independently replicated associations with infectious diseases.

Pattern Recognition Receptors and Innate Immunity

In 1992, Charles Janeway, Jr., advanced the field of innate immunity toward new horizons with his concept of selective recognition of conserved microbial structures by germline-encoded PRRs [14]. Indeed, it is nowadays well established that the first step in the development of an innate immune response implicates pathogen recognition by PRRs in an acute and conserved fashion [15]. Although there are substantial differences in the ways in which the multiple innate cell populations recognize specific pathogens, the overall framework is similar and involves the binding of conserved pathogen-associated molecular patterns (PAMPs) such as microbial cell wall constituents, nucleic acids, or metabolic products by PRRs. There are five major classes of receptors: Toll-like receptors (TLRs), C-type lectin receptors (CLRs), nucleotide-binding oligomerization domain (NOD) leucine-rich repeat containing receptors (NLRs), retinoic acid-inducible gene I protein (RIG-I) helicase receptors, and absent in melanoma 2 (AIM2)-like receptors (ALRs) [6]. Generally, by inducing the secretion of proinflammatory cytokines and chemokines, PRRs not only mediate downstream intracellular events related to pathogen clearance but also participate in complex and disparate processes of immunomodulation and activation of adaptive immunity through the coordination of T cell and B cell responses [16]. Pathogen recognition by the innate immune system is further supported by the opsonic activity of soluble PRRs, including collectins, ficolins, pentraxins, and complement components, which facilitate the interaction with phagocytes. On the other hand, PRRs are also able to respond to products released from damaged host cells during infection and other causes of injury (e.g., trauma and ischemia reperfusion), including nucleic acids and alarmin proteins, collectively known as danger-associated molecular patterns.

The role of TLRs in antimicrobial defense was first proposed in 1996 by Lemaitre and colleagues, following the observation that fruit flies lacking the hematocyte receptor Toll – which indirectly recognizes pathogens through the cytokine-like protein Spätzle – were highly susceptible to infection with fungi and Gram-negative bacteria [17]. This study was followed shortly by the discovery of TLRs expressed on cells of the mammalian immune system, and since then, 13 TLRs have been discovered. The extracellular domains of these receptors contain leucine-rich repeats that recognize PAMPs from all major classes of pathogens, whereas the amino acid sequence of the cytoplasmic domain is highly homologous to the sequences in the interleukin (IL)-1 and IL-18 receptors [18]. Ligand recognition by TLRs and intracellular signaling transduction by adaptor molecules that contain Toll-IL-1R (TIR) domains activate kinase cascades and promote the translocation of transcription factors to the nucleus, where they induce gene expression and downstream production of cytokines [15, 19] (Fig. 6.1).

The large family of CLRs includes members such as dectin-1, dectin-2, macrophage mannose receptor, dendritic cell-specific intercellular adhesion molecule 3-grabbing non-integrin (DC-SIGN), macrophage inducible C-type lectin (Mincle), macrophage C-type lectin (MCL), and dectin-2. These receptors have carbohydrate recognition domains and bind microbial polysaccharides commonly present in fungi and bacteria [20]. Dectin-1 was the first CLR to be identified and is currently the best described non-TLR receptor able to instruct activation of adaptive immunity. Following recognition of β-1,3-glucans, dectin-1 triggers different intracellular signaling pathways that, synergistically and through cross-regulatory mechanisms, regulate and fine-tune nuclear factor (NF)-κB activation and cytokine gene expression [21] (Fig. 6.2).

In addition to the mainly membrane-bound TLRs and CLRs, there are cytoplasmic receptors – NLRs and the DNA-sensing RIG-I helicase receptors – that are activated by pathogens when they invade a cell. NLRs recognize the peptidoglycans of the bacterial cell

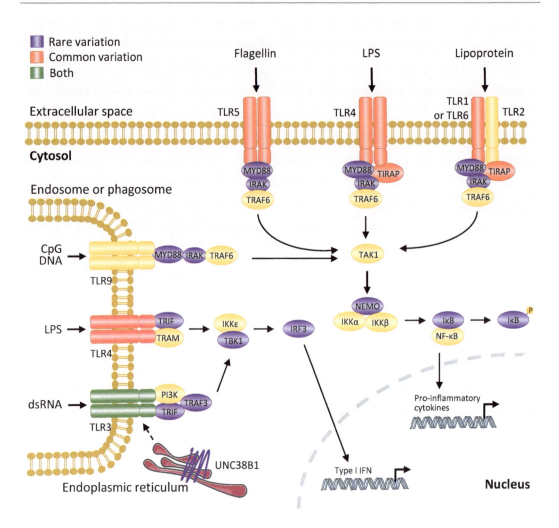

Fig. 6.1 Genetic defects affecting Toll-like receptor signaling and their role in susceptibility to infection. Toll-like receptors (TLRs) are present on the cell surface and in endosomes, where they detect pathogen-associated molecular patterns (PAMPs) such as lipopolysaccharide (LPS), lipoprotein, flagellin, CpG DNA, and double-stranded RNA. Upon stimulation, TLRs activate two disparate pathways that involve myeloid differentiation primary response 88 (MyD88) and/or Toll-interleukin (IL)-1 receptor (TIR) domain-containing adapter-inducing interferon (IFN)-β (TRIF). Crosstalk between TLR signaling cascades underlies the activation of different cellular processes, including the transcription of proinflammatory cytokines and chemokines and type I IFN. Major genetic variation in TLR signaling pathways implicated in susceptibility to infection is indicated in *purple* (rare), *red* (common), or *green* (evidence of both rare and common variation). *TIRAP* Toll-interleukin-1 receptor (TIR) domain-containing adaptor protein, *TRAM* TRIF-related adaptor molecule, *IRAK* IL-1 receptor-associated kinase, *TRAF* tumor necrosis factor receptor-associated factor, *UNC93B1* unc-93 homologue B1, *TAK1* transforming growth factor-β-activated kinase 1, *NF-κB* nuclear factor-κB, *NEMO* NF-κB essential modulator, *IKK* inhibitor of NF-κB kinase, *IκB* inhibitor of NF-κB, *IRF* IFN regulatory factor, *TBK1* TANK-binding kinase 1, *PI3K* phosphoinositide 3-kinase, *dsRNA* double-stranded RNA

wall and can activate inflammasomes, multimeric protein complexes that convert inactive pro-IL-1β and pro-IL-18 into bioactive cytokines [22]. The NLR family members NOD-containing receptors 1 (NOD1) and NOD2 recognize muramyl peptide moieties of the peptidoglycans of Gram-negative and Gram-positive bacteria, respectively [23, 24]. The RIG-I helicase receptors are known to recognize mainly viral nucleic acids and to activate inflammasome formation [25].

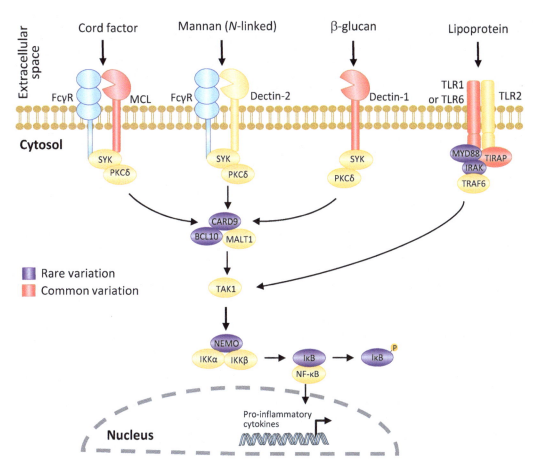

Fig. 6.2 Genetic defects affecting C-type lectin receptor signaling and their role in susceptibility to infection. The family of C-type lectin receptors (CLRs) recognizes microbial polysaccharides commonly present in fungi and bacteria. Cord factor is a commonly used term to refer to trehalose dimycolate, a glycolipid molecule found in the cell wall of *M. tuberculosis* and similar species. Upon stimulation, CLRs activate intracellular signaling pathways that, synergistically and through cross-regulatory mechanisms, regulate and fine-tune nuclear factor (NF)-κB activation and cytokine gene expression. Major genetic variation in CLR signaling pathways implicated in susceptibility to infection is indicated in *purple* (rare) or *red* (common). *FCγR* Fcγ receptor, *MCL* macrophage C-type lectin, *SYK* spleen tyrosine kinase, *PKCδ* protein kinase C-δ, *MyD88* myeloid differentiation primary response 88, *TIRAP* Toll-interleukin-1 receptor (TIR) domain-containing adaptor protein, *IRAK* IL-1 receptor-associated kinase, *TRAF* tumor necrosis factor receptor-associated factor, *CARD9* caspase recruitment domain-containing protein 9, *BCL10* B cell CLL/lymphoma 10, *MALT1* mucosa-associated lymphoid tissue lymphoma translocation protein 1, *NF-κB* nuclear factor-κB, *NEMO* NF-κB essential modulator, *TAK1* transforming growth factor-β-activated kinase 1, *IKK* inhibitor of NF-κB kinase

Ultimately, the coordinated regulation of the immune response will depend not only on the relative degree of stimulation of the individual receptors but also on the level of receptor cooperation and cellular localization. For example, synergy between TLRs and NOD2 is crucial for the activation of host defense against mycobacteria and staphylococci [26], and crosstalk between TLRs and CLRs is needed for optimal antifungal responses [27].

Genetic Defects in Pattern Recognition Receptors and Susceptibility to Infection

Genetic variants in the genes encoding PRRs can affect susceptibility to many infectious diseases. Importantly, genetic defects in these receptors or the downstream signaling pathways can cause immunodeficiency phenotypes rendering patients extremely susceptible to severe, life-threatening infections. We know of genetic defects across the different classes of PRRs, although in some cases (e.g., the NLR family) these have yet to be linked with susceptibility to infection. An overview of the genetic variants affecting PRRs reported in association with susceptibility to specific infectious diseases is presented in Table 6.1.

Genetic Variation in Toll-Like Receptor Signaling

Soon after the initial description of TLRs, genetic variability in these molecules was proposed to underlie differences in susceptibility to infectious and inflammatory diseases [28]. The first genetic variation to be described was polymorphisms in TLR4, specifically two amino acid changes reported to decrease the interaction of the receptor with lipopolysaccharide [29] and to increase susceptibility to Gram-negative bacterial sepsis [30]. During the subsequent decade and up until now, a multitude of studies described genetic variation in practically all TLRs (Fig. 6.1).

Myeloid differentiation primary response 88 (MyD88) is an adaptor molecule that transduces signals from TLRs (with the exception of TLR3 and the IL-1 and IL-18 receptors) [31]. The signaling involves a cascade of protein kinases which include the serine-threonine IL-1R-associated kinase 4 (IRAK4) [19]. The activation of the MyD88 and IRAK4 pathways has been deemed essential for the immune response to pyogenic bacteria based on the study of patients with rare mutations in these genes that resulted in invasive disease by *Streptococcus pneumoniae* and, to a lesser extent, by *Staphylococcus aureus*, *Pseudomonas aeruginosa*, or *Salmonella* species

[32, 33]. Several hypomorphic mutations have been identified in *MYD88* and *IRAK4* genes; two of them leading to MyD88 deficiency affecting amino acids in key positions for the interaction of the adaptor with IRAK4 [34]. Despite the manifest susceptibility to pyogenic bacteria, children with MyD88 and IRAK4 deficiency are typically resistant to other bacteria, mycobacteria, viruses, and fungi, and classically, their immunodeficiency improves with age, with less frequent and less severe forms of infection [35]. This may suggest that the development of protective T cell- or B cell-mediated immune responses after infancy compensates for the defective inflammatory reaction in the absence of proper TLR signaling [36].

Mutations in genes from the NF-κB pathway that interrupt multiple innate and adaptive pathways that signal to NF-κB, including TLR-mediated signaling, have also been identified [37–40]. In particular, hypomorphic mutations in NF-κB essential modulator (*NEMO*), which encodes the I-κB kinase regulatory subunit IKKγ, and IκBα inhibitor of NF-κB (*IKBA*) have been reported to underlie typically severe infections by a broad range of pathogens, including encapsulated bacteria, atypical mycobacteria, fungi, and viruses, and are also associated with ectodermal dysplasia [37–40].

In addition to the RIG-I helicase receptors, TLR3, TLR7, TLR8, and TLR9 bind to different microbial nucleic acids [15, 19]. Genetic defects in TLR3 [41] or proteins involved in the TLR3 pathway such as unc-93 homologue B1 (UNC93B1) [42] and TIR-domain-containing adapter-inducing interferon (IFN)-β (TRIF) [43] or tumor necrosis factor (TNF) receptor-associated factor 3 (TRAF3) [44] have been identified as rare causes of isolated susceptibility to recurrent, life-threatening encephalitis caused by herpes simplex virus-1 (HSV-1) in otherwise healthy children displaying normal resistance to other forms of HSV disease and indeed to other viruses. Herpes simplex encephalitis (HSE) has been linked to defects in the release of type I IFN, and importantly, blocking TLR3-dependent production of interferons in vitro enhanced viral replication leading to cell death, effects that were abrogated by recombinant IFN-β [41].

Table 6.1 Monogenic and polygenic defects in pattern recognition receptors and susceptibility to infectious diseases

PRR deficiency	Presumed defect(s)	Reported infection(s)	Frequency
TLR signaling			
MyD88	TLR signaling (Except TLR3)	Pyogenic bacteria	Very rare
IRAK4	TLR signaling (Except TLR3)	Pyogenic bacteria	Very rare
NEMO	TLR signaling	Pyogenic bacteria	Very rare
IKBA	TLR signaling	Pyogenic bacteria	Very rare
TLR3	dsRNA recognition	HSV	Very rare
	dsRNA recognition	*Aspergillus*	Common
UNC93B1	dsRNA recognition	HSV	Very rare
TRIF	TLR3 signaling	HSV	Very rare
TRAF3	TLR3 signaling	HSV	Very rare
TBK1	TLR3 signaling	HSV	Very rare
IRF3	TLR3 signaling	HSV	Very rare
IRF7	TLR7 and/or RIG-I signaling	Influenza virus	Very rare
TLR1	Lipopeptide recognition	Gram (+) bacteria, *Candida*	Common
TLR4	LPS recognition	Gram (−) bacteria, *Aspergillus*	Common
TLR5	Flagellin recognition	*Legionella*	Common
TIRAP	TLR2 and TLR4 signaling	*Mycobacterium*, gram (−) bacteria	Common
CLR signaling			
Dectin-1	β-Glucan recognition	*Candida, Trichophyton, Aspergillus*	Common
CARD9	CLR signaling	*Trichophyton, Exophiala*	Very rare
MCL	MCF recognition	*Mycobacterium*	Common
Soluble PRRs			
MBL	Opsonization	*Neisseria, Streptococcus*	Common
PTX3	Opsonization and fungicidal activity	*Aspergillus*	Common
PLG	Opsonization	*Aspergillus*	Common

PRR pattern recognition receptor, *TLR* Toll-like receptor, *CLR* C-type lectin receptor, *MyD88* myeloid differentiation primary response 88, *IRAK4* interleukin-1 receptor (IL-1R)-associated kinase 4, *NEMO* nuclear factor-κB (NF-κB) essential modulator, *IKBA* IκBα inhibitor of NF-κB, *UNC93B1*:unc-93 homologue B1, *TRIF* Toll-IL-1R (TIR) domain-containing adapter-inducing interferon β (IFNβ), *TRAF3* tumor necrosis factor receptor-associated factor 3, *TBK1* TRAF family member-associated NF-κB activator-binding kinase 1, *IRF* IFN regulatory factor, *TIRAP* TIR domain-containing adaptor protein, *CARD9* caspase recruitment domain-containing protein 9, *MCL* macrophage C-type lectin, *MBL* mannose-binding lectin, *PTX3* long pentraxin 3, *PLG* plasminogen, *dsRNA* double-stranded RNA, *RIG-I* retinoic acid-inducible gene I protein, *MCF* mycobacterial cord factor, *HSV* herpes simplex virus

Accordingly, children with HSE have been found to carry different heterozygous mutations in TRAF family member-associated NF-κB activator (TANK)-binding kinase 1 (*TBK1*), a kinase at the crossroads of multiple IFN-inducing signaling pathways [45]. Similar to TLR3 deficiency, fibroblasts from these patients displayed enhanced viral replication, whereas responses to TLR3-independent viruses were instead preserved. These findings were substantiated by the identification of a deficiency in the signal transducer and activator of transcription 1 (STAT1) protein, a signaling molecule in the type I IFN pathway, that resulted in the production of insufficient levels of type I IFN and susceptibility to HSE [46, 47].

A novel genetic etiology of HSE due to heterozygous loss-of-function in the IFN regulatory factor 3 (*IRF3*) gene – activated by several TLRs that bind viruses [48] – was also identified, providing the first description of a defect in an IFN-regulating transcription factor that confers increased susceptibility to viral infection of the human central nervous system [49]. Genetic susceptibility to other viruses, particularly influenza, among otherwise healthy children was also reported to result from compound heterozygous null mutations in *IRF7* [50]. In response to influenza virus, cells from these patients produced very little type I and III IFN while failing to control viral replication, suggesting that IRF7-dependent amplification of type I and III IFN is essentially required for protection against primary infection by influenza virus in humans.

Although the complete deficiencies in the TLR pathways have a large effect size, they are generally rare events (with the remarkable exception of TLR5 deficiency, discussed below) on the scale of an entire population. The genes encoding TLRs are however prominently polymorphic and encode many variant amino acid sites. Before the advent of genome-wide association studies (GWAS), polymorphisms in TLRs were considered outstanding, biologically plausible candidates for involvement in enhanced susceptibility to multiple infectious diseases [28]. Common polymorphisms in all TLRs have been described and a wealth of studies have reported their association with infection susceptibility. Excellent literature has already described those association studies in detail; therefore, we will focus mainly on discussing the most relevant studies evaluating TLR polymorphisms and their functional implications in the immunodeficient host.

As mentioned above, a TLR4 haplotype consisting of the D299G and T399I substitutions has been shown to be associated with an increased risk of sepsis [30] and is suggested to result in defective responses to lipopolysaccharide [29]. However, several other studies have failed to replicate these data at both genetic and functional levels [51], raising issues related to small sample sizes, population stratification, or the definition of case status. Interestingly, an enhanced production of TNF upon TLR4 stimulation has been demonstrated in cells from D299G, but not haplotype, carriers [52]. Nonetheless, the TLR4 haplotype was associated with the occurrence of infectious complications in HIV-1-infected patients – especially those with a history of low nadir CD4 cell counts [53] – and both sepsis and pneumonia in patients with acute myeloid leukemia following induction chemotherapy [54]. In addition, the

presence of these TLR4 variants in donors of stem cell transplantation has been disclosed as an important risk factor for developing invasive aspergillosis (IA) in the corresponding patients [55], a finding that was confirmed in two independent populations [56, 57]. Despite that the fungal ligand (or the host-derived molecule released in response to fungal infection) for TLR4 remains debated, the TLR4 haplotype was reported to underlie a delayed T cell and natural killer T cell immune reconstitution among stem cell transplant recipients [57]. The biological implications of these studies are further supported by the previous links of TLR4 variants with chronic aspergillosis in immunocompetent individuals [58] and fungal colonization in stem cell transplant recipients [59].

It is noteworthy that, in addition to TLR4, common genetic variation in other TLRs has also been proposed to influence the risk of infectious diseases. For example, genetic variation in TLR1 has been found to increase susceptibility to organ dysfunction and Gram-positive sepsis [60] and candidemia [61] and, most importantly, to impact the inflammatory response to bacterial lipopeptides [62]. On the other hand, a regulatory variant decreasing the expression of TLR3 was found to impair the recognition of fungal nucleic acids by dendritic cells and to compromise the efficient priming of protective memory CD8+ T cell responses, thereby rendering stem cell transplant recipients more prone to develop IA [63]. Ultimately, the evaluation of regulatory variation impacting adaptive immunity might help to enhance the discriminatory potential of recent immunodiagnostic strategies based on the evaluation of fungal-specific adaptive immune responses [64]. Specifically, patients suffering from IA display an enhanced in vitro expansion of IL-10-producing T cells following antigenic stimulation, and this has been proposed as a potential diagnostic approach in hematological patients [64]. However, we recently found that a regulatory variant in IL-10, and that underlies an increased risk of IA, regulated the expression of IL-10 and coordinated the activation of proinflammatory responses to the fungus [65]. This observation implies therefore that diagnostic (and immunotherapeutic) approaches are required to consider interindividual variability in immune function.

Other significant examples of variants affecting TLR signaling and associated with enhanced susceptibility to infectious disease are those in the adaptor Mal (encoded by *TIRAP*), which is part of the TLR2- and TLR4-dependent pathways [6]. Polymorphisms in TIRAP, particularly the S180L substitution, were initially shown to confer resistance to tuberculosis [66, 67] and septic shock [68], although a large meta-analysis failed to confirm this [69], ultimately reflecting the difficulties faced in ascribing host genetics to enhanced susceptibility to tuberculosis [13]. A similar case is also illustrated by the TLR5 deficiency. TLR5 is a receptor for flagellin, the PAMP present in the flagellum of flagellated bacteria [70]. Hawn and colleagues described a common polymorphism in TLR5 leading to the introduction of an early stop codon that was described to abrogate recognition of flagellin and leading to increased susceptibility to *Legionella* pneumonia [71]. Of note, this susceptibility phenotype is generally mild and affects the control of only certain flagellated pathogens. More recently, TLR5 deficiency was associated with increased risk of IA following stem cell transplantation [72], but further studies are warranted to identify the mechanism(s) by which TLR5 might influence susceptibility to fungal disease. In any case, the high and variable frequencies of this polymorphism, without forcing a severe primary immunodeficiency phenotype, suggest that it has a redundant role in host defense [73].

Genetic Variation in C-Type Lectin Receptor Signaling

In addition to TLRs, genetic variation in CLRs has been implicated in susceptibility to infectious diseases, namely, those caused by fungi (Fig. 6.2). Dectin-1 is the major PRR for β-1,3-glucan in the fungal cell wall [20], and it also recognizes components of *Mycobacterium tuberculosis* [74]. Genetic analysis of a family with recurrent vulvovaginal candidiasis and onychomycosis resulted in the identification of an early stop codon in *CLEC7A*, the gene encoding dectin-1 [75]. The truncated protein compromised the surface expression of dectin-1 in myeloid cells, thereby affecting their ability to bind β-glucan. This defect impaired the production of cytokines – namely, IL-6, TNF, and especially IL-17 – while it did not affect the ability of neutrophils to ingest and kill *Candida albicans* yeasts. This indicates that the contribution of dectin-1 deficiency to mucosal candidiasis likely relies on a defect in the activation of Th17-mediated immunity and not on activation of dectin-1 expressed on neutrophils.

The clinical phenotype of patients with dectin-1 deficiency is relatively mild and less severe than that of patients with classic chronic mucocutaneous candidiasis [76]. In fact, about 6 to 8% of Europeans are heterozygous for a disabling variant of the gene, and they do not, however, have an apparent immunodeficiency [75]. Yet, heterozygous carriers of the dectin-1 stop codon are more prone to develop IA [77, 78] and to be colonized with *C. albicans* [79] when undergoing stem cell transplantation. The fact that dectin-1 deficiency in both transplant donors and recipients synergizes toward risk of infection highlights the pivotal contribution of dectin-1 expression in multiple cell types to antifungal immunity. Thus, dectin-1 deficiency resembles a genetic polymorphism, which under specific circumstances (e.g., immunosuppression typical of certain clinical settings) is associated with susceptibility to fungal infection and/or colonization. Of note, a common polymorphism in another CLR, namely, MCL (encoded by *CLECSF8*), was recently associated with susceptibility to pulmonary tuberculosis, and a non-redundant role for this receptor in antimycobacterial immunity was proposed [80].

Several members of a family with mutations in caspase recruitment domain-containing protein 9 (*CARD9*), the adaptor molecule that mediates signaling induced by dectin-1 and other CLRs, have been found to display increased susceptibility to mucocutaneous fungal infections [81]. More recently, CARD9 deficiency was identified in patients suffering from deep dermatophytosis, a severe fungal infection caused by dermatophytes and characterized by extensive dermal and subcutaneous tissue invasion and by frequent dissemination to the lymph nodes and, occasionally, the central nervous system. Similar to dectin-1, patients with CARD9 mutations display a severe defect of IL-17 production [81, 82], a finding further supporting the pivotal role of the β-glucan recognition and Th17-mediated responses in antifungal immunity. Of note, individuals with inherited defects in B cell CLL/lymphoma 10 (BCL10), a protein that binds CARD9 to activate NF-κB signaling, displayed normal responses to a variety of PAMPs but impaired NF-κB-mediated functions [83]. The fact that susceptibility to infectious diseases was not reported highlights the selective role of dectin-1-/CARD9-dependent signaling in the immune response to fungal infection. Because multiple CLRs signal through CARD9, one can hypothesize that the more severe phenotypes of CARD9 deficiency are most likely due to antifungal immunity mechanisms that are independent of dectin-1 [84–86].

Defects of Soluble Pattern Recognition Receptors

Some components of the complement system have the capacity to interact with and bind to microbial polysaccharides without transducing intracellular signals, thereby functioning as soluble PRRs. One such molecule is the circulating mannose-binding lectin (MBL), which binds carbohydrate structures of microorganisms and activates the complement system [87]. MBL deficiency was initially reported in children with recurrent bacterial infections (especially *Neisseria meningitidis*), in addition to viral and fungal infections [88]. Subsequent studies showed however that polymorphisms in MBL drive a strong decrease in the levels of functional protein in as much as 8% of individuals in a given population, and yet, these do not display any obvious clinical consequences [89]. There is however evidence that MBL deficiency, although not being an outright immunodeficiency, acts as a risk factor for infection, especially in conditions of immunosuppression. For example, genetically

determined low serum concentrations of MBL were detected among immunocompromised patients suffering from IA [90], although the causal nature for this association remains unknown.

Another important molecule with opsonic activity is the long pentraxin 3 (PTX3), which has been shown to bind microbial moieties from a vast range of pathogens, including bacteria, viruses, and fungi [87]. Although no classic immunodeficiency phenotype related to PTX3 has been disclosed to date, common polymorphisms have been proposed as risk factors for multiple infectious diseases, most remarkably, urinary tract infections [91] and IA following stem cell transplantation [92]. The results from the latter study were confirmed by the validation of the association in a large, independent study [93]. The PTX3 deficiency was found to compromise the alveolar availability of the protein and, at a cellular level, its expression during the developmental programming of neutrophil precursors in the bone marrow, leading to defective antifungal effector mechanisms of mature cells [92]. Importantly, this association was recently replicated in recipients of lung transplant [94], highlighting a potential applicability of these markers in predicting fungal infection across patients with intrinsically different predisposing conditions. Alveolar levels of PTX3 have been demonstrated to discriminate microbiologically confirmed pneumonia in mechanically ventilated patients [95]. Given that these vary individually according to PTX3 genotypes [92], we can envisage the quantification of PTX3 in bronchoalveolar lavage fluids as a complementary surveillance measure in addition to the currently available diagnostic approaches. Finally, the fact that exogenous administration of PTX3 is able to revert the genetic defect in vitro, namely, by restoring the ability of neutrophils to adequately ingest and kill the fungus [92], further highlights the potential of PTX3-based immunotherapies to treat (or prevent) fungal infection [96].

Other relevant examples of genetic defects in soluble PRRs include the identification of a deleterious variant in plasminogen – a regulatory molecule with opsonic properties – as an important modulator of susceptibility to IA in humans using the genetic mapping analysis of survival data of animals subjected to experimental infection as discovery strategy [97]. Finally, microbial polysaccharides are also recognized by β_2-integrins such as complement receptor 3 (CD11b-CD18), which is required for neutrophil adhesion to endothelial cells and functions as a neutrophil β-glucan receptor [98]. The increased susceptibility to recurrent bacterial infections displayed by patients with leukocyte adhesion deficiency I is mainly due to defective processes of leukocyte adhesion.

Opportunities for Clinical Translation of Infectious Disease Genetics

Recent studies have clearly implicated genetic variation in PRRs and downstream signaling pathways in the susceptibility to infectious diseases. This is particularly true for several immunodeficiency syndromes, in which causal effects have been clearly defined and measures for patient-tailored management are now in place or under evaluation. Nevertheless, considerable further work is required in many cases to identify the causative alleles, their functional consequences, and the biological mechanisms by which they influence disease pathogenesis. A major challenge is to develop strategies for translating insights from the genetic basis of common infectious disease into improved patient outcomes. This objective has been hampered thus far by the size of the genotypic effect, which is often not sufficiently discriminatory to inform clinical decision-making. To enhance the predictive value of the genotypic information, future studies are expected to integrate it with other host and pathogen factors into combined predictive models to prospectively evaluate risk of and progression of disease, including treatment responses and durations, and adverse events.

It is plausible that the considerable genetic variation in PRR signaling may influence therapeutic strategies aimed at manipulating these pathways. Clinical trials that fail to take into account human genetic variation may omit relevant consequences on subgroups of individuals, such as those with extremes of inflammatory signaling. Indeed, such effects may partly account for the disappointing outcomes of clinical trials of anti-inflammatory agents for the treatment of sepsis. Thus, there is a need to identify the functional genetic variants controlling interindividual variation in PRR signaling and to stratify clinical trials of immunomodulatory agents by host genotypes.

The use of genetic information to predict risk of common infectious disease is unlikely to alter clinical practice in the near future, and the prognostic significance of genetic tools for risk assessment remains poor, even in more extensively studied, noninfectious disease traits. Clinical translation is more likely to result from the characterization of the molecular and cellular pathways involved in disease and the identification of novel targets for immunomodulatory drugs or vaccines, especially in the context of monogenic defects. Another interesting example regards the identification of the gene defect in PTX3 underlying IA, which raises the possibility to use recombinant PTX3 treatment to supplement antifungal agents, as demonstrated in animal models of infection [99, 100]. Furthermore, the application of systems biology to integrate genome-wide studies, including genomic, transcriptomic, proteomic, or metabolomic profiles, and their integration with clinical data may be a particularly powerful approach for identifying novel therapeutic targets [101]. Indeed, next-generation sequencing technologies now provide exciting avenues to pin down essential steps in host-pathogen interactions at a level of complexity previously unanticipated. Several GWAS exploring susceptibility to infection have been completed and provide unbiased insights into the genetic defects contributing to the development of disease. In this regard, recent functional genomics analyses have allowed the identification of new important players controlling susceptibility to candidemia in critical ill patients [102, 103]. These efforts are however centered on the fairly "static" role of the genetic variants. Physiological responses to infection require the coordinated regulation of gene expression, which may vary markedly between individuals and influence phenotypes such as protein levels, the immune cell morphology and function, and ultimately immunity to infection. Thus, genetic analysis of molecular traits such as the gene expression represents a powerful approach enabling insights into the human genomic landscape by generating expression maps useful for the functional interpretation of noncoding variants likely to arise from the ongoing genome-wide initiatives [104].

Conclusions and Perspectives

The clinical features of defects in PRRs are generally credited to an impaired cytokine response underlying increased susceptibility to infections (e.g., TLR3 and MyD88 deficiencies). Although genetic defects in NLRP3 are known to lead to an overwhelming release of proinflammatory cytokines, particularly IL-1β, these still remain to be associated with infectious diseases. Another critical point that deserves mention regards the clinical range of manifestations of PRR defects that range from severe (e.g., MyD88 and IRAK4 deficiencies) to mild (e.g., MBL, TLR5, and PTX3 deficiencies). In addition, the fact that several defects are associated with infection typically during infancy suggests that the maturation of proper adaptive immune responses may compensate for the innate immunity shortcomings. The field of primary immunodeficiencies has been shifting from research on rare familial defects in the adaptive immune system to studies of sporadic and selective disorders of the innate immunity; the defects in PRRs are an enlightening example of this change. By unraveling the functional consequences of these "experiments of nature," it has been possible to confer clinical relevance to immunologic pathways, which until now have been studied exclusively in the laboratory or using experimental models of infection.

The importance of the studies addressing polygenic susceptibility to common infectious diseases also deserves to be highlighted. Although the overall weight of the immune response is driven by adding effects of single genetic factors with modest effect sizes and their complex interactions with clinical immune dysfunctions, approaches based on individual genomics may warrant important clinical tools allowing discrimination of patients that might benefit from enhanced surveillance for infection or alternative therapies. By overcoming the limitations related to the study design discussed above, these approaches are expected to define the pathogenetic mechanisms at the basis of common infectious diseases and lay the foundations for well-designed prospective trials ultimately endorsing genetic testing in risk stratification approaches for infection, particularly among immunocompromised hosts. Perhaps more importantly, an improved understanding of the multiple pathways directly affected by host genetic variation will contribute to innovative strategies of immunotherapy. As shown for the PTX3 deficiency in stem cell transplant recipients [92], targeting cell function (e.g., exogenous administration of lacking or deficient factors) may prove an interesting approach to be validated in the future.

Acknowledgments This work was supported by the Northern Portugal Regional Operational Programme (NORTE 2020), under the Portugal 2020 Partnership Agreement, through the European Regional Development Fund (FEDER) (NORTE-01-0145-FEDER-000013), and the Fundação para a Ciência e Tecnologia (FCT) (IF/00735/2014 to A.C. and SFRH/BPD/96176/2013 to C.C.)

References

1. Alcais A, Abel L, Casanova JL. Human genetics of infectious diseases: between proof of principle and paradigm. J Clin Invest. 2009;119(9):2506–14. https://doi.org/10.1172/JCI38111.
2. Burgner D, Jamieson SE, Blackwell JM. Genetic susceptibility to infectious diseases: big is beautiful, but will bigger be even better? Lancet Infect Dis. 2006;6(10):653–63. https://doi.org/10.1016/S1473-3099(06)70601-6.
3. Chapman SJ, Hill AV. Human genetic susceptibility to infectious disease. Nat Rev Genet. 2012;13(3):175–88. https://doi.org/10.1038/nrg3114.

4. Hill AV. Aspects of genetic susceptibility to human infectious diseases. Annu Rev Genet. 2006;40:469–86. https://doi.org/10.1146/annurev.genet.40.110405.090546.

5. Netea MG, van der Meer JW. Immunodeficiency and genetic defects of pattern-recognition receptors. N Engl J Med. 2011;364(1):60–70. https://doi.org/10.1056/NEJMra1001976.

6. Netea MG, Wijmenga C, O'Neill LA. Genetic variation in Toll-like receptors and disease susceptibility. Nat Immunol. 2012;13(6):535–42. https://doi.org/10.1038/ni.2284.

7. van der Eijk EA, van de Vosse E, Vandenbroucke JP, van Dissel JT. Heredity versus environment in tuberculosis in twins: the 1950s United Kingdom Prophit Survey Simonds and Comstock revisited. Am J Respir Crit Care Med. 2007;176(12):1281–8. https://doi.org/10.1164/rccm.200703-435OC.

8. Sorensen TI, Nielsen GG, Andersen PK, Teasdale TW. Genetic and environmental influences on premature death in adult adoptees. N Engl J Med. 1988;318(12):727–32. https://doi.org/10.1056/NEJM198803243181202.

9. Gingles NA, Alexander JE, Kadioglu A, Andrew PW, Kerr A, Mitchell TJ, et al. Role of genetic resistance in invasive pneumococcal infection: identification and study of susceptibility and resistance in inbred mouse strains. Infect Immun. 2001;69(1):426–34. https://doi.org/10.1128/IAI.69.1.426-434.2001.

10. Allison AC. Protection afforded by sickle-cell trait against subtertian malarial infection. Br Med J. 1954;1(4857):290–4.

11. Casanova JL, Abel L. Primary immunodeficiencies: a field in its infancy. Science. 2007;317(5838):617–9. https://doi.org/10.1126/science.1142963.

12. Misch EA, Berrington WR, Vary JC Jr, Hawn TR. Leprosy and the human genome. Microbiol Mol Biol Rev: MMBR. 2010;74(4):589–620. https://doi.org/10.1128/MMBR.00025-10.

13. Stein CM. Genetic epidemiology of tuberculosis susceptibility: impact of study design. PLoS Pathog. 2011;7(1):e1001189. https://doi.org/10.1371/journal.ppat.1001189.

14. O'Neill LA, Bowie AG. The family of five: TIR-domain-containing adaptors in toll-like receptor signalling. Nat Rev Immunol. 2007;7(5):353–64. https://doi.org/10.1038/nri2079.

15. Akira S, Uematsu S, Takeuchi O. Pathogen recognition and innate immunity. Cell. 2006;124(4):783–801. https://doi.org/10.1016/j.cell.2006.02.015.

16. Iwasaki A, Medzhitov R. Regulation of adaptive immunity by the innate immune system. Science. 2010;327(5963):291–5. https://doi.org/10.1126/science.1183021.

17. Lemaitre B, Nicolas E, Michaut L, Reichhart JM, Hoffmann JA. The dorsoventral regulatory gene cassette spatzle/Toll/cactus controls the potent antifungal response in Drosophila adults. Cell. 1996;86(6):973–83.

18. Rock FL, Hardiman G, Timans JC, Kastelein RA, Bazan JF. A family of human receptors structurally related to Drosophila Toll. Proc Natl Acad Sci U S A. 1998;95(2):588–93.

19. Akira S, Takeda K. Toll-like receptor signalling. Nat Rev Immunol. 2004;4(7):499–511. https://doi.org/10.1038/nri1391.

20. Hardison SE, Brown GD. C-type lectin receptors orchestrate antifungal immunity. Nat Immunol. 2012;13(9):817–22. https://doi.org/10.1038/ni.2369.

21. Geijtenbeek TB, Gringhuis SI. Signalling through C-type lectin receptors: shaping immune responses. Nat Rev Immunol. 2009;9(7):465–79.

22. Guo H, Callaway JB, Ting JP. Inflammasomes: mechanism of action, role in disease, and therapeutics. Nat Med. 2015;21(7):677–87. https://doi.org/10.1038/nm.3893.

23. Girardin SE, Boneca IG, Carneiro LA, Antignac A, Jehanno M, Viala J, et al. Nod1 detects a unique muropeptide from gram-negative bacterial peptidoglycan. Science. 2003;300(5625):1584–7. https://doi.org/10.1126/science.1084677.

24. Girardin SE, Boneca IG, Viala J, Chamaillard M, Labigne A, Thomas G, et al. Nod2 is a general sensor of peptidoglycan through muramyl dipeptide (MDP) detection. J Biol Chem. 2003;278(11):8869–72. https://doi.org/10.1074/jbc.C200651200.

25. Kell AM, Gale M Jr. RIG-I in RNA virus recognition. Virology. 2015;479-480:110–21. https://doi.org/10.1016/j.virol.2015.02.017.

26. Ferwerda G, Girardin SE, Kullberg BJ, Le Bourhis L, de Jong DJ, Langenberg DM, et al. NOD2 and toll-like receptors are nonredundant recognition systems of Mycobacterium tuberculosis. PLoS Pathog. 2005;1(3):279–85. https://doi.org/10.1371/journal.ppat.0010034.

27. Netea MG, Joosten LA, van der Meer JW, Kullberg BJ, van de Veerdonk FL. Immune defence against Candida fungal infections. Nat Rev Immunol. 2015;15(10):630–42. https://doi.org/10.1038/nri3897.

28. Schroder NW, Schumann RR. Single nucleotide polymorphisms of Toll-like receptors and susceptibility to infectious disease. Lancet Infect Dis. 2005;5(3):156–64. https://doi.org/10.1016/S1473-3099(05)01308-3.

29. Arbour NC, Lorenz E, Schutte BC, Zabner J, Kline JN, Jones M, et al. TLR4 mutations are associated with endotoxin hyporesponsiveness in humans. Nat Genet. 2000;25(2):187–91. https://doi.org/10.1038/76048.

30. Lorenz E, Mira JP, Frees KL, Schwartz DA. Relevance of mutations in the TLR4 receptor in patients with gram-negative septic shock. Arch Intern Med. 2002;162(9):1028–32.

31. Adachi O, Kawai T, Takeda K, Matsumoto M, Tsutsui H, Sakagami M, et al. Targeted disruption of the MyD88 gene results in loss of IL-1- and IL-18-mediated function. Immunity. 1998;9(1):143–50.

32. Picard C, Puel A, Bonnet M, Ku CL, Bustamante J, Yang K, et al. Pyogenic bacterial infections in humans with IRAK-4 deficiency. Science. 2003;299(5615):2076–9. https://doi.org/10.1126/science.1081902.

33. von Bernuth H, Picard C, Jin Z, Pankla R, Xiao H, Ku CL, et al. Pyogenic bacterial infections in humans with MyD88 deficiency. Science. 2008;321(5889):691–6. https://doi.org/10.1126/science.1158298.

34. Lin SC, Lo YC, Wu H. Helical assembly in the MyD88-IRAK4-IRAK2 complex in TLR/IL-1R signalling. Nature. 2010;465(7300):885–90. https://doi.org/10.1038/nature09121.

35. Bousfiha A, Picard C, Boisson-Dupuis S, Zhang SY, Bustamante J, Puel A, et al. Primary immunodeficiencies of protective immunity to primary infections. Clin Immunol. 2010;135(2):204–9. https://doi.org/10.1016/j.clim.2010.02.001.

36. Ku CL, von Bernuth H, Picard C, Zhang SY, Chang HH, Yang K, et al. Selective predisposition to bacterial infections in IRAK-4-deficient children: IRAK-4-dependent TLRs are otherwise redundant in protective immunity. J Exp Med. 2007;204(10):2407–22. https://doi.org/10.1084/jem.20070628.

37. Courtois G, Smahi A, Reichenbach J, Doffinger R, Cancrini C, Bonnet M, et al. A hypermorphic IkappaBalpha mutation is associated with autosomal dominant anhidrotic ectodermal dysplasia and T cell immunodeficiency. J Clin Invest. 2003;112(7):1108–15. https://doi.org/10.1172/JCI18714.

38. Doffinger R, Smahi A, Bessia C, Geissmann F, Feinberg J, Durandy A, et al. X-linked anhidrotic ectodermal dysplasia with immunodeficiency is caused by impaired NF-kappaB signaling. Nat Genet. 2001;27(3):277–85. https://doi.org/10.1038/85837.

39. Janssen R, van Wengen A, Hoeve MA, ten Dam M, van der Burg M, van Dongen J, et al. The same IkappaBalpha mutation in two related individuals leads to completely different clinical syndromes. J Exp Med. 2004;200(5):559–68. https://doi.org/10.1084/jem.20040773.

40. Zonana J, Elder ME, Schneider LC, Orlow SJ, Moss C, Golabi M, et al. A novel X-linked disorder of immune deficiency and hypohidrotic ectodermal dysplasia is allelic to incontinentia pigmenti and due to mutations in IKK-gamma (NEMO). Am J Hum Genet. 2000;67(6):1555–62. https://doi.org/10.1086/316914.

41. Zhang SY, Jouanguy E, Ugolini S, Smahi A, Elain G, Romero P, et al. TLR3 deficiency in patients with herpes simplex encephalitis. Science. 2007;317(5844):1522–7. https://doi.org/10.1126/science.1139522.

42. Casrouge A, Zhang SY, Eidenschenk C, Jouanguy E, Puel A, Yang K, et al. Herpes simplex virus encephalitis in human UNC-93B deficiency. Science. 2006;314(5797):308–12. https://doi.org/10.1126/science.1128346.

43. Sancho-Shimizu V, Perez de Diego R, Lorenzo L, Halwani R, Alangari A, Israelsson E, et al. Herpes simplex encephalitis in children with autosomal recessive and dominant TRIF deficiency. J Clin Invest. 2011;121(12):4889–902. https://doi.org/10.1172/JCI59259.

44. Perez de Diego R, Sancho-Shimizu V, Lorenzo L, Puel A, Plancoulaine S, Picard C, et al. Human TRAF3 adaptor molecule deficiency leads to impaired Toll-like receptor 3 response and susceptibility to herpes simplex encephalitis. Immunity. 2010;33(3):400–11. https://doi.org/10.1016/j.immuni.2010.08.014.

45. Herman M, Ciancanelli M, Ou YH, Lorenzo L, Klaudel-Dreszler M, Pauwels E, et al. Heterozygous TBK1 mutations impair TLR3 immunity and underlie herpes simplex encephalitis of childhood. J Exp Med. 2012;209(9):1567–82. https://doi.org/10.1084/jem.20111316.

46. Chapgier A, Kong XF, Boisson-Dupuis S, Jouanguy E, Averbuch D, Feinberg J, et al. A partial form of recessive STAT1 deficiency in humans. J Clin Invest. 2009;119(6):1502–14. https://doi.org/10.1172/JCI37083.

47. Dupuis S, Jouanguy E, Al-Hajjar S, Fieschi C, Al-Mohsen IZ, Al-Jumaah S, et al. Impaired response to interferon-alpha/beta and lethal viral disease in human STAT1 deficiency. Nat Genet. 2003;33(3):388–91. https://doi.org/10.1038/ng1097.

48. Gonzalez-Navajas JM, Lee J, David M, Raz E. Immunomodulatory functions of type I interferons. Nat Rev Immunol. 2012;12(2):125–35. https://doi.org/10.1038/nri3133.

49. Andersen LL, Mork N, Reinert LS, Kofod-Olsen E, Narita R, Jorgensen SE, et al. Functional IRF3 deficiency in a patient with herpes simplex encephalitis. J Exp Med. 2015;212(9):1371–9. https://doi.org/10.1084/jem.20142274.

50. Ciancanelli MJ, Huang SX, Luthra P, Garner H, Itan Y, Volpi S, et al. Infectious disease. Life-threatening influenza and impaired interferon amplification in human IRF7 deficiency. Science. 2015;348(6233):448–53. https://doi.org/10.1126/science.aaa1578.

51. Ferwerda B, McCall MB, Verheijen K, Kullberg BJ, van der Ven AJ, Van der Meer JW, et al. Functional consequences of toll-like receptor 4 polymorphisms. Mol Med. 2008;14(5–6):346–52. https://doi.org/10.2119/2007-00135.Ferwerda.

52. Ferwerda B, McCall MB, Alonso S, Giamarellos-Bourboulis EJ, Mouktaroudi M, Izagirre N, et al. TLR4 polymorphisms, infectious diseases, and evolutionary pressure during migration of modern humans. Proc Natl Acad Sci U S A. 2007;104(42):16645–50. https://doi.org/10.1073/pnas.0704828104.

53. Papadopoulos AI, Ferwerda B, Antoniadou A, Sakka V, Galani L, Kavatha D, et al. Association of toll-like receptor 4 Asp299Gly and Thr399Ile polymorphisms with increased infection risk in patients

with advanced HIV-1 infection. Clin Infect Dis. 2010;51(2):242–7. https://doi.org/10.1086/653607.

54. Schnetzke U, Spies-Weisshart B, Yomade O, Fischer M, Rachow T, Schrenk K, et al. Polymorphisms of toll-like receptors (TLR2 and TLR4) are associated with the risk of infectious complications in acute myeloid leukemia. Genes Immun. 2015;16(1):83–8. https://doi.org/10.1038/gene.2014.67.

55. Bochud PY, Chien JW, Marr KA, Leisenring WM, Upton A, Janer M, et al. Toll-like receptor 4 polymorphisms and aspergillosis in stem-cell transplantation. N Engl J Med. 2008;359(17):1766–77. https://doi.org/10.1056/NEJMoa0802629.

56. de Boer MG, Jolink H, Halkes CJ, van der Heiden PL, Kremer D, Falkenburg JH, et al. Influence of polymorphisms in innate immunity genes on susceptibility to invasive aspergillosis after stem cell transplantation. PLoS One. 2011;6(4):e18403. https://doi.org/10.1371/journal.pone.0018403.

57. Koldehoff M, Beelen DW, Elmaagacli AH. Increased susceptibility for aspergillosis and post-transplant immune deficiency in patients with gene variants of TLR4 after stem cell transplantation. Transplant Infect Dis (An Official Journal of the Transplantation Society). 2013;15(5):533–9. https://doi.org/10.1111/tid.12115.

58. Carvalho A, Pasqualotto AC, Pitzurra L, Romani L, Denning DW, Rodrigues F. Polymorphisms in toll-like receptor genes and susceptibility to pulmonary aspergillosis. J Infect Dis. 2008;197(4):618–21. https://doi.org/10.1086/526500.

59. Carvalho A, Cunha C, Carotti A, Aloisi T, Guarrera O, Di Ianni M, et al. Polymorphisms in Toll-like receptor genes and susceptibility to infections in allogeneic stem cell transplantation. Exp Hematol. 2009;37(9):1022–9. https://doi.org/10.1016/j.exphem.2009.06.004.

60. Wurfel MM, Gordon AC, Holden TD, Radella F, Strout J, Kajikawa O, et al. Toll-like receptor 1 polymorphisms affect innate immune responses and outcomes in sepsis. Am J Respir Crit Care Med. 2008;178(7):710–20. https://doi.org/10.1164/rccm.200803-462OC.

61. Plantinga TS, Johnson MD, Scott WK, van de Vosse E, Velez Edwards DR, Smith PB, et al. Toll-like receptor 1 polymorphisms increase susceptibility to candidemia. J Infect Dis. 2012;205(6):934–43. https://doi.org/10.1093/infdis/jir867.

62. Hawn TR, Misch EA, Dunstan SJ, Thwaites GE, Lan NT, Quy HT, et al. A common human TLR1 polymorphism regulates the innate immune response to lipopeptides. Eur J Immunol. 2007;37(8):2280–9. https://doi.org/10.1002/eji.200737034.

63. Carvalho A, De Luca A, Bozza S, Cunha C, D'Angelo C, Moretti S, et al. TLR3 essentially promotes protective class I-restricted memory CD8(+) T-cell responses to Aspergillus fumigatus in hematopoietic transplanted patients. Blood. 2012;119(4):967–77. https://doi.org/10.1182/blood-2011-06-362582.

64. Potenza L, Vallerini D, Barozzi P, Riva G, Forghieri F, Beauvais A, et al. Characterization of specific immune responses to different Aspergillus antigens during the course of invasive Aspergillosis in hematologic patients. PLoS One. 2013;8(9):e74326. https://doi.org/10.1371/journal.pone.0074326.

65. Cunha C, Goncalves SM, Duarte-Oliveira C, Leite L, Lagrou K, Marques A, et al. IL-10 overexpression predisposes to invasive aspergillosis by suppressing antifungal immunity. J Allergy Clin Immunol. 2017;140(3):867–870.e9. https://doi.org/10.1016/j.jaci.2017.02.034.

66. Hawn TR, Dunstan SJ, Thwaites GE, Simmons CP, Thuong NT, Lan NT, et al. A polymorphism in Toll-interleukin 1 receptor domain containing adaptor protein is associated with susceptibility to meningeal tuberculosis. J Infect Dis. 2006;194(8):1127–34. https://doi.org/10.1086/507907.

67. Khor CC, Chapman SJ, Vannberg FO, Dunne A, Murphy C, Ling EY, et al. A Mal functional variant is associated with protection against invasive pneumococcal disease, bacteremia, malaria and tuberculosis. Nat Genet. 2007;39(4):523–8. https://doi.org/10.1038/ng1976.

68. Ferwerda B, Alonso S, Banahan K, McCall MB, Giamarellos-Bourboulis EJ, Ramakers BP, et al. Functional and genetic evidence that the Mal/TIRAP allele variant 180L has been selected by providing protection against septic shock. Proc Natl Acad Sci U S A. 2009;106(25):10272–7. https://doi.org/10.1073/pnas.0811273106.

69. Miao R, Li J, Sun Z, Xu F, Shen H. Meta-analysis on the association of TIRAP S180L variant and tuberculosis susceptibility. Tuberculosis. 2011;91(3):268–72. https://doi.org/10.1016/j.tube.2011.01.006.

70. Hayashi F, Smith KD, Ozinsky A, Hawn TR, Yi EC, Goodlett DR, et al. The innate immune response to bacterial flagellin is mediated by Toll-like receptor 5. Nature. 2001;410(6832):1099–103. https://doi.org/10.1038/35074106.

71. Hawn TR, Verbon A, Lettinga KD, Zhao LP, Li SS, Laws RJ, et al. A common dominant TLR5 stop codon polymorphism abolishes flagellin signaling and is associated with susceptibility to legionnaires' disease. J Exp Med. 2003;198(10):1563–72. https://doi.org/10.1084/jem.20031220.

72. Grube M, Loeffler J, Mezger M, Kruger B, Echtenacher B, Hoffmann P, et al. TLR5 stop codon polymorphism is associated with invasive aspergillosis after allogeneic stem cell transplantation. Med Mycol. 2013;51(8):818–25. https://doi.org/10.3109/13693786.2013.809630.

73. Wlasiuk G, Khan S, Switzer WM, Nachman MW. A history of recurrent positive selection at the toll-like receptor 5 in primates. Mol Biol Evol. 2009;26(4):937–49. https://doi.org/10.1093/molbev/msp018.

74. Yadav M, Schorey JS. The beta-glucan receptor dectin-1 functions together with TLR2 to mediate macrophage activation by mycobacteria. Blood.

2006;108(9):3168–75. https://doi.org/10.1182/blood-2006-05-024406.

75. Ferwerda B, Ferwerda G, Plantinga TS, Willment JA, van Spriel AB, Venselaar H, et al. Human dectin-1 deficiency and mucocutaneous fungal infections. N Engl J Med. 2009;361(18):1760–7. https://doi.org/10.1056/NEJMoa0901053.

76. Puel A, Doffinger R, Natividad A, Chrabieh M, Barcenas-Morales G, Picard C, et al. Autoantibodies against IL-17A, IL-17F, and IL-22 in patients with chronic mucocutaneous candidiasis and autoimmune polyendocrine syndrome type I. J Exp Med. 2010;207(2):291–7. https://doi.org/10.1084/jem.20091983.

77. Chai LY, de Boer MG, van der Velden WJ, Plantinga TS, van Spriel AB, Jacobs C, et al. The Y238X stop codon polymorphism in the human beta-glucan receptor dectin-1 and susceptibility to invasive aspergillosis. J Infect Dis. 2011;203(5):736–43. https://doi.org/10.1093/infdis/jiq102.

78. Cunha C, Di Ianni M, Bozza S, Giovannini G, Zagarella S, Zelante T, et al. Dectin-1 Y238X polymorphism associates with susceptibility to invasive aspergillosis in hematopoietic transplantation through impairment of both recipient- and donor-dependent mechanisms of antifungal immunity. Blood. 2010;116(24):5394–402. https://doi.org/10.1182/blood-2010-04-279307.

79. Plantinga TS, van der Velden WJ, Ferwerda B, van Spriel AB, Adema G, Feuth T, et al. Early stop polymorphism in human DECTIN-1 is associated with increased candida colonization in hematopoietic stem cell transplant recipients. Clin Infect Dis. 2009;49(5):724–32. https://doi.org/10.1086/604714.

80. Wilson GJ, Marakalala MJ, Hoving JC, van Laarhoven A, Drummond RA, Kerscher B, et al. The C-type lectin receptor CLECSF8/CLEC4D is a key component of anti-mycobacterial immunity. Cell Host Microbe. 2015;17(2):252–9. https://doi.org/10.1016/j.chom.2015.01.004.

81. Glocker EO, Hennigs A, Nabavi M, Schaffer AA, Woellner C, Salzer U, et al. A homozygous CARD9 mutation in a family with susceptibility to fungal infections. N Engl J Med. 2009;361(18):1727–35. https://doi.org/10.1056/NEJMoa0810719.

82. Lanternier F, Pathan S, Vincent QB, Liu L, Cypowyj S, Prando C, et al. Deep dermatophytosis and inherited CARD9 deficiency. N Engl J Med. 2013;369(18):1704–14. https://doi.org/10.1056/NEJMoa1208487.

83. Torres JM, Martinez-Barricarte R, Garcia-Gomez S, Mazariegos MS, Itan Y, Boisson B, et al. Inherited BCL10 deficiency impairs hematopoietic and nonhematopoietic immunity. J Clin Invest. 2014;124(12):5239–48. https://doi.org/10.1172/JCI77493.

84. Bugarcic A, Hitchens K, Beckhouse AG, Wells CA, Ashman RB, Blanchard H. Human and mouse macrophage-inducible C-type lectin (Mincle) bind Candida albicans. Glycobiology. 2008;18(9):679–85. https://doi.org/10.1093/glycob/cwn046.

85. Sato K, Yang XL, Yudate T, Chung JS, Wu J, Luby-Phelps K, et al. Dectin-2 is a pattern recognition receptor for fungi that couples with the Fc receptor gamma chain to induce innate immune responses. J Biol Chem. 2006;281(50):38854–66. https://doi.org/10.1074/jbc.M606542200.

86. Yamasaki S, Ishikawa E, Sakuma M, Hara H, Ogata K, Saito T. Mincle is an ITAM-coupled activating receptor that senses damaged cells. Nat Immunol. 2008;9(10):1179–88. https://doi.org/10.1038/ni.1651.

87. Foo SS, Reading PC, Jaillon S, Mantovani A, Mahalingam S. Pentraxins and Collectins: friend or foe during pathogen invasion? Trends Microbiol. 2015;23(12):799–811. https://doi.org/10.1016/j.tim.2015.09.006.

88. Eisen DP, Minchinton RM. Impact of mannose-binding lectin on susceptibility to infectious diseases. Clin Infect Dis. 2003;37(11):1496–505. https://doi.org/10.1086/379324.

89. Sprong T, van Deuren M. Mannose-binding lectin: ancient molecule, interesting future. Clin Infect Dis. 2008;47(4):517–8. https://doi.org/10.1086/590007.

90. Lambourne J, Agranoff D, Herbrecht R, Troke PF, Buchbinder A, Willis F, et al. Association of mannose-binding lectin deficiency with acute invasive aspergillosis in immunocompromised patients. Clin Infect Dis. 2009;49(10):1486–91. https://doi.org/10.1086/644619.

91. Jaillon S, Moalli F, Ragnarsdottir B, Bonavita E, Puthia M, Riva F, et al. The humoral pattern recognition molecule PTX3 is a key component of innate immunity against urinary tract infection. Immunity. 2014;40(4):621–32. https://doi.org/10.1016/j.immuni.2014.02.015.

92. Cunha C, Aversa F, Lacerda JF, Busca A, Kurzai O, Grube M, et al. Genetic PTX3 deficiency and aspergillosis in stem-cell transplantation. N Engl J Med. 2014;370(5):421–32. https://doi.org/10.1056/NEJMoa1211161.

93. Wojtowicz A, Lecompte TD, Bibert S, Manuel O, Rueger S, Berger C, et al. PTX3 polymorphisms and invasive mold infections after solid organ transplant. Clin Infect Dis. 2015;61(4):619–22. https://doi.org/10.1093/cid/civ386.

94. Cunha C, Monteiro AA, Oliveira-Coelho A, Kuhne J, Rodrigues F, Sasaki SD, et al. PTX3-based genetic testing for risk of aspergillosis after lung transplant. Clin Infect Dis. 2015;61(12):1893–4. https://doi.org/10.1093/cid/civ679.

95. Mauri T, Coppadoro A, Bombino M, Bellani G, Zambelli V, Fornari C, et al. Alveolar pentraxin 3 as an early marker of microbiologically confirmed pneumonia: a threshold-finding prospective observational study. Crit Care. 2014;18(5):562. https://doi.org/10.1186/s13054-014-0562-5.

96. Carvalho A, Cunha C, Bistoni F, Romani L. Immunotherapy of aspergillosis. Clin Microbiol Infect (The Official Publication of the European Society of Clinical Microbiology and Infectious Diseases). 2012;18(2):120–5. https://doi.org/10.1111/j.1469-0691.2011.03681.x.

97. Zaas AK, Liao G, Chien JW, Weinberg C, Shore D, Giles SS, et al. Plasminogen alleles influence susceptibility to invasive aspergillosis. PLoS Genet. 2008;4(6):e1000101. https://doi.org/10.1371/journal.pgen.1000101.

98. Notarangelo LD, Badolato R. Leukocyte trafficking in primary immunodeficiencies. J Leukoc Biol. 2009;85(3):335–43. https://doi.org/10.1189/jlb.0808474.

99. Lo Giudice P, Campo S, De Santis R, Salvatori G. Effect of PTX3 and voriconazole combination in a rat model of invasive pulmonary aspergillosis. Antimicrob Agents Chemother. 2012;56(12):6400–2. https://doi.org/10.1128/AAC.01000-12.

100. Marra E, Sousa VL, Gaziano R, Pacello ML, Arseni B, Aurisicchio L, et al. Efficacy of PTX3 and posaconazole combination in a rat model of invasive pulmonary aspergillosis. Antimicrob Agents Chemother. 2014;58(10):6284–6. https://doi.org/10.1128/AAC.03038-14.

101. Oliveira-Coelho A, Rodrigues F, Campos A Jr, Lacerda JF, Carvalho A, Cunha C. Paving the way for predictive diagnostics and personalized treatment of invasive aspergillosis. Front Microbiol. 2015;6:411. https://doi.org/10.3389/fmicb.2015.00411.

102. Kumar V, Cheng SC, Johnson MD, Smeekens SP, Wojtowicz A, Giamarellos-Bourboulis E, et al. Immunochip SNP array identifies novel genetic variants conferring susceptibility to candidaemia. Nat Commun. 2014;5:4675. https://doi.org/10.1038/ncomms5675.

103. Smeekens SP, Ng A, Kumar V, Johnson MD, Plantinga TS, van Diemen C, et al. Functional genomics identifies type I interferon pathway as central for host defense against Candida albicans. Nat Commun. 2013;4:1342. https://doi.org/10.1038/ncomms2343.

104. Fairfax BP, Knight JC. Genetics of gene expression in immunity to infection. Curr Opin Immunol. 2014;30C:63–71. https://doi.org/10.1016/j.coi.2014.07.001.

Defects of Innate Immunity

Jana P. Lovell and Steven M. Holland

White blood cells (WBCs) encompass a diversity of cells, which can be classified into two broad categories: lymphoid (T, B, NK, and NKT) and myeloid (neutrophils, eosinophils, basophils, and monocytes/macrophages, as well as those derived from the same progenitors, erythroid, and megakaryocytic). This chapter focuses primarily on neutrophils and monocytes and examines the disorders characterized by their quantitative and functional defects.

Neutrophil Disorders

Neutrophils arise from myeloid stem cells in the bone marrow over about 14 days. Mature neutrophils, containing primary, secondary, and tertiary granules, are released into the bloodstream and then migrate to infected or damaged tissues by chemotaxis. In the tissues, neutrophils function as the primary mediators of innate immunity against bacterial and fungal pathogens by phagocytosis of invaders, generation of toxic metabolites such as superoxide, mobilization of antimicrobial proteins, and formation of neutrophil extracellular traps (NETs). They also recruit other immune cells to sites of infection by the release of chemokines and cytokines.

Neutrophil disorders are divided into two broad categories: quantitative (neutrophilia or neutropenia) and qualitative (defects in motility, phagocytosis, granule synthesis and release, and killing). Neutrophilia is >7000 neutrophils/mcl in adults, while neutropenia is classified as mild (<1500 neutrophils per microliter), moderate (1500–1000 neutrophils per microliter), and severe (<500 neutrophils per microliter). Typically, neutrophilias result from extrinsic or iatrogenic causes (e.g., steroids, epinephrine, acute infections); however, intrinsic disorders can also be associated with neutrophilia (e.g., chronic idiopathic neutrophilia, leukocyte adhesion deficiencies, myeloproliferative diseases). Conversely, the causes of neutropenia are quite diverse, frequently due to iatrogenic events, such as drug allergies or cytotoxic chemotherapy. Intrinsic defects affecting neutrophils or their progenitors (Box 12-1) can be classified on the basis of decreased production (e.g., severe congenital neutropenia, cyclic neutropenia) or increased destruction (e.g., myelokathexis, immune neutropenias) of neutrophils or a combination of both processes.

Patients with recurrent, severe bacterial or fungal infections, particularly those caused by unusual organisms (e.g., *Chromobacterium violaceum*), should almost always be investigated for neutrophil disorders. Severe viral and parasitic

J. P. Lovell · S. M. Holland (✉)
Laboratory of Clinical Infectious Diseases, National Institute of Allergy and Infectious Diseases, NIH, Bethesda, MD, USA
e-mail: smh@nih.gov

© Springer International Publishing AG, part of Springer Nature 2018
B. H. Segal (ed.), *Management of Infections in the Immunocompromised Host*,
https://doi.org/10.1007/978-3-319-77674-3_7

infections are not typical of neutrophil disorders and suggest other immune defects. Repeated WBC counts with differentials and careful microscopic examination of neutrophils are the requisite starting points for evaluation of neutropenias. Flow cytometry helps quantify specific leukocyte markers (e.g., CD18). Functional assays such as for the neutrophil oxidative burst are commercially available, while others, such as phagocytosis, chemotaxis, and NET formation, are only available as research tests.

Neutropenia

Severe Congenital Neutropenia

Severe congenital neutropenia (SCN) encompasses a heterogeneous group of disorders with variable inheritance patterns that are all characterized by bone marrow granulocyte maturation arrest at the promyelocyte or myelocyte stage, severe chronic neutropenia (<200 neutrophils per microliter), and increased susceptibility to myelodysplastic syndrome (MDS) and acute myeloid leukemia (AML).

The clinical manifestations of SCN include omphalitis, upper and lower respiratory tract infections, and skin and liver abscesses. Patients with SCN develop symptoms shortly after birth; 50% of affected infants are symptomatic within the first month of life and 90% within the first 6 months of life [1].

Single allele mutations in the granulocyte-colony stimulating factor (G-CSF) receptor (*GCSFR*, 1p34.3) are associated with the development of MDS/AML in patients with SCN [2]. However, not all SCN patients develop mutations in the G-CSF receptor, suggesting that these mutations are somatic epiphenomena that occur in the setting of SCN [3].

The mainstay of therapy for most forms of SCN is subcutaneous recombinant G-CSF, which improves the lives of patients dramatically, reducing the number of infections and hospital days and increasing life expectancy [4]. However, given concern for increased risk for malignant transformation with prolonged G-CSF, patients with poor response to G-CSF or with MDS/AML are candidates for curative hematopoietic stem cell transplant (HSCT) [5]. Several of the genetic mutations associated with SCN are described below.

Autosomal Recessive SCN

HAX1 Deficiency (Kostmann Syndrome)

Homozygous mutations in the anti-apoptotic molecule *HAX1* (1q21.3) were initially identified in patients with autosomal recessive SCN [6–8]. HAX1 is critical for maintaining the inner mitochondrial membrane potential, protecting cells from apoptosis, and supporting signal transduction to the cytoskeleton. Patients with HAX1 deficiency may also have neurocognitive symptoms, including epilepsy and developmental delay. There are two isoforms of HAX1; patients with mutations affecting only isoform A only present with exclusively SCN, while patients with mutations affecting both isoforms A and B develop SCN with neurological symptoms [8, 9].

AK2 Deficiency (Reticular Dysgenesis)

Reticular dysgenesis is a rare autosomal recessive severe combined immunodeficiency characterized by early arrest of myeloid differentiation, profound neutropenia, lymphopenia, and associated sensorineural hearing loss. Reticular dysgenesis is caused by biallelic mutations in the adenylate kinase 2 gene (*AK2*, 1p35.1). AK2 is localized in the mitochondrial intermembrane space and is critical for the regulation of mitochondrial metabolism (similar to HAX1) [10–12]. AK2 deficiency causes premature apoptosis of myeloid and lymphoid cells that is not responsive to G-CSF; erythroid and megakaryocytic function are usually preserved [12]. Early hematopoietic stem cell transplantation is urgently required for survival, but does not repair the hearing loss [13].

G6PC3 Deficiency

Mutations in glucose-6-phosphatase catalytic subunit 3 (*G6PC3*) (17q21.31) also cause autosomal recessive SCN; however, this disorder is often associated with other congenital abnormalities, such as cardiac and urogenital malformations, inflammatory bowel disease, endocrine disorders, and abdominal wall venous angiectases [14, 15]. Increased neutrophil endoplasmic reticulum (ER) stress and apoptosis results in neutropenia; G6PC3 deficiency is also characterized by neutrophil and macrophage dysfunction [16, 17].

Autosomal Dominant SCN

Neutrophil Elastase (ELANE) Mutations

Neutrophil elastase (*ELANE*, 19p13.3) is a serine protease stored in the primary granules of neutrophils, from where it is delivered to phagolysosomes or outside the cell in the process of responding to intruders. Heterozygous mutations in *ELANE* are associated with both autosomal dominant and spontaneous SCN [18, 19], accounting for the majority of Caucasian patients with SCN [18]. The mechanisms by which neutrophil elastase mutations result in SCN are not fully understood, but may result from "the unfolded protein response" that can lead to apoptosis of myeloid progenitor cells [20]. *ELANE* mutations also result in cyclic neutropenia; however, the mutations causing cyclic neutropenia are usually clustered around the catalytically active site of neutrophil elastase, while the mutations associated with SCN are typically located elsewhere [20]. In general, SCN is more severe and has more complications than cyclic neutropenia. These conditions (SCN and cyclic neutropenia) are generally very responsive to G-CSF therapy, but hematopoietic stem cell transplantation may be required.

GFI1 Deficiency

Growth factor independent protein 1 (GFI1, 1p22.1) is a transcriptional repressor that controls the transcription of numerous genes involved in hematopoietic stem cell differentiation, including C/EBPε, ELANE, and the monocytopoietic cytokine, CSF1. Two families with SCN have been described with heterozygous mutations in GFI1 [21, 22]; GFI1's effects on multiple genes, including the expression of *ELANE*, confirm that this specific pathway affects multiple pathways of myeloid differentiation, resulting in congenital neutropenia.

X-Linked SCN

WASP Gain-of-Function

X-linked inheritance of SCN (X-linked neutropenia or XLN) has been associated with activating mutations in the Wiskott-Aldrich syndrome gene (WAS, Xp11.23) [23]. A specific mutation in WAS (L270P) results in a constitutively active mutant protein which causes neutropenia; in contrast, mutations causing reduced WASp expression are associated with classical Wiskott-Aldrich syndrome, characterized by eczema, thrombocytopenia, infections, and malignancies due to platelet and T cell defects. WASp is critical for the regulation of the actin cytoskeleton; constitutively active WASp may result in myeloid cell apoptosis due to aberrant actin polymerization [24]. Mild mutations affecting WASp activity can also cause X-linked thrombocytopenia (XLT), a less severe condition.

Cyclic Neutropenia/Cyclic Hematopoiesis

Cyclic neutropenia/cyclic hematopoiesis is commonly inherited in an autosomal dominant pattern. Mutations in *ELANE* (neutrophil elastase, 19p13.3), typically single-base heterozygous substitutions, have been identified in almost all patients [25]. Cyclic neutropenia/cyclic hematopoiesis is characterized by regular cyclic fluctuations in all hematopoietic lineages. The clinical manifestations of cyclic neutropenia appear in early childhood with painful oral ulcers, recurring fevers, and bacterial infections (e.g., pharyngitis/tonsillitis, cellulitis) [25]. Chronic gingivitis and periapical abscesses can result in early loss of permanent teeth [26]. These complications are associated with variations in neutrophil counts approximately every 21 days, with a range of 14–35 days. The periods of severe neutropenia

(<200 neutrophils per microliter) last 3–10 days [27, 28]. Bone marrow aspirates obtained during periods of neutropenia show maturation arrest at the myelocyte stage or, less frequently, bone marrow hypoplasia [29]. Unlike SCN, cyclic neutropenia is not generally associated with MDS/AML. The administration of G-CSF improves peripheral neutrophil counts and decreases morbidity. Patients typically respond to lower G-CSF doses than those required for SCN. The neutropenia may lessen naturally with age, and treatment may no longer be needed [26].

Adult-Onset Cyclic Neutropenia

Large granular lymphocytes (LGL) are activated clonal or oligoclonal lymphocytes, typically CD8+ T cells or NK cells. Adult-onset cyclic or sustained neutropenia can be due to LGL. LGL leukemia develops from the clonal expansion of CD8+ T cells and NK cells. The majority of LGL patients develop chronic neutropenia; however, cyclic neutropenia has been reported in a few patients [30, 31]. Patients may present with recurrent bacterial infections, including cellulitis, perirectal abscesses, and respiratory infections. The diagnosis is confirmed by the identification of clonal CD8+ T cells infiltrating the bone marrow. G-CSF or GM-CSF improves neutropenia in LGL patients but more directed therapy with antimetabolites or chemotherapy may be needed [30]. Large granular leukemias, also called LGL, can be very aggressive and treatment refractory, making cautious use of the term essential [30].

Warts, Hypogammaglobulinemia, Infections, and Myelokathexis (WHIM) Syndrome

The complex program of cell growth in the marrow, followed by release into the circulation, homing to lymph nodes or other sites, and return to the marrow are carefully orchestrated, in large part by chemokines (*chemo*attractant cyto*kines*). Central to hematopoiesis is the interaction of stromal derived factor-1 (SDF-1 or CXCL12) and its cognate receptor, CXCR4 (2q22.1). Heterozygous mutations of the intracellular

carboxy terminus of CXCR4 lead to exaggerated response to CXCL12, which is expressed on bone marrow stromal cells [32]. Enhanced CXCR4 activity leads to an exaggerated response to CXCL12, which is expressed on bone marrow stromal cells [32]. Delays in release of mature neutrophils from the bone marrow cause neutropenia and apoptosis of mature neutrophils in the marrow, or myelokathexis (from the Greek, meaning "retained in the bone marrow") [33, 34]. A significant number of patients with CXCR4 mutations have warts, hypogammaglobulinemia, infections, and myelokathexis (WHIM), with varying degrees of severity. Patients commonly have a history of recurrent pyogenic infections but also severe HPV infections, respiratory infections due to encapsulated bacteria, and recurrent otitis media [35]. During periods of infection, neutrophils typically increase relative to baseline levels. Monocytopenia, B and T cell lymphocytopenia, and hypogammaglobulinemia are also associated with WHIM. Bone marrow aspirates in WHIM patients show myeloid hypercellularity with increased numbers of granulocytes at all stages of differentiation. G-CSF or GM-CSF increase the number of neutrophils in the peripheral blood and decrease the number of infections [36]. The small-molecule CXCR4 antagonist, plerixafor, blocks CXCR4 retention of mature neutrophils in the marrow and has also been used to improve cell counts in WHIM syndrome [36, 37].

Immune-Mediated Neutropenias

Neonatal Alloimmune Neutropenia

Neonatal alloimmune neutropenia (NAN) is an immune-mediated neutropenia that results from the transplacental transfer of maternal antibodies against two isotopes of the immunoglobulin receptor FcγRIIIb, NA1 and NA2, leading to the immune destruction of neonatal neutrophils [38–42]. The development of maternal antibodies against NA1 and NA2 may result from the lack of expression of FcγRIIIb on maternal neutrophils and the concurrent expression of paternally encoded FcγRIIIb on fetal neutrophils. Antibody-coated neutrophils are phagocytosed in the reticuloendothelial system and removed from circulation, resulting in neutropenia. The mother is typically healthy and the course of pregnancy is uneventful.

Affected infants may present with omphalitis, cellulitis, and pneumonia in the setting of isolated neutropenia within the first 2 weeks of life. Complement-activating anti-neutrophil antibodies can be detected in 1 in 500 live births, suggesting the incidence of NAN is quite high. As such, NAN should be considered in all infants with isolated neutropenia, presenting with or without infection. Diagnosis can be confirmed by the detection of neutrophil-specific alloantibodies (e.g., anti-HNA-1a, anti-HNA-1b) in the maternal serum.

In the initial management of NAN, G-CSF and parenteral antibiotics should be initiated, even in the absence of signs of infection. NAN tends to spontaneously improve as maternal antibody levels decline; however, this waning may take several months [42].

Autoimmune Neutropenias

Autoimmune neutropenia (AIN) is a rare cause of neutropenia, caused by the peripheral destruction of neutrophils and/or their precursors by anti-neutrophil antibodies. AIN can be categorized as primary, when the neutropenia is an isolated clinical entity, or secondary, when the neutropenia is associated with another disease.

Primary Autoimmune Neutropenia
Primary AIN is the most common cause of chronic neutropenia (absolute neutrophil count <1500 per microliter for at least 6 months) in infancy and childhood. Primary AIN is ten-times more frequent than severe congenital neutropenia, with a reported incidence of 1:100,000 live births and a slight female predominance.

Patients typically present with skin or upper respiratory tract infections by 8 months of age. Less commonly, patients may develop severe infections, such as pneumonia, meningitis, or

sepsis. Patients may remain asymptomatic despite low neutrophil counts, delaying initial diagnosis. Neutrophil counts are usually below 1500 per microliter but above 500 per microliter at the time of diagnosis. During episodes of infection, neutrophils may transiently increase and then return to neutropenic levels following resolution. Bone marrow aspirates may reveal normal or hypercellularity.

The diagnosis of primary AIN requires the detection of anti-neutrophil antibodies, which may necessitate repeated testing [43]. Autoantibodies against NA1 and NA2 (the same targets associated with NAN) are present in about one-third of patients. Other reported autoantibodies are targeted against CD11b/CD18 (Mac-1), CD32 (FcγRII), and CD35 (C3b complement receptor).

Primary AIN is usually a self-limited disease, with spontaneous resolution of neutropenia within 7–24 months in 95% of patients following the disappearance of circulating autoantibodies. However, the clinical course of autoimmune neutropenia in older children tends to be more severe without spontaneous resolution. G-CSF should be reserved for the treatment of severe infections or in the setting of emergency surgery [43]. Otherwise, symptomatic treatment of infections with antibiotics is sufficient.

Secondary Autoimmune Neutropenia
Unlike primary AIN, secondary AIN more commonly presents in adults, although it can be seen at any age. Anti-neutrophil antibodies have pan-FcγRIII specificity, rather than specificity to the subunits, resulting in more severe neutropenia. Anti-CD18/11b antibodies have also been detected in some patients. Secondary AIN is often associated with autoimmune diseases (e.g., autoimmune hemolytic anemia, idiopathic thrombocytopenic purpura, systemic lupus erythematous, Sjogren's syndrome), hematologic and nonhematologic malignancies (e.g., LGL leukemia, hairy cell leukemia, Hodgkin lymphoma), and infections (Epstein-Barr virus, cytomegalovirus, HIV, parvovirus B19) [43, 44].

Patients may present with recurrent bacterial infections, including stomatitis, gingivitis, perirectal abscess, or cellulitis. Detecting neutrophil antibodies relies on a combination of granulocyte immunofluorescence test (GIFT) and granulocyte agglutination test (GAT). G-CSF is recommended for treatment in combination with treatment of the associated disease [43].

Defects of Granule Formation and Contents

Chediak-Higashi Syndrome

Chediak-Higashi syndrome (CHS) is a rare and life-threatening autosomal disease caused by mutations in the lysosomal trafficking regulator gene, *LYST* (1q42.3), also known as *CHS1*, resulting in failure to transport lysosomes and other intracellular granules appropriately [45, 46]. Giant granules are found in neutrophils, lymphocytes, and NK cells. Mild neutropenia may result from destruction within the bone marrow.

Patients develop frequent pyogenic bacterial infections of the skin, upper respiratory tract, and gingiva. Fungi are not part of the infectious spectrum. Partial oculocutaneous albinism results from giant and aberrant melanosomes, causing hypopigmentation of the skin, iris, and hair. A mild bleeding diathesis, as well as progressive peripheral neuropathies of the legs, cranial nerves, and autonomic nerves may complicate the disease. Seizures and impaired cognition are common symptoms.

Patients surviving childhood may develop hemophagocytic lymphohistiocytosis (HLH) during the "accelerated phase" of CHS. This form of HLH is clinical indistinguishable from other hemophagocytic syndromes and is similarly characterized by fever, hepatosplenomegaly, lymphadenopathy, cytopenias, hypertriglyceridemia, hypofibrinogenemia, hemophagocytosis, and tissue lymphohistiocytic infiltration. Treatment of the accelerated phase of CHS is similar to other cases of HLH, including dexamethasone, etoposide (VP16), cyclosporine A, and intrathecal methotrexate (when the CNS is involved). HSCT is the only curative treatment,

and in its absence, the accelerated phase usually recurs and is fatal [47].

Neutrophil-Specific Granule Deficiency

Neutrophil-specific granule deficiency is a rare, heterogeneous, autosomal recessive disease characterized by the profound reduction or absence of neutrophil-specific granules and their contents [48]. A homozygous, recessive mutation in *C/EBPε* (14q11.2) has been associated with this disease, although not all patients have this mutation, suggesting genetic heterogeneity [49]. C/EBPε is a member of the CCAAT/enhancer binding proteins, which are transcription factors critical for myelopoiesis and cellular differentiation [50].

Patients commonly develop pyogenic bacterial infections of the skin, ears, lungs, and lymph nodes. Blood smears reveal may a paucity of neutrophil-specific granules, bilobed neutrophils (pseudo-Pelger-Huët anomaly), and possible lack of eosinophils. Characteristically, neutrophils exhibit decreased specific granule contents (e.g., lactoferrin) and low or absent defensins, a primary granule product. Reduced levels of platelet-associated high-molecular-weight von Willebrand factor and platelet fibrinogen and fibronectin may result in bleeding abnormalities [51].

Aggressive diagnosis of infection, prolonged intravenous antibiotic therapy, and early use of surgical excision and debridement are critical. Unrelated HSCT corrected neutrophil-specific granule deficiency in a mutation-negative 13-month-old patient with intractable diarrhea and severe infections [52].

Defects of Oxidative Metabolism

Chronic Granulomatous Disease

Chronic granulomatous disease (CGD) is caused by defects in the NADPH oxidase, which is required for the formation of superoxide and its metabolites (e.g., hydrogen peroxide), which are in turn required for phagocytic killing [53, 54]. Mutations in any of the five genes of the NADPH oxidase (*CYBB*, gp91^{phox}; *CYBA*, p22 ^{phox}; *NCF1*, p47 ^{phox}; *NCF2*, p67 ^{phox}; *NCF4*, p40 ^{phox}) are associated with CGD. Mutations in the X-linked *CYBB* (Xp21.1) account for about two-thirds of cases in the absence of high rates of consanguineous marriage. Mutations in the other genes are autosomal recessive; there are no autosomal dominant cases of CGD [53]. The frequency of CGD in the Unites States is likely to be around 1:100,000.

The defective phagocyte killing makes patients susceptible to recurrent life-threatening infections caused by certain bacteria and fungi, as well as extensive granuloma formation. The clinical course of CGD is quite variable, although the majority of patients present as toddlers or young children with infections and/or granulomatous lesions [55]. The lung, skin, lymph nodes, and liver are the most frequent sites of infection. In North America, the majority of infections are caused by only five organisms: *Staphylococcus aureus*, *Burkholderia cepacia* complex, *Serratia marcescens*, *Nocardia* species, and *Aspergillus* species [55].

Staphylococcal liver abscesses characteristically are dense, caseous, and difficult to drain [56]. A combination of steroid and antibiotic therapy usually obviates the need for surgery [57].

Gastrointestinal (GI) inflammatory manifestations occur in up to 43% of X-linked and 11% of autosomal recessive cases [58]. Patients most commonly present with abdominal pain and less frequently with diarrhea, nausea, or vomiting. Chronic granulomatous lesions mimicking Crohn's-like inflammatory bowel disease (IBD), oral ulcers, esophagitis, gastric outlet obstruction, villous atrophy, intestinal strictures and fistulae, and perirectal abscesses can also occur. The extraintestinal manifestations of IBD (e.g., pyoderma, arthritis) are typically absent. GI manifestations are usually responsive to prednisone (1 mg/kg/day for several weeks followed by progressive tapering). However, relapses occur in nearly 70% of patients [58]. Low-dose maintenance prednisone may control symptoms without

an apparent increase in serious infections. Sulfasalazine, mesalamine, 6-mercaptopurine, azathioprine, and cyclosporine are effective second-line treatment options. Anecdotal use of TNF-alpha blocking antibodies in severe cases of CGD IBD has been reported to yield good symptom control but has been associated with severe and fatal infections with typical CGD pathogens. Therefore, TNF blockade should only be used in CGD with intensified vigilance and prophylaxis for intercurrent infections [59].

Genitourinary strictures and granulomas occur in up to 18% of CGD patients, more commonly in the *CYBA* and *CYBB* mutated patients [60]. Steroid therapy similar to that for CGD-IBD is usually effective [61, 62].

Inflammatory retinal involvement occurs in almost a quarter of X-linked CGD cases. Well-circumscribed asymptomatic "punched-out" retinal scars localized along the retinal vessels are typical and associated with pigment clumping. Notably, these lesions have also been identified in X-linked female carriers. Retinal involvement is typically nonprogressive and asymptomatic and requires no specific treatment; however, two patients had enucleation for painful retinal detachments [63, 64].

Autoimmune disorders are common in CGD patients. Discoid and systemic lupus erythematosus occur in CGD patients as well as in X-linked CGD female carriers [65, 66]. Idiopathic thrombocytopenic purpura and juvenile rheumatoid arthritis also occur more frequently in CGD patients than in the general public [55].

Diagnosis of CGD is made by direct measurement of superoxide production, ferricytochrome c reduction, chemiluminescence, nitroblue tetrazolium (NBT) reduction, or dihydrorhodamine (DHR) oxidation. DHR oxidation is the preferred test due to its ease of use, sensitivity to low numbers of functional neutrophils, and its ability to usually distinguish X-linked CGD from autosomal patterns on flow cytometry [67, 68].

Myeloperoxidase Deficiency

Myeloperoxidase (MPO) deficiency is the most common primary phagocytic disorder. It is an autosomal recessive disease with variable expressivity: 1 in 4000 individuals has complete MPO deficiency and 1 in 2000 has a partial defect [69]. Myeloperoxidase is synthesized in neutrophils and monocytes, packaged in azurophilic granules, and released into the phagosome or extracellular space where it catalyzes the conversion of hydrogen peroxide to hypohalous acid.

the P- and E-selectins on endothelial cells. While neutrophils are rolling along and sampling the endothelial surface, IL-8 release from infectious and inflammatory signals leads to upregulation of the CD18-dependent β2 integrins (LFA-1, MAC-1, p150,95), on the neutrophil surface, which then bind to endothelial ICAM-1 and ICAM-2, resulting in tight adhesion of the neutrophil to the vessel wall and facilitate opportunities for diapedesis into the surrounding tissue through engagement of PECAM-1.

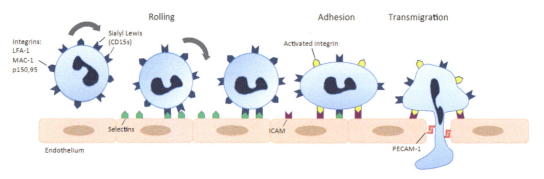

Clinically affected patients most commonly develop *Candida* infections, with cases of mucocutaneous, meningeal, and bone infections, as well as sepsis reported [70–73]. Diabetes mellitus is a significant comorbidity of *Candida* infections in the context of MPO deficiency.

Diagnosis is established by sequencing of the *MPO* gene (17q22) or histochemical staining of neutrophils for MPO. Therapy should be infection-specific and adequate control of diabetes is critical.

Defects of Chemotaxis

Leukocyte Adhesion Deficiencies

Leukocyte extravasation from the bloodstream to infected tissues requires interaction between glycoproteins expressed on the respective cell surfaces of neutrophils and endothelial cells. Light adhesion during neutrophil rolling results from the interaction of the carbohydrates in Sialyl-Lewis^X (CD15s) on the neutrophil surface with

Leukocyte Adhesion Deficiency, Type 1 (LAD1)

LAD1 is a rare autosomal recessive disorder caused by mutations in the *ITGB2* gene (21q22.3), which encodes CD18, the common chain of the β2 integrin family [74]. CD18 is required for the formation of the three β2 integrins expressed on the neutrophil surface: CD11a/CD18 (lymphocyte function-associated antigen-1, LFA-1), CD11b/CD18 (macrophage antigen-1, Mac-1, or complement receptor-3, CR3), and CD11c/CD18 (p150,95 or complement receptor-4, CR4). The interaction between the β2 integrins and the intercellular adhesion molecules 1 and 2 (ICAM-1 and ICAM-2) proteins on endothelial cells allow neutrophils to adhere tightly enough to be able to extravasate into the tissues, including to sites of infection. Nonfunctional or absent CD18, resulting in low to absent expression of the β2 integrins, reduces transmigration of neutrophils to normal and infected tissues [74]. Further, CD11b/CD18 (Mac-1) binds the complement factor iC3b on the surface of microbes, triggering phagocytosis.

The clinical phenotype of LAD1 ranges from severe, typically in patients with less than 1% of normal CD18 expression, to moderate, with up to 30% of normal CD18 expression [75]. The clinical manifestations of the severe phenotype include persistent leukocytosis (>15,000/uL), delayed umbilical stump separation, omphalitis, and severe, progressive gingivitis and periodontitis with associated loss of all dentition as well as alveolar bone. Skin, upper and lower respiratory tract, bowel, and perirectal infections are common, typically caused by *Staphylococcus aureus* or gram-negative bacilli; fungal infections are uncommon. Infections may be necrotic and progress to ulceration. Notably, pus is absent from lesions grossly, and histopathology reveals complete absence of neutrophil invasion despite circulating neutrophilia. Impaired healing of wounds is characteristic, and scars tend to exhibit a dystrophic "cigarette-paper" appearance. Patients with the moderate phenotype have less severe leukocytosis, more mild and delayed periodontal disease, and less severe delayed wound healing; however, patients with the moderate form typically present later in life, have normal umbilical separation, and have fewer severe infections [75].

Flow cytometry of blood samples confirms reduced expression of CD18 and its associated β2 integrins on neutrophils and other leukocytes and failure to upregulate CD18 in the presence of agonists like PMA/ionomycin. Since patients may express normal levels of nonfunctional CD18 protein, functional assays should be performed if the clinical suspicion for LAD1 remains high [76, 77].

Moderate LAD1 can be treated conservatively with infection-specific therapy, and patients may survive into adulthood. Early HSCT is recommended for severe LAD1, as patients can die early in infancy [78, 79]. Somatic reversion mutations involving CD18+ cytotoxic T lymphocytes has been reported in three adult patients; the effect of these reversion mutations on patient survival is unclear [80].

Leukocyte Adhesion Deficiency, Type 2 (LAD2), or Congenital Disorder of Glycosylation Type IIc (CDGIIc)

LAD2 is a very rare autosomal recessive disease caused by mutations of the GDP-fucose transporter gene, *SLC35C1* (11p11.2), resulting in absent expression of fucosylated proteins, including Sialyl-Lewis^X (CD15s) [81, 82]. Fucosylated proteins on the cell surface of leukocytes interact with selectins on endothelial cells (E-selectin), enabling neutrophil rolling and subsequent extravasation to infected tissues.

Clinical manifestations of LAD2 include skin, lung, and periodontal infections, leukocytosis, poor pus formation, development delay, short stature, dysmorphic facies, and the Bombay (hh) blood phenotype. The frequency and severity of infections tend to decline with age [83, 84]. Diagnosis is established by flow cytometry showing reduced expression of CD15s. Fucose supplementation has shown variable efficacy in LAD2 patients; otherwise, aggressive treatment of infections is appropriate [85, 86]. Patient survival into early adulthood has been reported.

Leukocyte Adhesion Deficiency, Type 3 (LAD3)

LAD3 (previously identified as LAD1 variant) is a rare autosomal recessive disease caused by mutations in *FERMT3* (11q13.1), the gene encoding kindlin-3, which is critical for β integrin activation and adhesive functions in leukocytes and platelets [87, 88].

Clinically, LAD3 may resemble LAD1 (e.g., recurrent nonpurulent infections, leukocytosis); however, LAD3 is associated with a Glanzmann thrombasthenia-like bleeding disorder due to defects in β3 integrin-mediated platelet aggregation. Osteopetrosis-like radiographic features have been reported in LAD3 patients [89]. Mortality is high, even with HSCT.

Rac2 Deficiency

Rac2 is a member of the Rho family of GTPases and is critical for phagocyte NADPH oxidase activation and regulation of the actin cytoskeleton. Rac2 deficiency has been described in four patients. Dominant negative mutations in *RAC2* (22q13.1) have been reported in two male infants. The clinical manifestations are a mixture of CGD and LAD1 pathologies. The first patient was a male infant who had delayed umbilical cord separation, perirectal abscesses, poor wound healing, and absent pus from lesions despite neutrophilia [90, 91]. Neutrophil chemotaxis, superoxide production, azurophilic granule release, and phagocytosis were impaired. The patient underwent a successful bone marrow transplantation. A second case was identified through newborn screening for T cell excision circles (TRECs) [92, 93]. Within the first 2 months of life, this patient developed omphalitis, leukocytosis, and a paratracheal abscess. Levels of CD18 and CD15 were normal, but neutrophil chemotaxis was impaired. This infant also underwent successful HSCT.

Autosomal recessive mutations in *RAC2* were reported in two children with common variable immunodeficiency (CVID) who were products of consanguineous parents [94]. They both had recurrent pneumonia and post-streptococcal glomerulonephritis. Unlike the patients with dominant negative mutations, these patients did not present with severe clinical manifestations in the neonatal period, but their neutrophils showed similar impaired chemotaxis and decreased numbers of granules.

Hyper IgE Syndrome

Autosomal Dominant HIES

Autosomal dominant Hyper-IgE syndrome (AD-HIES) is characterized by elevated serum IgE, eczema, recurrent skin and lung infections, and characteristic facies, scoliosis, and fractures [95–97]. AD-HIES results from dominant negative mutations in *STAT3* (17q21.2); heterozygous missense or in-frame deletions in the SH2 domain and DNA-binding domain have been reported. STAT3 deficiency is associated with impaired Th17 numbers, as well as variably decreased neutrophil numbers and chemotaxis [98].

Clinical manifestations of STAT3 deficiency typically begin with a newborn rash. Common infections include mucocutaneous candidiasis (e.g., oral thrush, vaginal candidiasis, onychomycosis), cutaneous *Staphylococcus aureus* "cold" abscesses, and recurrent pneumonias caused by *S. aureus*, *Streptococcus pneumoniae*, and *Haemophilus influenzae*. Pneumatoceles and bronchiectasis form during the healing process and usually persist, increasing susceptibility to gram-negative (e.g., *Pseudomonas*) and fungal (e.g., *Aspergillus* or *Scedosporium* spp.) pulmonary infections [95]. Thoracic surgical intervention for parenchymal abnormalities should be performed cautiously given the reported high complication rates [99]. Antimicrobial prophylaxis for *S. aureus* skin and lung infections may be broadened if gram-negative lung infections occur. Antifungal prophylaxis is effective to prevent mucocutaneous candidiasis; it remains unclear whether prophylaxis is effective for pulmonary aspergillosis.

The classical facies of AD-HIES is characterized by facial asymmetry, broad nose, deep-set eyes, and prominent forehead. Primary teeth are typically retained, resulting in layers of primary and secondary teeth [95, 100]. Vascular abnormalities include coronary artery aneurysms, dilatations, and tortuosities; carotid artery aneurysms; and early-onset MRI T2-weighted hyperintensities [101, 102]. Bone abnormalities include scoliosis, osteopenia, minimal trauma fractures, hyperextensibility, degenerative joint disease, craniosynostosis, and Chiari I malformations [100]. The mechanisms underlying these many complex bone abnormalities are unknown. Surgical correction is occasionally needed for craniosynostosis and Chiari I malformation; the use of bisphosphonates for osteoporosis and minimal trauma fractures in HIES is undefined.

HSCT has had variable results in AD-HIES and should be considered for patients with severe manifestations [103].

Autosomal Recessive HIES

Mutations in dedicator of cytokinesis 8 (*DOCK8*, 9p24.3), phosphoglucomutase 3 (*PGM3*, 6q14.1), and tyrosine kinase 2 (*TYK2*, 19p13.2) have been identified as causes of autosomal recessive HIES (AR-HIES) [104–108]. The autosomal recessive and autosomal dominant forms of HIES share several characteristics including eczema, sinopulmonary infections, and elevated IgE levels.

Patients with DOCK8 deficiency lack the parenchymal lung abnormalities, retained primary teeth, and minimal trauma fractures characteristic of autosomal HIES [103]. These patients may present with severe cutaneous viral infections and atopy. HSCT is recommended given the very high mortality in late childhood and adulthood.

Mutations in *PGM3* cause abnormal glycosylation of numerous proteins, including many that are essential to leukocytes. Motor and neurological deficits are more typical of PGM3 deficiency than DOCK8 deficiency; lack of pneumatoceles and retained teeth also differentiates PGM3 deficiency from AD-HIES [106, 107].

An HIES-type syndrome was described in one patient with complete TYK2 deficiency, who developed intracellular bacterial infections, chronic skin *Molluscum contagiosum* infections, and recurrent herpes simplex virus (HSV) [108]. Additional patients with *TYK2* mutations have developed intracellular bacterial and viral infections without classical signs of HIES and are thought to be more similar to the Mendelian susceptibility to mycobacterial disease group of diseases [109].

Disorders of Monocytes: Syndromes with Susceptibility to Environmental Mycobacteria

Host defense against mycobacteria relies on effective interaction between myeloid and lymphoid cells. Mycobacteria are phagocytosed by macrophages, causing the production and release of IL-12, which binds to the receptor formed by IL12Rβ1 and IL12Rβ2 on T cells and NK cells, stimulating the release of interferon (IFN)-γ.

Binding of IFN-γ to its receptor induces STAT1 phosphorylation, dimerization, and nuclear translocation to induce interferon-responsive genes, including IL-12 subunits, IFN-γ receptors, *STAT1*, *IRF8*, and *ISG15*.

Mutations at various points in this pathway resulting in increased susceptibility to mycobacteria and other intracellular pathogens have been identified: *IL12B* (IL-12p40; 5q33.1), *IFNGR1* (6q23.3), *IFNGR2* (21q22.11), *IL12RB1* (19p13.11), *STAT1* (2q32.2), *IRF8* (16q24.1), *ISG15* (1p36.33), and *GATA2* (3q21.3) are often collectively referred to as Mendelian susceptibility to mycobacterial disease (MSMD) [110–117]. IFN-γ receptor 1 and IL12Rβ1 deficiency account for almost 80% of reported cases of MSMD [117]. Patients with autosomal recessive mutations leading to complete deficiency of proteins in the IL-12/IFN-γ pathway tend to present in early childhood with severe and/or disseminated infections. In contrast, patients with dominant partial deficiencies typically present later with milder disease and have overall better treatment response and survival.

Flow cytometry is sufficient to detect most IFN-γ receptor 1 defects, whereas IFN-γ receptor 2 is more tightly controlled, and antibodies for its flow cytometric detection are few. Cell culture and proliferation are required for functional detection of IL-12 receptor defects, as the IL-12 receptor is not fully displayed on resting lymphocytes. Functional integrity of IFN-γ and IL-12 receptors can be determined indirectly via detection of intracellular phosphorylated STAT1 after IFN-γ stimulation or phosphorylated STAT4 after IL-12 stimulation, respectively. IL-12p40 deficiency can be diagnosed with direction detection of IL-12p40 or IL-12p80. Diagnosis of STAT1 defects requires research techniques. Overall, modern detection of defects in this and many of the discussed pathways should rely on genetic confirmation.

IFN-γ therapy is effective for autosomal dominant *IFNGR1* deficiency, the IL-12 defects, and the IL-12R defects; it is not effective for complete IFN-γ receptor deficiencies, as they will not allow any signal transduction. Long-term prophylaxis against environmental mycobacterial infections with a macrolide such as azithromycin is advisable, as is avoidance of BCG vaccination. HSCT is best performed before severe disseminated mycobacterial disease is present.

GATA2 Deficiency

GATA2 is a transcription factor required for the differentiation of hematopoietic stem cells as well as the development of blood vessels [118]. Haploinsufficiency for *GATA2* results in a variable-onset immunodeficiency characterized by disseminated nontuberculous mycobacterial, fungal, and viral (e.g., HPV, HSV) infections, often associated with diminished monocytes, B cells, and NK cells in the peripheral blood along with hypoplastic myelodysplasia. Along with monocytopenia, the phagocytic activity of monocytes may be impaired. Early HSCT is recommended.

NEMO Deficiency

The NFκB essential modulator (NEMO)-mediated pathway is also critical for immunity against mycobacteria. NEMO, encoded by the X-linked *IKBKG* (Xq28), is required for the activation of NF-κB, a transcription factor required for innate and adaptive immunity. NEMO responds to multiple signals, including IL-1, TNFα, LPS, and the endogenous ectodermal signal molecule, ectodysplasin [119]. Amorphic mutations in *IKBKG* result in male lethality in utero but cause *incontinentia pigmenti* in X-linked females [120]. Hypomorphic mutations resulting in reduced activation of NK-κB permit male survival but often cause ectodermal dysplasia, invasive pneumococcal diseases, severe viral infections, and disseminated nontuberculous mycobacterial infections [121]. Immunological profiles may include reduced NK cell cytotoxicity, variable hypogammaglobulinemia, and impaired function of the receptors of innate immunity [122].

Mucocutaneous Candidiasis

Isolated chronic mucocutaneous candidiasis (CMC) has been associated with genetic mutations. Mutations in dectin-1 (12p13.2), the cell surface receptor for fungal beta-D-glucan, have been identified in patients with severe vulvovaginal, oral, and nail infections [123]. Mutations in the gene encoding CARD9 (9q34.3), an adaptor protein downstream in the dectin-1 signaling pathway, have also been associated with cases of severe, invasive candidiasis, including meningitis [124]. Gain-of-function mutations in *STAT1* are the most common cause of CMC and should be considered in any case of CMC, especially in later childhood or adulthood [125].

Conclusions and Future Directions

Defects in innate immunity are being described at a dizzying rate. Molecular genetic studies are now attaching discrete genes to overlapping phenotypes, such as neutropenia and infection susceptibility. The emerging frontiers are the identification of the mechanisms of immunopathology and correction of the defects. In some cases these corrections will be with immunomodulation, while in others it will be correction at the level of the hematopoietic stem cell, either by gene therapy (replacement or correction) or hematopoietic stem cell transplantation. The future is very bright for patients with these disorders of innate immunity.

References

1. Celkan T, Koc BS. Approach to the patient with neutropenia in childhood. Turk Pediatri Arsivi. 2015;50:136–44. https://doi.org/10.5152/TurkPediatriArs.2015.2295.
2. Dong F, et al. Mutations in the gene for the granulocyte colony-stimulating-factor receptor in patients with acute myeloid leukemia preceded by severe congenital neutropenia. N Engl J Med. 1995;333:487–93. https://doi.org/10.1056/nejm199508243330804.
3. Germeshausen M, Skokowa J, Ballmaier M, Zeidler C, Welte K. G-CSF receptor mutations in patients with congenital neutropenia. Curr Opin

Hematol. 2008;15:332–7. https://doi.org/10.1097/MOH.0b013e328303b9f6.

4. Dale DC, et al. Severe chronic neutropenia: treatment and follow-up of patients in the Severe Chronic Neutropenia International Registry. Am J Hematol. 2003;72:82–93. https://doi.org/10.1002/ajh.10255.

5. Connelly JA, Choi SW, Levine JE. Hematopoietic stem cell transplantation for severe congenital neutropenia. Curr Opin Hematol. 2012;19:44–51. https://doi.org/10.1097/MOH.0b013e32834da96e.

6. Kostmann R. Infantile genetic agranulocytosis; agranulocytosis infantilis hereditaria. Acta Paediatr Suppl. 1956;45:1–78.

7. Klein C, et al. HAX1 deficiency causes autosomal recessive severe congenital neutropenia (Kostmann disease). Nat Genet. 2007;39:86–92. https://doi.org/10.1038/ng1940.

8. Germeshausen M, et al. Novel HAX1 mutations in patients with severe congenital neutropenia reveal isoform-dependent genotype-phenotype associations. Blood. 2008;111:4954–7. https://doi.org/10.1182/blood-2007-11-120667.

9. Roques G, et al. Neurological findings and genetic alterations in patients with Kostmann syndrome and HAX1 mutations. Pediatr Blood Cancer. 2014;61:1041–8. https://doi.org/10.1002/pbc.24964.

10. Pannicke U, et al. Reticular dysgenesis (aleukocytosis) is caused by mutations in the gene encoding mitochondrial adenylate kinase 2. Nat Genet. 2009;41:101–5. https://doi.org/10.1038/ng.265.

11. Lagresle-Peyrou C, et al. Human adenylate kinase 2 deficiency causes a profound hematopoietic defect associated with sensorineural deafness. Nat Genet. 2009;41:106–11. https://doi.org/10.1038/ng.278.

12. Six E, et al. AK2 deficiency compromises the mitochondrial energy metabolism required for differentiation of human neutrophil and lymphoid lineages. Cell Death Dis. 2015;6:e1856. https://doi.org/10.1038/cddis.2015.211.

13. Al-Zahrani D, Al-Ghonaium A, Al-Mousa H, Al-Kassar A, Roifman CM. Skeletal abnormalities and successful hematopoietic stem cell transplantation in patients with reticular dysgenesis. J Allergy Clin Immunol. 2013;132:993–6. https://doi.org/10.1016/j.jaci.2013.04.055.

14. Boztug K, et al. A syndrome with congenital neutropenia and mutations in G6PC3. N Engl J Med. 2009;360:32–43. https://doi.org/10.1056/NEJMoa0805051.

15. Banka S. GeneReviews is a registered trademark of the University of Washington, Seattle. In: Pagon, RA, et al., editors. GeneReviews(R). University of Washington, Seattle, University of Washington, Seattle. All rights reserved; 1993.

16. Jun HS, et al. Lack of glucose recycling between endoplasmic reticulum and cytoplasm underlies cellular dysfunction in glucose-6-phosphatase-beta-deficient neutrophils in a congenital neutropenia syndrome. Blood. 2010;116:2783–92. https://doi.org/10.1182/blood-2009-12-258491.

17. Jun HS, Cheung YY, Lee YM, Mansfield BC, Chou JY. Glucose-6-phosphatase-beta, implicated in a congenital neutropenia syndrome, is essential for macrophage energy homeostasis and functionality. Blood. 2012;119:4047–55. https://doi.org/10.1182/blood-2011-09-377820.

18. Horwitz MS, et al. Neutrophil elastase in cyclic and severe congenital neutropenia. Blood. 2007;109:1817–24. https://doi.org/10.1182/blood-2006-08-019166.

19. Dale DC, et al. Mutations in the gene encoding neutrophil elastase in congenital and cyclic neutropenia. Blood. 2000;96:2317–22.

20. Horwitz MS, Corey SJ, Grimes HL, Tidwell T. ELANE mutations in cyclic and severe congenital neutropenia: genetics and pathophysiology. Hematol Oncol Clin North Am. 2013;27:19–41., vii. https://doi.org/10.1016/j.hoc.2012.10.004.

21. Person RE, et al. Mutations in proto-oncogene GFI1 cause human neutropenia and target ELA2. Nat Genet. 2003;34:308–12. https://doi.org/10.1038/ng1170.

22. Zarebski A, et al. Mutations in growth factor independent-1 associated with human neutropenia block murine granulopoiesis through colony stimulating factor-1. Immunity. 2008;28:370–80. https://doi.org/10.1016/j.immuni.2007.12.020.

23. Devriendt K, et al. Constitutively activating mutation in WASP causes X-linked severe congenital neutropenia. Nat Genet. 2001;27:313–7. https://doi.org/10.1038/85886.

24. Ancliff PJ, et al. Two novel activating mutations in the Wiskott-Aldrich syndrome protein result in congenital neutropenia. Blood. 2006;108:2182–9. https://doi.org/10.1182/blood-2006-01-010249.

25. Makaryan V, et al. The diversity of mutations and clinical outcomes for ELANE-associated neutropenia. Curr Opin Hematol. 2015;22:3–11. https://doi.org/10.1097/moh.0000000000000105.

26. Palmer SE, Stephens K, Dale DC. Genetics, phenotype, and natural history of autosomal dominant cyclic hematopoiesis. Am J Med Genet. 1996;66:413–22. https://doi.org/10.1002/(sici)1096-8628(19961230)66:4<413::aid-ajmg5>3.0.co;2-l.

27. Wright DG, Dale DC, Fauci AS, Wolff SM. Human cyclic neutropenia: clinical review and long-term follow-up of patients. Medicine (Baltimore). 1981;60:1–13.

28. Dale DC, Hammond WPT. Cyclic neutropenia: a clinical review. Blood Rev. 1988;2:178–85.

29. Souid AK. Congenital cyclic neutropenia. Clin Pediatr. 1995;34:151–5.

30. Rose MG, Berliner N. T-cell large granular lymphocyte leukemia and related disorders. Oncologist. 2004;9:247–58.

31. Loughran TP Jr, Clark EA, Price TH, Hammond WP. Adult-onset cyclic neutropenia is associated with increased large granular lymphocytes. Blood. 1986;68:1082–7.

32. Hernandez PA, et al. Mutations in the chemokine receptor gene CXCR4 are associated with WHIM syndrome, a combined immunodeficiency disease. Nat Genet. 2003;34:70–4. https://doi.org/10.1038/ng1149.

33. Balabanian K, et al. WHIM syndromes with different genetic anomalies are accounted for by impaired CXCR4 desensitization to CXCL12. Blood. 2005;105:2449–57. https://doi.org/10.1182/blood-2004-06-2289.

34. Balabanian K, et al. Leukocyte analysis from WHIM syndrome patients reveals a pivotal role for GRK3 in CXCR4 signaling. J Clin Invest. 2008;118:1074–84. https://doi.org/10.1172/jci33187.

35. Al Ustwani O, Kurzrock R, Wetzler M. Genetics on a WHIM. Br J Haematol. 2014;164:15–23. https://doi.org/10.1111/bjh.12574.

36. McDermott DH, et al. A phase 1 clinical trial of long-term, low-dose treatment of WHIM syndrome with the CXCR4 antagonist plerixafor. Blood. 2014;123:2308–16. https://doi.org/10.1182/blood-2013-09-527226.

37. Dale DC, et al. The CXCR4 antagonist plerixafor is a potential therapy for myelokathexis WHIM syndrome. Blood. 2011;118:4963–6. https://doi.org/10.1182/blood-2011-06-360586.

38. Dale DC. Immune and idiopathic neutropenia. Curr Opin Hematol. 1998;5:33–6.

39. Huizinga TW, et al. Maternal genomic neutrophil FcRIII deficiency leading to neonatal isoimmune neutropenia. Blood. 1990;76:1927–32.

40. Stroncek DF, et al. Alloimmune neonatal neutropenia due to an antibody to the neutrophil Fc-gamma receptor III with maternal deficiency of CD16 antigen. Blood. 1991;77:1572–80.

41. Fromont P, et al. Frequency of the polymorphonuclear neutrophil Fc gamma receptor III deficiency in the French population and its involvement in the development of neonatal alloimmune neutropenia. Blood. 1992;79:2131–4.

42. Maheshwari A, Christensen RD, Calhoun DA. Immune-mediated neutropenia in the neonate. Acta Paediatr Suppl. 2002;91:98–103.

43. Akhtari M, Curtis B, Waller EK. Autoimmune neutropenia in adults. Autoimmun Rev. 2009;9:62–6. https://doi.org/10.1016/j.autrev.2009.03.006.

44. Farruggia P. Immune neutropenias of infancy and childhood. World J Pediatr: WJP. 2016;12:142–8. https://doi.org/10.1007/s12519-015-0056-9.

45. Barbosa MD, et al. Identification of the homologous beige and Chediak-Higashi syndrome genes. Nature. 1996;382:262–5. https://doi.org/10.1038/382262a0.

46. Nagle DL, et al. Identification and mutation analysis of the complete gene for Chediak-Higashi syndrome. Nat Genet. 1996;14:307–11. https://doi.org/10.1038/ng1196-307.

47. Eapen M, et al. Hematopoietic cell transplantation for Chediak-Higashi syndrome. Bone Marrow Transplant. 2007;39:411–5. https://doi.org/10.1038/sj.bmt.1705600.

48. Gallin JI, et al. Human neutrophil-specific granule deficiency: a model to assess the role of neutrophil-specific granules in the evolution of the inflammatory response. Blood. 1982;59:1317–29.

49. Lekstrom-Himes JA, Dorman SE, Kopar P, Holland SM, Gallin JI. Neutrophil-specific granule deficiency results from a novel mutation with loss of function of the transcription factor CCAAT/enhancer binding protein epsilon. J Exp Med. 1999;189:1847–52.

50. Lekstrom-Himes J, Xanthopoulos KG. Biological role of the CCAAT/enhancer-binding protein family of transcription factors. J Biol Chem. 1998;273:28545–8.

51. Gombart AF, Koeffler HP. Neutrophil specific granule deficiency and mutations in the gene encoding transcription factor C/EBP(epsilon). Curr Opin Hematol. 2002;9:36–42.

52. Wynn RF, et al. Intractable diarrhoea of infancy caused by neutrophil specific granule deficiency and cured by stem cell transplantation. Gut. 2006;55:292–3. https://doi.org/10.1136/gut.2005.081927.

53. Segal BH, Leto TL, Gallin JI, Malech HL, Holland SM. Genetic, biochemical, and clinical features of chronic granulomatous disease. Medicine (Baltimore). 2000;79:170–200.

54. Reeves EP, et al. Killing activity of neutrophils is mediated through activation of proteases by K+ flux. Nature. 2002;416:291–7. https://doi.org/10.1038/416291a.

55. Winkelstein JA, et al. Chronic granulomatous disease. Report on a national registry of 368 patients. Medicine (Baltimore). 2000;79:155–69.

56. Lublin M, et al. Hepatic abscess in patients with chronic granulomatous disease. Ann Surg. 2002;235:383–91.

57. Leiding JW, et al. Corticosteroid therapy for liver abscess in chronic granulomatous disease. Clin Infect Dis. 2012;54:694–700. https://doi.org/10.1093/cid/cir896.

58. Marciano BE, et al. Gastrointestinal involvement in chronic granulomatous disease. Pediatrics. 2004;114:462–8.

59. Uzel G, et al. Complications of tumor necrosis factor-alpha blockade in chronic granulomatous disease-related colitis. Clin Infect Dis. 2010;51:1429–34. https://doi.org/10.1086/657308.

60. Walther MM, et al. The urological manifestations of chronic granulomatous disease. J Urol. 1992;147:1314–8.

61. Chin TW, Stiehm ER, Falloon J, Gallin JI. Corticosteroids in treatment of obstructive lesions of chronic granulomatous disease. J Pediatr. 1987;111:349–52.

62. Quie PG, Belani KK. Corticosteroids for chronic granulomatous disease. J Pediatr. 1987;111:393–4.

63. Goldblatt D, Butcher J, Thrasher AJ, Russell-Eggitt I. Chorioretinal lesions in patients and carriers of chronic granulomatous disease. J Pediatr. 1999;134:780–3.

64. Kim SJ, Kim JG, Yu YS. Chorioretinal lesions in patients with chronic granulomatous disease. Retina (Philadelphia, Pa). 2003;23:360–5.

65. Manzi S, et al. Systemic lupus erythematosus in a boy with chronic granulomatous disease: case report and review of the literature. Arthritis Rheum. 1991;34:101–5.

66. Cale CM, Morton L, Goldblatt D. Cutaneous and other lupus-like symptoms in carriers of X-linked chronic granulomatous disease: incidence and autoimmune serology. Clin Exp Immunol. 2007;148:79–84. https://doi.org/10.1111/j.1365-2249.2007.03321.x.

67. Vowells SJ, et al. Genotype-dependent variability in flow cytometric evaluation of reduced nicotinamide adenine dinucleotide phosphate oxidase function in patients with chronic granulomatous disease. J Pediatr. 1996;128:104–7.

68. Vowells SJ, Sekhsaria S, Malech HL, Shalit M, Fleisher TA. Flow cytometric analysis of the granulocyte respiratory burst: a comparison study of fluorescent probes. J Immunol Methods. 1995;178:89–97.

69. Nauseef WM. Myeloperoxidase deficiency. Hematol Oncol Clin North Am. 1988;2:135–58.

70. Okuda T, Yasuoka T, Oka N. Myeloperoxidase deficiency as a predisposing factor for deep mucocutaneous candidiasis: a case report. J Oral Maxillofac Surg (Official Journal of the American Association of Oral and Maxillofacial Surgeons). 1991;49:183–6.

71. Ludviksson BR, Thorarensen O, Gudnason T, Halldorsson S. Candida albicans meningitis in a child with myeloperoxidase deficiency. Pediatr Infect Dis J. 1993;12:162–4.

72. Nguyen C, Katner HP. Myeloperoxidase deficiency manifesting as pustular candidal dermatitis. Clin Infect Dis. 1997;24:258–60.

73. Chiang AK, et al. Disseminated fungal infection associated with myeloperoxidase deficiency in a premature neonate. Pediatr Infect Dis J. 2000;19:1027–9.

74. Notarangelo LD, Badolato R. Leukocyte trafficking in primary immunodeficiencies. J Leukoc Biol. 2009;85:335–43. https://doi.org/10.1189/jlb.0808474.

75. Anderson DC, et al. The severe and moderate phenotypes of heritable Mac-1, LFA-1 deficiency: their quantitative definition and relation to leukocyte dysfunction and clinical features. J Infect Dis. 1985;152:668–89.

76. Kuijpers TW, et al. Leukocyte adhesion deficiency type 1 (LAD-1)/variant. A novel immunodeficiency syndrome characterized by dysfunctional beta2 integrins. J Clin Invest. 1997;100:1725–33. https://doi.org/10.1172/jci119697.

77. Hogg N, et al. A novel leukocyte adhesion deficiency caused by expressed but nonfunctional beta2 integrins Mac-1 and LFA-1. J Clin Invest. 1999;103:97–106. https://doi.org/10.1172/jci3312.

78. Thomas C, et al. Results of allogeneic bone marrow transplantation in patients with leukocyte adhesion deficiency. Blood. 1995;86:1629–35.

79. Qasim W, et al. Allogeneic hematopoietic stem-cell transplantation for leukocyte adhesion deficiency. Pediatrics. 2009;123:836–40. https://doi.org/10.1542/peds.2008-1191.

80. Uzel G, et al. Reversion mutations in patients with leukocyte adhesion deficiency type-1 (LAD-1). Blood. 2008;111:209–18. https://doi.org/10.1182/blood-2007-04-082552.

81. Lubke T, et al. Complementation cloning identifies CDG-IIc, a new type of congenital disorders of glycosylation, as a GDP-fucose transporter deficiency. Nat Genet. 2001;28:73–6. https://doi.org/10.1038/88299.

82. Luhn K, Wild MK, Eckhardt M, Gerardy-Schahn R, Vestweber D. The gene defective in leukocyte adhesion deficiency II encodes a putative GDP-fucose transporter. Nat Genet. 2001;28:69–72. https://doi.org/10.1038/88289.

83. Gazit Y, et al. Leukocyte adhesion deficiency type II: long-term follow-up and review of the literature. J Clin Immunol. 2010;30:308–13. https://doi.org/10.1007/s10875-009-9354-0.

84. Etzioni A, Gershoni-Baruch R, Pollack S, Shehadeh N. Leukocyte adhesion deficiency type II: long-term follow-up. J Allergy Clin Immunol. 1998;102:323–4.

85. Marquardt T, et al. Correction of leukocyte adhesion deficiency type II with oral fucose. Blood. 1999;94:3976–85.

86. Etzioni A, Tonetti M. Fucose supplementation in leukocyte adhesion deficiency type II. Blood. 2000;95:3641–3.

87. Mory A, et al. Kindlin-3: a new gene involved in the pathogenesis of LAD-III. Blood. 2008;112:2591. https://doi.org/10.1182/blood-2008-06-163162.

88. Kuijpers TW, et al. LAD-1/variant syndrome is caused by mutations in FERMT3. Blood. 2009;113:4740–6. https://doi.org/10.1182/blood-2008-10-182154.

89. Stepensky PY, et al. Leukocyte adhesion deficiency type III: clinical features and treatment with stem cell transplantation. J Pediatr Hematol Oncol. 2015;37:264–8. https://doi.org/10.1097/mph.0000000000000228.

90. Ambruso DR, et al. Human neutrophil immunodeficiency syndrome is associated with an inhibitory Rac2 mutation. Proc Natl Acad Sci U S A. 2000;97:4654–9. https://doi.org/10.1073/pnas.080074897.

91. Williams DA, et al. Dominant negative mutation of the hematopoietic-specific Rho GTPase, Rac2, is associated with a human phagocyte immunodeficiency. Blood. 2000;96:1646–54.

92. Routes JM, et al. Statewide newborn screening for severe T-cell lymphopenia. JAMA. 2009;302:2465–70. https://doi.org/10.1001/jama.2009.1806.

93. Accetta D, et al. Human phagocyte defect caused by a Rac2 mutation detected by means of neonatal

screening for T-cell lymphopenia. J Allergy Clin Immunol. 2011;127:535–538.e531-532. https://doi.org/10.1016/j.jaci.2010.10.013.

94. Alkhairy OK, et al. RAC2 loss-of-function mutation in 2 siblings with characteristics of common variable immunodeficiency. J Allergy Clin Immunol. 2015;135:1380–1384.e1381-1385. https://doi.org/10.1016/j.jaci.2014.10.039.

95. Grimbacher B, et al. Hyper-IgE syndrome with recurrent infections – an autosomal dominant multisystem disorder. N Engl J Med. 1999;340:692–702. https://doi.org/10.1056/nejm199903043400904.

96. Minegishi Y, et al. Dominant-negative mutations in the DNA-binding domain of STAT3 cause hyper-IgE syndrome. Nature. 2007;448:1058–62. https://doi.org/10.1038/nature06096.

97. Holland SM, et al. STAT3 mutations in the hyper-IgE syndrome. N Engl J Med. 2007;357:1608–19. https://doi.org/10.1056/NEJMoa073687.

98. Minegishi Y, et al. Molecular explanation for the contradiction between systemic Th17 defect and localized bacterial infection in hyper-IgE syndrome. J Exp Med. 2009;206:1291–301. https://doi.org/10.1084/jem.20082767.

99. Freeman AF, et al. Lung parenchyma surgery in autosomal dominant hyper-IgE syndrome. J Clin Immunol. 2013;33:896–902. https://doi.org/10.1007/s10875-013-9890-5.

100. Freeman AF, Holland SM. The hyper-IgE syndromes. Immunol Allergy Clin N Am. 2008;28:277–91., viii. https://doi.org/10.1016/j.iac.2008.01.005.

101. Ling JC, et al. Coronary artery aneurysms in patients with hyper IgE recurrent infection syndrome. Clin Immunol (Orlando, Fla). 2007;122:255–8. https://doi.org/10.1016/j.clim.2006.10.005.

102. Freeman AF, et al. Brain abnormalities in patients with hyperimmunoglobulin E syndrome. Pediatrics. 2007;119:e1121–5. https://doi.org/10.1542/peds.2006-2649.

103. Engelhardt KR, et al. The extended clinical phenotype of 64 patients with DOCK8 deficiency. J Allergy Clin Immunol. 2015;136:402–12. https://doi.org/10.1016/j.jaci.2014.12.1945.

104. Zhang Q, et al. Combined immunodeficiency associated with DOCK8 mutations. N Engl J Med. 2009;361:2046–55. https://doi.org/10.1056/NEJMoa0905506.

105. Engelhardt KR, et al. Large deletions and point mutations involving the dedicator of cytokinesis 8 (DOCK8) in the autosomal-recessive form of hyper-IgE syndrome. J Allergy Clin Immunol. 2009;124:1289–1302.e1284. https://doi.org/10.1016/j.jaci.2009.10.038.

106. Sassi A, et al. Hypomorphic, homozygous mutations in phosphoglucomutase 3 impair immunity and increase serum IgE levels. J Allergy Clin Immunol. 2014;133:1410–142013. https://doi.org/10.1016/j.jaci.2014.02.025.

107. Zhang Y, et al. Autosomal recessive PGM3 mutations link glycosylation defects to atopy,

immune deficiency, autoimmunity, and neurocognitive impairment. J Allergy Clin Immunol. 2014;133:1400–1409.e1405. https://doi.org/10.1016/j.jaci.2014.02.013.

108. Minegishi Y, et al. Human tyrosine kinase 2 deficiency reveals its requisite roles in multiple cytokine signals involved in innate and acquired immunity. Immunity. 2006;25:745–55. https://doi.org/10.1016/j.immuni.2006.09.009.

109. Kreins AY, et al. Human TYK2 deficiency: mycobacterial and viral infections without hyper-IgE syndrome. J Exp Med. 2015;212:1641–62. https://doi.org/10.1084/jem.20140280.

110. Bogunovic D, et al. Mycobacterial disease and impaired IFN-gamma immunity in humans with inherited ISG15 deficiency. Science. 2012;337:1684–8. https://doi.org/10.1126/science.1224026.

111. Hambleton S, et al. IRF8 mutations and human dendritic-cell immunodeficiency. N Engl J Med. 2011;365:127–38. https://doi.org/10.1056/NEJMoa1100066.

112. Haverkamp MH, van Dissel JT, Holland SM. Human host genetic factors in nontuberculous mycobacterial infection: lessons from single gene disorders affecting innate and adaptive immunity and lessons from molecular defects in interferon-gamma-dependent signaling. Microbes Infect. 2006;8:1157–66. https://doi.org/10.1016/j.micinf.2005.10.029.

113. Al-Muhsen S, Casanova JL. The genetic heterogeneity of mendelian susceptibility to mycobacterial diseases. J Allergy Clin Immunol. 2008;122:1043–51.; quiz 1052–1043. https://doi.org/10.1016/j.jaci.2008.10.037.

114. de Vor IC, et al. Deletion of the entire interferon-gamma receptor 1 gene causing complete deficiency in three related patients. J Clin Immunol. 2016;36:195–203. https://doi.org/10.1007/s10875-016-0244-y.

115. Prando C, et al. Inherited IL-12p40 deficiency: genetic, immunologic, and clinical features of 49 patients from 30 kindreds. Medicine (Baltimore). 2013;92:109–22. https://doi.org/10.1097/MD.0b013e31828a01f9.

116. Martinez-Barricarte R, et al. Mycobacterium simiae infection in two unrelated patients with different forms of inherited IFN-gammaR2 deficiency. J Clin Immunol. 2014;34:904–9. https://doi.org/10.1007/s10875-014-0085-5.

117. Wu UI, Holland SM. Host susceptibility to nontuberculous mycobacterial infections. Lancet Infect Dis. 2015;15:968–80. https://doi.org/10.1016/s1473-3099(15)00089-4.

118. Spinner MA, et al. GATA2 deficiency: a protean disorder of hematopoiesis, lymphatics, and immunity. Blood. 2014;123:809–21. https://doi.org/10.1182/blood-2013-07-515528.

119. Grabbe C, Husnjak K, Dikic I. The spatial and temporal organization of ubiquitin networks. Nat Rev Mol Cell Biol. 2011;12:295–307. https://doi.org/10.1038/nrm3099.

120. Smahi A, et al. Genomic rearrangement in NEMO impairs NF-kappaB activation and is a cause of incontinentia pigmenti. Int Incontinentia Pigmenti (IP) Consortium Nat. 2000;405:466–72.

121. Filipe-Santos O, et al. X-linked susceptibility to mycobacteria is caused by mutations in NEMO impairing CD40-dependent IL-12 production. J Exp Med. 2006;203:1745–59. https://doi.org/10.1084/jem.20060085.

122. Orange JS, et al. The presentation and natural history of immunodeficiency caused by nuclear factor kappaB essential modulator mutation. J Allergy Clin Immunol. 2004;113:725–33. https://doi.org/10.1016/j.jaci.2004.01.762.

123. Ferwerda B, et al. Human dectin-1 deficiency and mucocutaneous fungal infections. N Engl J Med. 2009;361:1760–7. https://doi.org/10.1056/NEJMoa0901053.

124. Glocker EO, et al. A homozygous CARD9 mutation in a family with susceptibility to fungal infections. N Engl J Med. 2009;361:1727–35. https://doi.org/10.1056/NEJMoa0810719.

125. Toubiana J, Okada S, Hiller J, et al. Heterozygous STAT1 gain-of-function mutations underlie an unexpectedly broad clinical phenotype. Blood. 2016;127(25):3154–64.

T Cell Defects

8

Morna J. Dorsey and Morton J. Cowan

Severe Combined Immunodeficiency (SCID)

SCID is a group of inheritable diseases occurring at a rate of 1/58,000 live births in the USA that results from defects in genes controlling lymphocyte development causing profound T cell deficiency [1, 2] (Table 8.1). As the most severe form of primary immunodeficiency (PID), typical SCID is generally fatal in the first year of life unless recognized and treated. Consequently, the treatment of choice is immune reconstitution through hematopoietic cell transplantation (HCT), enzyme replacement (in the case of adenosine deaminase deficiency), or experimental gene therapy (GT). Infants born with SCID are typically normal appearing and, unless diagnosed through NBS or by family history, are at high risk of serious infections after maternally transferred antibodies naturally decline and circulating antibody levels reach their nadir at 4–6 months of life. Common infections in the first year of life include opportunistic infections like *Pneumocystis jirovecii* and viral infections such as cytomegalovirus (CMV) as well as respiratory syncytial virus (RSV) and parainfluenza and

influenza viruses. Chronic diarrhea often with rotavirus vaccine strain occurs in SCID recipients of the oral rotavirus vaccine [3]. *Candida* infections are also common and recurrent, usually as oral thrush, and may be the reason for seeking medical attention; occasionally invasive disease such as meningitis may develop. Several of the specific gene defects that result in SCID can be associated with mild dysmorphia, but there are often no outward clues to the severity of the underlying diagnosis. The identification of infants with SCID has become a priority for states in the USA, and NBS for SCID is becoming more widespread. There are now several studies demonstrating that early transplantation leads to superior outcomes [4]. The rapid identification of patients with SCID and early HCT is of critical importance to successful treatment, in particular, because survival of >80% is seen in patients who have no active infection at the time of HCT regardless of age at HCT [4].

Definition

The definition of SCID is based on T cell lymphopenia and abnormal lymphocyte function. Table 8.2 highlights the current classification of SCID infants with low TRECS and is based on immune evaluation that includes total T cell numbers, lymphocyte responses to mitogens, and determination of presence or absence of maternal

M. J. Dorsey (✉) · M. J. Cowan
Allergy, Immunology, and Blood and Marrow
Transplant Division, Department of Pediatrics,
University of California, San Francisco, CA, USA
e-mail: Morna.dorsey@ucsf.edu; Mort.cowan@ucsf.
edu

© Springer International Publishing AG, part of Springer Nature 2018   151
B. H. Segal (ed.), *Management of Infections in the Immunocompromised Host*,
https://doi.org/10.1007/978-3-319-77674-3_8

Table 8.1 Summary of clinical and immunological features of SCID

Disease	Lymphocyte profile	Gene	Inheritance	Associated non-immunologic features
Impaired cytokine signaling and early lymphoid progenitor development				
IL2Rγ	T-B+NK-	IL2RG	X-linked	
JAK3 kinase	T-B+NK-	JAK3	AR	
IL-7Ra	T-B+NK-	IL7R	AR	
Defects in VDJ recombination				
RAG1	T-B-NK+	RAG1	AR	
RAG2	T-B-NK+	RAG2	AR	
Artemis	T-B-NK+	DCLRE1C	AR	Growth retardation, microcephaly
DNA-PKcs	T-B-NK+	PRKDC	AR	Growth retardation, dysmorphic facies, microcephaly
Ligase IV	T-B-NK+	LIG4	AR	Growth retardation, dysmorphic facies, microcephaly, bone marrow failure
Cernunnos	T-B-NK+	NHEJ	AR	Growth retardation, dysmorphic facies, microcephaly, bone marrow failure
Impaired signaling through TCR				
CD3δ	T-B+NK+	CD3D	AR	
CD3ε	T-B+NK+	CD3E	AR	
CD3ζ	T-B+NK+	CD3Z	AR	
CD45	T-B+NK+	PTPRC	AR	
Decreased lymphocyte survival, increased apoptosis, or impaired migration or function				
Reticular dysgenesis	T-B-NK-	AK2	AR	
ADA	T-B-NK-	ADA	AR	Skeletal abnormalities, pulmonary alveolar proteinosis, cognitive abnormalities

engraftment that can occur in 35–60% of cases of SCID [5, 6].

Pathogenesis of Selected SCID Genotypes

SCID and combined immunodeficiency (CID) comprise a spectrum of genetic disorders of the immune system that results in severe susceptibility to common opportunistic infections. Multiple gene defects have been identified as causing SCID, and these gene defects have illuminated the road to functional T cell development. While genetic testing is not essential in many cases to move forward with transplant, there are compelling reasons to pursue a genetic diagnosis. In some cases it will dictate the type of transplant performed, and inheritance pattern is important to determine recurrence risk in another child.

IL2Rγ Deficient SCID (X-SCID) The common γ chain (γc) (CD132) is a key component of the following cytokine receptors: IL-2, IL-4, IL-7, IL-9, IL-15, and IL-21. The absence of IL-7 signaling is likely the most deleterious effect of mutations as this is a critical T-lymphocyte development factor. Defective survival and function of early T cell progenitors in the thymus lead to extreme T cell lymphopenia. IL-4 and IL-21 are important for functional immunoglobulin production and B cell differentiation, and absent signaling results in the B cell defects seen in these patients. IL-15 is an important factor in natural killer (NK) cell development and its absence results in NK deficiency in X-SCID [7].

RAG Deficient SCID (RAG-SCID) Assembly of antigen receptor genes as part of the generation of T cell receptors (TCRs) and B cell receptors (BCRs) occurs through V(D)J recombination. Recombinase activating genes (RAG) are key

Table 8.2 Classification of infants with low TRECS and low T cells

Category	Definition of condition[a]
Typical SCID	<300 autologous T cells/uL, <10% of normal proliferation to PHA, frequently with maternal T cell engraftment and deleterious defect(s) in a known SCID gene
Leaky SCID	300–1499 autologous T cells/uL (or higher numbers of oligoclonal T cells), reduced proliferation to PHA, no maternal engraftment, generally with incomplete defect(s) in a known SCID gene
Omenn syndrome	Similar to leaky SCID but also with oligoclonal T cells, erythroderma, hepatosplenomegaly, eosinophilia, and elevated serum IgE levels
Syndrome with low T cells	Recognized genetic syndrome that includes low T cells within its spectrum of clinical findings
Secondary low T cells	Congenital malformation or disease process without intrinsic immunodeficiency that results in low circulating T cells
Preterm birth alone	Preterm infants with low T cells early that become normal over time
Idiopathic T cell lymphopenia	Persistently low T cells (300–1499/uL), functional T cell and/or B cell impairment, no defect in a typical SCID gene; etiology and clinical course undetermined

PHA phytohemagglutinin
[a]Definitions used by primary immunodeficiency treatment consortium
[b]When or if an etiology for low T cells is discovered, the affected individual is moved to the appropriate category

players in this assembly process. Recombination signal sequences (RSSs) flank each V, D, and J coding segment. RAG1/2 recombinase initiates recombination by introducing double-stranded breaks in the DNA between the RSS and coding segments. RAG gene mutations result in arrest of the V(D)J recombination process, with a resultant block in T and B cell differentiation [8].

ADA Deficient SCID (ADA-SCID) Adenosine deaminase (ADA) is an enzyme of the purine salvage pathway that is present in all cells. Activity is highest in the thymic T cells, lymphoid tissue, gastrointestinal tract, and brain [9]. ADA catalyzes the irreversible deamination of adenosine and deoxyadenosine to inosine and deoxyinosine [10]. As a result of ADA deficiency, increased concentrations of ADA substrates occur, particularly in the thymus, and induce apoptosis of immature thymic lymphocytes [11].

Artemis Deficient SCID (ART-SCID) DCLRE1C, which encodes Artemis protein, is mapped to chromosome 10 and is the gene responsible for radiation sensitive (RS)-SCID [12]. During the later steps of V(D)J recombination, the hairpin coding ends are opened prior to ligation by Artemis, which undergoes phosphorylation by DNA-PKcs to become an endonuclease [13].

IL-7Ra Deficient SCID IL-7 provides survival and proliferative signals through the IL-7 receptor and thus plays a critical role in early T cell development. The IL-7 receptor is composed of a unique alpha chain (CD127) and a gamma chain (CD132). B cell development in humans is independent of IL-7. NK cell numbers and function appear to be unaffected by IL-7Ra deficiency [14].

Clinical Presentation of Selected SCID Genotypes

If not identified by SCID NBS, infants with SCID typically present during the first months of life with recurrent and/or severe infections, such as oral candidiasis and pneumonias caused by *Pneumocystis jirovecii* or viral agents (e.g., CMV, RSV, adenovirus, herpes virus, parainfluenza), often concurrently. Persistent diarrhea with failure to thrive is also common; exposure to oral rotavirus vaccine can also be very problematic [3]. Occasionally, other intracellular organisms such as *Listeria monocytogenes* or *Legionella* species can lead to uncontrolled B cell proliferation. Live attenuated vaccines such as BCG, may lead to disseminated and even lethal infection [15, 16].

X-SCID T cells and NK cells are typically extremely low to absent in number, and B cell numbers are typically normal, but in up to 5% of patients, low B cells are seen (Buckley RH and Schiff RI). The presence of maternal T cells can be associated with a graft versus host (GVH) reaction that presents with an erythrodermic skin rash, eosinophilia, and hepatomegaly. See Table 8.1 for the lymphocyte profiles of SCID genotypes.

RAG-SCID The immunologic phenotype is characterized by severe lymphopenia with a virtual absence of T and B cells and presence of circulating NK cells. Hypomorphic mutations in RAG1 and/or RAG2 are the most frequent causes of Omenn syndrome (OS). Infants with OS present with varying degrees of eczematous rash that can be quite severe as well as diarrhea and enlarged lymph nodes and hepatosplenomegaly in severe cases [17]. When these manifestations are refractory to steroid treatment, calcineurin inhibitors or T cell-directed immunosuppression with anti-CD52 monoclonal antibody (alemtuzumab) or polyclonal rabbit antithymocyte globulin may be required before transplant. Some patients with leaky (less severe) RAG mutations are known to present later in childhood with a lifelong history of food allergy and eczematous skin or in adulthood with recurrent sinopulmonary infection and poor polysaccharide antibody responses [18, 19].

ADA-SCID Affected infants present with similar infectious manifestations as classical SCID. In addition to lymphopenia, infants often develop neutropenia that improves once life-saving ADA replacement therapy is initiated. In addition to hematologic aberrations, infants with ADA-SCID are susceptible to pulmonary alveolar proteinosis that can result in respiratory distress, typically manifesting with tachypnea and hypoxemia that improves with correction of the enzyme deficiency. Bony abnormalities can be seen on CXR with evidence of cupping of the anterior ribs and scapular spurring. Plaque-like or nodular skin dermatofibrosarcoma protuberans lesions are frequently seen in ADA deficiency [20]. In addition to cognitive and behavioral abnormalities, sensorineural hearing loss is frequently demonstrated [21]. Some patients are identified as late-onset ADA deficiency even into adulthood [22]. The most common presentation in these patients is lymphopenia and recurrent sinopulmonary disease [23].

ART-SCID The immunologic phenotype is characterized by profound T and B cell lymphopenia with the presence of circulating NK cells. This RS-SCID is very rare in the general population but is found with a high incidence among Athabascan-speaking Native Americans (1 in 2000 live births among Navajo Indians) [24]. Affected patients present early in life with recurrent and serious infection with opportunistic organisms. A classic clinical finding in affected infants is the presence of oral mucosal and urogenital ulcers that are painful and do not resolve until T cell immunity is reconstituted. Infants with hypomorphic Artemis mutations can present with symptoms similar to OS.

IL-7Ra deficient SCID Similar to X-SCID, maternal chimerism is seen frequently in this SCID genotype. T cells are profoundly low or absent and B cells are typically normal or increased in number. Hypomorphic mutations in the IL7Ra gene have been described in patients with erythroderma with evidence of oligoclonal, activated T cells consistent with OS. Polymorphisms in IL-7Ra have been shown to be a risk factor for a number of diseases that are autoimmune or involve excess immune and inflammatory responses including multiple sclerosis, type 1 diabetes, rheumatoid arthritis, and inflammatory bowel disease [25].

In addition to the classic SCID presentation described above, variants of each condition exist and can present in a number of different ways. This includes persistent lymphopenia, marrow failure, ill-defined autoimmunity, granulomas, and abnormal immunoglobulin production and function. The range of phenotypes associated with the variants is still not entirely clear, and infection is often not the major manifestation.

Diagnosis

Newborn screening for SCID utilizes a test based on quantification of T cell receptor excision circles (TRECS) produced during V(D)J recombination which is essential for T cell maturation in the thymus. TRECs correlate with production of naïve T cells. TRECs are very low in virtually all cases of SCID in which very low numbers of naïve T cells are generated. A typical evaluation for SCID includes determination of lymphocyte subsets including CD3, CD4, CD8, CD16/56, and CD19. Obtaining CD45RA/RO T cell markers is important for confirming the diagnosis and in assessing the likelihood of oligoclonal expansion of T cells, which is seen in transplacental maternal T cell engraftment (TME). In addition to conditions listed in Table 8.3, leaky ADA-SCID may not be identified by TREC NBS. Lymphocyte proliferation to mitogen is usually low to absent (<10% of the lower limit of normal for the lab) and confirms abnormal function. The presence of TME can be determined through studies of short tandem repeats (STR) analysis of infant and mother or fluorescence in situ hybridization (FISH) for X and Y chromosomes in male infants, the significance of which may influence the choice of donor and possible need for serotherapy or conditioning prior to HCT. The diagnosis of X-SCID should be considered in any male infant with severe lymphopenia. Immunoglobulin G levels at birth may be normal as the IgG present at birth is maternally derived. Based on the recent results of NBS in 11 states and the Navajo Nation as well as a study from California, the two most common forms of SCID in the USA are X-SCID (19%) and RAG-SCID (15%) followed by ADA-SCID (10%) [26]. A positive family history for SCID may be present and would enable diagnosis in the prenatal period, which could be performed by mutation detection in fetuses at risk using DNA obtained from chorionic villous biopsy performed at 8–10 weeks of pregnancy or amniotic fluid obtained somewhat later. Molecular confirmation can be obtained by sequencing the IL2RG gene. Flow cytometry analysis of CD132 (γc) cell surface expression can be challenging because of the presence of lymphopenia and the possibility of TME. In addition, missense mutations can result in normal γc expression further suggesting molecular identification as a means of identifying the gene defect. Genetic reversion events can lead to normal γc sequence and expression in lymphocytes requiring both somatic and peripheral lymphocyte DNA sequencing [27].

Other forms of SCID occurring in male patients can mimic the typical X-SCID phenotype and include JAK3 deficiency (Table 8.1) and IL-7Ra, although the latter generally presents with detectable peripheral blood NK cells. In males without the typical X-SCID phenotype, in affected females and when there may be consanguinity within a family, the differential diagnosis must include forms of autosomal recessive SCID including those with abnormal V(D)J recombination resulting from mutations in the recombinase activating genes, RAG1 or RAG2, or DCLRE1C genes as well as other causes of T-B-NK+ and T-B+NK+ SCID (Table 8.1). For patients with RS-SCID, because of their heightened sensitivity to radiation, imaging requiring radiation must be conducted judiciously and only if potential results would have significant impact on outcome. Additional features that may be helpful in focusing the diagnostic effort include microcephaly and marrow failure associated with some forms of RS-SCID, neutropenia, and/or pulmonary proteinosis seen with ADA-SCID (Table 8.1).

Enzyme assay of ADA activity can confirm deficiency using available cell lines including erythrocytes but may be unreliable in the setting

Table 8.3 Immune disorders and expectations for abnormally low TRECs at birth

SCID conditions proven to be identified by TREC NBS	CID conditions that have been identified by TREC NBS	Other conditions that have been identified by TREC NBS	Conditions in which TREC NBS would not be expected to identify affected infants
IL2Rγ, IL-7Ra, JAK3, ADA, CD3D, CD3E, CD3Z, CD45, RAG1, RAG2, Artemis, DNA-PKcs, Ligase IV, Reticular dysgenesis, Cernunnos	LCK, PNP, FOXN1, DOCK8, Coronin-1A, Cartilage-hair hypoplasia, combined ID with multiple intestinal atresia	RAC2, Nijmegen-breakage syndrome, Ataxia-telangiectasia, DiGeorge syndrome, CHARGE syndrome, Jacobsen syndrome, Trisomy 21, Trisomy 18, CLOVES, ECC, Fryns, TAR, Renpenning	ZAP-70, MHC class II, CD3G

CHARGE coloboma, heart defect, atresia choanae, retarded growth and development, genital and ear abnormality, *CLOVES* congenital lipomatous overgrowth, vascular malformations, epidermal nevi, and spinal/skeletal anomalies, *ECC* ectodermal dysplasia, ectrodactyly, and clefting, *TAR* thrombocytopenia and absent radius

of a recent blood transfusion. In those situations, studies in the parents can often demonstrate carrier status. Confirmation is typically conducted through genetic testing of the ADA gene.

Management

Parents of infants suspected to have SCID or leaky SCID based on NBS, or if identified by family history or clinical features, are given instructions regarding protective isolation precautions. However, in most instances, this is not easily attainable as an outpatient, and therefore, admission to the hospital is necessary. Infants should avoid live rotavirus vaccine, and the potential for CMV transmission from breastfeeding (if the mother is CMV seropositive) should be discussed with the parents. Caregivers of infants diagnosed with SCID have particular psychosocial vulnerability and are especially susceptible to postpartum depression and posttraumatic stress (M Dorsey, UCSF, personal communication). A social worker versed in SCID to identify needs for support of the family is an important part of the medical team. Infectious disease workup includes assessing for CMV by serum PCR, which may have been transmitted via breast milk prior to confirmation of SCID. Baseline immunologic function which includes lymphocyte proliferation to mitogens, immunoglobulin profile, as well as lymphocyte subset confirmation should be obtained, along with HLA testing of the infant and nuclear family members. Testing for maternal chimerism by DNA short tandem repeat marker analysis of the infant's whole blood and CD3-selected cells is the most sensitive method to demonstrate transplacentally transferred maternal T cells, the presence of which has implications for choice of a donor for HCT as well as GVHD prophylaxis (J Wahlstrom, UCSF, personal communication). An elevated proportion of CD45RO+ T cells suggests expansion of a limited repertoire of T cells of either infant or maternal origin. If an infant diagnosed with ADA-SCID has no matched sibling immediately available, PEG-ADA enzyme should be initiated while an unrelated donor search is underway or while awaiting gene therapy. If infection or respiratory distress due to pulmonary alveolar proteinosis (PAP) is present, PEG-ADA should not be delayed. Blood draws should be carefully planned to minimize discomfort and the smallest possible volumes drawn for each test to avoid iatrogenic anemia. Transfusions should be avoided to minimize risks of infection. If a transfusion is needed, only CMV-negative, irradiated, leukoreduced packed red cells should be given. Initiation of IgG replacement therapy should not be delayed. Introduction of prophylaxis with trimethoprim-sulfamethoxazole (TMP-SMX), acyclovir, and fluconazole can begin after the first month of life unless active infection is present, and providing the liver function tests is normal.

Multicenter collaborations, including the Primary Immunodeficiency Treatment Consortium (PIDTC), have begun to address unknowns regarding best practices and transplant outcomes for patients with mutations in specific genes by studying large numbers of patients enrolled from transplant centers across North America. The first PIDTC retrospective report on SCID showed that infants who received transplants at 3.5 months of age or younger had a 5-year survival rate of 94%, comparable to infants older than 3.5 months of age at the time of HCT and with no history of infection (90%) or whose infection had resolved by the time of HCT (82%) [4]. Children who were older than 3.5 months of age and had active infection at the time of HCT had the lowest survival (50%). HLA-matched sibling donors resulted in the best outcomes regardless of age or infection. While reduced intensity conditioning (RIC) or myeloablative conditioning (MAC) versus no or immunosuppression alone resulted in a higher likelihood of full T cell reconstitution and being free of immunoglobulin supplementation, the long-term effects of this therapy were not addressed in this study [4]. Autologous gene therapy has been successful for children with X-SCID and ADA-SCID [28]. The initial success in X-SCID was tempered by the development of insertional mutagenesis (IM) in 5 of the initial 20 recipients of cells transduced with Maloney retroviral vectors. Currently, there are ongoing trials using self-inactivating retroviral or lentiviral vectors, which appear to have a significantly lower risk of IM and potential risk of leukemia. In the early X-SCID trials, no conditioning was used resulting in T cell, but limited B and NK cell, reconstitution. The preliminary experience to date with low-dose busulfan and a lentiviral vector for ADA-SCID [29] and X-SCID [personal communication, H Malech, NIH-NIAID] suggests that B and NK cell reconstitution will be more likely.

Selected Combined Immunodeficiencies (CID)

CD40L Deficiency

Definition
CD40L deficiency is a class-switch recombination (CSR) defect that is characterized by normal or elevated IgM with other isotypes (IgG, IgA, IgE) low or absent (Table 8.4). Due to this typical laboratory phenotype and inheritance pattern, it is often referred to as X-linked hyper-IgM syndrome, estimated to occur at a rate of 1 in 500,000 male births [30].

Pathogenesis
CD40L (CD154) is a type II transmembrane protein with an extracellular domain that is a tumor necrosis factor (TNF) homologue. Expression on the mainly activated helper CD4+ T cell subset is transient, but CD40L is also known to be expressed by activated B cells, mast cells, and platelets [31]. T follicular helper (TFH) cells are known to express high levels of CD40L, and absence of interaction with CD40 on B cells results in absent germinal center formation with decreased B cell proliferation, class-switch recombination, and somatic hypermutation.

Interaction between CD40L expressed by the TFH cell subset and its receptor CD40 on B cells induces B cell proliferation, CSR, and somatic hypermutation (SHM). CD40 is constitutively expressed on B cells, and the CD40-CD40L signaling has an essential role in antibody

Table 8.4 Summary of immune and clinical features of combined immunodeficiencies

Disease	Immune profile	Gene	Inheritance	Associated features
Ligase IV	↓T and B cells, T cell proliferation	*LIG4,*	AR	Microcephaly, developmental delay, growth retardation
	↓Igs			
	Radiation sensitivity			
	Pancytopenia			
Cernunnos	↓T and B cells, T cell proliferation	*NHEJ1*	AR	Microcephaly, developmental delay, growth retardation
	↓Igs			
	Radiation sensitivity			
	Pancytopenia			
PNP	↓T cells, T cell proliferation	*PNP*	AR	Neurologic abnormalities
	Low uric acid and PNP activity			
CD8A	↓↓CD8 T cells	*CD8A*	AR	
	Normal T cell proliferation			
CD3γ	↓ or normal T cells but reduced TCR	CD3G	AR	
	Normal B cells			
ZAP70	↓↓CD8 T cells	*ZAP70*	AR	
	↓T cell proliferation			
CD40L	↑ or normal IgM	*CD40L*	X-linked	Neutropenia
	↓IgG and IgA			PJP, cryptosporidium
ORAI1, STIM1	↓T cell proliferation	*ORAI1*	AR	Abnormal dental enamel, ectodermal dysplasia, hypotonia, autoimmunity, and lymphoproliferation
	↓calcium influx with TCR stimulation	*STIM1*		
MHCI	↓MHCI expression	*MHCI*	AR	Necrotizing granulomas skin
MHCII	↓CD4 T cells, T cell proliferation to antigens	CIITA, RFXANK, RFX5, RFXAP	AR	Sclerosing cholangitis
	↓↓ MHCII expression			
FOXN1	↓↓MHCII expression	*FOXN1*	AR	Nail dystrophy, nail dystrophy
	↓T cell proliferation			
	↓↓TRECs			
MAGT1	↓CD4 T cells	*MAGT1*	X-linked	EBV lymphoma
	↓NKG2D expression on NK and CD8			
ITK	↓↓iNK T cells	*ITK*	AR	EBV lymphoma
	↓calcium influx with TCR stimulation			
IKAROS	↓B cell and NK cell	*IKAROS*	AD	Bone marrow aplasia
	Pancytopenia			
DOCK8	↓CD4 T cells	*DOCK8*	AR	Cutaneous viral and bacterial infection, lymphoma, squamous cell carcinoma
	↑IgE, eosinophils			

(continued)

Table 8.4 (continued)

Disease	Immune profile	Gene	Inheritance	Associated features
DOCK2	↓T cells, ↓NK cell function	*DOCK2*	AR	
	↓ TRECs			
	Poor PHA responses			
TYK2	↓Phosphorylation of STATs to IL-12, IL-23, IL-6, IL-10, type 1 IFN	*TYK2*	AR	Disseminated BCG
	↑IgE			
LCK	↓CD4 T cells, T cell proliferation	*LCK*	AR	Cytopenia, retinal vasculitis
	↓Antibody production			
CARD11	↓T cell proliferation	*CARD11*	AR	PJP, meningitis
	↓Igs			
MALT1	↓T and B cell proliferation	*MALT1*	AR	CMV, *Candida,* poor growth
	↓Functional antibodies			
IL-21R	↓Class switch recombination	*IL21R*	AR	PJP, cryptosporidium, *Candida*
	IgE			
	↓Phosphorylation of STATs to IL-21			
IL-21	Normal T cells	*IL21*	AR	Early-onset IBD
	↓ or normal T cell function			
LRBA	↓ or normal CD4 T cells	LRBA	AR	IBD, EBV
	↓ or normal B cells			
	↓IgG and IgA			
STK4 (MST1)	↓CD4 T cells, T cell proliferation	*STK4*	AR	Staph skin infections, mucocutaneous candidiasis, EBV, lymphoma
	↑IgE			
	↓IgM			
WAS	↓T cells, T cell proliferation	*WASP*	X-linked	Eczema, thrombocytopenia, small platelets, autoimmunity
	↓IgG and IgM			
	↑IgA and IgE			
	Post-vaccine titers			
Cartilage hair hypoplasia	↓CD4 and CD8 T cells, T cell proliferation	*RMRP*	AR	Hair hypoplasia, metaphyseal dysplasia, ligamentous laxity
	Anemia			
Combined immunodeficiency with multiple intestinal atresia	↓↓ or normal T cells	*TTC7A*	AR	Multiple intestinal atresia, can present with SCID
	Normal B cells			
Coronin-1A	↓↓ or normal T cells	*CORO1A*	AR	EBV, lymphoproliferation
	Normal B cells			

maturation and B cell proliferation and survival. Defects in the CD40L/CD40 interaction prevent the formation of germinal centers in the secondary lymphoid organs and thus impair CSR and SHM and an inability to generate memory B cells or mount IgG, IgA, or IgE responses to T cell-dependent antigens. CD40 is also expressed at the surface of monocytes, dendritic cells, and granulocyte progenitor cells, which may explain neutropenia commonly seen in these patients since GM-CSF and G-CSF are two important regulators of granulopoiesis that require CD40 activation on bone marrow stromal cells [32]. Defects in T cell and B cell interaction through CD40/CD40L result in impaired germinal center formation and an inability to generate memory B cells or mount IgG, IgA, or IgE responses to T cell-dependent antigens [33].

Clinical Presentation

Most CD40L-deficient patients suffer from upper and lower respiratory tract infections in the first few years of life. *Pneumocystis jiroveci* pneumonia (PjP) is often the presenting infection in affected children. Males with deficiency of CD40L exhibit defective humoral and cell-mediated immunity. Defects in antibody synthesis result in susceptibility to infections caused by *Haemophilus influenzae*, *Streptococcus pneumoniae*, *Streptococcus pyogenes*, and *Staphylococcus aureus*. These bacteria are resistant to destruction by phagocytic cells unless they are opsonized with antibody and complement. Defects in cell-mediated immunity due to abnormal T cell-mediated activation of macrophages result in susceptibility to opportunistic infections. *Giardia lamblia* and *Cryptosporidium* infections can be severe in these patients or can be chronic and subclinical [34]. Chronic *Cryptosporidium* infection can lead to sclerosing cholangitis, terminal liver damage, and cancer [35]. Although rare, enteroviral meningitis, skin infections, and soft tissue infections have been reported [36]. Neutropenia, seen in about 50% of cases, can be the initial presenting sign of the condition and is often associated with mouth ulcers.

Diagnosis

CD40L deficiency should be considered in male children with normal or elevated IgM and low IgG and IgA in the setting of recurrent infection. While total B cell counts are normal including CD19 B cells, there are typically low class switched memory B cells (CD19+CD27+IgD-IgM-) displaying a CSR defect. Infection with both common and opportunistic pathogens (e.g., PjP and *Cryptosporidium*) is common as is the

presence of neutropenia. Low T cell counts have been reported but this is more the exception than the rule. Absence or low level CD40L expression on in vitro-activated CD4+ T cells will aid in diagnosis. Genetic confirmation will likely identify mutations in exon 5 of CD40L gene, which shares the greatest degree of homology with TNF and where most mutations lie. In female carriers, random X-inactivation is observed.

Management

Immunoglobulin replacement and prophylaxis against PjP with TMP-SMX are the most important factors in reducing frequency and severity of infections. Patients with neutropenia may benefit from G-CSF. While infection can be mitigated with prophylactic therapy, infection and liver disease due to chronic sclerosing cholangitis are the main causes of death later in life [33]. Therefore, HCT should be considered early.

Wiskott-Aldrich Syndrome (WAS)

Definition

The Wiskott-Aldrich syndrome is an X-linked disorder characterized by a bleeding tendency, eczema, infections, high incidence of autoimmune disorders, and lymphoreticular neoplasia. The WAS protein (WASP) gene (*WAS*) has been mapped to the short arm of the X chromosome (Xp11.23) [37]. Mutations in *WAS* not only cause WAS but may also cause chronic or intermittent X-linked thrombocytopenia (XLT) and X-linked neutropenia (XLN). XLT is a milder form of WAS characterized by thrombocytopenia and small platelets and an increased risk of lymphoma. XLN is a rare WAS-associated disorder, which is clinically and biologically different, and is characterized by congenital neutropenia and an increased risk of myelodysplasia [38]. The incidence of the classic WAS phenotype has been estimated to be between one and ten in one million individuals [39].

Pathogenesis

WAS is expressed exclusively in all hematopoietic cells, including CD34+ stem cells, platelets, lymphocytes (including NK cells), neutrophils, monocytes and macrophages, and dendritic cells. The function of WASP includes actin polymerization, which plays an important role in T cell function. The cytoskeleton is linked to cell-surface receptors in the plasma membrane so that events occurring at the membrane can affect cytoskeleton reorganization. In cross-linking of T cell antigen receptors and co-receptors by antigen, MHC complexes lead to their aggregation at one pole of the T cell, with an accompanying concentration of the actin cytoskeleton at that point [40]. Many other T cell functions depend on the actin cytoskeleton including emigration from the thymus into the blood. T cells from patients with WAS are deficient in all of these normal cellular abilities and, in particular, seem unable to interact successfully with B cells and other target cells. T cells are morphologically abnormal in patients with WAS because the cells lose their surface microvilli and assume a characteristically bald appearance. In addition, because *WAS* is broadly expressed within the hematopoietic system, other blood cell lineages, in particular, platelets, are also affected.

Clinical Presentation

Patients with mutations in *WAS* can present with a spectrum of clinical manifestations. Strong phenotype-genotype correlations have been demonstrated, and most of the patients can be divided into two main categories: classic WAS where WASP is truncated or absent and X-linked thrombocytopenia (XLT) if the mutated WASP has normal size [41]. The classic clinical triad of WAS is infection, bleeding, and eczema with the most common characteristic finding being thrombocytopenia and small platelets. Patients with WAS have increased susceptibility to both pyogenic bacterial infections and opportunistic infections. Among the latter, severe varicella, herpes simplex, and molluscum contagiosum are often present. The increased susceptibility to viral infections may be at least partly due to the impaired cytotoxic function of CD8+ T cells and NK cells in WAS; the impairment seems to be in their inability to attach to target cells [42]. Antibody formation, particularly against carbo-

hydrate antigens, is defective and explains the increased susceptibility to sinopulmonary infections [43].

Diagnosis

The diagnosis of WAS or XLT should be considered in any male with congenital or early-onset thrombocytopenia and small platelets, especially with a family history of affected males. Infections and immunologic abnormalities (e.g., absent isohemagglutinin titers, absent responses to pneumococcal polysaccharide immunization, and low to absent T cell proliferative responses to anti-CD3) are characteristic of WAS but may be present or absent at various times across the trajectory of illness [44]. Patients with WAS are highly susceptible to autoimmune disease (cytopenias and renal disease) and malignancies, in particular, lymphomas. While small platelets are typically present in affected patients, the mean platelet volume (MPV) on the standard CBC is not reliable. Diagnosis can be made by intracytoplasmic WASP expression by flow cytometry and is a rapid screening tool. Abnormal WASP expression may indicate a variety of disease states including presence of disease, revertant states, and carrier status. Rare cases of females with WAS have been described involving a deleterious mutation of the paternally derived X chromosome and nonrandom inactivation of the maternally derived X chromosome [45]. The definitive diagnosis of WAS is made through sequencing of the *WAS* gene.

Management

Infection prophylaxis with TMP-SMX is needed to prevent PjP and acyclovir to prevent recurrent herpes simplex infections. Most practitioners agree that IgG replacement therapy at occasionally higher doses is needed given hypercatabolism of IgG. Splenectomy is often suggested for severe bleeding but significantly increases the risk of sepsis and is a risk factor for death in WAS following HCT [46]. HCT is the only curative therapy available for patients with WAS and should be performed as early as possible if an adequate donor is available. Matched sibling donors result in highly successful transplant with improved outcomes recently for matched unrelated donors. Gene therapy is an investigation therapy and may be an alternative strategy when an HLA-compatible donor is not available. However, insertional mutagenesis (IM) following gene therapy for WAS using a retroviral vector was very high in the initial patients treated [47]. Ongoing studies are using lentiviral vector constructs, which hopefully will have a lower tendency towards IM.

MHC Class II Deficiency

Definition

This form of bare lymphocyte syndrome (diseases resulting from mutations in genes required for MHC expression or function) causes severe susceptibility to bacterial, viral, and protozoal pathogens, accompanied by decreased CD4+ T cell numbers and impaired functions, including effects on T cell-dependent antibodies. MHC II deficiency is an autosomal recessive disease, which results from mutations in transcription factors required for the expression of MHC II genes. Mutations in any one of four regulatory genes (CIITA, RFXANK, RFX5, RFXAP) are responsible for the clinical presentation. Most have mutations in the RFXANK gene, due to a founder mutation c.752delG-25 in patients of North African origin [48].

Pathogenesis

During thymic development, expression of the MHC II genes in the HLA-DR, HLA-DP, and HLA-DQ loci is required for processing and presentation of exogenous antigens to CD4+ T cells and for the ability of mature peripheral CD4+ T cells to respond to antigens during infections. Loss of any one of the specific transcription factors causes defective constitutive expression of MHC-II molecules on dendritic cells, monocytes, and B cells as well as impaired IFN-γ-induced upregulation of MHC-II molecules on other cell types [49].

Clinical Presentation

Severe and recurrent infections of the respiratory tract are the most common presentation. Pathogens associated with infection include *Pneumocystis jirovecii*, CMV, adenovirus, RSV, *Haemophilus influenzae*, *Streptococcus pneumoniae*, *Staphylococcus aureus*, *Pseudomonas aeruginosa*, and *Moraxella catarrhalis*. Mucocutaneous candidiasis is common, and gastrointestinal infections can present with chronic diarrhea and are due to a variety of organisms including enteroviruses, *Salmonella enteritidis*, *Campylobacter jejuni*, adenovirus, *Escherichia coli*, *Klebsiella pneumonia*, *Staphylococcus aureus*, *Enterococcus* species, *Giardia lamblia*, and *Proteus mirabilis*. Sclerosing cholangitis, a condition resulting from chronic *Cryptosporidium parvum* infection, can result in liver failure. Viral central nervous system infections as well as orolabial HSV infections also occur [50].

Diagnosis

The immune profile of MHC-II patients is decreased CD4+ T cells or normal or decreased numbers of CD8+ T cells, B cells, and NK cells. Lymphocyte proliferation to mitogens is normal, but absent to antigens. Total immunoglobulin levels are usually low, and specific antibodies to protein antigens are absent. MHC class II expression on activated T cells and B cells during infection is typically absent or profoundly decreased and absent on monocytes. The diagnosis is confirmed by genotyping for the various MHCII regulatory genes.

Management

HCT does not improve CD4 T cell counts due to continued absence of MHC II expression on thymic epithelial cells [51, 52]. However, most patients die within the first decade of life due to infection unless they undergo HCT. Persistent viral infections appear to be associated with increased risk of GVHD. Despite this, with successful transplantation, patients clinically improve due to functional CD4 T cell proliferation to antigens and T cell-mediated B cell antibody production.

Future Directions

Advances in technology have improved detection of immune disorders. Through more widespread use of whole exome/genome sequencing, a growing appreciation of wide phenotypic variability for individual-specific genetic conditions exists. This variability highlights the complexity of PIDs with regards to immunologic and clinical presentation including increasingly observed immune dysregulation.

Significant advancement has also occurred in the treatment of PIDs. GT by gene edition using viral vector is currently under clinical trial investigation as an exciting treatment option for PID including X-SCID, ADA-SCID, WAS, chronic granulomatous disease, and leukocyte adhesion deficiency. Other forms of SCID including ART-SCID and RAG1/RAG2 SCID are currently under preclinical investigation with the goal of advancing to early-phase clinical trials. In addition to gene modification of hematopoietic stem cells using gene addition, new methods for gene editing through site-specific endonucleases such as zinc-finger nuclease (ZFN), transcription activator-like effector nuclease (TALEN), and clustered regularly interspaced short palindromic repeat (CRISPR) may allow for an alternative method of gene correction. By introducing a DNA break at essentially one site out of the entire genome, it is particularly attractive as it offers more precise regulation of expression.

References

1. Picard C, Al-Herz W, Bousfiha A, Casanova JL, Chatila T, Conley ME, et al. Primary immunodeficiency diseases: an update on the classification from the International Union of Immunological Societies Expert Committee for primary immunodeficiency 2015. J Clin Immunol. 2015;35(8):696–726.
2. Kwan A, Abraham RS, Currier R, Brower A, Andruszewski K, Abbott JK, et al. Newborn screening for severe combined immunodeficiency in 11 screening programs in the United States. JAMA. 2014;312(7):729–38.
3. Klinkenberg D, Blohm M, Hoehne M, Mas Marques A, Malecki M, Schildgen V, et al. Risk of rotavirus vaccination for children with SCID. Pediatr Infect Dis J. 2015;34(1):114–5.
4. Pai SY, Logan BR, Griffith LM, Buckley RH, Parrott RE, Dvorak CC, et al. Transplant outcomes for severe combined immunodeficiency, 2000–2009. N Engl J Med. 2014;371(5):434–46.
5. Shearer WT, Dunn E, Notarangelo LD, Dvorak CC, Puck JM, Logan BR, et al. Establishing diagnostic criteria for severe combined immunodeficiency disease (SCID), leaky SCID, and Omenn syndrome: the Primary Immune Deficiency Treatment Consortium experience. J Allergy Clin Immunol. 2014;133(4):1092–8.
6. Müller SM, Ege M, Pottharst A, Schulz AS, Schwarz K, Friedrich W. Transplacentally acquired maternal T lymphocytes in severe combined immunodeficiency: a study of 121 patients. Blood. 2001;98(6):1847–51.
7. Kovanen PE, Leonard WJ. Cytokines and immunodeficiency diseases: critical roles of the gamma(c)-dependent cytokines interleukins 2, 4, 7, 9, 15, and 21, and their signaling pathways. Immunol Rev. 2004;202:67–83.
8. Schatz DG, Ji Y. Recombination centres and the orchestration of V(D)J recombination. Nat Rev Immunol. 2011;11(4):251–63.
9. Hirschhorn R, Martiniuk F, Rosen FS. Adenosine deaminase activity in normal tissues and tissues from a child with severe combined immunodeficiency and adenosine deaminase deficiency. Clin Immunol Immunopathol. 1978;9(3):287–92.
10. Schrader WP, Stacy AR. Purification and subunit structure of adenosine deaminase from human kidney. J Biol Chem. 1977;252(18):6409–15.
11. Benveniste P, Cohen A. p53 expression is required for thymocyte apoptosis induced by adenosine deaminase deficiency. Proc Natl Acad Sci U S A. 1995;92(18):8373–7.
12. Cowan MJ, Gennery AR. Radiation-sensitive severe combined immunodeficiency: the arguments for and against conditioning before hematopoietic cell transplantation-what to do? J Allergy Clin Immunol. 2015;136(5):1178–85.
13. Ma Y, Pannicke U, Schwarz K, Lieber MR. Hairpin opening and overhang processing by an Artemis/DNA-dependent protein kinase complex in nonhomologous end joining and V (D) J recombination. Cell. 2002;108(6):781–94.
14. Puel A, Ziegler SF, Buckley RH, Leonard WJ. Defective IL-7R expression in T(2)B(1)NK(1) severe combined immunodeficiency. Nat Genet. 1998;20(4):394–7.
15. Buckley RH, Schiff RI, Schiff SE, Markert ML, Williams LW, Harville TO, et al. Human severe combined immunodeficiency: genetic, phenotypic, and functional diversity in one hundred eight infants. J Pediatr. 1997;130:378–87.
16. Stephan JL, Vlekova V, Le Deist F, Blanche S, Donadieu J, DeSaint-Basile G, et al. Severe combined immunodeficiency: a retrospective single-center study of clinical presentation and outcome in 117 patients. J Pediatr. 1993;123(4):564–71.

17. Omenn GS. Familial reticuloendotheliosis with eosinophilia. N Engl J Med. 1965;273:427–32.

18. Chan SK, Gelfand EW. Primary immunodeficiency masquerading as allergic disease. Immunol Allergy Clin N Am. 2015;35(4):767–78.

19. Geier CB, Piller A, Linder A, Sauerwein KM, Eibl MM, Wolf HM. Leaky RAG deficiency in adult patients with impaired antibody production against bacterial polysaccharide antigens. PLoS One. 2015;10(7):1–16.

20. Kesserwan C, Sokolic R, Cowen EW, Garabedian E, Heselmeyer-Haddad K, Lee CC, Pittaluga S, Ortiz C, Baird K, Lopez-Terrada D, Bridge J. Multicentric dermatofibrosarcoma protuberans in patients with adenosine deaminase–deficient severe combined immune deficiency. J Allergy Clin Immunol. 2012;129(3):762–9.

21. Albuquerque W, Gaspar HB. Bilateral sensorineural deafness in adenosine deaminase-deficient severe combined immunodeficiency. J Pediatr. 2004;144(2):278–80.

22. Shovlin CL, Hughes JM, Simmonds HA, Fairbanks L, Deacock S, Lechler R, et al. Adult presentation of adenosine deaminase deficiency. Lancet. 1993;341(8858):1471.

23. Ozsahin H, Arredondo-Vega FX, Santisteban I, Fuhrer H, Tuchschmid P, Jochum W, et al. Adenosine deaminase deficiency in adults. Blood. 1997;89(8):2849–55.

24. Li L, Moshous D, Zhou Y, Wang J, Xie G, Salido E, et al. A founder mutation in Artemis, an SNM1-like protein, causes SCID in Athabascan-speaking Native Americans. J Immunol. 2002;168(12):6323–9.

25. Mazzucchelli RI, Riva A, Durum SK. The human IL-7 receptor gene: deletions, polymorphisms and mutations. Semin Immunol. 2012;24(3):225–30.

26. Kwan A, Puck JM. History and current status of newborn screening for severe combined immunodeficiency. Semin Perinatol. 2015;39(3):194–205. WB Saunders

27. Speckmann C, Pannicke U, Wiech E, Schwarz K, Fisch P, Friedrich W, Niehues T, Gilmour K, Buiting K, Schlesier M, Eibel H. Clinical and immunologic consequences of a somatic reversion in a patient with X-linked severe combined immunodeficiency. Blood. 2008;112(10):4090–7.

28. Cicalese MP, Aiuti A. Clinical applications of gene therapy for primary immunodeficiencies. Hum Gene Ther. 2015;26(4):210–9.

29. Aiuti A, Cattaneo F, Galimberti S, Benninghoff U, Cassani B, Callegaro L, et al. Gene therapy for immunodeficiency due to adenosine deaminase deficiency. N Engl J Med. 2009;360(5):447–58.

30. Winkelstein JA, Marino MC, Ochs H, Fuleihan R, Scholl PR, Geha R, et al. The X-linked hyper-IgM syndrome: clinical and immunologic features of 79 patients. Medicine. 2003;82(6):373–84.

31. van Kooten C, Banchereau J. CD40-CD40 ligand. J Leukoc Biol. 2000;67(1):2–17.

32. Notarangelo LD, Duse MA, Ugazio AG. Immunodeficiency with hyper-IgM (HIM). Immunodefic Rev. 1991;3(2):101–21.

33. Levy J, Espanol-Boren T, Thomas C, Fischer A, Tovo P, Bordigoni P, Resnick I, Fasth A, Baer M, Gomez L, Sanders EA. Clinical spectrum of X-linked hyper-IgM syndrome. J Pediatr. 1997;131(1):47–54.

34. Harry W. Primary antibody deficiencies. Clin Immunol Princ Pract. 2012;26:421.

35. Hayward AR, Levy J, Facchetti F, Notarangelo L, Ochs HD, Etzioni A, et al. Cholangiopathy and tumors of the pancreas, liver, and biliary tree in boys with X-linked immunodeficiency with hyper-IgM. J Immunol. 1997;158(2):977–83.

36. Cunningham CK, Bonville CA, Ochs HD, Seyama K, John PA, Rotbart HA, Weiner LB. Enteroviral meningoencephalitis as a complication of X-linked hyper IgM syndrome. J Pediatr. 1999;134(5):584–8.

37. Kwan SP, Lehner T, Hagemann T, Lu B, Blaese M, Ochs H, et al. Localization of the gene for the Wiskott-Aldrich syndrome between two flanking markers, TIMP and DXS255, on Xp11. 22–Xp11. 3. Genomics. 1991;10(1):29–33.

38. Beel K, Vandenberghe P. G-CSF receptor (CSF3R) mutations in X-linked neutropenia evolving to acute myeloid leukemia or myelodysplasia. Haematologica. 2009;94(10):1449–52.

39. Ochs HD, Thrasher AJ. The Wiskott-Aldrich syndrome. J Allergy Clin Immunol. 2006;117(4):725–38.

40. Fuller CL, Braciale VL, Samelson LE. All roads lead to actin: the intimate relationship between TCR signaling and the cytoskeleton. Immunol Rev. 2003;191(1):220–36.

41. Zhu Q, Watanabe C, Liu T, Hollenbaugh D, Blaese RM, Kanner SB, Aruffo A, Ochs HD. Wiskott-Aldrich syndrome/X-linked thrombocytopenia: WASP gene mutations, protein expression, and phenotype. Blood. 1997;90(7):2680–9.

42. Orange JS. Formation and function of the lytic NK-cell immunological synapse. Nat Rev Immunol. 2008;8(9):713–25.

43. Ochs HD, Filipovich AH, Veys P, Cowan MJ, Kapoor N. Wiskott-Aldrich syndrome: diagnosis, clinical and laboratory manifestations, and treatment. Biol Blood Marrow Transpl. 2009;15(1):84–90.

44. Molina IJ, Sancho J, Terhorst C, Rosen FS, Remold-O'Donnell E. T cells of patients with the Wiskott-Aldrich syndrome have a restricted defect in proliferative responses. J Immunol. 1993;151(8):4383–90.

45. Naumova AK, Plenge RM, Bird LM, Leppert M, Morgan K, Willard HF, Sapienza C. Heritability of X chromosome-inactivation phenotype in a large family. Am J Hum Genet. 1996;58(6):1111.

46. Moratto D, Giliani S, Bonfim C, Mazzolari E, Fischer A, Ochs HD, et al. Long-term outcome and lineage-specific chimerism in 194 patients with Wiskott-Aldrich syndrome treated by hematopoietic cell transplantation in the period 1980–2009: an international collaborative study. Blood. 2011;118(6):1675–84.

47. Braun CJ, Boztug K, Paruzynski A, Witzel M, Schwarzer A, Rothe M, et al. Gene therapy for

Wiskott-Aldrich syndrome – long-term efficacy and genotoxicity. Sci Transl Med. 2014;6(227):227–33.

48. Ouederni M, Vincent QB, Frange P, Touzot F, Scerra S, Bejaoui M, et al. Major histocompatibility complex class II expression deficiency caused by a RFXANK founder mutation: a survey of 35 patients. Blood. 2011;118(19):5108–18.

49. Shrestha D, Szöllősi J, Jenei A. Bare lymphocyte syndrome: an opportunity to discover our immune system. Immunol Lett. 2012;141(2):147–57.

50. Hanna S, Etzioni A. MHC class I and II deficiencies. J Allergy Clin Immunol. 2014;134(2):269–75.

51. Picard C, Fischer A. Hematopoietic stem cell transplantation and other management strategies for MHC class II deficiency. Immunol Allergy Clin N Am. 2010;30(2):173–8.

52. Siepermann M, Gudowius S, Beltz K, Strier U, Feyen O, Troeger A, et al. MHC class II deficiency cured by unrelated mismatched umbilical cord blood transplantation: case report and review of 68 cases in the literature. Pediatr Transplant. 2011;15(4):E80–6.

Inflammatory Bowel Disease in Primary Immunodeficiencies

9

Abdul Aziz Elkadri and Aleixo Muise

Introduction

As the list of defined gene defects associated with primary immunodeficiency diseases (PID) grows, our understanding of the spectrum of phenotypes associated with these genetic defects grows too. One phenotype that is prevalent in a number of primary immunodeficiencies is the involvement of the gastrointestinal tract. This should not come as a surprise, as the bowel is the interface between the self and the outside world. It also hosts a large number of bacteria and viruses. Some estimates place the ratio of bacterial to human cells at 10:1 [1]. Yet bacteria are to a large extent tolerated in situations of normal health. As well, ingested foods in various states of digestion are also tolerated in healthy individuals with no systemic immune response.

The gastrointestinal system is the host for the gut-associated lymphoid tissue (GALT), which makes up 80% of the lymphoid tissue found in the body [2]. Our understanding of how the immune system interacts with the gastrointestinal tract has developed relatively recently with the discovery of specialized cells within the GALT,

such as microfold cells (M cells). These cells, along with mononuclear phagocytes that include dendritic cells and macrophages, are part of the interphase between the systemic circulation and the lumen of the gut involved in sampling and localized inflammatory response.

A model disease that highlights these issues is inflammatory bowel disease (IBD). This family of disorders includes Crohn's disease (CD) and ulcerative colitis. This group of diseases is differentiated mainly based on their clinical presentation and their disease behavior. Ulcerative colitis has involvement of the colonic mucosa starting from the rectum in a continuous retrograde manner, only involving the superficial mucosa of the colon. Crohn's disease, on the other hand, can involve any area of the gastrointestinal tract in a continuous or noncontinuous manner. It is also characterized by noncaseating granulomas on pathological examination of mucosal biopsies and can have transmural involvement of the wall of the gastrointestinal tract. These granulomas are not necessary for diagnosis and may be found in up to 48% of patients with Crohn's disease [3]. The transmural inflammation may lead to internal fistulous tracts between different portions of the intestine, requiring surgical correction. Another phenotypic subtype of Crohn's disease is perianal disease, characterized by fistulous tracts in the perianal area associated with abscesses and poorly heal-

A. A. Elkadri (✉)
Medical College of Wisconsin, Milwaukee, WI, USA
e-mail: aelkadri@mcw.edu

A. Muise
The Hospital for Sick Children, Inflammatory Bowel Disease Center, Toronto, Canada
e-mail: aleixo.muise@sickkids.ca

© Springer International Publishing AG, part of Springer Nature 2018
B. H. Segal (ed.), *Management of Infections in the Immunocompromised Host*,
https://doi.org/10.1007/978-3-319-77674-3_9

ing sinus tracts. This perianal disease may or may not mirror systemic disease severity.

Inflammatory bowel disease is believed to occur due to the contribution of four main factors: an underlying genetic predisposition, an environmental exposure or trigger, an abnormal immune response, and/or interactions with the microbiome (and more recently the intestinal virome). This topic is reviewed in detail by Sartor [4]. There has been an effort to create a model in the lab focusing on each of these main factors that cause IBD to develop. For example, a common method of inducing colitis involves exposure of mice to dextran sodium sulfate, or DSS, which induces an acute epithelial injury [5]. Interestingly, to highlight the interaction of these contributing factors, DSS-induced colitis worsens in the absence of bacteria in mice. In humans, there are examples of situations where specific genetic mutations cause disease resembling inflammatory bowel disease. A number of these genes have been identified as genetic mutations causing primary immunodeficiencies, yet the intestinal manifestations of these diseases have been relatively poorly described. In this chapter, we will review a number of genes and the known intestinal manifestations of mutations in these pathways in an attempt to better understand the intestine as an immune organ.

Technological Advances

Recent technological advances have allowed access to previously impossible or restricted techniques that study the genetics of patients presenting with an atypical phenotype. Taking the intestine as an example organ system, there has always been an understanding of the underlying contribution of genetics to disease development. The first evidence of such an underlying genetic cause was noted in studies of twin cohorts. The first Crohn's disease patients originally described in 1932 included a sibling pair presenting with the same disease manifestations at approximately the same age. Twin cohorts have shown between a 50% and 60% pairwise

concordance in Crohn's disease, while ulcerative colitis is less striking with a pairwise concordance closer to 18–20%. Building upon this idea of familial risk, families with multiply affected individuals were further studied using familial-based linkage analysis, or FBAT. From these, 9 loci, named IBD 1–9, were identified where there was overtransmission, suggesting involvement in inflammatory bowel disease. One of these genes, IBD1, was later identified as NOD2/CARD15 and is still the strongest known genetic risk loci in IBD.

The next advance came with the introduction of microarrays and a further mapping of the human genome. Chips containing a large number of loci could now be repeatedly produced with great accuracy at a reasonable price. One of these chips, called the Immunochip, was created in coordination between Illumina and the Wellcome Trust and gathered the known loci of 12 known immunologically mediated diseases, including rheumatoid arthritis, type I diabetes mellitus, celiac disease, and finally Crohn's disease and ulcerative colitis. As this chip was massively used around the world, it allowed for easier meta-analysis of multiple populations previously studied. In IBD, one such study identified 163 loci associated with disease, the largest set of loci identified to date. With microarrays, to allow for proper analysis, loci were required to be relatively common. This became an issue with more rare forms of disease of specific subphenotypic groups.

The next advance came with the introduction of next-generation sequencing, or NGS. This includes whole exome sequencing, or sequencing of the known exonic regions of genes, and whole genome sequencing, or sequencing of the whole genome from beginning to end. This technique has allowed for the identification of variants irrespective of whether or not they were common. As the technology has developed, cost has improved to the point where some commercial companies have offered the sequencing of the general public at an affordable price range. This technology has revolutionized the field of molecular genetics, as it has allowed detailed genetic examination of populations previously assumed to be part of other diseases. This was the case with inflammatory bowel disease, specifically regarding the youngest of individuals, or what is better known as very early-onset inflammatory bowel disease (VEOIBD). This group, usually described to be those presenting with IBD under the age of 6, is known to have a more severe disease course, disease extent, and lack of response to traditional medications [6].

Another development in technology that has aided in the investigation of patients with disease is tissue organoid technologies. This technique has allowed for the banking of intestinal stem cells and better characterization of the effect of mutations on the epithelial layer of the intestine. From biopsies taken from a patient, small spherical structures representing "mini-guts" can be formed. These "mini-guts" can be then maintained indefinitely in a culture system and have the potential for personalized therapies to be selected using available libraries of drugs.

A number of the genes identified to be associated with VEOIBD were also known as primary immunodeficiency disease genes. We will review a number of these genes here as they give us a window to the mechanisms of disease and an understanding to the mechanisms of immunity as a whole. Here, we will group the genes into those involved in the epithelial barrier, phagocytic defects, hyper- and auto-inflammatory disorders, T- and B-cell defects, and immunoregulatory defects. This list has been reviewed and is adapted from Uhlig et al. [7].

Review of Genes Associated with Gastrointestinal Involvement

Epithelial Barrier

The intestinal tract has been theorized to have a surface area of 32 m² [8], which is much greater than the skin, which is 2 m². This poses an issue of how this massive barrier to the outside world is maintained. Not surprisingly, defects of genes involved with this barrier lead to intestinal disease. Examples of disorders include epidermolysis bullosa, Kindler syndrome, and

incontinentia pigmenti or hypohidrotic ectodermal dysplasia. Though the manifestations of these diseases may not necessarily be considered typical of PID, defects within these genes pose a major issue with regard to therapeutic options. As the immune system is not directly involved, hematopoietic stem cell transplantation should not be considered, as the defect within the intestinal mucosa will remain, ultimately causing disease to reoccur.

Some of these disorders may have immunologic manifestations. X-linked ectodermal dysplasia (caused by mutations in IKBKG) is known to have low CD3 counts and increased B-cell counts. Phytohemagglutinin testing shows normal T-cell activation, and patients had circulating anti-centromere antibodies. With regard to their intestinal phenotype, these patients presented with perianal disease and colitis similar to patients with Crohn's disease [9]. Another example of mutations showing both an epithelial and immune phenotype is in patients presenting with TTC7A mutations. Two main phenotypes have been described: one with severe colitis with findings of apoptosis throughout the biopsy resembling graft versus host disease [10] and the other with multiple intestinal atresias with a component of severe combined immunodeficiency (SCID) phenotype in some patients [11]. In one case, HLA-matched cord blood transplantation was attempted, but unfortunately had recurrence of intestinal atresia. This underlies the need to identify whether mutations affect hematopoietic cells versus the epithelial layer only.

Phagocytic Defects

This category includes diseases such as chronic granulomatous disease or CGD (due to variants in CYBA, CYBB, NCF1, NCF2, NCF4), glycogen storage disease type 1b or GSD1b (due to mutations in SLC37A4), congenital neutropenia (due to mutations in G6PC3), and leukocyte adhesion deficiency type 1 or LAD1 (due to mutations in ITBG2). The inflammatory bowel disease features of CGD are almost indistinguishable from those of severe Crohn's disease, with some patients reaching adulthood with a misdiagnosis of Crohn's disease. A review of a British registry of patients with CGD found 37% of the patients had colitis resembling that of Crohn's disease [12] with granulomas and patchy disease in the colon. One differentiating factor on pathological examination is the presence of pigmented macrophages in patients with CGD. As well, patients with CGD will show an abnormal neutrophil oxidative burst index. They are also at risk for life-threatening infections and may respond well to antibiotic therapies. It is important to rule out CGD in patients with VEOIBD, as therapies targeting tumor necrosis factor alpha, which are commonly used in patients with IBD, may cause fatal complications in patients with CGD [13]. Another important issue is that earlier diagnosis provides a higher chance for better outcomes with curative hematopoietic stem cell transplantation, as lower age groups have a lower risk.

Hyper- and Auto-inflammatory Disorders

These disorders include mevalonate kinase deficiency, familial Mediterranean fever, familial cold auto-inflammatory syndrome (or cold urticarial, caused by PLCG2 mutations), Hermansky-Pudlak syndrome, X-linked lymphoproliferative syndrome, and familial hemophagocytic lymphohistiocytosis (HLH). Patients with these disorders have findings similar to severe IBD. One example of this is XIAP defects, which cause X-linked lymphoproliferative syndrome 2 (XLP2). There have been a number of case series published showing signs of VEOIBD, with severe fistulizing perianal disease in about 20% of patients [14–17]. One such patient carried a diagnosis of severe Crohn's disease for a number of years, with lack of response to therapy leading to colectomy, and severe fistulizing disease in the area of his stoma. He was identified via WES to carry a mutation in XIAP, leading to curative bone marrow transplantation. Interestingly, XLP1, caused by SH2D1A, is less associated with hemorrhagic colitis [16], though one study

found three patients with large deletions in SH2D1A and signs of gastritis and colitis [18]. Fifty-two percent of patients with XIAP had cytopenias not associated with active HLH, 87% had splenomegaly, and 23% had a fatal episode of HLH. Again, identification of this disorder allows for a quicker and earlier option of curative hematopoietic stem cell transplantation.

As XIAP is X-linked, it affects males predominantly. Interestingly, there have been recent studies showing functional assay defects in mothers of patients with XIAP. Aguilar et al. described two mothers diagnosed with Crohn's disease with boys diagnosed with XIAP [19]. Their hypothesis is that mosaicism of their hematopoietic system caused selective inactivation of the normal X chromosome, effectively giving them a pathway defect of a patient with XIAP. This has led to a widening of the possible patients with and phenotype carrying mutations in XIAP, as now female patients could also be considered. A number of groups retrospectively found a number of their adolescent and young adult patients with Crohn's disease patients to carry XIAP mutations.

XIAP ties in with the known genetics of Crohn's disease, as XIAP is a known E3 ubiquitin ligase that binds to RIPK2. NOD2, which is a key player in the detection of microbial peptidoglycans in the gastrointestinal tract, also interacts with RIPK2. It is one of the best studied genetic modifiers in Crohn's disease, with mutations associated with severe disease, earlier onset, and poorer surgical outcomes [20]. Functional assays exist for XIAP, and damaging mutations should be considered in recalcitrant cases of Crohn's disease with atypical features. Immunological testing may be relatively normal, with some patients showing normal CD56 levels and no elevation of traditional HLH markers (elevated ferritin, soluble CD163, soluble IL2 receptor).

T- and B-Cell Defects

Defects in T and B cells are known to lead to defects in immunity, but some of these mutations have been associated with inflammation involving the gastrointestinal tract resembling

IBD. Common variable immunodeficiency (CVID) is family of disorders which are likely polygenic, with a handful being caused by single-gene mutations. Hypogammaglobulinemia is a hallmark of CVID, along with defective or deficient antibody production. A number of these disorders are associated with a lower number of B cells, or functionally defective B cells, subsequently leading to lower immunoglobulin levels. Two genes have been identified as genes with intestinal involvement: ICOS [21], causing CVID type 1, and LRBA, causing CVID type 8 [22–24]. Interestingly, there has been a report of recurrence 1 year post-BMT in a patient with an LRBA defect [25], suggesting the possibility of a mixed system disorder involving not only the immune system.

Patients with abnormalities in immunoglobulin levels include agammaglobulinemia, caused by mutations in BTK [26, 27] and PIK3R1 [28], along with hyper-IgM syndrome, caused by CD40LG [29, 30] and AICDA [29, 31]. Intestinal disease in these patients has been described as Crohn's like, with very early onset. Interestingly, there is no clear genotype-phenotype correlation with many of these genes. Some patients may have an intermediate phenotype, with a slightly decreased or normal immunoglobulin level theorized to delay onset of disease. Another factor which hinders interpretation of the diagnostic phenotype is the frequent recurrent infections, with enteroviral infections leading to a severe neurological defect in some patients [32].

Wiskott-Aldrich syndrome, though typically associated with thrombocytopenia, recurrent infection, immune cell abnormality, arthritis, and vasculitis, is also known to have a gastrointestinal phenotype similar to ulcerative colitis. This colitis presents at a varying age of onset [33] and is not thought to be associated with the leukocytoclastic vasculitic process or due to the defect in platelets associated with the syndrome.

There have been many advances in diagnostics in the field of severe combined immunodeficiencies (SCID), with many jurisdictions providing routine newborn screening. This has led to long-term monitoring of these patients for manifestations and complications. Diarrhea is a known manifestation of atypical SCID. There are a number of genes that are associated with SCID: DCLRE1C [34], RAG2 [35], ZAP70 [36], IL2RG [37–39], and CD3G [40]. Many of these diseases resemble Crohn's disease, with oral-genital ulcers and lack of therapeutic responsiveness, though some have been noted to have only colonic disease. It is unclear to what extent the intestinal manifestations are to blame for the failure to thrive observed in these patients. Again, as this is an immunologically mediated disease, BMT should be curative.

Dyskeratosis congenita (due to DKC1 [41] and RTEL1 [42–44] mutations) is also associated with SCID and can be easily identified, as it is a multisystemic disorder with reticular skin hyperpigmentation, nail dystrophy, and leukoplakia. Patients have short stature and may develop bone marrow failure. They may also develop transient colitis of unclear etiology. It is important that these patients be monitored every few years with endoscopic evaluation for the development of adenomas in the colon, as there is a general increased predisposition for cancer. Unfortunately, bone marrow transplantation has not had much success in patients with dyskeratosis congenita.

DOCK8 mutations, with the typically elevated IgE associated with the disorder, are in some patients associated with diarrhea. A number of reports describe multiply affected families from Turkey [45] and the Middle East [46, 47], with one report of an Italian family [48]. Patients have been found to have granulomas on biopsies, with some patients having features consistent with primary sclerosing colitis, an immune-driven fibrosing bile duct disorder that leads to end-stage liver disease. Though this autosomal recessive disease is felt to be fully penetrant, prevalence of diarrhea was found to be around 14–17% [47], with some families completely affected [48].

Trichohepatoenteric syndrome, due to mutations in SKIV2L and TTC37, is associated with a syndrome of hypogammaglobulinemia, intractable diarrhea, hepatopathy, and trichorrhexis nodosa. A third of the patients with TTC37 [49] and half of the patients with SKIV2L [50] defects were reported to have colitis, though not all patients had endoscopic evaluation reported. Patients should be easily identifiable by their syndromic features of wooly hair and facial dysmorphism with hypertelorism and a prominent forehead. Diarrhea typically occurs within the first few weeks of life. Villous atrophy and colitis are described, with patients requiring long-term parenteral nutrition. This has led to some fatal liver disease complications, made worse by hepatic iron overload and intestinal failure-associated liver disease (IFALD). As treatment for the complications of long-term parenteral nutrition improve, the long-term follow-up and natural history remain to be seen. Recently, a patient with a compound heterozygous TTC37 mutation was reported at 12 years old with some intestinal symptoms where continual immunoglobulin supplementation has led to a decrease from continual antibiotic prophylaxis to intermittent antimicrobial therapy [51].

PTEN mutations cause hamartoma tumor syndrome, which has been associated with an increased risk of benign and malignant tumors of the thyroid, breast, and endometrium. In a few cases, PTEN mutations have been associated with autoimmunity and, specifically, colitis [52]. As mTORC1 signaling is upregulated, leading to reduced apoptosis in B cells, rapamycin therapy has been attempted, leading to an involution of the thymus in the case with colitis. They do not however report the response of the colitis to rapamycin therapy.

Defects in Immunoregulation

A model disorder of immune dysregulation is X-linked immune dysregulation, polyendocrinopathy, and enteropathy, or IPEX, caused by mutations in FOXP3 [53, 54] or IL2RA [55, 56]. It is associated with polyendocrinopathy, enteropathy, eczema, elevated IgE, multiple autoantibodies, and recurrent infections. Symptom onset is usually within the first few months of life, with the colitis noted to apparent within the first 2 years of life. There is subtotal or total villous atrophy with colitis, and the pattern of disease is similar to a severe celiac disease. In older patients, the colitis appears to be more clinically apparent. There is depletion of goblet cells, with the presence at times of an anti-goblet cell antibody. Anti-enterocyte antibody is an antibody reactive to protein produced by the epithelial cells of the intestinal lining. Positivity is highly suspicious for autoimmune enteropathy. Biopsies will usually be negative for staining of FOXP3-expressing T lymphocytes, but some FOXP3 expression may still be found. It is both X-linked and autosomal recessive. Though there have been some reported successes with other traditional IBD therapies such as anti-TNF and immunomodulatory medications, bone marrow transplantation should be considered, as it is curative.

One of the best examples of a mutation where the gastrointestinal system is involved in a mainly immunological process is that of IL10 pathway defects. IL10 is an anti-inflammatory cytokine which downregulates the TH1 response. The IL10 knockout mouse model has long been used as a model for colitis in basic research. As well, IL10RB has been associated with IBD in the large meta-GWAS analysis in IBD. The IL10 receptor complex is a heterodimer transmembrane protein made of IL10RA and IL10RB, with IL10 being required as the signal for the pathway to be stimulated. A defect in any one of these genes causes a highly penetrant syndrome characterized by folliculitis, diarrhea, recurrent fevers, colitis, perianal disease, recurrent septic episodes and, if the patient survives to an adolescent age, the development of non-Hodgkin's B-cell lymphoma. Symptoms develop relatively quickly within the first few months of life. A number of patients have been described around the world, with a growing number of patients effectively cured with allogenic BMT [57–62]. Measures taken to optimize nutrition via enteral formulas, along with early diversion of the fecal stream using a diversion ileostomy, appear to improve the general health of the patient while awaiting transplantation. Early antibiotic treatment for fevers and increased vigilance to the development of perianal abscesses are key as well.

Diagnostics

Patients with VEOIBD are some of the most difficult patients to manage. This stems from the rarity of the diagnosis, as well as the fact that these patients are by definition young. Due to the involvement of the gastrointestinal tract, absorption of medication may vary widely at different disease states. In general, due to the complexity and multisystemic nature of many of these patients with VEOIBD, a multidisciplinary team approach helps in dealing with the complex issues that may arise. As the pediatric age group has a relative paucity of randomized control trials, it's not surprising that VEOIBD has no randomized control trials. The vast majority of the literature consists of case reports or historic cross-sectional reviews. Due to this, there is a lack of long-term outcomes for most therapies attempted. Therefore, there are a wide variety of approaches to this disease subgroup.

As in most diseases, a thorough review of the history may reveal helpful hints toward the diagnosis of VEOIBD. The aim is to try and differentiate between infections and food intolerances, which may have an identical presentation to immune-mediated enteropathies and colitides. Food intolerances such as cow's milk protein intolerance (CMPI) are dramatically improved with removal of the offending protein epitope, whether it is cow's milk-like or soy-like. The vast majority of these patients improve within the span of 1 month. Reintroduction of the offending protein is not associated with a reoccurrence of symptoms after the age of one. In the rare case, diet modification may need to be used for a prolonged period of time, with symptoms only recurring with exposure to the offending epitope. No immunological or infectious abnormalities are found with this group of patients.

In attempting to take a history of diarrhea, one should focus on the measures of intestinal function of absorption. This includes descriptions of the onset (rapid versus gradual), stool consistency (formed, variably formed, or watery), presence of blood (absence, small amounts, or completely bloody), presence of tenesmus (a recurrent or continual feeling of needing to stool), rectal prolapse, or the presence of nocturnal stooling (if the child is potty-trained). Careful examination of the growth chart will help determine both the chronicity and the general severity of the disease, with growth lagging behind weight gain. A review of lab work may show microcytic anemia, thrombocytosis, hypoalbuminemia, and elevated acute-phase reactants or may even be relatively normal. Patients should have a complete immune workup performed, complete with measures of neutrophil function (NOBI), immune cell population (flow cytometry immunophenotyping), immunoglobulins (IgG, IgA, IgM, and IgE), and autoantibody markers (anti-enterocyte antibody, anti-neutrophil cytoplasmic antibody or ANCA, anti-tissue transglutaminase, anti-nuclear antibody and anti-*Saccharoymces cerevisiae* antibody). A positive ANCA suggests an auto-inflammatory etiology, as opposed to acute self-limiting colitis, which is a state of prolonged postinfectious inflammation that usually ceases after 1-month duration and has no long-term repercussions.

Radiological examination is helpful in the presence of inflammation to determine disease involvement. There should be an attempt to focus examination on the small bowel, as it may point to an enteropathy that requires closer monitoring and a different therapeutic approach. Due to the age group, many of the modalities are not currently possible, including magnetic resonance enterography, which requires the patient to ingest a large volume of contrast and remain still for image capture. Careful attention to the patient's growth and weight gain, along with monitoring of the presence and extent of diarrhea, will help determine whether there is subclinical inflammation present.

It is important to strive to examine and obtain tissue samples from both the large and small bowels as once therapy has been initiated, interpretation becomes difficult. Pinch biopsies taken from the duodenum, terminal ileum, and colon can be examined for the presence of FOXP3 positive cells, the absence of which suggests IPEX. Electron microscopy should be performed for patients where a diagnosis of enteropathy is being entertained. If available, providers should consider obtaining extra tissue biopsies, stored on dry ice, for future testing.

Therapeutics

The general aim of therapy is to induce a remission state, followed by a maintenance state to keep inflammation at bay. Each phase of therapy has specific therapeutic options. At the current time, there are few predictors of severe disease. A few examples of predictors include extremely early presentation, extensive disease involvement, multisystemic involvement, and/or a family history of similar disease or previous death of a sibling. In each of these cases, there are anecdotal examples where a patient presents with severe disease, only to have immediate responsiveness with therapy and have little or no future recurrence. A number of groups are attempting to find valid predictors of disease.

Steroids are a mainstay of the induction phase of therapy. The usual dose used is borrowed from the dosing used in acute colitis, which is 1–2 mg/kg. Exclusive enteral nutrition has been attempted in some cases, with efficacy at times in enteropathy cases equivalent to that of steroids. Though it may seem ideal, patients do usually not tolerate the volume required for the extensively hydrolyzed formula, and nasogastric administration is required. Another issue is the requirement for an exclusive enteral source of nutrition, which may lead to feeding aversion in the very young patients under age 1. Cost is also a major issue, along with the acceptance of the therapy by the family. In milder cases, sulfasalazine may be successfully used as an induction agent (more on sulfasalazine below).

In all cases, a proper maintenance therapy should be preselected and discussed with the family, as once the induction agent is weaned, disease should be expected to return. Initiation of the maintenance therapy at the initiation of the induction therapy allows time for transition of disease control from the induction agent to the maintenance agent. It also allows time to determine whether the patient will tolerate the therapy. A commonly used maintenance agent is sulfasalazine, a compound containing sulfapyradine and 5-aminosalicylic acid (5-ASA) bound by a disulfide bond. This bond is cleaved by the bacteria found in abundance within the colon and releases both medications. This accounts for the main site of action of sulfasalazine being the colon, as it contains the highest concentration of bacteria. Sulfapyradine is associated with most of the side effects of sulfasalazine: azoospermia (reversible), agranulocytosis (usually reversible), and headaches (which the patient becomes tolerant to within a week or two). The 5-ASA compound is the main active ingredient, acting as a local anti-inflammatory agent. Patients generally prefer sulfasalazine as it can be easily compounded in syrup form, allowing ease of administration and dosing. In those intolerant to sulfasalazine, other 5-ASA-only formulations with time and pH release vehicles, mainly Pentasa, are used. In rare cases, some patients are 5-ASA intolerant, presenting with severe watery diarrhea.

In patients with severe disease, immunomodulation is necessary to maintain remission. The two main agents usually used in VEOIBD are methotrexate and azathioprine. Methotrexate is usually used in patients with small bowel involvement, as the efficacy in colitis-only patients has not been shown to be ideal [63]. Azathioprine can be used in most cases, but has fallen out of favor in North America due to the association with fatal hepatosplenic T-cell lymphoma, mainly in young males. It can still be used, after testing for the presence of enzyme activity, or if unavailable, for the three major polymorphisms associated with increased levels of thioguanine metabolites. Elevated thioguanine metabolites are associated with severe myelosuppression and death. Often, azathioprine will still be used, as the benefits outweigh the risk of lack of disease control.

The next step in therapy is the biological class of medications. These specifically target anti-TNF alpha and have shown promising efficacy and safety in severe treatment resistant IBD. Two major forms exist: chimeric and humanized. Chimeric-based therapies are associated with an increased development of anti-biological antibodies, leading to an increased clearance of medication or a development of an anaphylactic reaction to therapy. Humanized anti-TNF alpha therapies have a lower rate of antibody formation but are relatively novel and have less long-term data. They also have been used in standardized subcutaneous dosages, whereas chimeric therapies are weight based and intravenous. As the pharmacokinetics of younger patients varies with subcutaneous administration, its use has been relatively limited in this group of diseases. Initiation of therapy requires continued administration to prevent antibody formation, and this would mean lifelong or at least prolonged uninterrupted therapy in this young group of patients. Efficacy of these therapies has not been determined in this age group. Other biological therapies are in the pipeline, but are still far from routine clinical use, especially in the youngest of patients.

Other immune modulators have been used sporadically, but usually carry an increased risk of side effects or are difficult to maintain at a therapeutic level. Medications such as FK506 strongly depend on the absorption in the small bowel. Whether the small bowel is involved or not, levels may decrease or increase levels. As increasing levels of therapy improves mucosal healing, this leads to a dramatic increase in absorption. Depending upon whether the factor of transit time or ability for absorption is more of an issue, levels may swing widely from subtherapeutic to super-therapeutic. Cyclosporine has been associated with mortality in historical trials in patients with severe colitis and hence has largely been avoided within the field of gastroenterology.

In cases of severe disease, treatment intolerance or failure, surgical options should be entertained. Prolonging the time a patient has untreated disease is in general not beneficial, as this leads to poorer nutritional status, prolonged steroid exposure, and continued patient suffering. Some factors, such as parental anxiety, should be tackled early on, allowing more time for the family to come to an acceptance of what is a very acceptable form of therapy.

With the identification of genes associated with PID, bone marrow transplantation has been used in situations where the immune system has been clearly identified as the culprit. In situations such as IL10 pathway defect, XIAP or IPEX, transplantation is curative. This is discussed further below. Transplantation should not, however, be used in all patients, as epithelial defects will likely recur, needlessly exposing the patient to a risky life-threatening procedure with minimal to no gain.

Translational Techniques

As more is understood about the molecular etiologies of early-onset inflammatory bowel disease, an attempt is being made at translating these findings to the bedside to benefit the patient. Personalized medicine is the goal of translational research, with therapies being targeted to patients who will benefit most, while minimizing risk involved. A number of examples exist where elucidating the molecular etiology leads to a clinical decision.

The first such example is in patients with a known mutation causing an immune-only effect. One example is with IL10 pathway mutations. These mutations are completely cured via bone marrow transplantation, with an acceptable risk versus benefit ratio. With the typical patient presentation of a patient with IL10 pathway mutations (in IL10RA, IL10RB, and IL10 genes) with diarrhea, folliculitis, recurrent fevers, and perianal disease, genetic testing can be done relatively rapidly. Functional assays looking at the downstream pathway can be done in specialized research laboratories, effectively confirming the defect. STAT3 phosphorylation is dependent upon the integrity of the IL10 receptor complex being formed by two copies of both the IL10RA and IL10RB gene, along with the presence of the IL10 signal. Absence of any of these components leads to the absence of STAT3 phosphorylation and confirmation of the defective pathway. The decision to proceed with a curative allogenic BMT is quickly and definitively reached.

The next example is in patients with an epithelial defect, which less likely to be cured by BMT. One specific example of this is patients with a TTC7A defect. There have been published reports of patients who have undergone BMT with TTC7A defects, only to have disease reoccur or progress. With TTC7A defects, intracellular trafficking becomes disrupted, causing issues with polarity to occur. Using the organoid system, researchers were able to determine that organoids grown from these patients showed a reversal of their polarity, effectively causing the organoids to grow inside out. These researchers focused on Rho kinase (ROCK) inhibitors due to their previous research on using ROCK inhibitors to reduce cell death in situations where cell-cell contacts were lost. When ROCK inhibitors were added, organoids were found to reverse polarity, effectively correcting the defect. This suggests that ROCK inhibitors may play a role in the therapeutic approach to patients with this life-threatening defect.

Gaps in Knowledge

Though there have been many recent advances in our understanding of the manifestations of PID within the intestinal tract, a few hurdles remain. At this time, a large number of the known genes associated with early-onset inflammatory bowel disease have few published reports describing the intestinal manifestations of disease. As these mutations are rare, some genes have only one published manuscript describing the clinical phenotype. As well, when the intestinal phenotype of PID-associated genes is described, some authors tend to naturally focus on the immune manifestations of disease, leaving a simple basic description of intestinal findings. This description may lack such things as the nutritional status of the child, the extent of disease, and a complete endoscopic evaluation or lack a pathological description of biopsies. In part, this may be due to the immunologic focus of both the authors and the journals. It may also be due to the lack of complete investigations in patients with PIDs with procedures such as colonoscopies and gas-troduodenoscopies and specialized imaging procedures such as magnetic resonance enterography and wireless capsule endoscopies. It may also stem from the difficulty in differentiating between the infectious diarrhea and an intestinal manifestation of the underlying disease in a patient with PID.

Another major hurdle is the ability to differentiate between epithelial defects and immune defects. As our ability to identify and characterize these disorders improves with better genetic diagnoses, the next natural question would be: "How are these diseases best treated?" In the case of barrier defects, stem cell transplantation may cure the immunological defect, but the intestinal defect remains. Disorders in TTC7A are an example of this. The result is a patient having undergone bone marrow transplantation, with all the risks associated with the procedure, along with the ongoing issue of the underlying intestinal manifestation of disease. Determining whether the genetic defect will be corrected with bone marrow transplantation is vital before proceeding with the potentially lifesaving therapy.

For cases where stem cell transplantation is not appropriate, proper therapeutic approaches have not been standardized. More and more, evidence is pointing to better outcomes in older patients with upfront aggressive therapeutic approaches in patients with IBD. Yet, these approaches may not be appropriate in patients with PID. As a large number of PID present at a younger age and are lifelong disorders, therapies initiated at an earlier stage will lead to a longer overall lifetime exposure to medications. This requires a better understanding of the long-term risks associated with a particular therapy. An example of this is antibiotic exposure. Antibiotics such as metronidazole are used for some patients with IBD in particular circumstances. Metronidazole has been associated with neurotoxicity after prolonged exposure in a few sporadic cases in the elderly. Antibiotic exposure, though it may be beneficial in patients with neutrophil defects, may lead to a selection of resistant organisms over a long period of time. The implications of this have not been investigated in a large enough cohort to account for such rare outcomes.

Next, though there have been many advances in the field of next-generation sequencing, the next big task is to develop better methods to interpret the data generated. As variants are defined as differences from the agreed upon reference sequence, frequencies of variants become important in deciding whether a variant is rare enough to account for the rare presentation of the patient being sequenced. This poses an issue in understudied populations, such as the Middle Eastern population and populations with sociopolitical or geographically driven bottlenecks (such as islands or mountain ranges), where background frequencies have not been determined. One method of accounting for these understudied groups is to sequence the parents and proband in a trio, effectively using the parents as an ethnic control at increased cost of sequencing. Another issue is the hypothesis surrounding whether multiple damaging variants across the same disease pathway leads to disease development. Though it appears plausible, there has been little in the way of examples of this type of disease inheritance pattern.

Finally, there remains a small group of patients who do not fit in the usual definition of either traditional PID or IBD. These patients may have some phenotypic aspects of an immunodeficiency, such as hypogammaglobulinemia resembling CVID. Yet, the loss of immune globulins is beyond the expected levels for patients with CVID. As well, due to the multisystemic nature of some of these patients, they do not fit the traditional IBD diagnosis either. Some patients will present with chronic interstitial lung disease, recurrent infections, serositis, hemophagocytic lymphohistiocytosis (HLH), or immune cell lineage abnormalities. Unfortunately, a significant number of these patients will not have an identifiable genetic variant. This group remains a difficult group to treat clinically and poses a challenging problem in that the therapeutic approaches of either group of patients may not be ideal or give suboptimal clinical response.

Future Directions

As our understanding of the intestinal tract as an immune organ increases, so will our need to better identify immune deficiencies with intestinal manifestations. As stated above, due to the rarity of a number of the known primary immunodeficiencies, reports have been mainly limited to the described phenotypic characteristics. Investigations of the gastrointestinal manifestations should be part of the workup for patients presenting with failure to thrive, diarrhea, nausea, abdominal pain, emesis, recurrent gastrointestinal infections, and unexplained anemia. In centers where biobanking is set up, creating and storing intestinal organoids will allow for genes and disorders to be studied at the intestinal epithelial level. As collaborations between immunologists and gastroenterologists grow, so too will our understanding of these patients and the immunology of the gastrointestinal tract.

As genetic testing becomes more commonplace, the number of identified mutations associated with a mainly intestinal phenotype will increase. There is a need for a meaningful categorization of patients with PIDs as we have attempted to do in this chapter. Better subgrouping will allow for grouping of cohorts in meaningful meta-analyses, possibly leading to new therapeutic approaches. It may also allow for multicenter trials of therapies in a case-control type of observational study. As heterogeneity is minimized, results will be easier to interpret. By the nature of the overlap between PID and IBD, therapeutic approaches in one disease may lead to different interventional strategies in the other.

As genetic underpinnings of inflammatory bowel disease become clearer, it is possible that there may be some specific high-yield gene targets for which gene-editing technologies may be more effective. Advances in genetic editing using Cas9/CRISPR and similar technologies may hold the key to correcting errors found in the genome of patients with severe disease. The off-target effects of this technology are thought to be much better than previous methods, which included lentiviral- and adenoviral-based methods. In those cases, patients had improvement of their diseases, only to develop lymphomas a few years later. Though the issues with off-target effects are real, a large hurdle remains in identifying proper vehicles for transporting and delivering the Cas9/CRISPR cassette to the target organ system and cell. An ideal vehicle would deliver the cassette to the tissue with high specificity and efficiency.

As a large number of the genes associated with VEOIBD are associated with immunodeficiencies, it is intuitive to think that replacement of the aberrant immune system with a "corrected" immune system will lead to correction of the underlying defect. As many of these diseases are inherited in a homozygous recessive manner, with two defective copies of the gene being required for disease manifestation. This has led to a modified approach to both the conditioning regiments for stem cell transplant, as well as the target for engraftment. As the parents of patients with a homozygous recessive disorder are both heterozygous for the defect, mosaicism will allow for at least 50% of the engrafted immune system to express the missing phenotype, essentially becoming functionally heterozygous in the process. As eradication of the host immune system is not necessary, conditioning with decreased intensity can be used. This allows for a safer induction for patients with conditions predisposing to infections and hopefully translates into less mortality and better outcomes. As patients are being identified at younger ages, lower risk stem cell transplantations can be considered as viable options. Better preparatory measures can be undertaken, including avoidance of infections, improvement of nutritional status, and more time for a better HLA identical match to be found.

References

1. Savage DC. Microbial ecology of the gastrointestinal tract. Annu Rev Microbiol. 1977;31:107–33. PubMed PMID: 334036
2. Castro GA, Arntzen CJ. Immunophysiology of the gut: a research frontier for integrative studies of the common mucosal immune system. Am J Phys. 1993;265(4 Pt 1):G599–610. PubMed PMID: 8238344
3. De Matos V, Russo PA, Cohen AB, Mamula P, Baldassano RN, Piccoli DA. Frequency and clinical correlations of granulomas in children with Crohn disease. J Pediatr Gastroenterol Nutr. 2008;46(4):392–8. PubMed PMID: 18367950
4. Sartor RB. Mechanisms of disease: pathogenesis of Crohn's disease and ulcerative colitis. Nat Clin Pract Gastroenterol Hepatol. 2006;3(7):390–407. PubMed PMID: 16819502. Epub 2006/07/05. eng
5. Rakoff-Nahoum S, Paglino J, Eslami-Varzaneh F, Edberg S, Medzhitov R. Recognition of commensal microflora by toll-like receptors is required for intestinal homeostasis. Cell. 2004;118(2):229–41. PubMed PMID: 15260992
6. Griffiths AM. Specificities of inflammatory bowel disease in childhood. Best Pract Res Clin Gastroenterol. 2004;18(3):509–23. PubMed PMID: 15157824. Epub 2004/05/26. eng
7. Uhlig HH, Schwerd T, Koletzko S, Shah N, Kammermeier J, Elkadri A, et al. The diagnostic approach to monogenic very early onset inflammatory bowel disease. Gastroenterology. 2014;147(5):990–1007 e3. PubMed PMID: 25058236
8. Helander HF, Fandriks L. Surface area of the digestive tract – revisited. Scand J Gastroenterol. 2014;49(6):681–9. PubMed PMID: 24694282
9. Mizukami T, Obara M, Nishikomori R, Kawai T, Tahara Y, Sameshima N, et al. Successful treatment with infliximab for inflammatory colitis in a patient with X-linked anhidrotic ectodermal dysplasia with immunodeficiency. J Clin Immunol. 2012;32(1):39–49. PubMed PMID: 21993693
10. Avitzur Y, Guo C, Mastropaolo LA, Bahrami E, Chen H, Zhao Z, et al. Mutations in tetratricopeptide repeat domain 7A result in a severe form of very early onset inflammatory bowel disease. Gastroenterology. 2014;146(4):1028–39. PubMed PMID: 24417819. Pubmed Central PMCID: 4002656
11. Bigorgne AE, Farin HF, Lemoine R, Mahlaoui N, Lambert N, Gil M, et al. TTC7A mutations disrupt intestinal epithelial apicobasal polarity. J Clin Invest. 2014;124(1):328–37. PubMed PMID: 24292712. Pubmed Central PMCID: 3871247
12. Jones LB, McGrogan P, Flood TJ, Gennery AR, Morton L, Thrasher A, et al. Special article: chronic granulomatous disease in the United Kingdom and Ireland: a comprehensive national patient-based registry. Clin Exp Immunol. 2008;152(2):211–8. PubMed PMID: 18410635. Pubmed Central PMCID: 2384093
13. Uzel G, Orange JS, Poliak N, Marciano BE, Heller T, Holland SM. Complications of tumor necrosis factor-alpha blockade in chronic granulomatous disease-related colitis. Clin Infect Dis: Off Publ Infect Dis Soc Am. 2010;51(12):1429–34. PubMed PMID: 21058909. Pubmed Central PMCID: 3106244
14. Rigaud S, Fondaneche MC, Lambert N, Pasquier B, Mateo V, Soulas P, et al. XIAP deficiency in humans causes an X-linked lymphoproliferative syndrome. Nature. 2006;444(7115):110–4. PubMed PMID: 17080092

15. Worthey EA, Mayer AN, Syverson GD, Helbling D, Bonacci BB, Decker B, et al. Making a definitive diagnosis: successful clinical application of whole exome sequencing in a child with intractable inflammatory bowel disease. Genet Med. 2011;13(3):255–62. PubMed PMID: 21173700. Epub 2010/12/22. eng

16. Pachlopnik Schmid J, Canioni D, Moshous D, Touzot F, Mahlaoui N, Hauck F, et al. Clinical similarities and differences of patients with X-linked lymphoproliferative syndrome type 1 (XLP-1/SAP deficiency) versus type 2 (XLP-2/XIAP deficiency). Blood. 2011;117(5):1522–9. PubMed PMID: 21119115

17. Yang X, Kanegane H, Nishida N, Imamura T, Hamamoto K, Miyashita R, et al. Clinical and genetic characteristics of XIAP deficiency in Japan. J Clin Immunol. 2012;32(3):411–20. PubMed PMID: 22228567. Epub 2012/01/10. eng

18. Booth C, Gilmour KC, Veys P, Gennery AR, Slatter MA, Chapel H, et al. X-linked lymphoproliferative disease due to SAP/SH2D1A deficiency: a multicenter study on the manifestations, management and outcome of the disease. Blood. 2011;117(1):53–62. PubMed PMID: 20926771. Pubmed Central PMCID: 3374620

19. Aguilar C, Lenoir C, Lambert N, Begue B, Brousse N, Canioni D, et al. Characterization of Crohn disease in X-linked inhibitor of apoptosis-deficient male patients and female symptomatic carriers. J Allergy Clin Immunol. 2014;134(5):1131–41 e9. PubMed PMID: 24942515

20. Van Limbergen J, Wilson DC, Satsangi J. The genetics of Crohn's disease. Annu Rev Genomics Hum Genet. 2009;10:89–116. PubMed PMID: 19453248. Epub 2009/05/21. eng

21. Takahashi N, Matsumoto K, Saito H, Nanki T, Miyasaka N, Kobata T, et al. Impaired CD4 and CD8 effector function and decreased memory T cell populations in ICOS-deficient patients. J Immunol. 2009;182(9):5515–27. PubMed PMID: 19380800. Epub 2009/04/22. eng

22. Burns SO, Zenner HL, Plagnol V, Curtis J, Mok K, Eisenhut M, et al. LRBA gene deletion in a patient presenting with autoimmunity without hypogammaglobulinemia. J Allergy Clin Immunol. 2012;130(6):1428–32. PubMed PMID: 22981790. Epub 2012/09/18. eng

23. Alangari A, Alsultan A, Adly N, Massaad MJ, Kiani IS, Aljebreen A, et al. LPS-responsive beige-like anchor (LRBA) gene mutation in a family with inflammatory bowel disease and combined immunodeficiency. J Allergy Clin Immunol. 2012;130(2):481–8 e2. PubMed PMID: 22721650. Epub 2012/06/23. eng

24. Lopez-Herrera G, Tampella G, Pan-Hammarstrom Q, Herholz P, Trujillo-Vargas CM, Phadwal K, et al. Deleterious mutations in LRBA are associated with a syndrome of immune deficiency and autoimmunity. Am J Hum Genet. 2012;90(6):986–1001. PubMed PMID: 22608502. Pubmed Central PMCID: 3370280. Epub 2012/05/23. eng

25. Seidel MG, Hirschmugl T, Gamez-Diaz L, Schwinger W, Serwas N, Deutschmann A, et al. Long-term remission after allogeneic hematopoietic stem cell transplantation in LPS-responsive beige-like anchor (LRBA) deficiency. J Allergy Clin Immunol. 2015;135(5):1384–90 e1-8. PubMed PMID: 25539626. Pubmed Central PMCID: 4429722

26. Agarwal S, Mayer L. Pathogenesis and treatment of gastrointestinal disease in antibody deficiency syndromes. J Allergy Clin Immunol. 2009;124(4):658–64. PubMed PMID: 19665769. Pubmed Central PMCID: 3882760

27. Maekawa K, Yamada M, Okura Y, Sato Y, Yamada Y, Kawamura N, et al. X-linked agammaglobulinemia in a 10-year-old boy with a novel non-invariant splice-site mutation in Btk gene. Blood Cells Mol Dis. 2010;44(4):300–4. PubMed PMID: 20122858

28. Conley ME, Dobbs AK, Quintana AM, Bosompem A, Wang YD, Coustan-Smith E, et al. Agammaglobulinemia and absent B lineage cells in a patient lacking the p85alpha subunit of PI3K. J Exp Med. 2012;209(3):463–70. PubMed PMID: 22351933. Pubmed Central PMCID: 3302225

29. Jesus AA, Duarte AJ, Oliveira JB. Autoimmunity in hyper-IgM syndrome. J Clin Immunol. 2008;28(Suppl 1):S62–6. PubMed PMID: 18246414. Epub 2008/02/05. eng

30. Levy J, Espanol-Boren T, Thomas C, Fischer A, Tovo P, Bordigoni P, et al. Clinical spectrum of X-linked hyper-IgM syndrome. J Pediatr. 1997;131(1 Pt 1):47–54. PubMed PMID: 9255191. Epub 1997/07/01. eng

31. Quartier P, Bustamante J, Sanal O, Plebani A, Debre M, Deville A, et al. Clinical, immunologic and genetic analysis of 29 patients with autosomal recessive hyper-IgM syndrome due to Activation-Induced Cytidine Deaminase deficiency. Clin Immunol. 2004;110(1):22–9. PubMed PMID: 14962793. Epub 2004/02/14. eng

32. Misbah SA, Spickett GP, Ryba PC, Hockaday JM, Kroll JS, Sherwood C, et al. Chronic enteroviral meningoencephalitis in agammaglobulinemia: case report and literature review. J Clin Immunol. 1992;12(4):266–70. PubMed PMID: 1512300

33. Mahlaoui N, Pellier I, Mignot C, Jais JP, Bilhou-Nabera C, Moshous D, et al. Characteristics and outcome of early-onset, severe forms of Wiskott-Aldrich syndrome. Blood. 2013;121(9):1510–6. PubMed PMID: 23264593

34. Rohr J, Pannicke U, Doring M, Schmitt-Graeff A, Wiech E, Busch A, et al. Chronic inflammatory bowel disease as key manifestation of atypical ARTEMIS deficiency. J Clin Immunol. 2010;30(2):314–20. PubMed PMID: 19967552. Epub 2009/12/08. eng

35. Chou J, Hanna-Wakim R, Tirosh I, Kane J, Fraulino D, Lee YN, et al. A novel homozygous mutation in recombination activating gene 2 in 2 relatives with different clinical phenotypes: Omenn syndrome and hyper-IgM syndrome. J Allergy Clin Immunol. 2012;130(6):1414–6. PubMed PMID: 22841008. Pubmed Central PMCID: 3511613

36. Parry D, Blumenthal J, Tomar R, Horowitz S, Elder M, Gern G. A 3-year-old boy with ZAP-70 deficiency, thrombocytopenia and ulcerative colitis. J Allergy Clin Immunol. 1996;97:390.

37. de Saint-Basile G, Le Deist F, Caniglia M, Lebranchu Y, Griscelli C, Fischer A. Genetic study of a new X-linked recessive immunodeficiency syndrome. J Clin Invest. 1992;89(3):861–6. PubMed PMID: 1347296. Pubmed Central PMCID: 442931

38. DiSanto JP, Rieux-Laucat F, Dautry-Varsat A, Fischer A, de Saint Basile G. Defective human interleukin 2 receptor gamma chain in an atypical X chromosome-linked severe combined immunodeficiency with peripheral T cells. Proc Natl Acad Sci U S A. 1994;91(20):9466–70. PubMed PMID: 7937790. Pubmed Central PMCID: 44833

39. Felgentreff K, Perez-Becker R, Speckmann C, Schwarz K, Kalwak K, Markelj G, et al. Clinical and immunological manifestations of patients with atypical severe combined immunodeficiency. Clin Immunol. 2011;141(1):73–82. PubMed PMID: 21664875

40. Ozgur TT, Asal GT, Cetinkaya D, Orhan D, Kilic SS, Usta Y, et al. Hematopoietic stem cell transplantation in a CD3 gamma-deficient infant with inflammatory bowel disease. Pediatr Transplant. 2008;12(8):910–3. PubMed PMID: 18482219

41. Sznajer Y, Baumann C, David A, Journel H, Lacombe D, Perel Y, et al. Further delineation of the congenital form of X-linked dyskeratosis congenita (Hoyeraal-Hreidarsson syndrome). Eur J Pediatr. 2003;162(12):863–7. PubMed PMID: 14648217

42. Ballew BJ, Joseph V, De S, Sarek G, Vannier JB, Stracker T, et al. A recessive founder mutation in regulator of telomere elongation helicase 1, RTEL1, underlies severe immunodeficiency and features of Hoyeraal Hreidarsson syndrome. PLoS Genet. 2013;9(8):e1003695. PubMed PMID: 24009516. Pubmed Central PMCID: 3757051

43. Deng Z, Glousker G, Molczan A, Fox AJ, Lamm N, Dheekollu J, et al. Inherited mutations in the helicase RTEL1 cause telomere dysfunction and Hoyeraal-Hreidarsson syndrome. Proc Natl Acad Sci U S A. 2013;110(36):E3408–16. PubMed PMID: 23959892. Pubmed Central PMCID: 3767560

44. Lamm N, Ordan E, Shponkin R, Richler C, Aker M, Tzfati Y. Diminished telomeric 3′ overhangs are associated with telomere dysfunction in Hoyeraal-Hreidarsson syndrome. PLoS One. 2009;4(5):e5666. PubMed PMID: 19461895. Pubmed Central PMCID: 2680952

45. Sanal O, Jing H, Ozgur T, Ayvaz D, Strauss-Albee DM, Ersoy-Evans S, et al. Additional diverse findings expand the clinical presentation of DOCK8 deficiency. J Clin Immunol. 2012;32(4):698–708. PubMed PMID: 22476911. Epub 2012/04/06. eng

46. Al-Herz W, Ragupathy R, Massaad MJ, Al-Attiyah R, Nanda A, Engelhardt KR, et al. Clinical, immunologic and genetic profiles of DOCK8-deficient patients in Kuwait. Clin Immunol. 2012;143(3):266–72. PubMed PMID: 22534316

47. Alsum Z, Hawwari A, Alsmadi O, Al-Hissi S, Borrero E, Abu-Staiteh A, et al. Clinical, immunological and molecular characterization of DOCK8 and DOCK8-like deficient patients: single center experience of twenty-five patients. J Clin Immunol. 2013;33(1):55–67. PubMed PMID: 22968740

48. Dinwiddie DL, Kingsmore SF, Caracciolo S, Rossi G, Moratto D, Mazza C, et al. Combined DOCK8 and CLEC7A mutations causing immunodeficiency in 3 brothers with diarrhea, eczema, and infections. J Allergy Clin Immunol. 2013;131(2):594–7 e1-3. PubMed PMID: 23374272. Pubmed Central PMCID: 3570814

49. Hartley JL, Zachos NC, Dawood B, Donowitz M, Forman J, Pollitt RJ, et al. Mutations in TTC37 cause trichohepatoenteric syndrome (phenotypic diarrhea of infancy). Gastroenterology. 2010;138(7):2388–98. 98 e1-2. PubMed PMID: 20176027. Pubmed Central PMCID: 3166659. Epub 2010/02/24. eng

50. Fabre A, Charroux B, Martinez-Vinson C, Roquelaure B, Odul E, Sayar E, et al. SKIV2L mutations cause syndromic diarrhea, or trichohepatoenteric syndrome. Am J Hum Genet. 2012;90(4):689–92. PubMed PMID: 22444670. Pubmed Central PMCID: 3322239. Epub 2012/03/27. eng

51. Rider NL, Boisson B, Jyonouchi S, Hanson EP, Rosenzweig SD, Cassanova JL, et al. Novel TTC37 mutations in a patient with immunodeficiency without diarrhea: extending the phenotype of trichohepatoenteric syndrome. Front Pediatr. 2015;3:2. PubMed PMID: 25688341. Pubmed Central PMCID: 4311608

52. Heindl M, Handel N, Ngeow J, Kionke J, Wittekind C, Kamprad M, et al. Autoimmunity, intestinal lymphoid hyperplasia, and defects in mucosal B-cell homeostasis in patients with PTEN hamartoma tumor syndrome. Gastroenterology. 2012;142(5):1093–6 e6. PubMed PMID: 22266152. Epub 2012/01/24. eng

53. Bennett CL, Christie J, Ramsdell F, Brunkow ME, Ferguson PJ, Whitesell L, et al. The immune dysregulation, polyendocrinopathy, enteropathy, X-linked syndrome (IPEX) is caused by mutations of FOXP3. Nat Genet. 2001;27(1):20–1. PubMed PMID: 11137993. Epub 2001/01/04. eng

54. Barzaghi F, Passerini L, Bacchetta R. Immune dysregulation, polyendocrinopathy, enteropathy, x-linked syndrome: a paradigm of immunodeficiency with autoimmunity. Front Immunol. 2012;3:211. PubMed PMID: 23060872. Pubmed Central PMCID: 3459184. Epub 2012/10/13. eng

55. Caudy AA, Reddy ST, Chatila T, Atkinson JP, Verbsky JW. CD25 deficiency causes an immune dysregulation, polyendocrinopathy, enteropathy, X-linked-like syndrome, and defective IL-10 expression from CD4 lymphocytes. J Allergy Clin Immunol. 2007;119(2):482–7. PubMed PMID: 17196245. Epub 2007/01/02. eng

56. Bezrodnik L, Caldirola MS, Seminario AG, Moreira I, Gaillard MI. Follicular bronchiolitis as phenotype

associated with Cd25 deficiency. Clin Exp Immunol. 2013;7. PubMed PMID: 24116927

57. Begue B, Verdier J, Rieux-Laucat F, Goulet O, Morali A, Canioni D, et al. Defective IL10 signaling defining a subgroup of patients with inflammatory bowel disease. Am J Gastroenterol. 2011;106(8):1544–55. PubMed PMID: 21519361. Epub 2011/04/27. eng

58. Engelhardt KR, Shah N, Faizura-Yeop I, Kocacik Uygun DF, Frede N, Muise AM, et al. Clinical outcome in IL-10- and IL-10 receptor-deficient patients with or without hematopoietic stem cell transplantation. J Allergy Clin Immunol. 2013;131(3):825–30 e9. PubMed PMID: 23158016. Epub 2012/11/20. eng

59. Glocker EO, Frede N, Perro M, Sebire N, Elawad M, Shah N, et al. Infant colitis – it's in the genes. Lancet. 2010;376(9748):1272. PubMed PMID: 20934598. Epub 2010/10/12. eng

60. Glocker EO, Kotlarz D, Boztug K, Gertz EM, Schaffer AA, Noyan F, et al. Inflammatory bowel disease and mutations affecting the interleukin-10 receptor. N Engl J Med. 2009;361(21):2033–45. PubMed PMID:

19890111. Pubmed Central PMCID: 2787406. Epub 2009/11/06. eng

61. Kotlarz D, Beier R, Murugan D, Diestelhorst J, Jensen O, Boztug K, et al. Loss of interleukin-10 signaling and infantile inflammatory bowel disease: implications for diagnosis and therapy. Gastroenterology. 2012;143(2):347–55. PubMed PMID: 22549091. Epub 2012/05/03. eng

62. Moran CJ, Walters TD, Guo CH, Kugathasan S, Klein C, Turner D, et al. IL-10R polymorphisms are associated with very-early-onset ulcerative colitis. Inflamm Bowel Dis. 2013;19(1):115–23. PubMed PMID: 22550014. Epub 2012/05/03. Eng

63. Carbonnel F, Colombel JF, Filippi J, Katsanos KH, Peyrin-Biroulet L, Allez M, et al. Methotrexate is not superior to placebo for inducing steroid-free remission, but induces steroid-free clinical remission in a larger proportion of patients with ulcerative colitis. Gastroenterology. 2016;150(2):380–8 e4. PubMed PMID: 26632520

Infections in Cancer

Andrea J. Zimmer and Alison G. Freifeld

Introduction

Infections are an important cause of morbidity and mortality in the oncology population. Individual's risk of various infections is dependent on a multitude factors, particularly the type of cancer, sites involved, treatment regimen, procedures, and neutropenia. Preexisting comorbidities such as obesity, diabetes, and lung, kidney, and liver disease are also important factors to take into consideration, as are age, malnutrition, and deconditioning. Neutropenia remains the most important risk factor, with increased depth and duration associated with higher incidence of infection. In this chapter, we will be discussing infections in patients with solid tumors and hematologic malignancies, with the exception of hematopoietic stem cell transplant (HSCT) recipients, as this population will be discussed in a separate chapter.

Risks for Infection

Numerous factors contribute to the increased infection risk in cancer patients, such as age, underlying tumor, type of chemotherapy or transplant, nutritional status, and the presence of comorbid medical conditions including diabetes and renal or liver insufficiency. The overall infection risk level is related to the severity and accumulated frequency of factors in a given patient [1]. For example, cytotoxic chemotherapy has been the mainstay of many cancer treatments for the past 60 years, and its association with increased risk of infection has been firmly established [2]. Many cytotoxic agents interfere with tumor cell survival and replication, but they simultaneously act on myeloproliferative cells of the bone marrow, resulting in neutropenia, defined as an absolute neutrophil count (ANC) of 500 neutrophils/μl or fewer (in contrast, the normal range for the ANC in peripheral blood is about 1500–8000 neutrophils/μl). Neutrophils play a vital role in the innate immune response to invading pathogens, primarily bacteria and fungi, and their main functions include directly attacking bacterial cells or fungal hyphae and releasing cytokines to recruit a cascade of inflammatory responses at the site of infection [3]. Risk of infection is inversely proportional to the depth and duration of neutropenia with rates of infection incrementally increasing when the absolute neutrophil count (ANC) falls below 1000 cells/

A. J. Zimmer (✉) · A. G. Freifeld
Internal Medicine, Division of Infectious Diseases,
University of Nebraska Medical Center,
Omaha, NE, USA
e-mail: andreaj.zimmer@unmc.edu; afreifeld@unmc.edu

© Springer International Publishing AG, part of Springer Nature 2018
B. H. Segal (ed.), *Management of Infections in the Immunocompromised Host*,
https://doi.org/10.1007/978-3-319-77674-3_10

mm³, 500 cells/mm³, and 100 cells/mm³, respectively. Likewise, increasing durations of neutropenia of 7 days or longer are associated with higher rates of infectious complications due to bacterial and fungal pathogens [2, 4]. Typically, the onset of neutropenia occurs approximately 1 week following delivery of cytotoxic chemotherapy. Patients receiving chemotherapy for solid tumors will generally have neutropenia that lasts less than 7 days and, therefore, typically have relatively low risk of infection compared to those with hematologic malignancies. Neutropenia in patients undergoing hematopoietic stem cell transplant with conditioning therapy or receiving chemotherapy for hematologic malignancies may last 14 days or more, with an attendant increase in infection risk.

The underlying malignancy itself can predispose patients to infection. In particular, patients with hematologic malignancies are at an increased risk for infection, given the nature of the cells involved. Typically, there is unregulated proliferation of abnormal cells from an individual cell line, which may result in impaired function in these cells; specific examples will be discussed in further detail later in the chapter. Solid organ tumors can also leave patients vulnerable to infections. Masses that involve or invade into non-sterile sites or that cause obstruction of normally patent lumens are potential sources of infection. For example, tumors involving or in close proximity to the biliary tree, causing biliary obstruction, may lead to cholangitis. Malignancies invading through gut lumen allow bacteria to spill into sterile spaces, such as the peritoneum. Bronchial obstruction causing postobstructive pneumonia may be a sequela of lung cancer. Tumors obstructing the urinary tract can be associated with upper tract urinary infections.

Both chemotherapy and radiation can damage the cells lining the mouth and gastrointestinal track, causing mucosal barrier injury (MBI) or mucositis. MBI itself can cause fevers as the tissue destruction and cell death elicits a robust inflammatory response. In combination with neutropenia, MBI also creates an opportunity for bacterial translocation and localized infections or bacteremia with organisms that colonize the mouth and gastrointestinal (GI) tract [5]. MBI typically manifests approximately 7–10 days after receiving cytotoxic chemotherapy [6]. Other integument or mucosal barrier breeches are common in this population either as a result of recent biopsy procedure, tumor debulking surgery, or the presence of a central venous catheter.

Fever and Neutropenia

Febrile neutropenia is defined as a onetime oral temperature of $\geq 38.3°$ or a sustained oral of $\geq 38°$ for an hour or longer in a patient with an ANC of <500 cell/mm³ or who is predicted to have an ANC of <500 cell/mm³ within a 48 h period [4]. The first cycle of chemotherapy has the highest likelihood of causing neutropenic fever [7–9]. Other factors associated with increased risk of febrile neutropenia include age greater than 65 years, renal dysfunction, cardiovascular disease, preexisting anemia, and high-intensity chemotherapy [10]. Various studies have shown overall mortality in patients with neutropenic fever to be 8–15%, with higher mortality seen in patients with documented Gram-negative bacteremia and/or tissue-invasive infections such as pneumonia [1, 11]. An infectious etiology is only identified in 40–50% of episodes with 10–20% having bacteremia [3, 7, 12–14]. However, as the inflammatory response in this population is attenuated, fever may be the only sign or symptom of infection. In the absence of neutrophils, localizing signs and symptoms of infection, may be very subtle, if present at all [15]. In studies from the 1960s to 1970s, when cytotoxic chemotherapy was being introduced for treatment of acute leukemia, it was demonstrated that a very high mortality rate occurred in febrile neutropenic patients who did not receive prompt empiric antibiotic therapy. Many of these episodes resulted from enteric Gram-negative bloodstream infections (*E. coli*, *Enterobacter*, and *Klebsiella* species primarily) as well as *Pseudomonas aeruginosa*, which was linked to especially high rates of mortality when empiric treatment was delayed in the setting of neutropenia. Based on these observations, the standard of care for more than 40 years is that episodes of neutropenic fever require immediate treatment with empiric antibiotics, with coverage against *Pseudomonas* and Gram-negative enteric pathogens [11, 12, 16]. Although Gram-positive bacteremias have become more common in the last 30 years, they rarely cause rapid demise in febrile neutropenic patients. Accordingly, for stable patients without sepsis, pneumonia, mucositis, or evidence of line infection, there is no benefit to empirically adding vancomycin to the initial empiric regimen used for management of febrile neutropenia (FN) [17, 18]. In these stable FN patients, monotherapy with antipseudomonal agents such as ceftazidime, cefepime, piperacillin-tazobactam, or an antipseudomonal carbapenem (imipenem or meropenem) is currently recommended for empiric coverage. Several clinical practice guidelines exist to help with management of these populations [4, 19].

Many centers use antimicrobial prophylaxis in patients who are at high risk for infection, particularly due to prolonged neutropenia. In a randomized double-blinded prospective study, levofloxacin prophylaxis reduced the incidence of infections and rates of febrile neutropenia in patients receiving chemotherapy for hematologic malignancies or undergoing stem cell transplant with an anticipated neutropenia of at least 7 days [20]. Reductions in frequency of febrile neutropenia and of Gram-negative bacteremia were demonstrated, but there were no differences in mortality between those who received prophylaxis compared to those who did not. Of concern, the results did demonstrate a slight increase of levofloxacin-resistant organisms in patients who received levofloxacin prophylaxis [20]. Clinical guidelines suggest consideration of antibacterial prophylaxis in patients with expected neutropenia of ≤ 100 cells/mm^3 for at least 7 days [4, 21]. Following the implementation of fluoroquinolone prophylaxis, there has been a rise in the incidence of antimicrobial drug resistance in some centers [22, 23]. Of particular concern, increasing rates of multidrug-resistant (MDR) Gram-negative organisms are being reported, including *Enterobacteriaceae* (e.g., *E. coli* and *Klebsiella* and *Enterobacter* species) and *Pseudomonas* species., prompting some centers to change their empiric regimen for febrile neutropenia to a carbapenem-based regimen until susceptibilities are available [24, 25]. Fluoroquinolone prophylaxis is also associated with increased risk for methicillin-resistant *Staphylococcus aureus* (MRSA) and vancomycin-resistant *Enterococcus* (VRE) colonization and infection [22, 26].

For patients who are unable to tolerate fluoroquinolones, third-generation cephalosporins, such as oral cefpodoxime, have been sometimes used as an alternative. As they do not have activity against *Pseudomonas* spp., a randomized trial showed that rates of infections with this organism were higher compared to patients receiving levofloxacin prophylaxis (16% versus 1.8%) [27]. Most of the breakthrough infections due to *Enterobacteriaceae* had some degree of resistance to fluoroquinolones obviating that class of agents for empirical therapy, but all the isolates remained susceptible to cefepime and meropenem [27].

Recombinant granulocyte colony-stimulating factor (G-CSF) is a synthesized glycoprotein that stimulates proliferation of granulocytic progenitor cells in the bone marrow and release of granulocytes into the bloodstream to elevate the peripheral blood neutrophil count. G-CSF can shorten the duration of neutropenia associated with many chemotherapy regimens and has been shown to reduce incidence of fever and infections in settings where neutropenia is most profound and prolonged. Since it is a rather expensive agent, its use is restricted to regimens causing longer duration of neutropenia and specifically to those patients who are at increased risk for neutropenic fever. G-CSF is typically recommended for use in patients with a risk $\geq 20\%$ of febrile neutropenia or those with a previous history of FN, according to current guidelines [4, 9]. They are not generally recommended for treatment of established febrile neutropenia, except in instances where a life-threatening infection is identified; in those cases, it is hoped – but not proven – to be beneficial.

Risk Assessment and Treatment of Febrile Neutropenia

The Multinational Association for Supportive Care in Cancer (MASCC) risk index score was published in 2000 with a goal of identifying those patients who, on presentation with FN, are at low risk for mortality and other serious complications during the subsequent course of neutropenia [28]. With early identification of those at low versus high risk for complications, it is possible to develop less intensive empiric antibiotic management schemes for the low-risk group, i.e., oral and/or outpatient antibiotics. Factors comprising this weighted MASCC scoring system include degree of symptoms attributable to febrile neutropenia at presentation, hypotension, history of pulmonary disease, history of fungal infection, dehydration, age, and whether the patient is an outpatient or inpatient at the time of onset of the febrile neutropenia (see Table 10.1). Patients with a score of >21 are at low risk for serious complications. This algorithm has been validated by numerous studies, with sensitivities and specificities ranging from 71–95% to 40–95%, respectively [29–31]. Many centers use these criteria to determine whether a patient with febrile neutropenia requires hospitalization or can be managed as an outpatient with oral antibiotic therapy. Oral

Table 10.1 The Multinational Association for Supportive Care in Cancer (MASCC) score

Characteristic	Weight (# of points)
Burden of febrile neutropenia	
No or mild symptoms	5
Moderate symptoms	3
Severe symptoms or moribund	0
No hypotension (SBP >90 mmHg)	5
No COPD	4
Solid tumor OR HM w/o previous fungal infection	4
No dehydration requiring parenteral fluids	3
Outpatient status	3
Age <60	2

Applicable points are added to create a cumulative score. The maximum score is 26, and a score of >20 has a predicted low risk (<10%) for serious medical complications during the course of the febrile neutropenia

options include oral ciprofloxacin plus amoxicillin/clavulanic acid versus moxifloxacin with the coverage spectrum to include both Gram-negative and Gram-positive organisms [13, 32, 33]. However, patients who are already receiving an oral fluoroquinolone as prophylaxis are not candidates for treatment with oral agents [33].

Pathogens

Bacteria

Gram-negative organisms were historically the most common pathogens isolated in neutropenic patients, but due to antimicrobial prophylaxis and empiric therapy, infections due to Gram-positive bacteria have become more common [34]. Gram-positive organisms now account for more than 50% of bacteremias in febrile neutropenia with coagulase-negative *Staphylococcus* species and *Streptococcus* species being the most common [14, 35]. Up to 10–15% of bacteremias are polymicrobial, most commonly occurring in patients with enteric or lower respiratory sources of infection [14]. *Enterobacteriaceae* are the most common Gram-negative organisms isolated in neutropenic patients, with *E. coli* and *Klebsiella* species topping the list [3]. *Pseudomonas aeruginosa* accounts for about 20% of Gram-negative infections but has a high mortality rate.

Viridans group *Streptococcus* is an increasingly common cause of bacteremia and can cause severe sepsis in neutropenic patients and typically arises from mucositis or enteric translocation. They are often susceptible to beta-lactams, but resistant organisms have been increasing with some studies reporting up to 30–40% of isolates with resistance to cephalosporins and extended spectrum beta-lactams [36, 37]. Therefore, clinical guidelines do recommend the addition of vancomycin in patients with signs of clinical instability due to sepsis associated with neutropenic fevers to cover possible VGS bacteremia [4, 38]. Factors associated with penicillin resistance include beta-lactam prophylaxis, recent treatment with beta-lactam antibiotics, or nosocomial onset of infection [39, 40].

Infections with multidrug-resistant organisms, particularly VRE, extended-spectrum beta-lactamase (ESBL)-producing Gram-negative infections, and carbapenem-resistant *Enterobacteriaceae* (CRE) are on the rise and associated with increased morbidity and mortality as well as inadequate initial antibiotic therapy. The prevalence of these organisms varies globally and among different institutions. Prolonged hospitalization and antibiotic use, including as prophylaxis, are associated with colonization and infection with resistant organisms such as VRE, ESLB, and CRE [35, 41–45]. Treatment of febrile neutropenia in patients at high for resistant organisms should be tailored based on local antibiograms and on the susceptibility patterns of prior infections.

Viruses

Reactivation of herpes simplex virus (HSV) and varicella zoster virus (VZV) is relatively common in patients receiving chemotherapy for solid tumors or hematologic malignancies [46]. Regimens that cause prolonged suppression of cell-mediated immunity or neutropenia, particularly those used for hematologic malignancies, are associated with increased risk of viral reactivation, and prophylaxis with acyclovir, valacyclovir, or famciclovir can be considered in patients who are seropositive for HSV and/or VZV [21, 46–48]. In particular, agents such as alemtuzumab, bortezomib, fludarabine, antithymocyte globulin (ATG), and high-dose steroids are associated with high risk of viral reactivation. Clinically significant infections due to cytomegalovirus (CMV) or Epstein-Barr virus (EBV) are uncommon in the non-transplant population.

Yearly vaccination with the inactivated influenza vaccine is routinely recommended in patients undergoing cancer treatment. Depending on their chemotherapy regimen and underlying disease, some patients may have suboptimal immunologic response, but studies have shown that a significant number do have documented seroconversion. Strategies, such as using the high-dose influenza vaccine and timing vaccination between chemotherapy cycles, likely increase response [4, 49, 50]. It is also recommended that caregivers and household contacts receive yearly influenza vaccination. Patients with documented or suspected infection due to influenza should be promptly treated with effective therapy with a neuraminidase inhibitor such as oseltamivir, zanamivir, or peramivir. Infections due to other respiratory viruses are common in this population, and patients should be advised to try to avoid sick contacts. Treatment is supportive care, including for RSV, as treatment with ribavirin and/or immunotherapy is generally not recommended outside the posttransplant population.

Fungi

Current guidelines recommend empiric antifungal therapy if febrile neutropenia recurs or persists for 4–7 days despite broad-spectrum antibiotic therapy. Since fungal infections are the culprit in only 5–10% of those cases, empiric antifungal therapy, by design, results in overuse of antifungal therapy [4]. Factors increasing risk for invasive fungal infection (IFI) include increased depth and duration of neutropenia (with most mold IFI's occurring when neutropenia lasts longer than 2 weeks), refractory hematologic disease, prolonged steroid use, and multiple previous cytotoxic treatments [51]. *Candida* species commonly colonize the GI tract and can cause a spectrum of infections in patients with cancer, ranging from mucocutaneous lesions (thrush), candidemia, or even tissue-invasive infections such as hepatosplenic candidiasis. The risk of disseminated candidiasis is increased in patients with prolonged neutropenia, high-dose steroid use, indwelling central catheters, total parenteral nutrition (TPN), and MBI. Invasive candidiasis is associated with significant morbidity and mortality, and, therefore, patients considered to be at high risk are often placed on antifungal prophylaxis. This practice has led to a dramatic decrease in both superficial and disseminated candida infections in this patient population [52, 53].

Patients with profound neutropenia lasting more than 10–14 days are at increased risk for invasive mold infections due to organisms such as *Aspergillus* spp. and zygomycetes. Therefore, azoles with anti-mold activity, such as posaconazole or voriconazole, are used at many centers for prophylaxis in patients with acute myelogenous leukemia (AML) or myelodysplastic syndrome (MDS) who are receiving induction/reinduction and consolidation chemotherapy [21, 54, 55]. These agents are also recommended in patients with graft-versus-host-disease (GVHD) following allogeneic stem cell transplant (SCT), a population that is discussed in great detail in another chapter [21].

The diagnosis of invasive fungal disease (IFD) can be challenging as clinical symptoms, radiographic test, and cultures have low sensitivity and specificity. Biopsy of affected tissue may demonstrate invasive hyphae, which confirms the diagnosis, even if cultures are negative. However, due to frequent thrombocytopenia in this patient population, we are often not able to obtain a biopsy without significant risk. The use of fungal biomarkers, such as galactomannan (GM), beta-D-glucan, and polymerase chain reaction (PCR) tests may also be useful in the diagnostic evaluation [56, 57]. Galactomannan is a polysaccharide that constitutes a majority of *Aspergillus* species cell walls as well as the cell walls of other mold species, with the exception of zygomycetes which include *Mucor*, *Rhizomucor*, and *Cunninghamella* species. There is a commercial assay that uses a double-sandwich enzyme immunoassay (EIA) to detect the presence of this polysaccharide in clinical specimens, including serum, bronchoalveolar lavage (BAL) fluid, and CSF of high-risk populations [57]. In serum, serial GM testing may identify patients with invasive aspergillosis earlier than CT scanning of the chest or sinuses, but the sensitivity varies considerably in different studies. However, the GM test for BAL fluid is typically associated with at least 80% sensitivity for detection of invasive pulmonary aspergillosis. 1, 3-Beta-D-glucan is also a cell wall component that is present in a variety of fungal organisms, including *Candida*, *Pneumocystis*, and *Aspergillus* species, but not *Cryptococcus* species and zygomycetes [58–60]. The use of fungal biomarkers in preemptive therapy in high-risk populations is currently under investigation [61, 62].

Clinical Syndromes in Neutropenic Patients

Pulmonary Infiltrates

Pulmonary infiltrates occur in up to 25% of patient with neutropenia lasting for 10 days or more and account for up to 40% of infections in neutropenic fever [3, 63]. The infectious differential is broad and includes common bacterial pathogens and respiratory viruses, as well as fungal and mycobacterial infections. Noninfectious etiologies, including drug toxicity, alveolar hemorrhage, and radiation pneumonitis, should be considered. Radiographic appearance can be helpful in stratifying most likely causes. Consolidations or nodular lesions with cavities, "air crescent sign," or "halo sign" are concerning for infection due to filamentous fungi. A "reversed halo sign" is a classic finding in neutropenic patients with infections due to zygomycetes species, but it is not specific to this process [56]. Diffuse bilateral infiltrates, particularly with ground glass opacities, may be suggestion of infection due to *Pneumocystis*. Infections due to mycobacteria or *Nocardia* can also be seen in these populations, but bacterial organisms are the most common cause of pneumonia. Bronchoscopy with BAL can be helpful in obtaining a microbiologic diagnosis, but it can be nondiagnostic in over half of cases, particularly if patients have already received empiric treatment. Histopathology with invasive hyphae is diagnostic for invasive fungal infection and can be seen even when cultures are negative. However, if patients are also thrombocytopenic, biopsies are associated with increased risk of bleeding or other complications.

Central Line-Associated Infections

Due to the need for frequent blood draws and administration of intravenous medications and because of the caustic effect of some agents on smaller vessels, many patients receiving chemotherapy will have an indwelling central venous catheter. Accordingly, central line-associated bloodstream infections (CLABSI) account for some of the most common infections identified in patients with febrile neutropenia. In order to determine whether the catheter is the source of the infection, blood cultures should be obtained from a peripheral venous puncture and from each catheter lumen. If the time to positivity differential is 2 h or more from the catheter as compared to the peripheral set, it suggests the catheter is the source of the blood stream infection [64]. Gram-positive organisms, particularly coagulase-negative staphylococci and *Staphylococcus aureus*, are the most common pathogens to cause CLABSI. Gram-negative organisms and *Candida* species are also identified fairly frequently. Whether the catheter needs to be removed depends on the clinical presentation (i.e., whether the patient is hemodynamically unstable), type of catheter, and organisms identified. In general infections due to *S. aureus*, *Pseudomonas* spp. or *Candida* spp. require catheter removal. The catheter should be removed if signs of tunnel infection occur.

Typhlitis and Colitis

Typhlitis or neutropenic enterocolitis is a disease process unique to neutropenic patients and typically occurs in patients who have received cytotoxic chemotherapy, leading to disruption of mucosal integrity. Onset occurs 2–3 weeks on average after receiving chemotherapy [65]. The compromised mucosa in combination with neutropenia allows enteric organisms to invade intestinal tissue, which is thought to elicit inflammatory processes including cytokine activation. Oftentimes patients will have concomitant blood stream infections from bacterial translocation. Patients typically have complaints of fevers, abdominal pain, cramping, or diarrhea, but symptoms may be blunted in comparison to the severity of disease. Computed tomography (CT) is the preferred diagnostic imaging study, and classic findings include bowel wall thickening with mesenteric stranding, particularly involving the ileocecal region. This process can result in significant bowel necrosis with pneumatosis or even perforation, which may require surgical invention and resection. In the absence of these severe features, management is typically medical and includes bowel rest, adequate hydration, and antibiotics targeting enteric Gram-negative organisms as well as anaerobes. G-CSF may be used as adjunctive treatment [66, 67]. Colitis due to *Clostridium difficile* can also present similarly, but typically with a more predominant diarrheal illness. This infection is not limited to the neutropenic population, but the disease may be more severe or protracted compared to normal hosts [68]. Cancer patients are at risk for *Clostridium difficile* colitis and relapsed disease for a number of reasons, including immunosuppression due to chemotherapy and disease; need for close contact with the healthcare system, including hospitalizations; and frequent antimicrobial therapy.

Infections in Hematologic Malignancies

Patients with hematologic malignancies may have abnormal counts or functions of certain leukocyte cell lines depending on the underlying disease. Patients with treatment refractory or relapsed disease are at a much higher risk for infectious complications than those who have rapid and sustained response to therapy [21]. As some of these diseases are more prevalent in older adults, therefore immunologic impair caused by malignancy may be compounded with waning immune function related to aging.

Myelogenous leukemias involve the uncontrolled clonal proliferation of myeloid cells (cell line that normally differentiates into granulocytes, monocytes, erythrocytes, and megakaryocytes), giving rise to cells with abnormal antimicrobial activity or "functional neutropenia" [69, 70]. Acute leukemias are life threatening and generally require aggressive chemotherapy, often with the goal of SCT if remission can be achieved after induction therapy and multiple cycles of consolidation therapy. Induction therapy typically results in 3–6 weeks of profound neutropenia, and during that time, bacterial and fungal mold infections are not uncommon. Myelodysplastic syndromes are a constellation of malignant hematopoietic stem cell disorders with dysplastic and abnormal cell production with may cause neutropenia, anemia, and/or thrombocytopenia. Patients with MDS are at increased risk for infection if they have leukopenia or granulocyte dysfunction. MDS also has the potential to transform to a more aggressive leukemia [71–73].

The hallmark of chronic lymphocytic leukemia (CLL) is the progressive accumulation of dysfunctional monoclonal lymphocytes. This disease process leads to multifaceted immunologic impairments, including hypogammaglobulinemia, and impaired cellular immunity due to quantitative and qualitative lymphocyte abnormalities, both of which generally worsen over time. Advanced disease may result in neutropenia due to marrow replacement [74]. Patients with CLL are therefore at increased risk for numerous infectious complications even if they are not receiving chemotherapy. Bacterial infections involving the skin, respiratory system, and urinary tract are most common, and reactivation of herpes virus, particularly with HSV and VZV, also frequently occur [75, 76].

The risk of infections in CLL is both a function of the severity of the disease and response to therapy as well as treatment-related immunosuppression. Treatment-related infections are problematic in this population as chemotherapy regimens may include myelosuppressing and lymphocyte-depleting purine analogs such as fludarabine, cladribine, or pentostatin. Other agents used in CLL include alemtuzumab and rituximab, which are monoclonal antibodies

that target specific immune populations (described in "Targeted Cancer Therapies and Infection") and predispose to a number of infectious complications [74]. These opportunistic infections include *Pneumocystis*, *Aspergillus*, CMV, *Cryptococcus*, and *Listeria*, among others [76–78]. Concomitant use of corticosteroids increases infection risk [79].

Multiple myeloma is characterized by a monoclonal proliferation of plasma cells, which are derived from B cells. As a result, patients with multiple myeloma often have hypogammaglobulinemia, causing impaired humoral immunity, and are therefore at higher risk for infections due to viruses and encapsulated bacterial pathogens, such as *Streptococcus pneumoniae* and *Haemophilus influenzae* [80]. It is important that these patients are kept up to date on recommended vaccinations, including pneumococcus and annual influenza, although it should be noted that levels of protection may be inadequate due to impaired B-cell responses. In addition, dysfunctions of the complement system, dendritic cells, NK cells, and T cells have been described [81]. Advanced disease and treatment can result in organ dysfunction with nephrotic syndrome, respiratory compromise, and transfusion-related iron overload, all of which are also associated with infectious risk [80].

Targeted Cancer Therapies and Infection

New therapies with more targeted sites of action are being developed for many cancer types with the hope of having fewer side effects and less bone marrow toxicity and, accordingly, less frequent and profound neutropenic periods. Experience with some of these agents is limited to date, but, depending on their cellular targets of action, some of these agents can cause immunologic impairment and increased risk of certain types of infection. Rituximab, for example, is a monoclonal antibody that targets CD20-positive cells, thereby making it an effective treatment of CLL and lymphoma. However, it does have activity against both malignant and normal B cells, and therefore, its use results in prolonged suppression of humoral immunity. Rituximab has been associated with reactivation of hepatitis B as well as other viral infections, including *Herpesviridae* and JC virus infection [82]. Alemtuzumab is an anti-CD52 monoclonal antibody sometimes used for the treatment of chronic lymphocytic leukemia as it causes destruction of B and T lymphocytes as well as natural killer cells. As such its use results in prolonged immunosuppression with increased risk of bacterial, viral, and fungal infections [83]. Bortezomib is a proteasome inhibitor used to treat multiple myeloma and some lymphomas. Its use causes cell-mediated immunity impairment and frequently results in reactivation of VZV and HSV [80]. Bevacizumab is a monoclonal antibody that targets vascular endothelial growth factor (VEGF) and is used to treat a wide array of solid tumors, including non-small cell lung cancer, colorectal cancer, and ovarian cancer. Its use may cause delayed wound healing or dehiscence, and therefore it is recommended to discontinue at least a month preoperatively and not to resume until the wound is fully healed [84, 85]. Cases of abscesses and fistula formation associated with bevacizumab have also been reported [85]. As new targeted agents become available, their side effect profiles should be monitored for infectious complications.

References

1. Kuderer NM, et al. Mortality, morbidity, and cost associated with febrile neutropenia in adult cancer patients. Cancer. 2006;106(10):2258–66.
2. Bodey GP, et al. Quantitative relationships between circulating leukocytes and infection in patients with acute leukemia. Ann Intern Med. 1966;64(2):328–40.
3. Nesher L, Rolston KV. The current spectrum of infection in cancer patients with chemotherapy related neutropenia. Infection. 2014;42(1):5–13.
4. Freifeld AG, et al. Clinical practice guideline for the use of antimicrobial agents in neutropenic patients with cancer: 2010 update by the infectious diseases society of america. Clin Infect Dis. 2011;52(4):e56–93.
5. van der Velden WJ, et al. Mucosal barrier injury, fever and infection in neutropenic patients with cancer: introducing the paradigm febrile mucositis. Br J Haematol. 2014;167(4):441–52.
6. Epstein JB, et al. Oral complications of cancer and cancer therapy: from cancer treatment to survivorship. CA Cancer J Clin. 2012;62(6):400–22.
7. Crawford J, Dale DC, Lyman GH. Chemotherapy-induced neutropenia: risks, consequences, and new directions for its management. Cancer. 2004;100(2):228–37.
8. Crawford J, et al. Risk and timing of neutropenic events in adult cancer patients receiving chemotherapy: the results of a prospective nationwide study of oncology practice. J Natl Compr Cancer Netw. 2008;6(2):109–18.
9. Lyman GH, et al. Predicting individual risk of neutropenic complications in patients receiving cancer chemotherapy. Cancer. 2011;117(9):1917–27.
10. Lyman GH, Lyman CH, Agboola O. Risk models for predicting chemotherapy-induced neutropenia. Oncologist. 2005;10(6):427–37.
11. Paul M, et al. Empirical antibiotic monotherapy for febrile neutropenia: systematic review and meta-analysis of randomized controlled trials. J Antimicrob Chemother. 2006;57(2):176–89.
12. Schimpff SC. Empiric antibiotic therapy for granulocytopenic cancer patients. Am J Med. 1986;80(5C):13–20.
13. Freifeld A, et al. A double-blind comparison of empirical oral and intravenous antibiotic therapy for low-risk febrile patients with neutropenia during cancer chemotherapy. N Engl J Med. 1999;341(5):305–11.
14. Klastersky J, et al. Bacteraemia in febrile neutropenic cancer patients. Int J Antimicrob Agents. 2007;30(Suppl 1):S51–9.
15. Schimpff SC. Overview of empiric antibiotic therapy for the febrile neutropenic patient. Rev Infect Dis. 1985;7(Suppl 4):S734–40.
16. Paul M, et al. Anti-pseudomonal beta-lactams for the initial, empirical, treatment of febrile neutropenia: comparison of beta-lactams. Cochrane Database Syst Rev. 2010;11:CD005197.
17. Cometta A, et al. Vancomycin versus placebo for treating persistent fever in patients with neutropenic cancer receiving piperacillin-tazobactam monotherapy. Clin Infect Dis. 2003;37(3):382–9.
18. Vancomycin added to empirical combination antibiotic therapy for fever in granulocytopenic cancer patients. European Organization for Research and Treatment of Cancer (EORTC) International Antimicrobial Therapy Cooperative Group and the National Cancer Institute of Canada-Clinical Trials Group. J Infect Dis. 1991;163(5):951–8.
19. de Naurois J, et al. Management of febrile neutropenia: ESMO clinical practice guidelines. Ann Oncol. 2010;21(Suppl 5):v252–6.
20. Bucaneve G, et al. Levofloxacin to prevent bacterial infection in patients with cancer and neutropenia. N Engl J Med. 2005;353(10):977–87.

21. Baden LR, et al. Prevention and treatment of cancer-related infections. J Natl Compr Cancer Netw. 2012;10(11):1412–45.

22. Rangaraj G, et al. Perils of quinolone exposure in cancer patients: breakthrough bacteremia with multidrug-resistant organisms. Cancer. 2010;116(4):967–73.

23. Trecarichi EM, Tumbarello M. Antimicrobial-resistant Gram-negative bacteria in febrile neutropenic patients with cancer: current epidemiology and clinical impact. Curr Opin Infect Dis. 2014;27(2):200–10.

24. Nguyen AD, et al. A single-center evaluation of the risk for colonization or bacteremia with piperacillin-tazobactam- and cefepime-resistant bacteria in patients with acute leukemia receiving fluoroquinolone prophylaxis. J Oncol Pharm Pract. 2016;22(2):303–7.

25. Garnica M, et al. Ciprofloxacin prophylaxis in high risk neutropenic patients: effects on outcomes, antimicrobial therapy and resistance. BMC Infect Dis. 2013;13:356.

26. Bow EJ. Fluoroquinolones, antimicrobial resistance and neutropenic cancer patients. Curr Opin Infect Dis. 2011;24(6):545–53.

27. Wojenski DJ, et al. Cefpodoxime for antimicrobial prophylaxis in neutropenia: a retrospective case series. Clin Ther. 2014;36(6):976–81.

28. Klastersky J, et al. The multinational association for supportive care in cancer risk index: a multinational scoring system for identifying low-risk febrile neutropenic cancer patients. J Clin Oncol. 2000;18(16):3038–51.

29. Baskaran ND, Gan GG, Adeeba K. Applying the Multinational Association for Supportive Care in Cancer risk scoring in predicting outcome of febrile neutropenia patients in a cohort of patients. Ann Hematol. 2008;87(7):563–9.

30. Innes H, et al. Management of febrile neutropenia in solid tumours and lymphomas using the Multinational Association for Supportive Care in Cancer (MASCC) risk index: feasibility and safety in routine clinical practice. Support Care Cancer. 2008;16(5):485–91.

31. Uys A, Rapoport BL, Anderson R. Febrile neutropenia: a prospective study to validate the Multinational Association of Supportive Care of Cancer (MASCC) risk-index score. Support Care Cancer. 2004;12(8):555–60.

32. Kern WV, et al. Oral antibiotics for fever in low-risk neutropenic patients with cancer: a double-blind, randomized, multicenter trial comparing single daily moxifloxacin with twice daily ciprofloxacin plus amoxicillin/clavulanic acid combination therapy – EORTC infectious diseases group trial XV. J Clin Oncol. 2013;31(9):1149–56.

33. Flowers CR, et al. Antimicrobial prophylaxis and outpatient management of fever and neutropenia in adults treated for malignancy: American Society of Clinical Oncology clinical practice guideline. J Clin Oncol. 2013;31(6):794–810.

34. Bodey GP, et al. Fever and infection in leukemic patients: a study of 494 consecutive patients. Cancer. 1978;41(4):1610–22.

35. Ortega M, et al. Epidemiology and outcome of bacteraemia in neutropenic patients in a single institution from 1991–2012. Epidemiol Infect. 2015;143(4):734–40.

36. Han SB, et al. Clinical characteristics and antibiotic susceptibility of viridans streptococcal bacteremia in children with febrile neutropenia. Infection. 2013;41(5):917–24.

37. Han SB, et al. Clinical characteristics and antimicrobial susceptibilities of viridans streptococcal bacteremia during febrile neutropenia in patients with hematologic malignancies: a comparison between adults and children. BMC Infect Dis. 2013;13:273.

38. Freifeld AG, Razonable RR. Viridans group streptococci in febrile neutropenic cancer patients: what should we fear? Clin Infect Dis. 2014;59(2):231–3.

39. Shelburne SA 3rd, et al. Development and validation of a clinical model to predict the presence of beta-lactam resistance in viridans group streptococci causing bacteremia in neutropenic cancer patients. Clin Infect Dis. 2014;59(2):223–30.

40. Marron A, et al. High rates of resistance to cephalosporins among viridans-group streptococci causing bacteraemia in neutropenic cancer patients. J Antimicrob Chemother. 2001;47(1):87–91.

41. Ford CD, et al. Frequency, risk factors, and outcomes of vancomycin-resistant Enterococcus colonization and infection in patients with newly diagnosed acute leukemia: different patterns in patients with acute myelogenous and acute lymphoblastic leukemia. Infect Control Hosp Epidemiol. 2015;36(1):47–53.

42. Vigil KJ, et al. Multidrug-resistant *Escherichia coli* bacteremia in cancer patients. Am J Infect Control. 2009;37(9):741–5.

43. Gudiol C, et al. Bacteraemia due to multidrug-resistant Gram-negative bacilli in cancer patients: risk factors, antibiotic therapy and outcomes. J Antimicrob Chemother. 2011;66(3):657–63.

44. Gudiol C, et al. Bacteraemia due to extended-spectrum beta-lactamase-producing *Escherichia coli* (ESBL-EC) in cancer patients: clinical features, risk factors, molecular epidemiology and outcome. J Antimicrob Chemother. 2010;65(2):333–41.

45. De Rosa FG, et al. Epidemiology of bloodstream infections in patients with acute myeloid leukemia undergoing levofloxacin prophylaxis. BMC Infect Dis. 2013;13:563.

46. Sandherr M, et al. Antiviral prophylaxis in patients with solid tumours and haematological malignancies – update of the Guidelines of the Infectious Diseases Working Party (AGIHO) of the German Society for Hematology and Medical Oncology (DGHO). Ann Hematol. 2015;94(9):1441–50.

47. Bergmann OJ, et al. Acyclovir given as prophylaxis against oral ulcers in acute myeloid leukaemia: randomised, double blind, placebo controlled trial. BMJ. 1995;310(6988):1169–72.

48. Aoki T, et al. Efficacy of continuous, daily, oral, ultra-low-dose 200 mg acyclovir to prevent herpes zoster events among bortezomib-treated patients:

a report from retrospective study. Jpn J Clin Oncol. 2011;41(7):876–81.

49. Pollyea DA, Brown JM, Horning SJ. Utility of influenza vaccination for oncology patients. J Clin Oncol. 2010;28(14):2481–90.

50. Safdar A, et al. Dose-related safety and immunogenicity of baculovirus-expressed trivalent influenza vaccine: a double-blind, controlled trial in adult patients with non-Hodgkin B cell lymphoma. J Infect Dis. 2006;194(10):1394–7.

51. Takaoka K, et al. A novel scoring system to predict the incidence of invasive fungal disease in salvage chemotherapies for malignant lymphoma. Ann Hematol. 2014;93(10):1637–44.

52. Vehreschild JJ, et al. A double-blind trial on prophylactic voriconazole (VRC) or placebo during induction chemotherapy for acute myelogenous leukaemia (AML). J Infect. 2007;55(5):445–9.

53. Rotstein C, et al. Randomized placebo-controlled trial of fluconazole prophylaxis for neutropenic cancer patients: benefit based on purpose and intensity of cytotoxic therapy. The Canadian Fluconazole Prophylaxis Study Group. Clin Infect Dis. 1999;28(2):331–40.

54. Cornely OA, et al. Posaconazole vs. fluconazole or itraconazole prophylaxis in patients with neutropenia. N Engl J Med. 2007;356(4):348–59.

55. Barreto JN, et al. The incidence of invasive fungal infections in neutropenic patients with acute leukemia and myelodysplastic syndromes receiving primary antifungal prophylaxis with voriconazole. Am J Hematol. 2013;88(4):283–8.

56. De Pauw B, et al. Revised definitions of invasive fungal disease from the European Organization for Research and Treatment of Cancer/Invasive Fungal Infections Cooperative Group and the National Institute of Allergy and Infectious Diseases Mycoses Study Group (EORTC/MSG) Consensus Group. Clin Infect Dis. 2008;46(12):1813–21.

57. Pfeiffer CD, Fine JP, Safdar N. Diagnosis of invasive aspergillosis using a galactomannan assay: a meta-analysis. Clin Infect Dis. 2006;42(10):1417–27.

58. Koo S, et al. Diagnostic performance of the (1-->3)-beta-D-glucan assay for invasive fungal disease. Clin Infect Dis. 2009;49(11):1650–9.

59. Marty FM, et al. (1->3) beta-D-glucan assay positivity in patients with Pneumocystis (carinii) jiroveci pneumonia. Ann Intern Med. 2007;147(1):70–2.

60. Karageorgopoulos DE, et al. Beta-D-glucan assay for the diagnosis of invasive fungal infections: a meta-analysis. Clin Infect Dis. 2011;52(6):750–70.

61. Fung M, et al. Meta-analysis and cost comparison of empirical versus pre-emptive antifungal strategies in hematologic malignancy patients with high-risk febrile neutropenia. PLoS One. 2015;10(11):e0140930.

62. Wingard JR, et al. Randomized, double-blind trial of fluconazole versus voriconazole for prevention of invasive fungal infection after alloge-

neic hematopoietic cell transplantation. Blood. 2010;116(24):5111–8.

63. Maschmeyer G, et al. Diagnosis and antimicrobial therapy of lung infiltrates in febrile neutropenic patients (allogeneic SCT excluded): updated guidelines of the Infectious Diseases Working Party (AGIHO) of the German Society of Hematology and Medical Oncology (DGHO). Ann Oncol. 2015;26(1):21–33.

64. Safdar N, Fine JP, Maki DG. Meta-analysis: methods for diagnosing intravascular device-related bloodstream infection. Ann Intern Med. 2005;142(6):451–66.

65. Bow EJ, Meddings JB. Intestinal mucosal dysfunction and infection during remission-induction therapy for acute myeloid leukaemia. Leukemia. 2006;20(12):2087–92.

66. Nesher L, Rolston KV. Neutropenic enterocolitis, a growing concern in the era of widespread use of aggressive chemotherapy. Clin Infect Dis. 2013;56(5):711–7.

67. Gomez L, Martino R, Rolston KV. Neutropenic enterocolitis: spectrum of the disease and comparison of definite and possible cases. Clin Infect Dis. 1998;27(4):695–9.

68. Aksoy DY, et al. Diarrhea in neutropenic patients: a prospective cohort study with emphasis on neutropenic enterocolitis. Ann Oncol. 2007;18(1):183–9.

69. Dohner H, Weisdorf DJ, Bloomfield CD. Acute myeloid leukemia. N Engl J Med. 2015;373(12):1136–52.

70. Faderl S, et al. The biology of chronic myeloid leukemia. N Engl J Med. 1999;341(3):164–72.

71. Woll PS, et al. Myelodysplastic syndromes are propagated by rare and distinct human cancer stem cells in vivo. Cancer Cell. 2014;25(6):794–808.

72. Pang WW, et al. Hematopoietic stem cell and progenitor cell mechanisms in myelodysplastic syndromes. Proc Natl Acad Sci U S A. 2013;110(8):3011–6.

73. Papaemmanuil E, et al. Clinical and biological implications of driver mutations in myelodysplastic syndromes. Blood. 2013;122(22):3616–27. quiz 3699

74. Ravandi F, O'Brien S. Immune defects in patients with chronic lymphocytic leukemia. Cancer Immunol Immunother. 2006;55(2):197–209.

75. Freeman JA, et al. Immunoglobulin G subclass deficiency and infection risk in 150 patients with chronic lymphocytic leukemia. Leuk Lymphoma. 2013;54(1):99–104.

76. Hamblin AD, Hamblin TJ. The immunodeficiency of chronic lymphocytic leukaemia. Br Med Bull. 2008;87:49–62.

77. Abkur TM, et al. Pneumocystis jiroveci prophylaxis in patients undergoing Bendamustine treatment: the need for a standardized protocol. Clin Case Rep. 2015;3(4):255–9.

78. Morrison VA. Infectious complications in patients with chronic lymphocytic leukemia: pathogenesis, spectrum of infection, and approaches to prophylaxis. Clin Lymphoma Myeloma. 2009;9(5):365–70.

79. Morrison VA. Management of infectious complications in patients with chronic lymphocytic leukemia. Hematol Am Soc Hematol Educ Program. 2007:332–8.
80. Nucci M, Anaissie E. Infections in patients with multiple myeloma in the era of high-dose therapy and novel agents. Clin Infect Dis. 2009;49(8):1211–25.
81. Costa DB, Shin B, Cooper DL. Pneumococcemia as the presenting feature of multiple myeloma. Am J Hematol. 2004;77(3):277–81.
82. Lanini S, et al. Risk of infection in patients with lymphoma receiving rituximab: systematic review and meta-analysis. BMC Med. 2011;9:36.
83. Martin SI, et al. Infectious complications associated with alemtuzumab use for lymphoproliferative disorders. Clin Infect Dis. 2006;43(1):16–24.
84. Scappaticci FA, et al. Surgical wound healing complications in metastatic colorectal cancer patients treated with bevacizumab. J Surg Oncol. 2005;91(3):173–80.
85. Eveno C, et al. Bevacizumab doubles the early postoperative complication rate after cytoreductive surgery with hyperthermic intraperitoneal chemotherapy (HIPEC) for peritoneal carcinomatosis of colorectal origin. Ann Surg Oncol. 2014;21(6):1792–800.

Nikolaos G. Almyroudis

Immune Reconstitution and Timing of Infections After Hematopoietic Stem Cell Transplantation

Hematopoietic stem cell transplantation (HSCT) is a well-established therapy for a number of hematologic malignancies and disorders. Immune recovery after HSCT occurs gradually [1]. Bone marrow engraftment, defined as an absolute neutrophil count of $> 0.5 \times 10^9$/L for 3 consecutive days, occurs between days 10 and 25 after transplant. Following engraftment, innate immunity recovers faster than adaptive immunity [2]. The cells of innate immunity to appear initially are monocytes followed shortly by granulocytes and NK cells. Although NK-cell function recovers right away [3], neutrophil function, measured as chemotaxis, superoxide production, and phagocytic-bactericidal activity, may take up to 4 months to recover [4] and monocyte function up to a year. Finally, mucositis due to conditioning resolves with engraftment, but mucositis associated with graft-versus-host disease (GvHD) of the gastrointestinal tract may recur.

With the exception of CD4+ T cells, lymphocyte subsets and total lymphocyte counts recover within the first 2–3 months after transplant. However, despite numerical T-lymphocyte recovery, T-cell responses remain defective for a long period after transplant [5]. Though CD8+ T-cell recovery occurs within the first 2–3 months post HSCT, these cells are predominantly derived by clonal expansion of the donor's cells and are characterized by limited repertoire diversity [6]. Effective T-cell responses recover when normal thymopoiesis is reestablished, by seeding of the thymus by donor's hematopoietic progenitors [6]. Overall, CD4+ cell function and consequently T-cell function recovery depends significantly on the presence of a functional thymus [7], rendering the age of the recipient a crucial factor for immune reconstitution. Graft-versus-host disease (GvHD) and immunosuppressive therapy to treat GvHD are the major barriers to reconstitution of T-cell immunity.

B cells achieve normal values 6 months after autologous HSCT and 9 months after allogeneic HSCT [8, 9]. Despite reaching adequate numbers, antibody responses remain defective due to lack of T-cell interaction and GvHD and its treatments [9, 10]. As a result, B-cell function and antibody repertoire are limited during the early transplant period and further delayed by GvHD.

Infections after allogeneic HSCT occur during three well-defined time periods (Fig. 11.1). These include the pre-engraftment period that extends from the day of transplant (day 0) to bone marrow

N. G. Almyroudis (✉)
Jacobs School of Medicine and Biomedical Sciences, State University of New York at Buffalo, Division of Infectious Diseases, Roswell Park Comprehensive Cancer Center, Buffalo, NY, USA
e-mail: Nikolaos.Almyroudis@RoswellPark.org

© Springer International Publishing AG, part of Springer Nature 2018
B. H. Segal (ed.), *Management of Infections in the Immunocompromised Host*,
https://doi.org/10.1007/978-3-319-77674-3_11

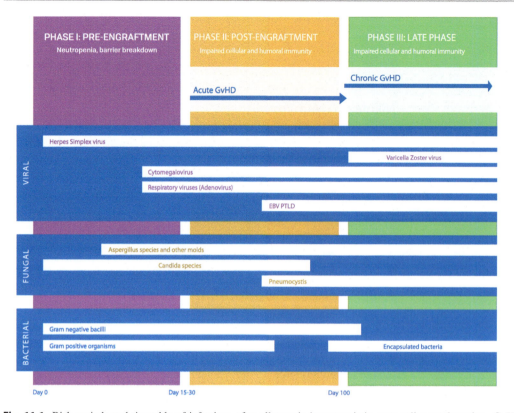

Fig. 11.1 Risk periods and timetable of infections after allogeneic hematopoietic stem cell transplantation. *GvHD* graft-versus-host disease, *EBV* Epstein-Barr virus, *PTLD* posttransplant lymphoproliferative disorder

engraftment (day +30), the early post-engraftment period (engraftment until day +100), and the late post-engraftment period (day +100 onward) [11]. The pre-engraftment period is dominated by neutropenia, compromised mucosal immunity as a result of preparative chemotherapy, and compromised skin barrier as a result of vascular access. The early post-engraftment period is characterized by impaired cell-mediated immunity due to immunosuppression and acute GvHD and its treatments. Infections during the late post-engraftment period are the result of impaired cell- and humoral-mediated immunity [11]. A timetable of infections is provided in Fig. 11.1. By contrast, autologous HSCT does not require immunosuppression after HSCT, and immune recovery is faster and commonly completed within 9 months after transplant.

The degree of HLA disparity between donor and recipient correlates with GvHD and immunosuppression used for GvHD, which in turn drive the risk of infectious complications. Risk of infections is greater for recipients who use alternative sources of stem cells such as unrelated donors, cord blood stem cells, or haploidentical donors. Infection rates are higher in recipients of matched unrelated donor transplants than in recipients of matched related donor transplants [12]. Cord blood transplants are characterized by slow engraftment due to the low number of stem cells infused. As a result they may be complicated by prolonged neutropenia that can last up to 6 weeks, leading to high incidence of bacterial and fungal infections [13]. In addition, due to lack of antigen-specific memory T cells that can expand in a thymus-independent fashion, cord blood transplants are associated with severe late viral and fungal infections [14]. Haploidentical HSCT are complicated by a considerable rate of infections [15] although one study found no increased risk over matched unrelated transplants [12].

In addition to immunosuppressive therapy, in vitro or in vivo manipulation of the graft to prevent GvHD may lead to a greater risk of infections. T-cell depletion through either CD34+ selection or in vivo by administration of alemtuzumab or anti-thymocyte globulin leads to profound and frequently prolonged T-cell immunodeficiency further associated with an increased risk for viral and fungal infections [16, 17].

Exposure to multiple rounds of chemotherapy (e.g., for relapsed or refractory malignancy) preceding transplant or more than one transplant are significant risk factors for posttransplant infectious complications. They may affect not only the incidence and severity of infections but also the epidemiology as demonstrated in one study where there was a shift in the etiology of invasive mold infections from *Aspergillus* species to zygomycetes and other rare molds among patients who received multiple transplants [18].

Several immune deficits may occur simultaneously or sequentially, and patients may experience the immune defect of the underlying condition, complication of transplants (i.e., GvHD), and iatrogenic immunosuppression to prevent or treat GvHD. Although HSCT is associated with profound immune defects, appropriate prophylactic and treatment strategies decrease significantly the infection-related morbidity and mortality.

Bacterial Infections

Bacterial Infections Associated with Neutropenia and Mucositis

Bacterial infections are the most common infections encountered after HSCT, and bacteremia is the most serious manifestation. Early after transplant and during periods of acute and chronic GvHD, causative pathogens originate from the patient's own flora, as pathogenesis involves compromised cutaneous and mucosal barriers from the conditioning regimen and GvHD [11]. Community-acquired infections occur after the transplant recipients leave the hospital. The management of neutropenic febrile episodes is guided by the same principles and guidelines as in other neutropenic hosts [19]. When a specific organism has been isolated, targeted antibiotic therapy is administered following standards applied to general population.

Due to the presence of central venous catheters, infections due to coagulase-negative *Staphylococcus* species are the leading cause of bacteremia among HSCT recipients [20], while infections due to *Staphylococcus aureus* are less common [21]. Infections due to methicillin-resistant *Staphylococcus aureus* are even less frequent [21] and are associated with high mortality rates [22]. Early removal of the central venous catheter when feasible for patients with *S. aureus* bacteremia is strongly recommended.

Bacteremia due to *Streptococcus viridans* or *Enterococcus* species typically originates from the gastrointestinal tract. *Streptococcus viridans* species are frequently resistant to penicillins and fluoroquinolones in patients with malignancies [23]. Empiric treatment with vancomycin is therefore advised until susceptibilities are available. Similarly, the majority of enterococcal isolates are resistant to ampicillin and vancomycin [24]. Empiric treatment with antibiotics with activity against vancomycin-resistant *Enterococcus* is not recommended because of potential for development of resistance [19]. Targeted therapy may include linezolid, daptomycin, or quinupristin-dalfopristin [19, 25–30]. It should be noted that although daptomycin has activity against vancomycin-resistant *Enterococcus* it is not FDA approved for this indication and that quinupristin-dalfopristin is active only against *Enterococcus faecium* species. Quinupristin-dalfopristin can be associated with severe myalgias and, in our practice, is not used as first-line therapy.

Enterobacteriaceae (e.g., *E. coli*, *Klebsiella* species, and *Enterobacter* species), *Pseudomonas*, and *Acinetobacter* species are the predominant

Gram-negative pathogens encountered after transplant [21]. The wide use of prophylactic or therapeutic antibiotics before transplant or in the early posttransplant period may select for resistant isolates. Extended-spectrum beta-lactamase (ESBL) and carbapenemase producing Gram-negative organisms are being reported with increasing frequency [21, 31, 32] and may significantly complicate the course of transplantation. Infections due to these bacteria are treated as in other hosts except that in transplant recipients, severe immune impairment and comorbidities predispose to refractory infections and mortality.

Considerable attention is given to prevention of bacterial infections after transplant. Levofloxacin was shown to prevent bacterial infections in patients with prolonged (more than 7 days duration) and profound neutropenia when compared to placebo [33] although the same study failed to show a survival benefit. A meta-analysis showed that fluoroquinolones significantly decrease the incidence of Gram-negative infections without affecting the incidence of Gram-positive infections or infection-related mortality [34]. These studies involved patients with cancer and chemotherapy-induced neutropenia of varying durations, and not specifically HSCT recipients; however, results can be reasonably extrapolated to HSCT recipients with neutropenia following conditioning. Disadvantages of fluoroquinolone prophylaxis are potential toxicity, potential for emergence of quinolone resistance, *Streptococcus viridans* breakthrough bacteremias [35, 36], and development of *Clostridium difficile* colitis [37]. Antibacterial prophylaxis with a fluoroquinolone is recommended for expected neutropenia of at least 7 days duration after autologous as well as allogeneic HSCT [19].

Efficacy of intravenous immunoglobulin (IvIg) in preventing bacterial infections and reducing mortality has not been established [38]. Many centers use intravenous immunoglobulin (IvIg) in transplant recipients with severe hypogammaglobulinemia (serum IgG level <400 mg/dL) [39]. Dose for adolescents and adults is 500 mg/kg/month, and frequency should be adjusted to achieve serum trough levels >400 mg/dL.

Bacterial Infections Associated with Impaired Cellular Immunity

Listeria monocytogenes

T-cell deficiency predisposes the allogeneic transplant recipients to infections due to *Listeria* [40]. Infections due to *Listeria monocytogenes* in HSCT recipients present as bacteremia, often accompanied by meningitis [41]. Infections predominantly occur early after HSCT or during periods of augmented immunosuppression [42]. Antibiotics of choice are high dose ampicillin or penicillin G [43–45]. Because *Listeria* is an intracellular pathogen and permeability and bactericidal activity of ampicillin and penicillin G are suboptimal, addition of gentamicin for synergy is recommended, especially in the immunocompromised setting and central nervous system (CNS) infections [46, 47]. Alternative therapy for patients allergic to penicillins includes high-dose trimethoprim-sulfamethoxazole [43, 44, 48]. Imipenem-cilastatin and meropenem are also effective against *Listeria* but are characterized by inferior bactericidal activity than ampicillin [45, 49]. Although vancomycin is active against *Listeria* [44], its minimal inhibitory concentration is higher than ampicillin [45], and penetration into the CNS is suboptimal. Due to high risk for recurrence, recommended duration is 3 weeks for bacteremia and meningitis and longer for brain abscess. Transplant recipients are advised to avoid unpasteurized milk, soft cheese, and luncheon meat as they have been associated with *Listeria* infections [43]. Trimethoprim-sulfamethoxazole prophylaxis against *Pneumocystis* is thought to provide protection against *Listeria* [48].

Nocardia spp.

The overall incidence of *Nocardia* infections after HSCT is low, between 0.3% and 1.7% according to two studies [50, 51]. They occur almost exclusively in allogeneic transplant recipients after engraftment and primarily during the first year after transplant [50, 51]. Clinical manifestations of nocardiosis in transplant recipients include pulmonary, cutaneous, CNS, and disseminated disease [52]. Trimethoprim-sulfamethoxazole is the agent of choice for the treatment of *Nocardia* [50, 53]. Because of its potential for resistance development [54, 55], some experts recommend combination of trimethoprim-sulfamethoxazole with a second agent. Combination of imipenem-cilastatin along with amikacin was shown to be superior in a mouse model of CNS disease [56]. Alternative antimicrobials with activity against *Nocardia* include imipenem, meropenem, ceftriaxone, cefotaxime, amikacin, and minocycline [57]. Ertapenem is significantly less active against *Nocardia* species than imipenem and should be avoided [57]. Linezolid has in vitro activity against *Nocardia* [58]; however, its use is limited by its duration-dependent potential for myelosuppression and peripheral neuropathy. Susceptibility data can guide antimicrobial selection. Recommended duration of treatment for pulmonary or cutaneous disease is 4–6 months and for CNS or disseminated disease 12 months or longer. Finally, trimethoprim-sulfamethoxazole at prophylactic doses to prevent *Pneumocystis jirovecii* is not consistently protective against *Nocardia* species, and breakthrough infections have been reported [50, 51].

Tuberculosis and Nontuberculous Mycobacteriosis

Tuberculosis after HSCT usually occurs in recipients who have resided in a country with high prevalence of tuberculosis [59]. Although the majority of cases have been observed in allogeneic HSCT recipients, 20% have occurred in recipients of autologous transplants. Besides exposure history, screening of HSCT recipients for latent tuberculosis can be performed with either tuberculin skin test or with an ex vivo interferon-gamma release assay [39]. However, there is disagreement among experts on the value of routine screening, as sensitivity of either test is diminished in the immunocompromised setting

and prior BCG vaccination may complicate interpretation of tuberculin skin test. Interferon-gamma release assay does not cross-react with prior BCG vaccination and is recommended in this setting [60].

Latent tuberculosis is not a contraindication for HSCT. All patients with pretransplant positive screening or history of positive screen should be evaluated for active tuberculosis [39, 60]. Chemoprophylaxis is recommended for all HSCT candidates or recipients with positive interferon-gamma release assay or tuberculin skin test regardless of prior BCG vaccination [39]. It is also recommended for those with documented exposure to an individual with active infectious pulmonary or laryngeal tuberculosis regardless the tuberculin skin test or interferon-gamma release assay [39]. If chemoprophylaxis cannot be completed before HSCT, it is advised to be provided after transplant [61]. Chemoprophylaxis with isoniazid and pyridoxine should be continued for at least 9 months and longer in the presence of augmented immunosuppressive therapy [39]. Shortcomings of isoniazid prophylaxis are the potential for liver toxicity [62] and neuropathy [63], drug interactions with other medications such as cyclosporine and tacrolimus [64], and selection of isoniazid-resistant strains. Chemoprophylaxis with rifampin is not suitable in the posttransplant setting because of significant drug interactions [65]. Chemoprophylaxis with pyrazinamide and rifampin should be avoided due to substantial hepatotoxic potential [66]. Finally, 3 months of rifapentine in combination with isoniazid was as effective as a 9-month course of isoniazid in the general population [67] in HIV-infected individuals [68] and in renal transplant recipients [69].

Although treatment of active tuberculosis in HSCT recipients is guided by the same principles as in the general population [64], there is no consensus on the duration of antituberculous therapy. Common practice is a longer duration, usually 12–18 months. Drug interactions with rifampin may lead to sub-therapeutic levels of cyclosporine and tacrolimus [64, 65].

Treatment of nontuberculous mycobacteriosis in the posttransplant setting follows the guidelines of general population and, to a large degree, is guided by the susceptibility of the isolate [70]. Similarly, there is no consensus on duration of treatment, and physicians tend to treat at least until resolution of signs of infection and resolution or scarring of lesions are seen on imaging.

Bacterial Infections Associated with Impaired Humoral Immunity and Functional Asplenia

Recipients of allogeneic HSCT are at a considerable risk for sepsis due to encapsulated bacteria, *Streptococcus pneumoniae*, *Haemophilus influenzae*, and *Neisseria meningitidis*, due to impaired B-cell immunity, functional asplenia, and GvHD [71]. *Streptococcus pneumoniae* is the most important pathogen of the encapsulated bacteria in HSCT recipients and can cause life-threatening pneumonia and sepsis. The majority of infections due to *Streptococcus pneumoniae* occur in the late post-engraftment period, from 3 months to several years after transplant, with chronic GvHD as the major risk factor [72, 73]. Therefore, prophylaxis with penicillin is recommended for allogeneic HSCT recipients from 3 months after HSCT to at least a year, until immunosuppression is discontinued, and longer if chronic GvHD develops [19, 39]. Recommended dose of penicillin is 500 mg twice daily (or 750 mg for individuals over 60 kg). Penicillin prophylaxis is recommended regardless of previous pneumococcal vaccination. Shortcomings of this approach are selection and breakthrough infections due to penicillin-resistant *Streptococcus pneumoniae* [74]. In communities with considerable penicillin-resistant *Streptococcus pneumoniae*, alternative agents such as TMP/SMX should be considered. The CDC recommends immunization with the 13-valent *Streptococcus pneumoniae* conjugate vaccine (PCV13; Prevnar 13, Wyeth Pharmaceuticals, Inc.) followed by 23-valent polysaccharide pneumococcal vaccine (PPSV23; Pneumovax 23, Merck & Co. Inc.) 8 weeks later

in the general population [75]. In allogeneic HSCT recipients, the optimal timing of administration isn't established since vaccination is unlikely to be effective prior to reconstitution of B-cell immunity and in the setting of GvHD. One approach involves vaccination with the conjugated 13-valent vaccine 6–12 months after HSCT or the polysaccharide pneumococcal vaccine at 1 year after cessation of immunosuppression, followed by revaccination after 5 years [19].

Fungal Infections

Fungal infections after HSCT are associated with significant morbidity and mortality [76, 77]. The most clinically significant fungal pathogenic organisms include yeast (mainly *Candida*), molds (*Aspergillus*, zygomycetes, and rare molds), endemic fungi, *Cryptococcus*, and *Pneumocystis*.

Mucocutaneous and Invasive Candidiasis Syndromes

According to two large multicenter surveillance studies on invasive fungal infections in HSCT recipients in North America [77, 78], invasive candidiasis was the second most common fungal infection after invasive aspergillosis. Median time of onset was 61 days posttransplant, and invasive candidiasis was much more frequent after allogeneic than autologous HSCT [78]. In both studies, the majority of cases were due to non-*albicans* species [77, 78], and in one of these studies [78], the most commonly isolated species was *Candida glabrata* (33%) with *Candida albicans* causing only 20% of infections [78]. These findings are important because of the variable sensitivity of *C. glabrata* to azoles. This shift in epidemiology has been attributed to the widespread use of azoles as prophylaxis [79, 80].

Risk factors for invasive *Candida* infections after HSCT include compromised mucosal or cutaneous barriers. In the normal host, reservoir for *Candida* is the gastrointestinal tract, while in the ill state, it tends to colonize the skin. The first line of defense against *Candida* infections is the mucosal barriers of the gastrointestinal tract and the integrity of the cutaneous tissues. After HSCT, the gastrointestinal mucosa is compromised by the conditioning regimen and subsequently by gastrointestinal GvHD [11]. Similarly, skin integrity is compromised by implantable central venous catheter or cutaneous GvHD. Therefore, common sources of invasive candidiasis after HSCT are the gastrointestinal tract and the site of implantable central venous catheters.

The most common manifestations of mucosal candidiasis are oral mucocutaneous (oral thrush), esophageal, and vaginal candidiasis. Candidemia is the most common form of invasive candidiasis and can lead to hematogenous dissemination with involvement of the skin, eyes, central nervous system, and visceral organs. Chronic hepatosplenic candidiasis, the most frequent form of chronic disseminated candidiasis, is principally a complication of gastrointestinal mucosal disruption. The use of yeast-active antifungal prophylaxis has reduced the overall incidence of mucosal and invasive candidiasis but at the expense of a shift to more candida infections that are resistant to azoles and other antifungals.

Although for mild cases of oropharyngeal candidiasis (thrush) clotrimazole troches [81] or miconazole mucoadhesive buccal tablets [82] for 7–14 days are acceptable, fluconazole is an appropriate agent for moderate to severe disease [83]. Voriconazole, posaconazole, or echinocandins can be used for fluconazole-refractory cases, although cross-resistance is observed among azoles as a class [84–86]. The advantage of echinocandins is their efficacy against fluconazole-resistant *Candida* species such as *C. krusei* and *C. glabrata* [87].

Treatment of esophageal candidiasis includes oral fluconazole or intravenous fluconazole or an echinocandin if the patient is unable to tolerate oral therapy [86, 88, 89]. As echinocandins have been associated with higher relapse rates compared to fluconazole, micafungin was approved at 150 mg intravenous daily [90].

Duration of treatment should be at least 14 days and not infrequently may need to be extended to 21 days depending on the severity of illness and clinical response [91]. Treatment should be followed by chronic secondary prevention with an oral azole.

Antifungal therapy is recommended for all patients with candidemia regardless of the source of infection [92]. Early initiation of appropriate treatment and source control are essential [93–95]. Initial therapy with an echinocandin is recommended [19, 91]. Antifungal treatment can be modified based on species and susceptibilities but also the need for mold prophylaxis. As HSCT recipients frequently require prophylaxis against mold, a mold-active azole is favored over fluconazole [91]. Duration of therapy in neutropenic patients is not well defined, but a minimum 2-week course of systemic antifungals after clearance of the bloodstream should be the shortest treatment duration for nondisseminated candidiasis [91]. Antifungal therapy should be continued throughout neutropenia. Early during therapy a thorough ophthalmologic examination should be performed to investigate for endophthalmitis [91, 96]. After neutrophil recovery, management may include an ultrasound or preferably CT imaging of the liver and spleen with intravenous contrast to detect chronic hepatosplenic candidiasis [97].

Removal of central venous catheter in neutropenic patients has been debated as source in these patients is commonly the gastrointestinal tract. Currently, guidelines of the Infectious Diseases Society of America (IDSA) support removal of central venous catheter when it is considered the potential source of candidemia in non-neutropenic patients and removal on an individual basis on neutropenic patients as the source in these patients is commonly the gastrointestinal tract [91]. However, even in the presence of an alternative source, catheters can be secondarily infected, and the risk of recurrent candidemia and associated complications (i.e., dissemination) is a significant consideration in profoundly immunocompromised HSCT recipients. Therefore, clinical judgment and low threshold for catheter removal is advised.

Lipid formulations of amphotericin B 3–5 mg/kg/day or an echinocandin remain the antifungal agent of choice for initial therapy of chronic disseminated candidiasis (hepatosplenic candidiasis) [98–101]. After several weeks, transition to oral fluconazole 400 mg daily can be considered for fluconazole-susceptible *Candida* isolates [102, 103]. Duration of treatment is prolonged and usually for several months and throughout the period of immunosuppression. Short course of NSAIDs or corticosteroids (oral prednisone 0.5–1 mg/kg daily tapering dose) can be administered to patients with persistent fever and intense inflammatory response [104, 105].

Prevention of Invasive Candida Syndromes

Prophylaxis against invasive candidiasis after HSCT is reserved for high-risk groups and in particular those with significant mucositis and prolonged neutropenia and allogeneic HSCT recipients with GvHD [19]. In particular, for autologous HSCT without mucositis, no prophylaxis is required. In contrast, the presence of significant mucositis after autologous HSCT increases substantially the risk for invasive candidiasis, and therefore prophylaxis with fluconazole [106–108] or micafungin [109] is advised [19]. As prolonged neutropenia or significant GvHD is associated with a substantial risk for invasive aspergillosis [16] and infections due to other molds [18], prophylaxis with a mold-active azole, such as posaconazole [110, 111] or voriconazole [112], micafungin [109], or an amphotericin B formulation [113] is recommended.

Invasive Aspergillosis

Aspergillus is a hyaline mold ubiquitous in nature, found in decaying material, soil, air, and water. Invasive aspergillosis is associated with significant morbidity and mortality after HSCT. In two large multicenter cohorts, invasive aspergillosis was the most common fungal infection representing 43% [78] and 59.2% [77] of total fungal infections. *Aspergillus fumigatus*

was the most frequently isolated pathogenic species followed by *A. niger*, *A. flavus*, *A. terreus*, and other species [78].

Although the principal risk factor for invasive aspergillosis is prolonged neutropenia, several other risk factors may occur after HSCT. These include acute and chronic GvHD and its treatment (steroids, T-cell lymphocyte antibodies, and other immunosuppressants), HLA mismatched or unrelated donor transplants, and T-cell depletion of the graft [16]. As a result, the epidemiology of invasive aspergillosis and other molds after HSCT is bimodal, with more infections occurring during the late post-engraftment period associated with GvHD and its treatments rather than during the neutropenic phase of the early pre-engraftment period [16]. Finally, cumulative incidence of invasive aspergillosis is higher after allogeneic rather than autologous HSCT [78].

In contrast to *Candida* species that are members of the normal human flora, *Aspergillus* and other molds are acquired through environmental exposure. More specifically the conidial concentration in the air is estimated to be 1–100 conidia/m^3, and an average individual inhales more than 100 conidia of *Aspergillus fumigatus* in a day [114]. Respiratory mucosal epithelial cells form an anatomical barrier against fungal invasion and promote mucociliary clearance [115]. Alveolar macrophages constitute the first line of phagocytic host defense against inhaled conidia [116]. Following tissue invasion, neutrophils and peripheral blood monocytes are recruited and represent the principal line of host defense against hyphae [116]. Finally, dendritic cells activate a protective immune response guided by Th1 CD4+ T lymphocytes [117, 118]. Therefore, periods at high risk for invasive mold infection after HSCT are neutropenia and periods of significant acute or chronic GvHD.

As the usual source of invasive aspergillosis is the respiratory tract, most frequent clinical manifestations include pulmonary disease followed by sinusitis [119]. Another portal of entry can be the gastrointestinal tract, and invasive aspergillosis can disseminate to other organs such as the brain, liver, and skin [120].

Treatment of Invasive Aspergillosis

Voriconazole, a second-generation triazole, is the drug of choice for treatment of documented invasive aspergillosis [121]. Voriconazole was compared to amphotericin B deoxycholate in a double-blind randomized noninferiority clinical trial [122]. Initial therapy with voriconazole was associated with better responses and improved survival and resulted in fewer severe side effects. Based on these data, voriconazole is now the treatment of choice for invasive aspergillosis. Dosing schedule includes loading with 6 mg/kg every 12 h followed by 4 mg/kg every 12 h. Amphotericin B lipid formulations are acceptable alternatives to voriconazole [121]. Lipid formulations of amphotericin B are characterized by improved toxicity profile over amphotericin B deoxycholate. Liposomal amphotericin B at 3 mg/kg/day is the established dose based on a study that compared low dose to 10 mg/kg/day and found no additional benefit and higher rates of nephrotoxicity of the higher dose [123]. Isavuconazole is also an acceptable alternative [121, 124]. Echinocandins are reserved for patients in whom use of azoles or amphotericin B formulations is contraindicated or associated with significant toxicity.

Combination antifungal therapy is advised for refractory or progressive disease. Clinical studies suggest a beneficial effect when a polyene or azoles are combined with an echinocandin [125–127]. Surgery is reserved for cases complicated by intractable hemoptysis or for centrally located lesions infiltrating large vessels [128, 129].

Immune Augmentation

Reduction in immunosuppression is important but not always feasible. Colony-stimulating factors such as granulocyte colony-stimulating factor (G-CSF) or granulocyte macrophage colony-stimulating factor (GM-CSF) accelerate neutrophil recovery and stimulate macrophages and monocytes. They have been the standard of care in diminishing the period of neutropenia and preventing neutropenic fever events [130]. Their role as an adjunct to treatment of documented fungal infections is not clearly defined. Preclinical data support their use in neutropenic patients with fungal infections [131].

A randomized trial of granulocyte transfusions in neutropenic patients with severe infections failed to demonstrate benefit [132]. In addition, granulocyte transfusion is associated with major adverse events such as acute lung injury [133] and likely alloimmunization causing graft failure. Therefore, granulocyte transfusions are not recommended. Data to support the use of recombinant interferon gamma (IFN-γ) in the treatment of invasive aspergillosis is inadequate. In addition there is a concern that IFN-γ may exacerbate graft-versus-host disease after HSCT, although a small study suggested that IFN-γ is safe in this setting [134].

Assessing Response to Treatment

Response to treatment is evidenced by improvement or resolution of symptoms and radiologic and mycologic improvement. Radiologic response should be evaluated with repeat CT scan imaging 7–10 days after initiation of antifungal treatment. Serial galactomannan levels can be followed in patients with elevated values upon diagnosis of invasive aspergillosis as data suggest that a falling level predicts treatment success and a rising level predicts failure [135]. Inadequate data exist to support the use of (1→3)-β-D-glucan assay to predict response to treatment.

Susceptibility Testing and Therapeutic Drug Monitoring

Susceptibility testing is useful in patients with azole-refractory disease to guide therapy [121] but is generally not performed routinely in all cases. Preliminary data support therapeutic drug monitoring for voriconazole, posaconazole suspension, and itraconazole [136, 137] to maximize efficacy and minimize toxicity. Sub-therapeutic serum concentrations have been correlated with treatment failure and drug toxicity in small studies [138–140]. Therapeutic drug monitoring is recommended in refractory cases, if toxicity is suspected [19] or if a drug known to interact with voriconazole is co-administered [121]. Serum levels should be measured at steady state that is achieved at least 4 days after initiating treatment. Therapeutic concentration for itraconazole is a trough of 0.5–1 µg/L (measured by HPLC/mass spectrometry) and for voriconazole a trough of 1–5.5 µg/mL [137]. For posaconazole, although a level of 0.7 µg/mL is acceptable for prophylaxis, a trough of at least 1 µg/mL is considered therapeutic [137].

Azoles and Drug Interactions

Voriconazole, posaconazole, and itraconazole are potent inhibitors of the cytochrome P450 3A4 [141] isoenzymes and may reduce efficacy or increase the potential for toxicity of other drugs. Effect on cytochrome P450 3A4 is less potent for isavuconazole [142] and fluconazole [143]. Fluconazole and voriconazole are inhibitors of the CYP2C9 and CYP2C19 enzymes [144, 145], and voriconazole is subject to significant variability of genetic CYP2C19 allelic polymorphisms [146, 147]. Itraconazole and posaconazole can further affect drug levels by inhibiting the P-glycoprotein transport system [148]. Commonly used drugs that have the potential for interaction with azoles include calcineurin inhibitors (i.e., cyclosporine and tacrolimus), sirolimus, corticosteroids [141, 149], antibiotics, chemotherapeutic agents, and acid-suppressive therapies [141], and pertinent data are presented in Table 11.1.

HSCT in Patients with Presumed or Definitive Invasive Aspergillosis

Presumed or definitive invasive aspergillosis is not a contraindication for transplantation [150, 151]. No specific guidelines exist, but an adequate course of antifungals (at least 2 weeks) followed by evidence of symptomatic, radiologic, and mycologic response (i.e., a downtrend in galactomannan if elevated) is necessary before the transplant candidate can receive the conditioning regimen and enter safely the periods of neutropenia and subsequent acute GvHD. Uninterrupted mold-active antifungal therapy throughout conditioning and subsequent transplantation is recommended. The duration of antifungal therapy preceding transplant should be decided collectively among the infectious diseases and transplant services and should take into consideration the benefits of delay in HSCT to increase the odds of controlling the fungal infection pre-HSCT versus the increased risk of malignancy relapse by delaying HSCT.

Mucormycosis (Zygomycosis), Fusariosis, and Infections due to Other Molds

Mucormycosis (zygomycosis) is the second most common mold and the third invasive fungal infection after invasive aspergillosis and invasive candidiasis in HSCT recipients with overall incidence of 8% [19]. Treatment of mucormycosis includes amphotericin B, either deoxycholate 1 mg/kg/day or preferably one of the lipid formulations at dose 5 mg/kg/day. Posaconazole is an alternative to amphotericin B for intolerant cases to amphotericin B or in the salvage setting [152, 153]. Isavuconazole outcomes in patients with invasive mucormycosis (zygomycosis) were comparable to amphotericin B-treated historical controls [154]. Initial treatment with an amphotericin B formulation with transition to oral posaconazole or isavuconazole maintenance after response is a reasonable approach.

Fusariosis and rare molds afflict HSCT recipients more rarely than zygomycetes. Treatment options for *Fusarium* infections include voriconazole [155] and posaconazole [156]. Amphotericin B formulations have variable activity against *Fusarium* species.

Prevention of Invasive Aspergillosis and Other Molds

Prevention of invasive aspergillosis and other molds includes placement of patients in a protected environment that includes a positive pressure room, a high-efficiency particulate air (HEPA) filtration [157], and/or a laminar flow [158], when admitted to the hospital. Avoiding construction or renovation sites, gardening, spreading mulch, mowing the lawn, or vacuum

Table 11.1 Interactions between antifungal agents and commonly used medications during hematopoietic stem cell transplantation

Antifungal agent	Medication	Pharmacologic effect of combination	Clinical effect of combination	Recommendation
Polyenes	Calcineurin inhibitors (CNI)	Additive nephrotoxicity	Kidney injury	Monitor CNI concentrations and kidney function
Polyenes	mTOR inhibitors (sirolimus)	Additive nephrotoxicity	Kidney injury	Monitor sirolimus concentration and kidney function
Azoles	Calcineurin inhibitors (CNI)	Increases CNI levels	Potential for CNI toxicity	Decrease CNI by 30–50%
Azoles	mTOR inhibitors (sirolimus)	Increases sirolimus levels	Potential for sirolimus toxicity	Decrease sirolimus dose
Azoles	Corticosteroids	Increases steroid levels	Excessive steroid exposure	Monitor for toxicity of methylprednisolone
Azoles	Cyclophosphamide	Increases cyclophosphamide levels	Hepatic, renal, urinary toxicity	Administer with caution Monitor for toxicity
Azoles	Vincristine and vinca alkaloids	Unknown	Neurotoxicity, seizures, peripheral neuropathy	Avoid co-administration
Azoles	Rifampin/rifabutin	Increases rifampin levels Decreased azole levels	Hepatic toxicity Decreases azole efficacy	Avoid co-administration Monitor for toxicity if given Monitor azole efficacy
Azoles[a]	Macrolide antibiotics	QTc prolongation	Torsades de pointes, cardiac arrhythmias	Administer with caution Assess risk for arrhythmia
Azoles[a]	Fluoroquinolones	QTc prolongation	Torsades de pointes, cardiac arrhythmias	Administer with caution Assess risk for arrhythmia

[a]All azoles prolong the QTc except isavuconazole that shortens the QTc interval

cleaning [159] are also recommended to reduce exposure to conidia. Continuous surveillance of invasive aspergillosis and other mold infections is also recommended.

Mold-active prophylaxis after HSCT targets the periods of high risk and in particular neutropenia and periods of significant acute and chronic GvHD and its treatment such as significant steroid use, lymphocyte-depleting agents, or tumor necrosis factor-α (TNF-α) inhibitors [19, 121]. Better-studied mold-active antifungals for prophylaxis in HSCT recipients are posaconazole [111] and voriconazole [112, 160, 161]. The critical benefit of posaconazole over voriconazole prophylaxis is its broader antifungal spectrum that includes *Zygomycetes* [162–164]. Recommended prophylactic dose of posaconazole delayed-release tablets is 300 mg daily (after a loading dose of 300 mg twice daily

on day 1) with food and for the oral suspension is 200 mg three times daily with meals, nutritional supplement, or acidic carbonated beverage [111]. Prophylactic dose of oral voriconazole is 200 mg twice daily [121]. Micafungin [109] and one of the lipid formulations of amphotericin B [113] are acceptable alternatives, while the erratic absorption [165] and toxicity profile of itraconazole prohibit its use.

Cryptococcosis

Management of cryptococcal meningoencephalitis, acute pulmonary cryptococcosis, or disseminated disease in HSCT recipients should include induction with a lipid formulation of amphotericin B (liposomal amphotericin B 3–4 mg/kg daily or amphotericin B lipid complex 5 mg/kg daily) ideally with oral 5-flucytosine (100 mg/kg daily divided in four doses), for a minimum of 2 weeks [166, 167]. Drug level monitoring of 5-flucytosine is recommended to prevent hematologic toxicities (leucopenia and thrombocytopenia) [168] as well as hepatic toxicity. For those intolerant to 5-flucytosine, induction with amphotericin B lipid formulation should be extended to 4–6 weeks, or fluconazole 800 mg daily can be added to amphotericin B formulation. Transition to oral fluconazole 6–12 mg/kg daily (400–800 mg daily) for 8 weeks is feasible after sterilization of cerebrospinal fluid has been documented in repeat cerebrospinal fluid sampling [169]. This should be followed by maintenance therapy with oral fluconazole 3–6 mg/kg daily (200–400 mg daily) for 6–12 months to avoid relapse [169]. Pulmonary disease of mild to moderate severity can be treated with oral fluconazole 400 mg daily [170]. Management of elevated intracranial pressure (≥25 cm or consistent symptoms) should include repeat lumbar punctures for decompression. Management of refractory cases includes temporary lumbar drains, ventriculostomy, and permanent ventriculoperitoneal shunt in persistent cases. Primary prophylaxis against cryptococcosis is not advised in HSCT recipients [170], although azoles used as anti-candidal and anti-*Aspergillus* prophylaxis are expected to be effective as prophylaxis against cryptococcal infection. Routine screening of HSCT recipients with cryptococcal antigen is not recommended.

Endemic Mycoses

Amphotericin B is the recommended treatment for severe pulmonary histoplasmosis in HSCT recipients [171]. Liposomal amphotericin B 3–5 mg/kg daily or another lipid formulation of amphotericin B is preferred over deoxycholate due to their reduced nephrotoxic potential [172]. After clinical improvement is documented, antifungals can be changed to oral itraconazole 200 mg twice daily after a loading dose of 200 mg three times daily for 3 days [171]. Posaconazole and voriconazole are active in vitro against *H. capsulatum*, but clinical data is limited

[173–175]. They represent reasonable alternatives in those intolerant to itraconazole or when broader mold activity is desired. Duration of antifungal treatment should be at least 12 months. Treatment with an azole is an option for milder cases of pulmonary histoplasmosis. Although solid evidence is lacking, it is reasonable to continue secondary suppression during periods of profound immunosuppression to avoid relapse. There is no evidence to support antifungal prophylaxis in HSCT candidates with radiographic evidence (calcified pulmonary or splenic lesions) or serologic evidence of previous histoplasmosis [176].

Treatment of pulmonary coccidioidomycosis in HSCT recipients includes fluconazole 400 mg orally daily after a loading dose of 800 mg [177], unless severe, rapidly progressing, or disseminated disease. In such cases a lipid formulation of amphotericin B at 3–5 mg/kg daily is preferred as initial therapy [178] followed by oral azole after clinical response has been documented. Following treatment of acute infection, chronic suppressive therapy is advised to prevent relapses. However, large randomized studies in HSCT recipients are lacking. Azole prophylaxis during the first 6–12 months after HSCT is recommended in all HSCT recipients in endemic areas [177]. Although voriconazole, posaconazole, and isavuconazole are active in vitro against *Coccidioides* species, clinical data are limited, and therefore these agents aren't typically used as initial therapy [179].

Treatment of blastomycosis in HSCT recipients should include a lipid formulation of amphotericin B (liposomal amphotericin B 3–5 mg/kg daily or amphotericin B lipid complex) [180]. Transition to oral itraconazole (200 mg orally three times daily for 2 days followed by 200 mg orally twice daily) [181] is recommended after clinical response is documented or radiologic response if applicable. Although clinical evidence is limited, a mold-active azole such as voriconazole, posaconazole, or isavuconazole can be tried instead. Treatment should be continued for at least 12 months. Long-term secondary suppression is advised throughout the immunodeficiency state [180].

Pneumocystis jirovecii

Pneumocystis jirovecii pneumonia is an infrequent infection after HSCT as a result of effective prophylaxis. In a prospective surveillance study in HSCT recipients (TRANSNET), incidence of pneumocystis infections was 2% [78]. Preferred agent for prophylaxis against *Pneumocystis* is trimethoprim-sulfamethoxazole as it is highly effective [182, 183] and provides additional coverage against *Nocardia*, *Toxoplasma*, and *Listeria* (Table 11.2). Desensitization is advised in HSCT

Table 11.2 Prophylaxis and treatment regimens for *Pneumocystis jirovecii*

Prophylactic regimens	
First choice	Trimethoprim-sulfamethoxazole one double-strength tablet once daily
	Trimethoprim-sulfamethoxazole one single-strength tablet once daily
Alternative regimens	Trimethoprim-sulfamethoxazole one double-strength tablet three times per week
	Dapsone 100 mg tablet once daily or dapsone 50 mg tablet twice daily
	Atovaquone oral suspension 1500 mg daily with food
	Aerosolized pentamidine 300 mg monthly
Treatment regimens	
First choice	Trimethoprim-sulfamethoxazole IV 15–20 mg/kg/day of trimethoprim component divided to 3 or 4 doses
	Trimethoprim-sulfamethoxazole DS 2 tablets orally every 8 h daily for milder cases
Alternative regimens	Trimethoprim 5 mg/kg/orally three times daily plus dapsone 100 mg orally once daily
	Primaquine 30 mg orally once daily plus clindamycin 900 mg IV every 8 h or 600 mg orally every 8 h daily
	Atovaquone oral suspension 750 mg orally twice daily (with food)
	Pentamidine 4 mg/kg IV once daily
Adjuvant steroids	
	Prednisone 40 mg orally twice daily for 5 days followed by Prednisone 40 mg orally once daily for 5 days followed by Prednisone 20 mg orally once daily for 11 days or the equivalent dose of intravenous methylprednisolone

IV intravenous

recipients with history of allergic reaction to trimethoprim-sulfamethoxazole. However, the bone marrow suppressive potential of trimethoprim-sulfamethoxazole is a frequent problem limiting its use after HSCT. Alternative agents include atovaquone oral suspension [184] that provides coverage against *Pneumocystis* and *Toxoplasma gondii*, aerosolized pentamidine [185], and oral dapsone [186] that only target *Pneumocystis*. Prophylaxis against *Pneumocystis* is recommended from engraftment to at least 6 months after allogeneic HSCT and during periods of immunosuppression and for 3–6 months after autologous HSCT [19].

Treatment of *Pneumocystis* pneumonia consists of trimethoprim-sulfamethoxazole at 15–20 mg/kg of trimethoprim component divided in three or four equal doses [187]. Alternative regimens include primaquine-clindamycin, atovaquone oral suspension, trimethoprim-dapsone, or intravenous atovaquone (Table 11.2). Adjuvant steroids are indicated for those with a PaO2 <70 mmHg on room air, alveolar-arterial (A-a) oxygen gradient ≥35 mmHg, or evidence of hypoxemia [187]. Steroids should be given in a fast tapering scheme, either oral prednisone or intravenous methylprednisolone (Table 11.2) [187].

Viral Infections

Herpes Simplex Virus and Varicella Zoster Virus

Herpes simplex virus reactivation commonly manifests as mucocutaneous disease after transplantation. Prior to the introduction of acyclovir prophylaxis, incidence of herpes simplex virus (HSV) disease among HSCT recipients was about 70% [188], with most cases occurring early after transplantation. With the introduction of acyclovir prophylaxis, this incidence has dramatically decreased. In one retrospective study on autologous and allogeneic HSCT recipients, the 2-year probability of HSV disease was 31.6% when prophylaxis was administered the first 30 days posttransplant [189]. The 2-year probability dropped to 3.2%

when prophylaxis was administered for 1 year and to 0% when prophylaxis was given for an even more extended period. Oral acyclovir 400–800 mg twice daily or oral valacyclovir 500 mg twice daily or intravenous acyclovir 5 mg/kg every 12 h provides adequate prophylaxis against HSV [19, 39, 188, 189]. When ganciclovir or foscarnet is administered for prevention or treatment of CMV, concomitant acyclovir prophylaxis is not necessary as these agents provide adequate activity against HSV [19]. Prophylaxis should be administered from the conditioning regimen or transplantation day until engraftment or day 30+ whichever occurs first [39]. However, ongoing prophylaxis against varicella zoster virus (VZV) at later periods efficiently prevents HSV disease. Treatment of mucocutaneous HSV disease consists of intravenous acyclovir 5 mg/kg every 8 h for 7–10 days [190], while for disseminated HSV disease, higher-dose acyclovir at 10 mg/kg every 8 h is preferred. Options for acyclovir-resistant HSV are foscarnet [191] and cidofovir [192].

The 1-year probability of VZV disease after HSCT was 30% before acyclovir was introduced [193]. Eighty percent of cases occurred the first 9 months after transplant and were associated with significant mortality [193]. The rate significantly decreases with acyclovir prophylaxis [194]. Therefore, long-term prophylaxis is recommended for seropositive autologous and allogeneic HSCT recipients [194] for the first year after transplant and longer if chronic GvHD or if systemic immunosuppression continues [39]. Prophylactic regimens include oral acyclovir 800 mg orally twice daily [19, 195] and oral valacyclovir 500 mg twice daily or three times daily [19, 196]. Acyclovir or valacyclovir can be held in transplant recipients who receive ganciclovir, valganciclovir, or foscarnet for management of CMV, considering the efficacy of these agents against VZV [39, 197, 198]. Treatment of herpes zoster limited to one dermatome includes oral acyclovir 800 mg five times daily, oral valacyclovir 1 g three times daily, or intravenous acyclovir 10 mg/kg q 8 h for 7–14 days [19, 199]. Transition to an oral agent should be considered when clinical response is documented. In contrast, disseminated zoster or visceral disease including encephalitis is treated with intravenous acyclovir 10 mg/kg every 8 h for 14–21 days. Resistant VZV disease should be treated with foscarnet [198].

Postexposure prophylaxis should be given to all HSCT recipients who have close contact with an individual with chicken pox or shingles reactivation with a course of acyclovir or valacyclovir for 3 weeks [39].

Since the available vaccines against VZV contain live attenuated virus, they are contraindicated to immunocompromised individuals. However, transplant recipients would benefit from vaccination of household members who can potentially be a source for virus transmission [39]. If the individual develops a vaccine-associated rash, he/she should avoid contact with the transplant recipient. Finally, a recombinant vaccine is undergoing clinical investigation.

Cytomegalovirus Infection and Disease

Cytomegalovirus is a herpesvirus (human herpesvirus 5). Similar to other herpesviruses, cytomegalovirus (CMV) establishes latency after primary infection and reactivates during periods of profound T-cell immunodeficiency after transplantation (Fig. 11.1). Primary infection is usually transmitted through the graft in CMV-negative recipients. CMV disease is rare after autologous HSCT [200]. CD8+ and CD4+ T-cell responses are crucial in maintaining latency and controlling infection by CMV [201, 202]. The role of innate immunity is also important through production of inflammatory cytokines [203, 204]. Manifestations include CMV infection and CMV disease. CMV infection refers to detection of CMV replication in plasma or whole blood by pp65 antigenemia or DNA or messenger RNA PCR [205]. CMV disease is defined by the presence of end-organ involvement and refers to CMV pneumonia, gastrointestinal disease, hepatitis, retinitis, or CNS disease [205].

Prevention of CMV Infection and Disease in Allogeneic HSCT Recipients

Prevention of CMV infection and disease starts with selection of appropriate donor. A CMV-seronegative donor is preferred for a CMV-seronegative recipient if available; however, HLA-antigen match will be the primary criterion for donor selection. In the myeloablative setting, selection of a CMV-seropositive unrelated donor for a CMV-positive recipient is associated with a survival advantage [206]. In addition, the use of blood products from CMV-seronegative donors and leukocyte-depleted filtered blood products further decreased the risk [207]. The use of intravenous immunoglobulin is not recommended as its preventive effect is modest and a survival benefit has not been documented [38, 39].

The preventive potential of ganciclovir prophylaxis on CMV infection and disease, administered from engraftment until day +100, was demonstrated in two double-blind placebo-controlled clinical trials [208, 209]. Ganciclovir prophylaxis was frequently associated with neutropenia in both studies. Literature on valganciclovir prophylaxis is more limited. An unintended consequence of prophylaxis is late CMV disease and in particular pneumonia, following cessation of prophylaxis after day +100 [210]. Letermovir effectively prevents CMV reactivation and disease and is characterized by a more favorable side effect profile although its long-term adverse effects have not been studied [211]. The available agents for prophylaxis and treatment of CMV infection and disease are provided in Table 11.3.

Preemptive therapy is an approach for prevention of CMV disease that circumvents prophylaxis, thus preventing drug exposure and its consequences, as well as late CMV disease [212]. Preemptive therapy includes detection of viral replication and initiation of effective antiviral therapy at an early stage, before end-organ involvement has occurred [39, 213]. It entails weekly or more frequent monitoring of transplant recipients with sensitive tests detecting CMV elements on plasma or whole blood [213].

Preemptive strategy is initiated early after transplant until day +100 or longer for high-risk individuals [192, 213]. The most widely used assays to detect CMV are pp65 antigenemia and quantitative CMV PCR with the latter being more sensitive [214]. Uniformly accepted cutoffs for initiation of antiviral treatment have not been established due to variation in assays and lack of standardization of quantitative PCR. Detection of mRNA by nucleic acid sequence-based amplification (NASBA) is as effective as pp65 antigenemia assay and CMV DNA PCR [215].

Ganciclovir is preferred over foscarnet for preemptive therapy due to the unfavorable side effect profile of the latter [216, 217] (Table 11.3). Valganciclovir can be used when oral therapy is appropriate in the absence of significant gastrointestinal GvHD [19, 218]. These agents are used at induction doses for 1–2 weeks and until the qPCR is trending down. Maintenance therapy is continued until CMV is undetectable by PCR or under the predefined limit. When pp65 antigenemia is used to guide preemptive therapy, antivirals are continued until two negative measurements are documented, at least 1 week apart. A rise in the titer within 1 week after initiation of appropriate treatment is not uncommon and should not prompt changes in antiviral regimen [219]. The available agents for prophylaxis and treatment of CMV infection and disease are provided in Table 11.3.

Another strategy for CMV prevention posttransplant is vaccination of the donor or recipient. A DNA vaccine consisting of immunogenic proteins gB and pp65 [220] and a CMV peptide vaccine designed to induce pp65-specific cytotoxic T-cell responses [221] are undergoing clinical evaluation with promising results.

Intensive monitoring of cytotoxic CD8+ T lymphocytes and/or CD4+ CMV-specific T cells by means of tetramer detection or determination of peptide-specific lymphocyte responses is being studied with the aim to identify high-risk transplant recipients [222–225]. However, it has not been adopted for routine use in clinical practice yet.

Table 11.3 Antiviral agents for prevention and treatment of cytomegalovirus infection and disease

Prophylaxis

	Dose and route of administration	Side effects
Valganciclovir	900 mg PO once daily	Bone marrow suppression
Letermovir	480 mg PO or IV once daily (or 240 mg per day in patients on cyclosporine)	Nausea, vomiting, diarrhea, peripheral edema

Treatment

	Dose and route of administration		Side effects
	Induction	Maintenance	
Ganciclovir	5 mg/kg IV twice daily	5 mg/kg IV once daily	Bone marrow suppression
Valganciclovir	900 mg PO twice daily (for weight ≥40 kg)	900 mg PO once daily (for weight ≥40 kg)	Bone marrow suppression
Foscarnet	90 mg/kg IV twice daily	90 mg/kg IV once daily	Nephrotoxicity, electrolyte imbalance, anemia
Cidofovir	5 mg/kg/week IV	5 mg/kg IV every 2 weeks	Nephrotoxicity, ocular toxicity, Fanconi's syndrome

IV intravenous, *PO* oral

Treatment of CMV Disease

As a principal, reduction of immunosuppression when feasible should be attempted. Moreover, treatment of invasive CMV disease differs from preemptive therapy in that duration of induction and maintenance therapy is longer.

CMV pneumonia is the most severe manifestation of CMV disease associated with high mortality rates. Treatment of CMV pneumonia includes induction doses continued for at least 3–4 weeks followed by longer courses of maintenance. First-line antiviral agent for treatment of CMV disease remains intravenous ganciclovir [217]. Foscarnet is an alternative for patients' refractory infection or intolerance to ganciclovir [216]. Limited data support the use of intravenous immunoglobulin as an adjunct in the treatment of CMV pneumonia [226–228]. Studies are hampered by small number of participants and lack of contemporaneous controls. For this indication intravenous immunoglobulin is usually administered every other day for three to five doses. CMV-specific immunoglobulin does not offer any specific advantage over pooled immunoglobulin. Immunoglobulin is currently recommended only as an adjunct in the treatment of CMV pneumonia.

Gastrointestinal CMV disease is treated with ganciclovir induction for at least 2–3 weeks, followed by several weeks of maintenance therapy. Foscarnet is an alternative when neutropenia has complicated the patient's course [216]. If recurrence is documented, prophylaxis with valganciclovir or ganciclovir may be necessary to prevent further relapses.

CMV retinitis occurs during the late post-engraftment period, is frequently bilateral (in half of the cases), and can lead to irreversible visual loss [229]. Treatment of CMV retinitis includes systemic ganciclovir or foscarnet along with intraocular ganciclovir injections or implants [230]. Duration of treatment is prolonged and not precisely defined.

Discontinuation of antivirals is guided by resolution of clinical symptoms and signs of CMV disease and documentation of cessation of viral replication but more importantly when profound immunosuppression has been withdrawn allowing for some degree of immune restoration. When intense immunosuppression cannot be reduced, transplant recipients may benefit from secondary prophylaxis.

Drug-Resistant CMV

CMV resistance to antivirals is infrequent in allogeneic HSCT recipients [231, 232] and occurs in the setting of profound immunodeficiency and prolonged antiviral drug exposure. It is most commonly reported in association to ganciclovir and its prodrug valganciclovir, as these are the most extensively used antiviral drugs.

Although within the first 2 weeks after initiation of antiviral treatment the viral load or antigenemia level may increase due to the immunosuppression [219], any increase after that should raise concerns for CMV antiviral resistance, especially if the patient was previously exposed to the antiviral drug. In that case a sample should be tested for genotypic resistance [233]. Standard for detection of resistance is DNA sequencing considering the slow turnaround time of phenotypic assays. Sensitivity increases for viral loads of 1000 IU/mL and higher. Deep sequencing techniques may detect resistant subpopulations [234] that would otherwise be missed resulting in false negative [235]. Changing to another antiviral class is recommended before results of resistance testing are available.

Mutations in the UL97 phosphotransferase gene, which encodes for the UL97 kinase and mediates the initial phosphorylation of ganciclovir, confer resistance to ganciclovir and its prodrug valganciclovir [236]. Foscarnet and cidofovir are unaffected by the UL97 mutations. In contrast, mutations in the UL54 gene that encodes for DNA polymerase confer resistance to ganciclovir, its prodrug valganciclovir, foscarnet, and cidofovir, as all these antivirals inhibit DNA polymerase.

In patients exposed to ganciclovir, the first mutation to appear is usually on the UL97 gene [232], allowing for empiric treatment with foscarnet until genotyping results become available. Due to its nephrotoxic potential, experience with cidofovir in this setting is limited. UL54 gene mutations usually follow the development of UL97 resistance [237], and besides its multiclass effect, it confers additional resistance against ganciclovir to that guided by UL97 mutation [238].

Although supportive clinical data are limited, combination of foscarnet with ganciclovir has been used when resistance is traced to single UL97 mutation that conveys resistance exclusively to ganciclovir [239, 240]. Reasoning for that is that ganciclovir may retain part of its antiviral activity in the presence of a single UL97 mutation [241], and ganciclovir in combination with foscarnet has demonstrated at least an additive effect against sensitive CMV strains in vitro [242, 243].

The level of resistance to ganciclovir varies depending on the UL97 codon mutated. Based on that, high-dose ganciclovir from 7.5 to 10 mg/kg every 12 h has been used [244] when resistance is traced to mutations in C592G codon that confers low-level resistance [236]. However, available clinical experience is limited, and other mutations that confer additive resistance may coexist or accumulate rendering ganciclovir inactive [236]. We therefore reserve this therapeutic option for patients who are not candidates for alternative antivirals, have no CMV disease and whose condition is not severe.

For CMV-resistant virus that carries the UL54 mutation, therapeutic options are limited. Maribavir [245] and letermovir [246] have in vitro activity against resistant CMV. Sirolimus has an inhibitory effect on CMV replication, thus reducing the risk for CMV reactivation after HSCT when part of the immunosuppressive regimen [247]. Adoptive transfer of CMV-specific T lymphocytes is an investigational therapy for resistant CMV infection or disease [201, 248]. Finally, reduction in immunosuppression is crucial in the outcome of drug-resistant CMV infection or disease.

Newer Agents Under Development

Maribavir inhibits UL97 kinase and CMV replication in vitro [249] and is active against isolates resistant to ganciclovir, foscarnet, and cidofovir [245]. Although its prophylactic potential continues to be under clinical investigation [250], it may have a role in the treatment of resistant CMV [251, 252], and a clinical trial is ongoing (ClinicalTrials.gov NCT01611974). Brincidofovir, a lipid conjugate of cidofovir, lacks the potent nephrotoxic properties of cidofovir [253]. Letermovir is a new promising agent that is undergoing evaluation in the treatment of CMV [211, 246]. The potential of leflunomide and artesunate against CMV has been studied, but their activity appears to be modest.

Adoptive Immunotherapy

Adoptive immunotherapy refers to the transfer of CMV-reactive cytotoxic T lymphocytes to treat CMV infection or disease [201, 248]. Although it continues to undergo intense clinical investigation, it can be used for treatment of refractory or recurrent disease when all other options have been exhausted. It is extensively discussed in a dedicated chapter of this book.

Human Herpesvirus 6

Human herpesvirus 6 (HHV-6) reactivation has been reported up to 70% of recipients of allogeneic HSCT [254] with the majority of episodes manifested as asymptomatic viremia occurring between the second and fourth week after transplant [255]. Etiologic association between encephalitis, bone marrow suppression, and HHV-6 is well documented [254, 256]. Less consistent association has been described with pneumonitis and GvHD.

Treatment recommendations are based on in vitro studies and small case series that lack comparator arm. Antivirals of choice include foscarnet 60 mg/kg intravenously every 8 h or 90 mg/kg intravenously every 12 h or ganciclovir 5 mg/kg every 12 h [257, 258]. Cidofovir has activity against HHV-6; however, its nephrotoxic potential limits its use [216, 259]. Duration of treatment is not independently defined; however, most experts recommend a 21-day course.

Epstein-Barr Virus

Epstein-Barr virus (EBV) in allogeneic transplant recipients is associated with posttransplant lymphoproliferative disorder (PTLD) that encompasses a spectrum of lymphoid and plasmacytic proliferation [260, 261]. Although not always related to EBV, PTLD in allogeneic HSCT recipients is usually donor derived and presumably involves the proliferation of the EBV-infected B cells that escape the dysregulated T-cell surveillance [262]. Although acyclovir and ganciclovir have in vitro activity against EBV, they have no role in the treatment of PTLD, as they require phosphorylation by viral enzymes that are not available. Their preventive value is also unclear [262]. Treatment includes rituximab (for CD20+ expressing PTLD), chemotherapy, and adoptive transfer of EBV-specific cytotoxic T cells or donor lymphocyte infusion [261].

Adenovirus Infections

Adenovirus disease is more common in pediatric transplant recipients than in adults and in allogeneic transplant recipients compared to recipients of autologous grafts [263]. Disease usually occurs during the early post-engraftment period following HSCT (Fig. 11.1). Clinical manifestations of adenovirus disease in transplant recipients include asymptomatic viremia, upper respiratory tract infection, pneumonia, gastroenteritis, hemorrhagic cystitis, disseminated disease with multiorgan failure, nephritis, hepatitis, and encephalitis [264]. Severity of disease varies from mild to fatal [263, 265].

Asymptomatic shedding of adenovirus in the upper respiratory tract, feces, and urine does not correlate with clinical disease [266]. Therefore, positive results should be interpreted as diagnostic only in the presence of compatible clinical and radiologic findings. Moreover, tissue diagnosis is frequently necessary to confirm invasive disease and exclude asymptomatic shedding.

Rising levels of viremia have been associated with development of invasive adenovirus disease, and severe disease is invariably associated with viremia [266]. Despite that, the benefit of preemptive therapy for adenovirus infection is not established as asymptomatic viremia can be self-limited and the available treatments option (cidofovir) has significant nephrotoxic potential [259]. Further studies are needed to investigate the potential benefit of preemptive therapy in high-risk patients, such as pediatric recipients of T-cell-depleted grafts or those with graft-versus-host disease.

Adenovirus is susceptible in vitro to cidofovir [267], and cidofovir is currently the standard of care for adenovirus disease. It is characterized by long half-life allowing for weekly dosing. Induction dose consists of 5 mg/kg/week followed by maintenance of 5 mg/kg every 2 weeks. However, major limitation is its nephrotoxic potential [259]. Prehydration and concurrent use of probenecid have been successful in mitigating renal toxicity. A modified dosing regimen consisting of cidofovir 1 mg/kg three times per week is probably associated with less nephrotoxicity [268], but reliable conclusions on efficacy cannot be made as published studies included small numbers of patients [268, 269]. It can be used as an alternative in patients with history of renal insufficiency or on other nephrotoxic medications. Other side effects of cidofovir are neutropenia, ocular side effects including uveitis, and Fanconi's syndrome [270]. Brincidofovir was well tolerated and effective in controlling adenoviremia in pediatric recipients of allogeneic HSCT [271]. Adenovirus is variably susceptible to ribavirin in vitro, and susceptibility appears to be species specific [267]. Ribavirin failed to demonstrate reliable responses in small series of pediatric patients [272, 273].

Pooled intravenous immunoglobulin can be used as an adjunct to antivirals [265]. Because delayed recovery of adenovirus-specific T cell correlates with increased risk for adenovirus disease [274], adoptive transfer of adenovirus-specific donor T cells led to viral clearance in a small study of children with adenovirus disease [275].

Influenza, Parainfluenza, and Respiratory Syncytial Virus

Although antiviral treatment for influenza is most beneficial if started within 48 h of onset of symptoms, in hematopoietic transplant recipients, treatment should be initiated even if the patient presented after 2 days of symptom onset [276, 277]. First-line therapy for treatment of influenza is oseltamivir 75 mg orally twice daily due to its broader spectrum that includes influenza A and B and superior side effect profile [278]. Recommended duration of treatment is 10 days [276, 279] considering the longer replication period in immunocompromised individuals. There is no specific antiviral therapy available for parainfluenza virus. Intravenous immunoglobulin has been used for severe disease [280]. Finally treatment options for lower respiratory tract infection due to respiratory syncytial virus include aerosolized ribavirin [281] and oral ribavirin [282, 283] with or without intravenous immunoglobulin [284].

Disease due to Human Polyomavirus

BK Virus Cystitis and Nephropathy

BK virus is a polyomavirus that has the potential to cause hemorrhagic cystitis and rarely nephropathy in the posttransplant setting. Diagnosis of hemorrhagic cystitis is made by a positive PCR for BK virus in a urine sample, in the presence of signs and symptoms suggestive of hemorrhagic cystitis. Randomized clinical trials are lacking, and treatment recommendations are driven by limited clinical studies. Intravenous cidofovir 5 mg/kg every 2 weeks or at 1 mg/kg three times per week or intravesicular cidofovir 5 mg/kg in 60–100 mL appears to be effective, although evidence from randomized controlled trials is lacking [285, 286]. Ciprofloxacin or levofloxacin has activity against BK virus in vitro [287]. The clinical efficacy however is not established [288, 289]. Intravenous immunoglobulin can be used as an adjunct [290]. Finally leflunomide appears to have activity against BK virus in vitro [291].

Progressive Multifocal Leukoencephalopathy

Progressive multifocal leukoencephalopathy (PML) is a demyelinating disease of the central nervous system, caused by JC virus [292]. Cidofovir and cytarabine have been tried with disappointing results [293, 294]. The role of serotonin reuptake inhibitor such as mirtazapine and risperidone [295, 296], mefloquine [297, 298], and interleukin-7 [299] is under investigation. Reduction in immunosuppression appears to be crucial in the outcome of this disease.

Infections due to Parasites

Toxoplasmosis

Toxoplasma gondii is an intracellular protozoan parasite that has the potential to cause primary disease or reactivate in allogeneic HSCT recipients [300]. In contrast to other T-cell-deficient individuals (i.e., solid organ transplant or AIDS), disease due to *Toxoplasma* is uncommon among allogeneic HSCT recipients and extremely rare in autologous HSCT recipients [301]. Incidence was 2% among allogeneic seropositive transplant recipients [300] and 2.2% among T-cell-depleted allogeneic HSCT recipients [302]. Incidence varies significantly by geographic region probably reflecting the diverse seroprevalence in the general population worldwide [303]. In HSCT recipients, it can manifest as brain abscess, encephalitis, pneumonitis, cardiac disease, and more rarely chorioretinitis [302, 304] with potentially fatal outcome.

Treatment of choice consists of sulfadiazine along with pyrimethamine. The dose of oral sulfadiazine is 1000–1500 mg four times daily and is weight based, and dose of oral pyrimethamine is 200 mg loading dose once, followed by weight-based dose of 50–75 mg orally per day [305]. Pyrimethamine exerts its effect on folate biosynthesis by inhibiting dihydrofolate reductase and therefore can cause hematologic toxicity. To prevent that, patients should be on supplemental folinic acid (leucovorin) 10–25 mg orally daily, and blood counts should be monitored frequently. For those intolerant to sulfadiazine, alternative regimens include pyrimethamine (and leucovorin) along with clindamycin (600 mg oral or intravenous every 6 h) or oral azithromycin 900–1200 mg once daily or atovaquone 1500 mg twice daily [305]. Trimethoprim-sulfamethoxazole 5 mg/kg of trimethoprim compound every 12 h orally or intravenously has been studied in HIV/AIDS patients with toxoplasmic encephalitis and appears to be effective [306].

Duration of treatment is 4–6 weeks until complete resolution of clinical microbiological and radiologic findings. Treatment should be followed by long-term secondary suppression during continued immunosuppression.

Prevention of toxoplasmosis after transplantation starts with pretransplant serologic screen that should be performed in all allogeneic transplant candidates [39]. However, disease due to toxoplasmosis has been reported in transplant recipients who were seronegative pretransplant [300, 302]. Trimethoprim-sulfamethoxazole prophylaxis prevents toxoplasmosis although breakthrough infections in HSCT recipients have been reported at the dose used for *Pneumocystis jirovecii* prophylaxis [300]. Alternative prophylactic regimen would include oral atovaquone 1500 mg daily.

Finally all transplant recipients should avoid exposure to cat feces and consumption of undercooked meat [39] that are well-documented sources of transmission of *Toxoplasma gondii*.

Strongyloidiasis

Strongyloides stercoralis is a nematode parasite endemic in the tropic and subtropic regions although sporadic acquisition has been reported in other areas of the world (Southeastern USA and Southern Europe). Infections are acquired during travel in endemic areas. *Strongyloides stercoralis* is capable of completing its cycle within a single host leading to autoinfection, thus establishing permanent presence in the host [307]. In particular, during initial infection, filariform larvae penetrate the skin after direct exposure and reach the lungs through the circulation. Through respiratory secretions, they ascend to the pharynx, are swallowed, and reach the intestine, where they develop to adult worms. Autoinfection ensues as female worms produce eggs that hatch into rhabditiform larvae that transform into the infective filariform larvae that penetrate the intestinal mucosa and migrate to the lungs [307].

The majority of infected immunocompetent individuals are asymptomatic or may have asymptomatic eosinophilia and may have acquired the infection several decades previously.

In immunocompromised individuals, clinical manifestations are associated with the migration of the larvae through the intestinal mucosa (i.e., abdominal pain, diarrhea, gastrointestinal bleeding, or obstruction) and lungs (cough, wheezing, dyspnea, etc.) but also bacteremia due to Gram-negative rods and other enteric florae, presumed to enter the circulation carried by the larvae [308]. An accelerated conversion of the rhabditiform to the infective filariform larvae may occur in transplant recipients termed *Strongyloides* hyperinfection syndrome [309].

Treatment of choice for uncomplicated strongyloidiasis is two doses of ivermectin 200 mcg/kg either administered for 2 consecutive days or 1 week apart [310, 311]. Due to each inferior efficacy, albendazole 400 mg orally twice daily for 3–7 days is recommended as alternative [312].

Approach to the Patient with Posttransplant Complications

Considering the unique features of hematopoietic transplant recipients, several principles guide the management of posttransplant complications. Differential diagnosis of infectious complications is wide and includes noninfectious conditions, empiric regimens consist of multiple agents that are potentially toxic, and duration of therapy is frequently prolonged and often requires lifelong secondary suppression. Therefore, pursuing a definitive diagnosis is highly advised. On the other hand, diagnostic tests may be insensitive (e.g., serology in the posttransplant setting can be falsely negative), diagnosis frequently requires invasive diagnostic procedures that may not be feasible because of the patient's condition (e.g., advanced respiratory failure that renders bronchoscopy a high-risk procedure, poor wound healing due to cutaneous GvHD that prevents biopsy, platelet-refractory thrombocytopenia, etc.), and samples for cultures may not be available before initiation of antibiotics.

Unless specimens for cultures or a diagnostic procedure can be done promptly, our approach includes initiation of broad empirical antimicrobial coverage that targets the likely and most virulent pathogens while awaiting results of noninvasive diagnostic workup (blood tests, sputum cultures, etc.). If the initial workup is inconclusive and the condition progresses, we pursue the diagnosis employing a procedure, assuming the patient understands the risk involved and their condition allows. The invasive procedure can be performed earlier if the patient's condition progresses rapidly enough to make it unfeasible or high risk.

Approach to the Transplant Recipient with Pulmonary Infiltrates

Development of pulmonary infiltrates is a common complication after transplantation. Several factors weigh in in selecting empirical antimicrobial coverage. Timing of infection after transplant is important as well as the underlying immunodeficiency. Invasive mold infections usually occur after at least 10 days of profound neutropenia. CMV reactivation or *Pneumocystis* pneumonia occurs during the period of T-cell immune deficiency and is unlikely in the pre-engraftment period.

Ongoing prophylaxis is also essential in defining the empiric regimen. While TMP/SMX is effective in preventing infections due to *Pneumocystis jirovecii*, *Toxoplasma gondii*, *Nocardia* species, and *Listeria*, oral atovaquone is effective only against *Pneumocystis* and *Toxoplasma gondii* and inhaled pentamidine only against *Pneumocystis*, therefore widening the differential diagnosis. Cases of invasive zygomycosis (mucormycosis) have been reported breaking through voriconazole prophylaxis as the antifungal spectrum of voriconazole does not include zygomycetes.

The type of infiltrates is suggestive of the etiology and can be used to modify the empirical antimicrobial coverage. Bilateral ground glass infiltrates that start perihilar and expand peripherally are suggestive of *Pneumocystis jirovecii* pneumonia. Diffuse bilateral interstitial infiltrates are suggestive of viral pneumonia and in particular CMV as well as community-acquired respiratory viruses (e.g., influenza, parainfluenza, adenovirus, RSV, and human metapneumovirus). Pulmonary nodules with or without a halo sign and cavitary lesions are highly suggestive of infections due to mold. Infiltrates due to congestive heart failure follow the gravity and are usually accompanied by pleural effusions, while pulmonary GvHD frequently has a peribronchial distribution.

Every attempt should be made to obtain respiratory samples for bacterial, viral, fungal, and acid-fast bacilli cultures, and other studies (PCR, etc.) before empirical antibiotic coverage are initiated. However, this is not always feasible. If the initial workup is inconclusive and there is no response to empirical antibiotic coverage, we proceed with diagnostic bronchoscopy or percutaneous biopsy, depending on the differential diagnosis and distribution of the infiltrates.

Finally, many of the noninfectious pulmonary complications (e.g., diffuse alveolar hemorrhage and pulmonary GvHD) are potentially steroid-responsive. This question usually arises when noninvasive evaluation for infections (e.g., cultures, antigen testing, PCR) is negative and a noninfectious process is highly suspected. In the absence of clinical or radiologic response to antimicrobials, a trial of steroids can be considered when there is a high clinical suspicion for steroid-responsive conditions and an invasive procedure (e.g., lung biopsy) carries substantial risk of complications or is unfeasible. Due to the additive immunosuppressive effect of steroids, adequate and uninterrupted antifungal and pneumocystis prophylaxis should be provided.

Future Directions

The field of transplant infectious diseases is constantly evolving. Several areas of intensive research are worth mentioning. Better insight and understanding of the interplay of native and adaptive immunity can help optimize preventive and therapeutic strategies. Innovations in transplantation such as donor selection, manipulation of the graft, and new immunosuppressive agents for prevention and treatment of GvHD expand the spectrum of host characteristics and the epidemiology of infections posttransplantation. The ever-evolving epidemiology of bacterial resistance and the emergence of resistance in yeast or mold mandate the adoption of new preventive and therapeutic strategies [21, 31, 32, 313, 314].

The role of microbiota in transplant outcomes and the potential of microbiome manipulation has been the subject of intense investigation. Higher abundance of *Eubacterium limosum* and other bacteria was associated with lower risk for relapse of malignancy [315]. Low diversity correlated with mortality after allogeneic transplantation [316]. Increased bacterial diversity and bacteria belonging to the genus *Blautia* were associated with reduced GvHD-related mortality [317]. These data suggest that maintenance of certain bacterial phyla after transplantation may be beneficial to the recipient.

There are also opportunities for immunotherapy for specific infections. A promising strategy for CMV prevention posttransplant is vaccination of the donor or recipient. A DNA vaccine consisting of immunogenic proteins gB and pp65 [220] and a CMV peptide vaccine designed to induce pp65-specific cytotoxic T-cell responses [221] are undergoing clinical evaluation with promising results.

Adoptive immunotherapy for the treatment of infections is a matter of intense research. Adoptive transfer of CMV-specific T lymphocytes for the treatment of resistant CMV infection or disease is undergoing clinical investigation [201, 248]. Adoptive transfer of EBV-specific cytotoxic T cells [261] and adenovirus-specific donor T cells [275] has been studied in the treatment of PTLD and adenovirus disease, respectively.

In addition, we are learning genetic risk factors for specific transplant-associated infections that may lead to more refined risk stratification. Genetic polymorphism of donor or recipient may predict the risk of infections posttransplantation. Recipients with mutation in the mannose-binding lectin gene appear to have an increased risk for infections following neutrophil recovery after myeloablative transplant [318]. Donor haplotypes of toll-like receptor 4 (TLR4) genes may lead to an increased risk of invasive aspergillosis [319]. Certain donors' activated killer immunoglobulin-like receptor haplotypes may be protective against CMV reactivation [320]. Preliminary data are promising, but further investigation is needed before this information translates into clinical practice.

References

1. Storek J. Immunological reconstitution after hematopoietic cell transplantation – its relation to the contents of the graft. Expert Opin Biol Ther. 2008;8(5):583–97.
2. Storek J, Geddes M, Khan F, Huard B, Helg C, Chalandon Y, et al. Reconstitution of the immune system after hematopoietic stem cell transplantation in humans. Semin Immunopathol. 2008;30(4):425–37.
3. Jacobs R, Stoll M, Stratmann G, Leo R, Link H, Schmidt RE. CD16- CD56+ natural killer cells after bone marrow transplantation. Blood. 1992;79(12):3239–44.
4. Zimmerli W, Zarth A, Gratwohl A, Speck B. Neutrophil function and pyogenic infections in bone marrow transplant recipients. Blood. 1991;77(2):393–9.
5. Storek J, Gooley T, Witherspoon RP, Sullivan KM, Storb R. Infectious morbidity in long-term survivors of allogeneic marrow transplantation is associated with low CD4 T cell counts. Am J Hematol. 1997;54(2):131–8.
6. Hakim FT, Gress RE. Reconstitution of thymic function after stem cell transplantation in humans. Curr Opin Hematol. 2002;9(6):490–6.
7. Hakim FT, Memon SA, Cepeda R, Jones EC, Chow CK, Kasten-Sportes C, et al. Age-dependent incidence, time course, and consequences of thymic renewal in adults. J Clin Invest. 2005;115(4):930–9.
8. Storek J. B-cell immunity after allogeneic hematopoietic cell transplantation. Cytotherapy. 2002;4(5):423–4.
9. Small TN, Keever CA, Weiner-Fedus S, Heller G, O'Reilly RJ, Flomenberg N. B-cell differentiation following autologous, conventional, or T-cell depleted bone marrow transplantation: a recapitulation of normal B-cell ontogeny. Blood. 1990;76(8):1647–56.
10. Storek J, Wells D, Dawson MA, Storer B, Maloney DG. Factors influencing B lymphopoiesis after allogeneic hematopoietic cell transplantation. Blood. 2001;98(2):489–91.
11. Wingard JR, Hsu J, Hiemenz JW. Hematopoietic stem cell transplantation: an overview of infection risks and epidemiology. Infect Dis Clin N Am. 2010;24(2):257–72.
12. Srinivasan A, Wang C, Srivastava DK, Burnette K, Shenep JL, Leung W, et al. Timeline, epidemiology, and risk factors for bacterial, fungal, and viral infections in children and adolescents after allogeneic hematopoietic stem cell transplantation. Biol Blood Marrow Transplant. 2013;19(1):94–101.
13. Safdar A, Rodriguez GH, De Lima MJ, Petropoulos D, Chemaly RF, Worth LL, et al. Infections in 100 cord blood transplantations: spectrum of early and late posttransplant infections in adult and pediatric patients 1996–2005. Medicine (Baltimore). 2007;86(6):324–33.
14. Martino R, Bautista G, Parody R, Garcia I, Esquirol A, Rovira M, et al. Severe infections after single umbilical cord blood transplantation in adults with or without the co-infusion of CD34+ cells from a third-party donor: results of a multicenter study from the Grupo Espanol de Trasplante Hematopoyetico (GETH). Transpl Infect Dis. 2015;17(2):221–33.
15. Slade M, Goldsmith S, Romee R, DiPersio JF, Dubberke ER, Westervelt P, et al. Epidemiology of infections following haploidentical peripheral blood hematopoietic cell transplantation. Transpl Infect Dis. 2017;19(1). doi: 10.1111/tid.12629
16. Marr KA, Carter RA, Boeckh M, Martin P, Corey L. Invasive aspergillosis in allogeneic stem cell transplant recipients: changes in epidemiology and risk factors. Blood. 2002;100(13):4358–66.
17. Myers GD, Krance RA, Weiss H, Kuehnle I, Demmler G, Heslop HE, et al. Adenovirus infection rates in pediatric recipients of alternate donor allogeneic bone marrow transplants receiving either antithymocyte globulin (ATG) or alemtuzumab (Campath). Bone Marrow Transplant. 2005;36(11):1001–8.
18. Marr KA, Carter RA, Crippa F, Wald A, Corey L. Epidemiology and outcome of mould infections in hematopoietic stem cell transplant recipients. Clin Infect Dis. 2002;34(7):909–17.
19. Baden LR, Swaminathan S, Almyroudis NG, Angarone M, Blouin G, Camins BC, et al. Prevention and treatment of cancer-related infections, version 1.2018, NCCN clinical practice guidelines in oncology 2018 [cited 2018 January 11, 2018]. Available from: https://www.nccn.org/professionals/physician_gls/pdf/infections.pdf.
20. Cappellano P, Viscoli C, Bruzzi P, Van Lint MT, Pereira CA, Bacigalupo A. Epidemiology and risk factors for bloodstream infections after allogeneic hematopoietic stem cell transplantation. New Microbiol. 2007;30(2):89–99.
21. Mikulska M, Viscoli C, Orasch C, Livermore DM, Averbuch D, Cordonnier C, et al. Aetiology and resistance in bacteraemias among adult and paediatric haematology and cancer patients. J Infect. 2014;68(4):321–31.

22. Shaw BE, Boswell T, Byrne JL, Yates C, Russell NH. Clinical impact of MRSA in a stem cell transplant unit: analysis before, during and after an MRSA outbreak. Bone Marrow Transplant. 2007;39(10):623–9.

23. Han XY, Kamana M, Rolston KV. Viridans streptococci isolated by culture from blood of cancer patients: clinical and microbiologic analysis of 50 cases. J Clin Microbiol. 2006;44(1):160–5.

24. Kamboj M, Chung D, Seo SK, Pamer EG, Sepkowitz KA, Jakubowski AA, et al. The changing epidemiology of vancomycin-resistant Enterococcus (VRE) bacteremia in allogeneic hematopoietic stem cell transplant (HSCT) recipients. Biol Blood Marrow Transplant. 2010;16(11):1576–81.

25. Chuang YC, Wang JT, Lin HY, Chang SC. Daptomycin versus linezolid for treatment of vancomycin-resistant enterococcal bacteremia: systematic review and meta-analysis. BMC Infect Dis. 2014;14:687.

26. Balli EP, Venetis CA, Miyakis S. Systematic review and meta-analysis of linezolid versus daptomycin for treatment of vancomycin-resistant enterococcal bacteremia. Antimicrob Agents Chemother. 2014;58(2):734–9.

27. Whang DW, Miller LG, Partain NM, McKinnell JA. Systematic review and meta-analysis of linezolid and daptomycin for treatment of vancomycin-resistant enterococcal bloodstream infections. Antimicrob Agents Chemother. 2013; 57(10):5013–8.

28. Britt NS, Potter EM, Patel N, Steed ME. Comparison of the effectiveness and safety of linezolid and daptomycin in vancomycin-resistant enterococcal bloodstream infection: a National Cohort Study of Veterans Affairs Patients. Clin Infect Dis. 2015;61(6):871–8.

29. Raad I, Hachem R, Hanna H, Afif C, Escalante C, Kantarjian H, et al. Prospective, randomized study comparing quinupristin-dalfopristin with linezolid in the treatment of vancomycin-resistant Enterococcus faecium infections. J Antimicrob Chemother. 2004;53(4):646–9.

30. Poutsiaka DD, Skiffington S, Miller KB, Hadley S, Snydman DR. Daptomycin in the treatment of vancomycin-resistant Enterococcus faecium bacteremia in neutropenic patients. J Infect. 2007;54(6):567–71.

31. Sood P, Seth T, Kapil A, Sharma V, Dayama A, Sharma S, et al. Emergence of multidrug resistant acinetobacter blood stream infections in febrile neutropenia patients with haematological cancers and bone marrow failure syndromes. J Indian Med Assoc. 2012;110(7):439–44.

32. Satlin MJ, Calfee DP, Chen L, Fauntleroy KA, Wilson SJ, Jenkins SG, et al. Emergence of carbapenem-resistant Enterobacteriaceae as causes of bloodstream infections in patients with hematologic malignancies. Leuk Lymphoma. 2013;54(4):799–806.

33. Bucaneve G, Micozzi A, Menichetti F, Martino P, Dionisi MS, Martinelli G, et al. Levofloxacin to prevent bacterial infection in patients with cancer and neutropenia. N Engl J Med. 2005;353(10):977–87.

34. Engels EA, Lau J, Barza M. Efficacy of quinolone prophylaxis in neutropenic cancer patients: a meta-analysis. J Clin Oncol. 1998;16(3):1179–87.

35. Razonable RR, Litzow MR, Khaliq Y, Piper KE, Rouse MS, Patel R. Bacteremia due to viridans group Streptococci with diminished susceptibility to levofloxacin among neutropenic patients receiving levofloxacin prophylaxis. Clin Infect Dis. 2002;34(11):1469–74.

36. Elting LS, Bodey GP, Keefe BH. Septicemia and shock syndrome due to viridans streptococci: a case-control study of predisposing factors. Clin Infect Dis. 1992;14(6):1201–7.

37. Loo VG, Poirier L, Miller MA, Oughton M, Libman MD, Michaud S, et al. A predominantly clonal multi-institutional outbreak of Clostridium difficile-associated diarrhea with high morbidity and mortality. N Engl J Med. 2005;353(23):2442–9.

38. Raanani P, Gafter-Gvili A, Paul M, Ben-Bassat I, Leibovici L, Shpilberg O. Immunoglobulin prophylaxis in hematopoietic stem cell transplantation: systematic review and meta-analysis. J Clin Oncol. 2009;27(5):770–81.

39. Tomblyn M, Chiller T, Einsele H, Gress R, Sepkowitz K, Storek J, et al. Guidelines for preventing infectious complications among hematopoietic cell transplantation recipients: a global perspective. Biol Blood Marrow Transplant. 2009;15(10):1143–238.

40. Zenewicz LA, Shen H. Innate and adaptive immune responses to Listeria monocytogenes: a short overview. Microbes Infect. 2007;9(10):1208–15.

41. Skogberg K, Syrjanen J, Jahkola M, Renkonen OV, Paavonen J, Ahonen J, et al. Clinical presentation and outcome of listeriosis in patients with and without immunosuppressive therapy. Clin Infect Dis. 1992;14(4):815–21.

42. Chang J, Powles R, Mehta J, Paton N, Treleaven J, Jameson B. Listeriosis in bone marrow transplant recipients: incidence, clinical features, and treatment. Clin Infect Dis. 1995;21(5):1289–90.

43. Clauss HE, Lorber B. Central nervous system infection with Listeria monocytogenes. Curr Infect Dis Rep. 2008;10(4):300–6.

44. Lorber B. Listeriosis. Clin Infect Dis. 1997;24(1):1–9. quiz 10-1

45. Safdar A, Armstrong D. Antimicrobial activities against 84 Listeria monocytogenes isolates from patients with systemic listeriosis at a comprehensive cancer center (1955–1997). J Clin Microbiol. 2003;41(1):483–5.

46. Hof H, Nichterlein T, Kretschmar M. Management of listeriosis. Clin Microbiol Rev. 1997;10(2):345–57.

47. Drevets DA, Canono BP, Leenen PJ, Campbell PA. Gentamicin kills intracellular Listeria monocytogenes. Infect Immun. 1994;62(6):2222–8.

48. Winslow DL, Pankey GA. In vitro activities of tri-methoprim and sulfamethoxazole against *Listeria monocytogenes*. Antimicrob Agents Chemother. 1982;22(1):51–4.

49. Kim KS. In vitro and in vivo studies of imipenem-cilastatin alone and in combination with gentamicin against *Listeria monocytogenes*. Antimicrob Agents Chemother. 1986;29(2):289–93.

50. Choucino C, Goodman SA, Greer JP, Stein RS, Wolff SN, Dummer JS. Nocardial infections in bone marrow transplant recipients. Clin Infect Dis. 1996;23(5):1012–9.

51. van Burik JA, Hackman RC, Nadeem SQ, Hiemenz JW, White MH, Flowers ME, et al. Nocardiosis after bone marrow transplantation: a retrospective study. Clin Infect Dis. 1997;24(6):1154–60.

52. Beaman BL, Beaman L. Nocardia species: host-parasite relationships. Clin Microbiol Rev. 1994;7(2):213–64.

53. Wallace RJ Jr, Septimus EJ, Williams TW Jr, Conklin RH, Satterwhite TK, Bushby MB, et al. Use of trimethoprim-sulfamethoxazole for treatment of infections due to Nocardia. Rev Infect Dis. 1982;4(2):315–25.

54. Uhde KB, Pathak S, McCullum I Jr, Jannat-Khah DP, Shadomy SV, Dykewicz CA, et al. Antimicrobial-resistant nocardia isolates, United States, 1995–2004. Clin Infect Dis. 2010;51(12):1445–8.

55. Brown-Elliott BA, Biehle J, Conville PS, Cohen S, Saubolle M, Sussland D, et al. Sulfonamide resistance in isolates of Nocardia spp. from a US multicenter survey. J Clin Microbiol. 2012;50(3):670–2.

56. Gombert ME, Aulicino TM, duBouchet L, Silverman GE, Sheinbaum WM. Therapy of experimental cerebral nocardiosis with imipenem, amikacin, trimethoprim-sulfamethoxazole, and minocycline. Antimicrob Agents Chemother. 1986;30(2):270–3.

57. Cercenado E, Marin M, Sanchez-Martinez M, Cuevas O, Martinez-Alarcon J, Bouza E. In vitro activities of tigecycline and eight other antimicrobials against different Nocardia species identified by molecular methods. Antimicrob Agents Chemother. 2007;51(3):1102–4.

58. Brown-Elliott BA, Ward SC, Crist CJ, Mann LB, Wilson RW, Wallace RJ Jr. In vitro activities of linezolid against multiple Nocardia species. Antimicrob Agents Chemother. 2001;45(4):1295–7.

59. Erdstein AA, Daas P, Bradstock KF, Robinson T, Hertzberg MS. Tuberculosis in allogeneic stem cell transplant recipients: still a problem in the 21st century. Transpl Infect Dis. 2004;6(4):142–6.

60. Lewinsohn DM, Leonard MK, LoBue PA, Cohn DL, Daley CL, Desmond E, et al. Official American Thoracic Society/Infectious Diseases Society of America/Centers for Disease Control and Prevention clinical practice guidelines: diagnosis of tuberculosis in adults and children. Clin Infect Dis. 2017;64(2):111–5.

61. Ahmed P, Anwar M, Khan B, Altaf C, Ullah K, Raza S, et al. Role of isoniazid prophylaxis for prevention of tuberculosis in haemopoietic stem cell transplant recipients. J Pak Med Assoc. 2005;55(9):378–81.

62. Saukkonen JJ, Cohn DL, Jasmer RM, Schenker S, Jereb JA, Nolan CM, et al. An official ATS statement: hepatotoxicity of antituberculosis therapy. Am J Respir Crit Care Med. 2006;174(8):935–52.

63. Lubing HN. Peripheral neuropathy in tuberculosis patients treated with isoniazid. Am Rev Tuberc. 1953;68(3):458–61.

64. Nahid P, Dorman SE, Alipanah N, Barry PM, Brozek JL, Cattamanchi A, et al. Executive summary: official American Thoracic Society/Centers for Disease Control and Prevention/Infectious Diseases Society of America clinical practice guidelines: treatment of drug-susceptible tuberculosis. Clin Infect Dis. 2016;63(7):853–67.

65. Finch CK, Chrisman CR, Baciewicz AM, Self TH. Rifampin and rifabutin drug interactions: an update. Arch Intern Med. 2002;162(9):985–92.

66. Centers for Disease C, Prevention, American Thoracic S. Update: adverse event data and revised American Thoracic Society/CDC recommendations against the use of rifampin and pyrazinamide for treatment of latent tuberculosis infection–United States, 2003. MMWR Morb Mortal Wkly Rep. 2003;52(31):735–9.

67. Sterling TR, Villarino ME, Borisov AS, Shang N, Gordin F, Bliven-Sizemore E, et al. Three months of rifapentine and isoniazid for latent tuberculosis infection. N Engl J Med. 2011;365(23):2155–66.

68. Sterling TR, Scott NA, Miro JM, Calvet G, La Rosa A, Infante R, et al. Three months of weekly rifapentine and isoniazid for treatment of Mycobacterium tuberculosis infection in HIV-coinfected persons. AIDS. 2016;30(10):1607–15.

69. Simkins J, Abbo LM, Camargo JF, Rosa R, Morris MI. Twelve-week rifapentine plus isoniazid versus 9-month isoniazid for the treatment of latent tuberculosis in renal transplant candidates. Transplantation. 2017;101(6):1468–72.

70. Griffith DE, Aksamit T, Brown-Elliott BA, Catanzaro A, Daley C, Gordin F, et al. An official ATS/IDSA statement: diagnosis, treatment, and prevention of nontuberculous mycobacterial diseases. Am J Respir Crit Care Med. 2007;175(4):367–416.

71. Engelhard D, Cordonnier C, Shaw PJ, Parkalli T, Guenther C, Martino R, et al. Early and late invasive pneumococcal infection following stem cell transplantation: a European Bone Marrow Transplantation survey. Br J Haematol. 2002;117(2):444–50.

72. Youssef S, Rodriguez G, Rolston KV, Champlin RE, Raad II, Safdar A. Streptococcus pneumoniae infections in 47 hematopoietic stem cell transplantation recipients: clinical characteristics of infections and vaccine-breakthrough infections, 1989-2005. Medicine (Baltimore). 2007;86(2):69–77.

73. Kulkarni S, Powles R, Treleaven J, Riley U, Singhal S, Horton C, et al. Chronic graft versus host disease is associated with long-term risk for pneumococcal infections in recipients of bone marrow transplants. Blood. 2000;95(12):3683–6.

74. Kumashi P, Girgawy E, Tarrand JJ, Rolston KV, Raad II, Safdar A. Streptococcus pneumoniae bacteremia in patients with cancer: disease characteristics and outcomes in the era of escalating drug resistance (1998–2002). Medicine (Baltimore). 2005;84(5):303–12.

75. Centers for Disease C, Prevention. Use of 13-valent pneumococcal conjugate vaccine and 23-valent pneumococcal polysaccharide vaccine for adults with immunocompromising conditions: recommendations of the Advisory Committee on Immunization Practices (ACIP). MMWR Morb Mortal Wkly Rep. 2012;61(40):816–9.

76. Pfaller M, Neofytos D, Diekema D, Azie N, Meier-Kriesche HU, Quan SP, et al. Epidemiology and outcomes of candidemia in 3648 patients: data from the Prospective Antifungal Therapy (PATH Alliance(R)) registry, 2004–2008. Diagn Microbiol Infect Dis. 2012;74(4):323–31.

77. Neofytos D, Horn D, Anaissie E, Steinbach W, Olyaei A, Fishman J, et al. Epidemiology and outcome of invasive fungal infection in adult hematopoietic stem cell transplant recipients: analysis of Multicenter Prospective Antifungal Therapy (PATH) Alliance registry. Clin Infect Dis. 2009;48(3):265–73.

78. Kontoyiannis DP, Marr KA, Park BJ, Alexander BD, Anaissie EJ, Walsh TJ, et al. Prospective surveillance for invasive fungal infections in hematopoietic stem cell transplant recipients, 2001-2006: overview of the Transplant-Associated Infection Surveillance Network (TRANSNET) Database. Clin Infect Dis. 2010;50(8):1091–100.

79. van Burik JH, Leisenring W, Myerson D, Hackman RC, Shulman HM, Sale GE, et al. The effect of prophylactic fluconazole on the clinical spectrum of fungal diseases in bone marrow transplant recipients with special attention to hepatic candidiasis. An autopsy study of 355 patients. Medicine (Baltimore). 1998;77(4):246–54.

80. Singh N. Impact of current transplantation practices on the changing epidemiology of infections in transplant recipients. Lancet Infect Dis. 2003;3(3):156–61.

81. Pons V, Greenspan D, Debruin M. Therapy for oropharyngeal candidiasis in HIV-infected patients: a randomized, prospective multicenter study of oral fluconazole versus clotrimazole troches. The Multicenter Study Group. J Acquir Immune Defic Syndr. 1993;6(12):1311–6.

82. Vazquez JA, Patton LL, Epstein JB, Ramlachan P, Mitha I, Noveljic Z, et al. Randomized, comparative, double-blind, double-dummy, multicenter trial of miconazole buccal tablet and clotrimazole troches for the treatment of oropharyngeal candidiasis:

study of miconazole Lauriad(R) efficacy and safety (SMiLES). HIV Clin Trials. 2010;11(4):186–96.

83. Phillips P, De Beule K, Frechette G, Tchamouroff S, Vandercam B, Weitner L, et al. A double-blind comparison of itraconazole oral solution and fluconazole capsules for the treatment of oropharyngeal candidiasis in patients with AIDS. Clin Infect Dis. 1998;26(6):1368–73.

84. Hegener P, Troke PF, Fatkenheuer G, Diehl V, Ruhnke M. Treatment of fluconazole-resistant candidiasis with voriconazole in patients with AIDS. AIDS. 1998;12(16):2227–8.

85. Skiest DJ, Vazquez JA, Anstead GM, Graybill JR, Reynes J, Ward D, et al. Posaconazole for the treatment of azole-refractory oropharyngeal and esophageal candidiasis in subjects with HIV infection. Clin Infect Dis. 2007;44(4):607–14.

86. Villanueva A, Gotuzzo E, Arathoon EG, Noriega LM, Kartsonis NA, Lupinacci RJ, et al. A randomized double-blind study of caspofungin versus fluconazole for the treatment of esophageal candidiasis. Am J Med. 2002;113(4):294–9.

87. Pfaller MA, Boyken L, Hollis RJ, Kroeger J, Messer SA, Tendolkar S, et al. In vitro susceptibility of invasive isolates of Candida spp. to anidulafungin, caspofungin, and micafungin: six years of global surveillance. J Clin Microbiol. 2008;46(1):150–6.

88. Villanueva A, Arathoon EG, Gotuzzo E, Berman RS, DiNubile MJ, Sable CA. A randomized double-blind study of caspofungin versus amphotericin for the treatment of candidal esophagitis. Clin Infect Dis. 2001;33(9):1529–35.

89. Krause DS, Simjee AE, van Rensburg C, Viljoen J, Walsh TJ, Goldstein BP, et al. A randomized, double-blind trial of anidulafungin versus fluconazole for the treatment of esophageal candidiasis. Clin Infect Dis. 2004;39(6):770–5.

90. de Wet NT, Bester AJ, Viljoen JJ, Filho F, Suleiman JM, Ticona E, et al. A randomized, double blind, comparative trial of micafungin (FK463) vs. fluconazole for the treatment of oesophageal candidiasis. Aliment Pharmacol Ther. 2005;21(7):899–907.

91. Pappas PG, Kauffman CA, Andes DR, Clancy CJ, Marr KA, Ostrosky-Zeichner L, et al. Clinical practice guideline for the management of candidiasis: 2016 update by the Infectious Diseases Society of America. Clin Infect Dis. 2016;62(4):e1–50.

92. Lecciones JA, Lee JW, Navarro EE, Witebsky FG, Marshall D, Steinberg SM, et al. Vascular catheter-associated fungemia in patients with cancer: analysis of 155 episodes. Clin Infect Dis. 1992;14(4):875–83.

93. Labelle AJ, Micek ST, Roubinian N, Kollef MH. Treatment-related risk factors for hospital mortality in Candida bloodstream infections. Crit Care Med. 2008;36(11):2967–72.

94. Garey KW, Rege M, Pai MP, Mingo DE, Suda KJ, Turpin RS, et al. Time to initiation of fluconazole therapy impacts mortality in patients with candidemia: a multi-institutional study. Clin Infect Dis. 2006;43(1):25–31.

95. Morrell M, Fraser VJ, Kollef MH. Delaying the empiric treatment of candida bloodstream infection until positive blood culture results are obtained: a potential risk factor for hospital mortality. Antimicrob Agents Chemother. 2005;49(9):3640–5.

96. Bennett JE. Echinocandins for candidemia in adults without neutropenia. N Engl J Med. 2006;355(11):1154–9.

97. Kontoyiannis DP, Luna MA, Samuels BI, Bodey GP. Hepatosplenic candidiasis. A manifestation of chronic disseminated candidiasis. Infect Dis Clin N Am. 2000;14(3):721–39.

98. De Castro N, Mazoyer E, Porcher R, Raffoux E, Suarez F, Ribaud P, et al. Hepatosplenic candidiasis in the era of new antifungal drugs: a study in Paris 2000-2007. Clin Microbiol Infect. 2012;18(6):E185–7.

99. Rammaert B, Desjardins A, Lortholary O. New insights into hepatosplenic candidosis, a manifestation of chronic disseminated candidosis. Mycoses. 2012;55(3):e74–84.

100. Sallah S, Semelka RC, Sallah W, Vainright JR, Philips DL. Amphotericin B lipid complex for the treatment of patients with acute leukemia and hepatosplenic candidiasis. Leuk Res. 1999;23(11):995–9.

101. Masood A, Sallah S. Chronic disseminated candidiasis in patients with acute leukemia: emphasis on diagnostic definition and treatment. Leuk Res. 2005;29(5):493–501.

102. Kauffman CA, Bradley SF, Ross SC, Weber DR. Hepatosplenic candidiasis: successful treatment with fluconazole. Am J Med. 1991;91(2):137–41.

103. Anaissie E, Bodey GP, Kantarjian H, David C, Barnett K, Bow E, et al. Fluconazole therapy for chronic disseminated candidiasis in patients with leukemia and prior amphotericin B therapy. Am J Med. 1991;91(2):142–50.

104. Legrand F, Lecuit M, Dupont B, Bellaton E, Huerre M, Rohrlich PS, et al. Adjuvant corticosteroid therapy for chronic disseminated candidiasis. Clin Infect Dis. 2008;46(5):696–702.

105. Chaussade H, Bastides F, Lissandre S, Blouin P, Bailly E, Chandenier J, et al. Usefulness of corticosteroid therapy during chronic disseminated candidiasis: case reports and literature review. J Antimicrob Chemother. 2012;67(6):1493–5.

106. Goodman JL, Winston DJ, Greenfield RA, Chandrasekar PH, Fox B, Kaizer H, et al. A controlled trial of fluconazole to prevent fungal infections in patients undergoing bone marrow transplantation. N Engl J Med. 1992;326(13):845–51.

107. Rotstein C, Bow EJ, Laverdiere M, Ioannou S, Carr D, Moghaddam N. Randomized placebo-controlled trial of fluconazole prophylaxis for neutropenic cancer patients: benefit based on purpose and intensity of cytotoxic therapy. The Canadian Fluconazole Prophylaxis Study Group. Clin Infect Dis. 1999;28(2):331–40.

108. Slavin MA, Osborne B, Adams R, Levenstein MJ, Schoch HG, Feldman AR, et al. Efficacy and safety of fluconazole prophylaxis for fungal infections after marrow transplantation–a prospective, randomized, double-blind study. J Infect Dis. 1995;171(6):1545–52.

109. van Burik JA, Ratanatharathorn V, Stepan DE, Miller CB, Lipton JH, Vesole DH, et al. Micafungin versus fluconazole for prophylaxis against invasive fungal infections during neutropenia in patients undergoing hematopoietic stem cell transplantation. Clin Infect Dis. 2004;39(10):1407–16.

110. Cornely OA, Maertens J, Winston DJ, Perfect J, Ullmann AJ, Walsh TJ, et al. Posaconazole vs. fluconazole or itraconazole prophylaxis in patients with neutropenia. N Engl J Med. 2007;356(4):348–59.

111. Ullmann AJ, Lipton JH, Vesole DH, Chandrasekar P, Langston A, Tarantolo SR, et al. Posaconazole or fluconazole for prophylaxis in severe graft-versus-host disease. N Engl J Med. 2007;356(4):335–47.

112. Wingard JR, Carter SL, Walsh TJ, Kurtzberg J, Small TN, Baden LR, et al. Randomized, double-blind trial of fluconazole versus voriconazole for prevention of invasive fungal infection after allogeneic hematopoietic cell transplantation. Blood. 2010;116(24):5111–8.

113. Koh LP, Kurup A, Goh YT, Fook-Chong SM, Tan PH. Randomized trial of fluconazole versus low-dose amphotericin B in prophylaxis against fungal infections in patients undergoing hematopoietic stem cell transplantation. Am J Hematol. 2002;71(4):260–7.

114. Brakhage AA, Langfelder K. Menacing mold: the molecular biology of Aspergillus fumigatus. Annu Rev Microbiol. 2002;56:433–55.

115. Margalit A, Kavanagh K. The innate immune response to Aspergillus fumigatus at the alveolar surface. FEMS Microbiol Rev. 2015;39(5):670–87.

116. Schaffner A, Douglas H, Braude A. Selective protection against conidia by mononuclear and against mycelia by polymorphonuclear phagocytes in resistance to Aspergillus. Observations on these two lines of defense in vivo and in vitro with human and mouse phagocytes. J Clin Invest. 1982;69(3):617–31.

117. Chai LY, van de Veerdonk F, Marijnissen RJ, Cheng SC, Khoo AL, Hectors M, et al. Anti-Aspergillus human host defence relies on type 1 T helper (Th1), rather than type 17 T helper (Th17), cellular immunity. Immunology. 2010;130(1):46–54.

118. Cenci E, Mencacci A, Fe d'Ostiani C, Del Sero G, Mosci P, Montagnoli C, et al. Cytokine- and T helper-dependent lung mucosal immunity in mice with invasive pulmonary aspergillosis. J Infect Dis. 1998;178(6):1750–60.

119. Segal BH. Aspergillosis. N Engl J Med. 2009;360(18):1870–84.

120. Denning DW. Invasive aspergillosis. Clin Infect Dis. 1998;26(4):781–803. quiz 4-5

121. Patterson TF, Thompson GR 3rd, Denning DW, Fishman JA, Hadley S, Herbrecht R, et al. Practice guidelines for the diagnosis and management of aspergillosis: 2016 update by the Infectious

Diseases Society of America. Clin Infect Dis. 2016;63(4):e1–e60.

122. Herbrecht R, Denning DW, Patterson TF, Bennett JE, Greene RE, Oestmann JW, et al. Voriconazole versus amphotericin B for primary therapy of invasive aspergillosis. N Engl J Med. 2002;347(6):408–15.

123. Cornely OA, Maertens J, Bresnik M, Ebrahimi R, Ullmann AJ, Bouza E, et al. Liposomal amphotericin B as initial therapy for invasive mold infection: a randomized trial comparing a high-loading dose regimen with standard dosing (AmBiLoad trial). Clin Infect Dis. 2007;44(10):1289–97.

124. Maertens JA, Raad II, Marr KA, Patterson TF, Kontoyiannis DP, Cornely OA, et al. Isavuconazole versus voriconazole for primary treatment of invasive mould disease caused by Aspergillus and other filamentous fungi (SECURE): a phase 3, randomised-controlled, non-inferiority trial. Lancet. 2016;387(10020):760–9.

125. Kontoyiannis DP, Ratanatharathorn V, Young JA, Raymond J, Laverdiere M, Denning DW, et al. Micafungin alone or in combination with other systemic antifungal therapies in hematopoietic stem cell transplant recipients with invasive aspergillosis. Transpl Infect Dis. 2009;11(1):89–93.

126. Maertens J, Glasmacher A, Herbrecht R, Thiebaut A, Cordonnier C, Segal BH, et al. Multicenter, noncomparative study of caspofungin in combination with other antifungals as salvage therapy in adults with invasive aspergillosis. Cancer. 2006;107(12):2888–97.

127. Denning DW, Marr KA, Lau WM, Facklam DP, Ratanatharathorn V, Becker C, et al. Micafungin (FK463), alone or in combination with other systemic antifungal agents, for the treatment of acute invasive aspergillosis. J Infect. 2006;53(5):337–49.

128. Bernard A, Caillot D, Couaillier JF, Casasnovas O, Guy H, Favre JP. Surgical management of invasive pulmonary aspergillosis in neutropenic patients. Ann Thorac Surg. 1997;64(5):1441–7.

129. Salerno CT, Ouyang DW, Pederson TS, Larson DM, Shake JP, Johnson EM, et al. Surgical therapy for pulmonary aspergillosis in immunocompromised patients. Ann Thorac Surg. 1998;65(5):1415–9.

130. Kuderer NM, Dale DC, Crawford J, Lyman GH. Impact of primary prophylaxis with granulocyte colony-stimulating factor on febrile neutropenia and mortality in adult cancer patients receiving chemotherapy: a systematic review. J Clin Oncol. 2007;25(21):3158–67.

131. Quezada G, Koshkina NV, Zweidler-McKay P, Zhou Z, Kontoyiannis DP, Kleinerman ES. Intranasal granulocyte-macrophage colony-stimulating factor reduces the Aspergillus burden in an immunosuppressed murine model of pulmonary aspergillosis. Antimicrob Agents Chemother. 2008;52(2):716–8.

132. Price TH, Boeckh M, Harrison RW, McCullough J, Ness PM, Strauss RG, et al. Efficacy of transfusion with granulocytes from G-CSF/dexamethasone-treated donors in neutropenic patients with infection. Blood. 2015;126(18):2153–61.

133. Wright DG, Robichaud KJ, Pizzo PA, Deisseroth AB. Lethal pulmonary reactions associated with the combined use of amphotericin B and leukocyte transfusions. N Engl J Med. 1981;304(20):1185–9.

134. Safdar A, Rodriguez G, Ohmagari N, Kontoyiannis DP, Rolston KV, Raad II, et al. The safety of interferon-gamma-1b therapy for invasive fungal infections after hematopoietic stem cell transplantation. Cancer. 2005;103(4):731–9.

135. Maertens J, Buve K, Theunissen K, Meersseman W, Verbeken E, Verhoef G, et al. Galactomannan serves as a surrogate endpoint for outcome of pulmonary invasive aspergillosis in neutropenic hematology patients. Cancer. 2009;115(2):355–62.

136. Andes D, Pascual A, Marchetti O. Antifungal therapeutic drug monitoring: established and emerging indications. Antimicrob Agents Chemother. 2009;53(1):24–34.

137. Ashbee HR, Barnes RA, Johnson EM, Richardson MD, Gorton R, Hope WW. Therapeutic drug monitoring (TDM) of antifungal agents: guidelines from the British Society for Medical Mycology. J Antimicrob Chemother. 2014;69(5):1162–76.

138. Smith J, Safdar N, Knasinski V, Simmons W, Bhavnani SM, Ambrose PG, et al. Voriconazole therapeutic drug monitoring. Antimicrob Agents Chemother. 2006;50(4):1570–2.

139. Tan K, Brayshaw N, Tomaszewski K, Troke P, Wood N. Investigation of the potential relationships between plasma voriconazole concentrations and visual adverse events or liver function test abnormalities. J Clin Pharmacol. 2006;46(2):235–43.

140. Lerolle N, Raffoux E, Socie G, Touratier S, Sauvageon H, Porcher R, et al. Breakthrough invasive fungal disease in patients receiving posaconazole primary prophylaxis: a 4-year study. Clin Microbiol Infect. 2014;20(11):O952–9.

141. Bruggemann RJ, Alffenaar JW, Blijlevens NM, Billaud EM, Kosterink JG, Verweij PE, et al. Clinical relevance of the pharmacokinetic interactions of azole antifungal drugs with other coadministered agents. Clin Infect Dis. 2009;48(10):1441–58.

142. Miceli MH, Kauffman CA. Isavuconazole: a new broad-spectrum triazole antifungal agent. Clin Infect Dis. 2015;61(10):1558–65.

143. Humphrey MJ, Jevons S, Tarbit MH. Pharmacokinetic evaluation of UK-49,858, a metabolically stable triazole antifungal drug, in animals and humans. Antimicrob Agents Chemother. 1985;28(5):648–53.

144. Hyland R, Jones BC, Smith DA. Identification of the cytochrome P450 enzymes involved in the N-oxidation of voriconazole. Drug Metab Dispos. 2003;31(5):540–7.

145. Black DJ, Kunze KL, Wienkers LC, Gidal BE, Seaton TL, McDonnell ND, et al. Warfarin-fluconazole. II. A metabolically based drug interaction: in vivo studies. Drug Metab Dispos. 1996;24(4):422–8.

146. Zonios D, Yamazaki H, Murayama N, Natarajan V, Palmore T, Childs R, et al. Voriconazole metabolism, toxicity, and the effect of cytochrome P450 2C19 genotype. J Infect Dis. 2014;209(12):1941–8.

147. Ikeda Y, Umemura K, Kondo K, Sekiguchi K, Miyoshi S, Nakashima M. Pharmacokinetics of voriconazole and cytochrome P450 2C19 genetic status. Clin Pharmacol Ther. 2004;75(6):587–8.

148. Wang EJ, Lew K, Casciano CN, Clement RP, Johnson WW. Interaction of common azole antifungals with P glycoprotein. Antimicrob Agents Chemother. 2002;46(1):160–5.

149. Dodds-Ashley E. Management of drug and food interactions with azole antifungal agents in transplant recipients. Pharmacotherapy. 2010;30(8):842–54.

150. Martino R, Parody R, Fukuda T, Maertens J, Theunissen K, Ho A, et al. Impact of the intensity of the pretransplantation conditioning regimen in patients with prior invasive aspergillosis undergoing allogeneic hematopoietic stem cell transplantation: a retrospective survey of the Infectious Diseases Working Party of the European Group for Blood and Marrow Transplantation. Blood. 2006;108(9):2928–36.

151. Maziarz RT, Brazauskas R, Chen M, McLeod AA, Martino R, Wingard JR, et al. Pre-existing invasive fungal infection is not a contraindication for allogeneic HSCT for patients with hematologic malignancies: a CIBMTR study. Bone Marrow Transplant. 2016;52:270–8.

152. Greenberg RN, Mullane K, van Burik JA, Raad I, Abzug MJ, Anstead G, et al. Posaconazole as salvage therapy for zygomycosis. Antimicrob Agents Chemother. 2006;50(1):126–33.

153. van Burik JA, Hare RS, Solomon HF, Corrado ML, Kontoyiannis DP. Posaconazole is effective as salvage therapy in zygomycosis: a retrospective summary of 91 cases. Clin Infect Dis. 2006;42(7):e61–5.

154. Marty FM, Ostrosky-Zeichner L, Cornely OA, Mullane KM, Perfect JR, Thompson GR 3rd, et al. Isavuconazole treatment for mucormycosis: a single-arm open-label trial and case-control analysis. Lancet Infect Dis. 2016;16(7):828–37.

155. Perfect JR, Marr KA, Walsh TJ, Greenberg RN, DuPont B, de la Torre-Cisneros J, et al. Voriconazole treatment for less-common, emerging, or refractory fungal infections. Clin Infect Dis. 2003;36(9):1122–31.

156. Raad II, Hachem RY, Herbrecht R, Graybill JR, Hare R, Corcoran G, et al. Posaconazole as salvage treatment for invasive fusariosis in patients with underlying hematologic malignancy and other conditions. Clin Infect Dis. 2006;42(10):1398–403.

157. Hahn T, Cummings KM, Michalek AM, Lipman BJ, Segal BH, McCarthy PL Jr. Efficacy of high-efficiency particulate air filtration in preventing aspergillosis in immunocompromised patients with hematologic malignancies. Infect Control Hosp Epidemiol. 2002;23(9):525–31.

158. Partridge-Hinckley K, Liddell GM, Almyroudis NG, Segal BH. Infection control measures to prevent invasive mould diseases in hematopoietic stem cell transplant recipients. Mycopathologia. 2009;168(6):329–37.

159. Kontoyiannis DP. Preventing fungal disease in chronically immunosuppressed outpatients: time for action? Ann Intern Med. 2013;158(7):555–6.

160. Gergis U, Markey K, Greene J, Kharfan-Dabaja M, Field T, Wetzstein G, et al. Voriconazole provides effective prophylaxis for invasive fungal infection in patients receiving glucocorticoid therapy for GVHD. Bone Marrow Transplant. 2010;45(4):662–7.

161. Molina JR, Serrano J, Sanchez-Garcia J, Rodriguez-Villa A, Gomez P, Tallon D, et al. Voriconazole as primary antifungal prophylaxis in children undergoing allo-SCT. Bone Marrow Transplant. 2012;47(4):562–7.

162. Trifilio SM, Bennett CL, Yarnold PR, McKoy JM, Parada J, Mehta J, et al. Breakthrough zygomycosis after voriconazole administration among patients with hematologic malignancies who receive hematopoietic stem-cell transplants or intensive chemotherapy. Bone Marrow Transplant. 2007;39(7):425–9.

163. Kontoyiannis DP, Lionakis MS, Lewis RE, Chamilos G, Healy M, Perego C, et al. Zygomycosis in a tertiary-care cancer center in the era of Aspergillus-active antifungal therapy: a case-control observational study of 27 recent cases. J Infect Dis. 2005;191(8):1350–60.

164. Almyroudis NG, Sutton DA, Fothergill AW, Rinaldi MG, Kusne S. In vitro susceptibilities of 217 clinical isolates of zygomycetes to conventional and new antifungal agents. Antimicrob Agents Chemother. 2007;51(7):2587–90.

165. Lazo de la Vega S, Volkow P, Yeates RA, Pfaff G. Administration of the antimycotic agents fluconazole and itraconazole to leukaemia patients: a comparative pharmacokinetic study. Drugs Exp Clin Res. 1994;20(2):69–75.

166. van der Horst CM, Saag MS, Cloud GA, Hamill RJ, Graybill JR, Sobel JD, et al. Treatment of cryptococcal meningitis associated with the acquired immunodeficiency syndrome. National Institute of Allergy and Infectious Diseases Mycoses Study Group and AIDS Clinical Trials Group. N Engl J Med. 1997;337(1):15–21.

167. Day JN, Chau TT, Wolbers M, Mai PP, Dung NT, Mai NH, et al. Combination antifungal therapy for cryptococcal meningitis. N Engl J Med. 2013;368(14):1291–302.

168. Vermes A, Guchelaar HJ, Dankert J. Prediction of flucytosine-induced thrombocytopenia using creatinine clearance. Chemotherapy. 2000;46(5):335–41.

169. Singh N, Lortholary O, Alexander BD, Gupta KL, John GT, Pursell KJ, et al. Antifungal management practices and evolution of infection in organ transplant recipients with *cryptococcus neoformans* infection. Transplantation. 2005;80(8):1033–9.

170. Perfect JR, Dismukes WE, Dromer F, Goldman DL, Graybill JR, Hamill RJ, et al. Clinical practice guidelines for the management of cryptococcal disease: 2010 update by the infectious diseases society of america. Clin Infect Dis. 2010;50(3):291–322.

171. Wheat LJ, Freifeld AG, Kleiman MB, Baddley JW, McKinsey DS, Loyd JE, et al. Clinical practice guidelines for the management of patients with histoplasmosis: 2007 update by the Infectious Diseases Society of America. Clin Infect Dis. 2007;45(7):807–25.

172. Johnson PC, Wheat LJ, Cloud GA, Goldman M, Lancaster D, Bamberger DM, et al. Safety and efficacy of liposomal amphotericin B compared with conventional amphotericin B for induction therapy of histoplasmosis in patients with AIDS. Ann Intern Med. 2002;137(2):105–9.

173. Restrepo A, Tobon A, Clark B, Graham DR, Corcoran G, Bradsher RW, et al. Salvage treatment of histoplasmosis with posaconazole. J Infect. 2007;54(4):319–27.

174. Freifeld AG, Iwen PC, Lesiak BL, Gilroy RK, Stevens RB, Kalil AC. Histoplasmosis in solid organ transplant recipients at a large Midwestern university transplant center. Transpl Infect Dis. 2005;7(3–4):109–15.

175. Freifeld A, Proia L, Andes D, Baddour LM, Blair J, Spellberg B, et al. Voriconazole use for endemic fungal infections. Antimicrob Agents Chemother. 2009;53(4):1648–51.

176. Vail GM, Young RS, Wheat LJ, Filo RS, Cornetta K, Goldman M. Incidence of histoplasmosis following allogeneic bone marrow transplant or solid organ transplant in a hyperendemic area. Transpl Infect Dis. 2002;4(3):148–51.

177. Galgiani JN, Ampel NM, Blair JE, Catanzaro A, Geertsma F, Hoover SE, et al. 2016 Infectious Diseases Society of America (IDSA) clinical practice guideline for the treatment of coccidioidomycosis. Clin Infect Dis. 2016;63(6):e112–46.

178. Galgiani JN, Ampel NM, Blair JE, Catanzaro A, Johnson RH, Stevens DA, et al. Coccidioidomycosis. Clin Infect Dis. 2005;41(9):1217–23.

179. Kim MM, Vikram HR, Kusne S, Seville MT, Blair JE. Treatment of refractory coccidioidomycosis with voriconazole or posaconazole. Clin Infect Dis. 2011;53(11):1060–6.

180. Chapman SW, Dismukes WE, Proia LA, Bradsher RW, Pappas PG, Threlkeld MG, et al. Clinical practice guidelines for the management of blastomycosis: 2008 update by the Infectious Diseases Society of America. Clin Infect Dis. 2008;46(12):1801–12.

181. Dismukes WE, Bradsher RW Jr, Cloud GC, Kauffman CA, Chapman SW, George RB, et al. Itraconazole therapy for blastomycosis and histoplasmosis. NIAID Mycoses Study Group. Am J Med. 1992;93(5):489–97.

182. Green H, Paul M, Vidal L, Leibovici L. Prophylaxis of Pneumocystis pneumonia in immunocompromised non-HIV-infected patients: systematic review and meta-analysis of randomized controlled trials. Mayo Clin Proc. 2007;82(9):1052–9.

183. Hughes WT, Rivera GK, Schell MJ, Thornton D, Lott L. Successful intermittent chemoprophylaxis for Pneumocystis carinii pneumonitis. N Engl J Med. 1987;316(26):1627–32.

184. Madden RM, Pui CH, Hughes WT, Flynn PM, Leung W. Prophylaxis of Pneumocystis carinii pneumonia with atovaquone in children with leukemia. Cancer. 2007;109(8):1654–8.

185. Marras TK, Sanders K, Lipton JH, Messner HA, Conly J, Chan CK. Aerosolized pentamidine prophylaxis for Pneumocystis carinii pneumonia after allogeneic marrow transplantation. Transpl Infect Dis. 2002;4(2):66–74.

186. Sangiolo D, Storer B, Nash R, Corey L, Davis C, Flowers M, et al. Toxicity and efficacy of daily dapsone as Pneumocystis jirovecii prophylaxis after hematopoietic stem cell transplantation: a case-control study. Biol Blood Marrow Transplant. 2005;11(7):521–9.

187. Thomas CF Jr, Limper AH. Pneumocystis pneumonia. N Engl J Med. 2004;350(24):2487–98.

188. Saral R, Burns WH, Laskin OL, Santos GW, Lietman PS. Acyclovir prophylaxis of herpes-simplex-virus infections. N Engl J Med. 1981;305(2):63–7.

189. Erard V, Wald A, Corey L, Leisenring WM, Boeckh M. Use of long-term suppressive acyclovir after hematopoietic stem-cell transplantation: impact on herpes simplex virus (HSV) disease and drug-resistant HSV disease. J Infect Dis. 2007;196(2):266–70.

190. Meyers JD, Wade JC, Mitchell CD, Saral R, Lietman PS, Durack DT, et al. Multicenter collaborative trial of intravenous acyclovir for treatment of mucocutaneous herpes simplex virus infection in the immunocompromised host. Am J Med. 1982;73(1A):229–35.

191. Naik HR, Siddique N, Chandrasekar PH. Foscarnet therapy for acyclovir-resistant herpes simplex virus 1 infection in allogeneic bone marrow transplant recipients. Clin Infect Dis. 1995;21(6):1514–5.

192. Zaia J, Baden L, Boeckh MJ, Chakrabarti S, Einsele H, Ljungman P, et al. Viral disease prevention after hematopoietic cell transplantation. Bone Marrow Transplant. 2009;44(8):471–82.

193. Locksley RM, Flournoy N, Sullivan KM, Meyers JD. Infection with varicella-zoster virus after marrow transplantation. J Infect Dis. 1985;152(6):1172–81.

194. Boeckh M, Kim HW, Flowers ME, Meyers JD, Bowden RA. Long-term acyclovir for prevention of varicella zoster virus disease after allogeneic hematopoietic cell transplantation – a randomized double-blind placebo-controlled study. Blood. 2006;107(5):1800–5.

195. Erard V, Guthrie KA, Varley C, Heugel J, Wald A, Flowers ME, et al. One-year acyclovir prophylaxis for preventing varicella-zoster virus disease after hematopoietic cell transplantation: no evidence of rebound varicella-zoster virus disease after drug discontinuation. Blood. 2007;110(8):3071–7.

196. Ljungman P, de la Camara R, Milpied N, Volin L, Russell CA, Crisp A, et al. Randomized study of valacyclovir as prophylaxis against cytomegalovirus reactivation in recipients of allogeneic bone marrow transplants. Blood. 2002;99(8):3050–6.

197. Steer CB, Szer J, Sasadeusz J, Matthews JP, Beresford JA, Grigg A. Varicella-zoster infection after allogeneic bone marrow transplantation: incidence, risk factors and prevention with low-dose aciclovir and ganciclovir. Bone Marrow Transplant. 2000;25(6):657–64.

198. Hatchette T, Tipples GA, Peters G, Alsuwaidi A, Zhou J, Mailman TL. Foscarnet salvage therapy for acyclovir-resistant varicella zoster: report of a novel thymidine kinase mutation and review of the literature. Pediatr Infect Dis J. 2008;27(1):75–7.

199. Meyers JD, Wade JC, Shepp DH, Newton B. Acyclovir treatment of varicella-zoster virus infection in the compromised host. Transplantation. 1984;37(6):571–4.

200. Bilgrami S, Aslanzadeh J, Feingold JM, Bona RD, Clive J, Dorsky D, et al. Cytomegalovirus viremia, viruria and disease after autologous peripheral blood stem cell transplantation: no need for surveillance. Bone Marrow Transplant. 1999;24(1):69–73.

201. Einsele H, Roosnek E, Rufer N, Sinzger C, Riegler S, Loffler J, et al. Infusion of cytomegalovirus (CMV)-specific T cells for the treatment of CMV infection not responding to antiviral chemotherapy. Blood. 2002;99(11):3916–22.

202. Tormo N, Solano C, Benet I, Nieto J, de la Camara R, Lopez J, et al. Reconstitution of CMV pp65 and IE-1-specific IFN-gamma CD8(+) and CD4(+) T-cell responses affording protection from CMV DNAemia following allogeneic hematopoietic SCT. Bone Marrow Transplant. 2011;46(11):1437–43.

203. Fietze E, Prosch S, Reinke P, Stein J, Docke WD, Staffa G, et al. Cytomegalovirus infection in transplant recipients. The role of tumor necrosis factor. Transplantation. 1994;58(6):675–80.

204. Humar A, St Louis P, Mazzulli T, McGeer A, Lipton J, Messner H, et al. Elevated serum cytokines are associated with cytomegalovirus infection and disease in bone marrow transplant recipients. J Infect Dis. 1999;179(2):484–8.

205. Ljungman P, Griffiths P, Paya C. Definitions of cytomegalovirus infection and disease in transplant recipients. Clin Infect Dis. 2002;34(8):1094–7.

206. Ljungman P, Brand R, Hoek J, de la Camara R, Cordonnier C, Einsele H, et al. Donor cytomegalovirus status influences the outcome of allogeneic stem cell transplant: a study by the European group for blood and marrow transplantation. Clin Infect Dis. 2014;59(4):473–81.

207. Ljungman P, Larsson K, Kumlien G, Aschan J, Barkholt L, Gustafsson-Jernberg A, et al. Leukocyte depleted, unscreened blood products give a low risk for CMV infection and disease in CMV seronegative allogeneic stem cell transplant recipients with seronegative stem cell donors. Scand J Infect Dis. 2002;34(5):347–50.

208. Goodrich JM, Bowden RA, Fisher L, Keller C, Schoch G, Meyers JD. Ganciclovir prophylaxis to prevent cytomegalovirus disease after allogeneic marrow transplant. Ann Intern Med. 1993;118(3):173–8.

209. Winston DJ, Ho WG, Bartoni K, Du Mond C, Ebeling DF, Buhles WC, et al. Ganciclovir prophylaxis of cytomegalovirus infection and disease in allogeneic bone marrow transplant recipients. Results of a placebo-controlled, double-blind trial. Ann Intern Med. 1993;118(3):179–84.

210. Nguyen Q, Champlin R, Giralt S, Rolston K, Raad I, Jacobson K, et al. Late cytomegalovirus pneumonia in adult allogeneic blood and marrow transplant recipients. Clin Infect Dis. 1999;28(3):618–23.

211. Marty FM, Ljungman P, Chemaly RF, Maertens J, Dadwal SS, Duarte RF, et al. Letermovir prophylaxis for cytomegalovirus in hematopoietic-cell transplantation. N Engl J Med. 2017;377(25):2433–44.

212. Ljungman P, Aschan J, Lewensohn-Fuchs I, Carlens S, Larsson K, Lonnqvist B, et al. Results of different strategies for reducing cytomegalovirus-associated mortality in allogeneic stem cell transplant recipients. Transplantation. 1998;66(10):1330–4.

213. Boeckh M, Gooley TA, Myerson D, Cunningham T, Schoch G, Bowden RA. Cytomegalovirus pp65 antigenemia-guided early treatment with ganciclovir versus ganciclovir at engraftment after allogeneic marrow transplantation: a randomized double-blind study. Blood. 1996;88(10):4063–71.

214. Drew WL. Laboratory diagnosis of cytomegalovirus infection and disease in immunocompromised patients. Curr Opin Infect Dis. 2007;20(4):408–11.

215. Gerna G, Lilleri D, Baldanti F, Torsellini M, Giorgiani G, Zecca M, et al. Human cytomegalovirus immediate-early mRNAemia versus pp65 antigenemia for guiding pre-emptive therapy in children and young adults undergoing hematopoietic stem cell transplantation: a prospective, randomized, open-label trial. Blood. 2003;101(12):5053–60.

216. Reusser P, Einsele H, Lee J, Volin L, Rovira M, Engelhard D, et al. Randomized multicenter trial of foscarnet versus ganciclovir for preemptive therapy of cytomegalovirus infection after allogeneic stem cell transplantation. Blood. 2002;99(4):1159–64.

217. Goodrich JM, Mori M, Gleaves CA, Du Mond C, Cays M, Ebeling DF, et al. Early treatment with ganciclovir to prevent cytomegalovirus disease after allogeneic bone marrow transplantation. N Engl J Med. 1991;325(23):1601–7.

218. van der Heiden PL, Kalpoe JS, Barge RM, Willemze R, Kroes AC, Schippers EF. Oral valganciclovir as pre-emptive therapy has similar efficacy on cytomegalovirus DNA load reduction as intravenous ganciclovir in allogeneic stem cell transplantation recipients. Bone Marrow Transplant. 2006;37(7):693–8.

219. Nichols WG, Corey L, Gooley T, Drew WL, Miner R, Huang M, et al. Rising pp65 antigenemia during preemptive anticytomegalovirus therapy after allogeneic hematopoietic stem cell transplantation: risk factors, correlation with DNA load, and outcomes. Blood. 2001;97(4):867–74.

220. Kharfan-Dabaja MA, Boeckh M, Wilck MB, Langston AA, Chu AH, Wloch MK, et al. A novel therapeutic cytomegalovirus DNA vaccine in allogeneic haemopoietic stem-cell transplantation: a randomised, double-blind, placebo-controlled, phase 2 trial. Lancet Infect Dis. 2012;12(4):290–9.

221. La Rosa C, Longmate J, Lacey SF, Kaltcheva T, Sharan R, Marsano D, et al. Clinical evaluation of safety and immunogenicity of PADRE-cytomegalovirus (CMV) and tetanus-CMV fusion peptide vaccines with or without PF03512676 adjuvant. J Infect Dis. 2012;205(8):1294–304.

222. Krause H, Hebart H, Jahn G, Muller CA, Einsele H. Screening for CMV-specific T cell proliferation to identify patients at risk of developing late onset CMV disease. Bone Marrow Transplant. 1997;19(11):1111–6.

223. Reusser P, Riddell SR, Meyers JD, Greenberg PD. Cytotoxic T-lymphocyte response to cytomegalovirus after human allogeneic bone marrow transplantation: pattern of recovery and correlation with cytomegalovirus infection and disease. Blood. 1991;78(5):1373–80.

224. Hakki M, Riddell SR, Storek J, Carter RA, Stevens-Ayers T, Sudour P, et al. Immune reconstitution to cytomegalovirus after allogeneic hematopoietic stem cell transplantation: impact of host factors, drug therapy, and subclinical reactivation. Blood. 2003;102(8):3060–7.

225. Ljungman P, Aschan J, Azinge JN, Brandt L, Ehrnst A, Hammarstrom V, et al. Cytomegalovirus viraemia and specific T-helper cell responses as predictors of disease after allogeneic marrow transplantation. Br J Haematol. 1993;83(1):118–24.

226. Erard V, Guthrie KA, Seo S, Smith J, Huang M, Chien J, et al. Reduced mortality of cytomegalovirus pneumonia after hematopoietic cell transplantation due to antiviral therapy and changes in transplantation practices. Clin Infect Dis. 2015;61(1):31–9.

227. Reed EC, Bowden RA, Dandliker PS, Lilleby KE, Meyers JD. Treatment of cytomegalovirus pneumonia with ganciclovir and intravenous cytomegalovirus immunoglobulin in patients with bone marrow transplants. Ann Intern Med. 1988;109(10):783–8.

228. Alexander BT, Hladnik LM, Augustin KM, Casabar E, McKinnon PS, Reichley RM, et al. Use of cytomegalovirus intravenous immune globulin for the adjunctive treatment of cytomegalovirus in hematopoietic stem cell transplant recipients. Pharmacotherapy. 2010;30(6):554–61.

229. Crippa F, Corey L, Chuang EL, Sale G, Boeckh M. Virological, clinical, and ophthalmologic features of cytomegalovirus retinitis after hematopoietic stem cell transplantation. Clin Infect Dis. 2001;32(2):214–9.

230. Chang M, Dunn JP. Ganciclovir implant in the treatment of cytomegalovirus retinitis. Expert Rev Med Devices. 2005;2(4):421–7.

231. Shmueli E, Or R, Shapira MY, Resnick IB, Caplan O, Bdolah-Abram T, et al. High rate of cytomegalovirus drug resistance among patients receiving preemptive antiviral treatment after haploidentical stem cell transplantation. J Infect Dis. 2014;209(4):557–61.

232. Hantz S, Garnier-Geoffroy F, Mazeron MC, Garrigue I, Merville P, Mengelle C, et al. Drug-resistant cytomegalovirus in transplant recipients: a French cohort study. J Antimicrob Chemother. 2010;65(12):2628–40.

233. Hall Sedlak R, Castor J, Butler-Wu SM, Chan E, Cook L, Limaye AP, et al. Rapid detection of human cytomegalovirus UL97 and UL54 mutations directly from patient samples. J Clin Microbiol. 2013;51(7):2354–9.

234. Chou S, Ercolani RJ, Sahoo MK, Lefterova MI, Strasfeld LM, Pinsky BA. Improved detection of emerging drug-resistant mutant cytomegalovirus subpopulations by deep sequencing. Antimicrob Agents Chemother. 2014;58(8):4697–702.

235. Chou S, Erice A, Jordan MC, Vercellotti GM, Michels KR, Talarico CL, et al. Analysis of the UL97 phosphotransferase coding sequence in clinical cytomegalovirus isolates and identification of mutations conferring ganciclovir resistance. J Infect Dis. 1995;171(3):576–83.

236. Lurain NS, Chou S. Antiviral drug resistance of human cytomegalovirus. Clin Microbiol Rev. 2010;23(4):689–712.

237. El Chaer F, Shah DP, Chemaly RF. How I treat resistant cytomegalovirus infection in hematopoietic cell transplantation recipients. Blood. 2016;128(23):2624–36.

238. Smith IL, Cherrington JM, Jiles RE, Fuller MD, Freeman WR, Spector SA. High-level resistance of cytomegalovirus to ganciclovir is associated with alterations in both the UL97 and DNA polymerase genes. J Infect Dis. 1997;176(1):69–77.

239. Bacigalupo A, Bregante S, Tedone E, Isaza A, Van Lint MT, Moro F, et al. Combined foscarnet -ganciclovir treatment for cytomegalovirus infections after allogeneic hemopoietic stem cell transplantation (Hsct). Bone Marrow Transplant. 1996;18(Suppl 2):110–4.

240. Mylonakis E, Kallas WM, Fishman JA. Combination antiviral therapy for ganciclovir-resistant cytomegalovirus infection in solid-organ transplant recipients. Clin Infect Dis. 2002;34(10):1337–41.

241. Emery VC, Griffiths PD. Prediction of cytomegalovirus load and resistance patterns after antiviral chemotherapy. Proc Natl Acad Sci U S A. 2000;97(14):8039–44.

242. Manion DJ, Vibhagool A, Chou TC, Kaplan J, Caliendo A, Hirsch MS. Susceptibility of human cytomegalovirus to two-drug combinations in vitro. Antivir Ther. 1996;1(4):237–45.

243. Manischewitz JF, Quinnan GV Jr, Lane HC, Wittek AE. Synergistic effect of ganciclovir and foscarnet on cytomegalovirus replication in vitro. Antimicrob Agents Chemother. 1990;34(2):373–5.

244. Gracia-Ahufinger I, Gutierrez-Aroca J, Cordero E, Vidal E, Cantisan S, del Castillo D, et al. Use of

high-dose ganciclovir for the treatment of cytomegalovirus replication in solid organ transplant patients with ganciclovir resistance-inducing mutations. Transplantation. 2013;95(8):1015–20.

245. Drew WL, Miner RC, Marousek GI, Chou S. Maribavir sensitivity of cytomegalovirus isolates resistant to ganciclovir, cidofovir or foscarnet. J Clin Virol. 2006;37(2):124–7.

246. Lischka P, Hewlett G, Wunberg T, Baumeister J, Paulsen D, Goldner T, et al. In vitro and in vivo activities of the novel anticytomegalovirus compound AIC246. Antimicrob Agents Chemother. 2010;54(3):1290–7.

247. Marty FM, Bryar J, Browne SK, Schwarzberg T, Ho VT, Bassett IV, et al. Sirolimus-based graft-versus-host disease prophylaxis protects against cytomegalovirus reactivation after allogeneic hematopoietic stem cell transplantation: a cohort analysis. Blood. 2007;110(2):490–500.

248. Heslop HE, Leen AM. T-cell therapy for viral infections. Hematology Am Soc Hematol Educ Program. 2013;2013:342–7.

249. Biron KK, Harvey RJ, Chamberlain SC, Good SS, Smith AA 3rd, Davis MG, et al. Potent and selective inhibition of human cytomegalovirus replication by 1263W94, a benzimidazole L-riboside with a unique mode of action. Antimicrob Agents Chemother. 2002;46(8):2365–72.

250. Marty FM, Ljungman P, Papanicolaou GA, Winston DJ, Chemaly RF, Strasfeld L, et al. Maribavir prophylaxis for prevention of cytomegalovirus disease in recipients of allogeneic stem-cell transplants: a phase 3, double-blind, placebo-controlled, randomised trial. Lancet Infect Dis. 2011;11(4):284–92.

251. Avery RK, Marty FM, Strasfeld L, Lee I, Arrieta A, Chou S, et al. Oral maribavir for treatment of refractory or resistant cytomegalovirus infections in transplant recipients. Transpl Infect Dis. 2010;12(6):489–96.

252. Alain S, Revest M, Veyer D, Essig M, Rerolles JP, Rawlinson W, et al. Maribavir use in practice for cytomegalovirus infection in French transplantation centers. Transplant Proc. 2013;45(4):1603–7.

253. Williams-Aziz SL, Hartline CB, Harden EA, Daily SL, Prichard MN, Kushner NL, et al. Comparative activities of lipid esters of cidofovir and cyclic cidofovir against replication of herpesviruses in vitro. Antimicrob Agents Chemother. 2005;49(9):3724–33.

254. Ogata M, Satou T, Kadota J, Saito N, Yoshida T, Okumura H, et al. Human herpesvirus 6 (HHV-6) reactivation and HHV-6 encephalitis after allogeneic hematopoietic cell transplantation: a multicenter, prospective study. Clin Infect Dis. 2013;57(5):671–81.

255. Yoshikawa T, Asano Y, Ihira M, Suzuki K, Ohashi M, Suga S, et al. Human herpesvirus 6 viremia in bone marrow transplant recipients: clinical features and risk factors. J Infect Dis. 2002;185(7):847–53.

256. Isomura H, Yamada M, Yoshida M, Tanaka H, Kitamura T, Oda M, et al. Suppressive effects of human herpesvirus 6 on in vitro colony formation of hematopoietic progenitor cells. J Med Virol. 1997;52(4):406–12.

257. Tunkel AR, Glaser CA, Bloch KC, Sejvar JJ, Marra CM, Roos KL, et al. The management of encephalitis: clinical practice guidelines by the Infectious Diseases Society of America. Clin Infect Dis. 2008;47(3):303–27.

258. Zerr DM, Gupta D, Huang ML, Carter R, Corey L. Effect of antivirals on human herpesvirus 6 replication in hematopoietic stem cell transplant recipients. Clin Infect Dis. 2002;34(3):309–17.

259. Ljungman P, Ribaud P, Eyrich M, Matthes-Martin S, Einsele H, Bleakley M, et al. Cidofovir for adenovirus infections after allogeneic hematopoietic stem cell transplantation: a survey by the Infectious Diseases Working Party of the European Group for Blood and Marrow Transplantation. Bone Marrow Transplant. 2003;31(6):481–6.

260. Patton DF, Wilkowski CW, Hanson CA, Shapiro R, Gajl-Peczalska KJ, Filipovich AH, et al. Epstein-Barr virus–determined clonality in posttransplant lymphoproliferative disease. Transplantation. 1990;49(6):1080–4.

261. Rouce RH, Louis CU, Heslop HE. Epstein-Barr virus lymphoproliferative disease after hematopoietic stem cell transplant. Curr Opin Hematol. 2014;21(6):476–81.

262. Funch DP, Walker AM, Schneider G, Ziyadeh NJ, Pescovitz MD. Ganciclovir and acyclovir reduce the risk of post-transplant lymphoproliferative disorder in renal transplant recipients. Am J Transplant. 2005;5(12):2894–900.

263. Baldwin A, Kingman H, Darville M, Foot AB, Grier D, Cornish JM, et al. Outcome and clinical course of 100 patients with adenovirus infection following bone marrow transplantation. Bone Marrow Transplant. 2000;26(12):1333–8.

264. Ison MG. Adenovirus infections in transplant recipients. Clin Infect Dis. 2006;43(3):331–9.

265. Neofytos D, Ojha A, Mookerjee B, Wagner J, Filicko J, Ferber A, et al. Treatment of adenovirus disease in stem cell transplant recipients with cidofovir. Biol Blood Marrow Transplant. 2007;13(1):74–81.

266. Lion T, Baumgartinger R, Watzinger F, Matthes-Martin S, Suda M, Preuner S, et al. Molecular monitoring of adenovirus in peripheral blood after allogeneic bone marrow transplantation permits early diagnosis of disseminated disease. Blood. 2003;102(3):1114–20.

267. Morfin F, Dupuis-Girod S, Frobert E, Mundweiler S, Carrington D, Sedlacek P, et al. Differential susceptibility of adenovirus clinical isolates to cidofovir and ribavirin is not related to species alone. Antivir Ther. 2009;14(1):55–61.

268. Hoffman JA, Shah AJ, Ross LA, Kapoor N. Adenoviral infections and a prospective trial

of cidofovir in pediatric hematopoietic stem cell transplantation. Biol Blood Marrow Transplant. 2001;7(7):388–94.

269. Anderson EJ, Guzman-Cottrill JA, Kletzel M, Thormann K, Sullivan C, Zheng X, et al. High-risk adenovirus-infected pediatric allogeneic hematopoietic progenitor cell transplant recipients and preemptive cidofovir therapy. Pediatr Transplant. 2008;12(2):219–27.

270. ViSTIDE® (cidofovir injection) – Package Insert 2000, June 20, 2017. Available from: https://www.accessdata.fda.gov/drugsatfda_docs/label/1999/020638s003lbl.pdf.

271. Hiwarkar P, Amrolia P, Sivaprakasam P, Lum SH, Doss H, O'Rafferty C, et al. Brincidofovir is highly efficacious in controlling adenoviremia in pediatric recipients of hematopoietic cell transplant. Blood. 2017;129(14):2033–7.

272. Lankester AC, Heemskerk B, Claas EC, Schilham MW, Beersma MF, Bredius RG, et al. Effect of ribavirin on the plasma viral DNA load in patients with disseminating adenovirus infection. Clin Infect Dis. 2004;38(11):1521–5.

273. Gavin PJ, Katz BZ. Intravenous ribavirin treatment for severe adenovirus disease in immunocompromised children. Pediatrics. 2002;110(1 Pt 1):e9.

274. Myers GD, Bollard CM, Wu MF, Weiss H, Rooney CM, Heslop HE, et al. Reconstitution of adenovirus-specific cell-mediated immunity in pediatric patients after hematopoietic stem cell transplantation. Bone Marrow Transplant. 2007;39(11):677–86.

275. Feuchtinger T, Matthes-Martin S, Richard C, Lion T, Fuhrer M, Hamprecht K, et al. Safe adoptive transfer of virus-specific T-cell immunity for the treatment of systemic adenovirus infection after allogeneic stem cell transplantation. Br J Haematol. 2006;134(1):64–76.

276. Khanna N, Steffen I, Studt JD, Schreiber A, Lehmann T, Weisser M, et al. Outcome of influenza infections in outpatients after allogeneic hematopoietic stem cell transplantation. Transpl Infect Dis. 2009;11(2):100–5.

277. Choi SM, Boudreault AA, Xie H, Englund JA, Corey L, Boeckh M. Differences in clinical outcomes after 2009 influenza A/H1N1 and seasonal influenza among hematopoietic cell transplant recipients. Blood. 2011;117(19):5050–6.

278. Nicholson KG, Aoki FY, Osterhaus AD, Trottier S, Carewicz O, Mercier CH, et al. Efficacy and safety of oseltamivir in treatment of acute influenza: a randomised controlled trial. Neuraminidase Inhibitor Flu Treatment Investigator Group. Lancet. 2000;355(9218):1845–50.

279. Chemaly RF, Shah DP, Boeckh MJ. Management of respiratory viral infections in hematopoietic cell transplant recipients and patients with hematologic malignancies. Clin Infect Dis. 2014;59(Suppl 5):S344–51.

280. Renaud C, Englund JA. Antiviral therapy of respiratory viruses in haematopoietic stem cell transplant recipients. Antivir Ther. 2012;17(1 Pt B):175–91.

281. Waghmare A, Campbell AP, Xie H, Seo S, Kuypers J, Leisenring W, et al. Respiratory syncytial virus lower respiratory disease in hematopoietic cell transplant recipients: viral RNA detection in blood, antiviral treatment, and clinical outcomes. Clin Infect Dis. 2013;57(12):1731–41.

282. Marcelin JR, Wilson JW, Razonable RR, Mayo Clinic HO, Transplant Infectious Diseases S. Oral ribavirin therapy for respiratory syncytial virus infections in moderately to severely immunocompromised patients. Transpl Infect Dis. 2014;16(2):242–50.

283. Avetisyan G, Mattsson J, Sparrelid E, Ljungman P. Respiratory syncytial virus infection in recipients of allogeneic stem-cell transplantation: a retrospective study of the incidence, clinical features, and outcome. Transplantation. 2009;88(10):1222–6.

284. De Vincenzo JP, Leombruno D, Soiffer RJ, Siber GR. Immunotherapy of respiratory syncytial virus pneumonia following bone marrow transplantation. Bone Marrow Transplant. 1996;17(6):1051–6.

285. Cesaro S, Hirsch HH, Faraci M, Owoc-Lempach J, Beltrame A, Tendas A, et al. Cidofovir for BK virus-associated hemorrhagic cystitis: a retrospective study. Clin Infect Dis. 2009;49(2):233–40.

286. Vats A, Shapiro R, Singh Randhawa P, Scantlebury V, Tuzuner A, Saxena M, et al. Quantitative viral load monitoring and cidofovir therapy for the management of BK virus-associated nephropathy in children and adults. Transplantation. 2003;75(1):105–12.

287. Rinaldo CH, Hirsch HH. Antivirals for the treatment of polyomavirus BK replication. Expert Rev Anti-Infect Ther. 2007;5(1):105–15.

288. Lee BT, Gabardi S, Grafals M, Hofmann RM, Akalin E, Aljanabi A, et al. Efficacy of levofloxacin in the treatment of BK viremia: a multicenter, double-blinded, randomized, placebo-controlled trial. Clin J Am Soc Nephrol. 2014;9(3):583–9.

289. Leung AY, Chan MT, Yuen KY, Cheng VC, Chan KH, Wong CL, et al. Ciprofloxacin decreased polyoma BK virus load in patients who underwent allogeneic hematopoietic stem cell transplantation. Clin Infect Dis. 2005;40(4):528–37.

290. Sener A, House AA, Jevnikar AM, Boudville N, McAlister VC, Muirhead N, et al. Intravenous immunoglobulin as a treatment for BK virus associated nephropathy: one-year follow-up of renal allograft recipients. Transplantation. 2006;81(1):117–20.

291. Farasati NA, Shapiro R, Vats A, Randhawa P. Effect of leflunomide and cidofovir on replication of BK virus in an in vitro culture system. Transplantation. 2005;79(1):116–8.

292. Shitrit D, Lev N, Bar-Gil-Shitrit A, Kramer MR. Progressive multifocal leukoencephalopathy in transplant recipients. Transpl Int. 2005;17(11):658–65.

293. De Luca A, Ammassari A, Pezzotti P, Cinque P, Gasnault J, Berenguer J, et al. Cidofovir in addition to antiretroviral treatment is not effective for AIDS-associated progressive multifocal leukoencephalopathy: a multicohort analysis. AIDS. 2008;22(14):1759–67.

294. Hall CD, Dafni U, Simpson D, Clifford D, Wetherill PE, Cohen B, et al. Failure of cytarabine in progressive multifocal leukoencephalopathy associated with human immunodeficiency virus infection. AIDS Clinical Trials Group 243 Team. N Engl J Med. 1998;338(19):1345–51.

295. Jamilloux Y, Kerever S, Ferry T, Broussolle C, Honnorat J, Seve P. Treatment of progressive multifocal leukoencephalopathy with mirtazapine. Clin Drug Investig. 2016;36(10):783–9.

296. Verma S, Cikurel K, Koralnik IJ, Morgello S, Cunningham-Rundles C, Weinstein ZR, et al. Mirtazapine in progressive multifocal leukoencephalopathy associated with polycythemia vera. J Infect Dis. 2007;196(5):709–11.

297. Clifford DB, Nath A, Cinque P, Brew BJ, Zivadinov R, Gorelik L, et al. A study of mefloquine treatment for progressive multifocal leukoencephalopathy: results and exploration of predictors of PML outcomes. J Neurovirol. 2013;19(4):351–8.

298. Brickelmaier M, Lugovskoy A, Kartikeyan R, Reviriego-Mendoza MM, Allaire N, Simon K, et al. Identification and characterization of mefloquine efficacy against JC virus in vitro. Antimicrob Agents Chemother. 2009;53(5):1840–9.

299. Sospedra M, Schippling S, Yousef S, Jelcic I, Bofill-Mas S, Planas R, et al. Treating progressive multifocal leukoencephalopathy with interleukin 7 and vaccination with JC virus capsid protein VP1. Clin Infect Dis. 2014;59(11):1588–92.

300. Slavin MA, Meyers JD, Remington JS, Hackman RC. Toxoplasma gondii infection in marrow transplant recipients: a 20 year experience. Bone Marrow Transplant. 1994;13(5):549–57.

301. Geissmann F, Derouin F, Marolleau JP, Gisselbrecht C, Brice P. Disseminated toxoplasmosis following autologous bone marrow transplantation. Clin Infect Dis. 1994;19(4):800–1.

302. Small TN, Leung L, Stiles J, Kiehn TE, Malak SA, O'Reilly RJ, et al. Disseminated toxoplasmosis following T cell-depleted related and unrelated bone marrow transplantation. Bone Marrow Transplant. 2000;25(9):969–73.

303. Derouin F, Gluckman E, Beauvais B, Devergie A, Melo R, Monny M, et al. Toxoplasma infection after human allogeneic bone marrow transplantation: clinical and serological study of 80 patients. Bone Marrow Transplant. 1986;1(1):67–73.

304. Mele A, Paterson PJ, Prentice HG, Leoni P, Kibbler CC. Toxoplasmosis in bone marrow transplantation: a report of two cases and systematic review of the literature. Bone Marrow Transplant. 2002;29(8):691–8.

305. Katlama C, De Wit S, O'Doherty E, Van Glabeke M, Clumeck N. Pyrimethamine-clindamycin vs. pyrimethamine-sulfadiazine as acute and long-term therapy for toxoplasmic encephalitis in patients with AIDS. Clin Infect Dis. 1996;22(2):268–75.

306. Torre D, Casari S, Speranza F, Donisi A, Gregis G, Poggio A, et al. Randomized trial of trimethoprim-sulfamethoxazole versus pyrimethamine-sulfadiazine for therapy of toxoplasmic encephalitis in patients with AIDS. Italian Collaborative Study Group. Antimicrob Agents Chemother. 1998;42(6):1346–9.

307. Liu LX, Weller PF. Strongyloidiasis and other intestinal nematode infections. Infect Dis Clin N Am. 1993;7(3):655–82.

308. Roxby AC, Gottlieb GS, Limaye AP. Strongyloidiasis in transplant patients. Clin Infect Dis. 2009;49(9):1411–23.

309. Wirk B, Wingard JR. Strongyloides stercoralis hyperinfection in hematopoietic stem cell transplantation. Transpl Infect Dis. 2009;11(2):143–8.

310. Zaha O, Hirata T, Uchima N, Kinjo F, Saito A. Comparison of anthelmintic effects of two doses of ivermectin on intestinal strongyloidiasis in patients negative or positive for anti-HTLV-1 antibody. J Infect Chemother. 2004;10(6):348–51.

311. Zaha O, Hirata T, Kinjo F, Saito A, Fukuhara H. Efficacy of ivermectin for chronic strongyloidiasis: two single doses given 2 weeks apart. J Infect Chemother. 2002;8(1):94–8.

312. Marti H, Haji HJ, Savioli L, Chwaya HM, Mgeni AF, Ameir JS, et al. A comparative trial of a single-dose ivermectin versus three days of albendazole for treatment of Strongyloides stercoralis and other soil-transmitted helminth infections in children. Am J Trop Med Hyg. 1996;55(5):477–81.

313. Sanguinetti M, Posteraro B, Lass-Florl C. Antifungal drug resistance among Candida species: mechanisms and clinical impact. Mycoses. 2015;58(Suppl 2):2–13.

314. Wiederhold NP, Patterson TF. Emergence of azole resistance in aspergillus. Semin Respir Crit Care Med. 2015;36(5):673–80.

315. Peled JU, Devlin SM, Staffas A, Lumish M, Khanin R, Littmann ER, et al. Intestinal microbiota and relapse after hematopoietic-cell transplantation. J Clin Oncol. 2017;35(15):1650–9.

316. Taur Y, Jenq RR, Perales MA, Littmann ER, Morjaria S, Ling L, et al. The effects of intestinal tract bacterial diversity on mortality following allogeneic hematopoietic stem cell transplantation. Blood. 2014;124(7):1174–82.

317. Jenq RR, Taur Y, Devlin SM, Ponce DM, Goldberg JD, Ahr KF, et al. Intestinal Blautia is associated with reduced death from graft-versus-host disease. Biol Blood Marrow Transplant. 2015;21(8):1373–83.

318. Mullighan CG, Heatley SL, Danner S, Dean MM, Doherty K, Hahn U, et al. Mannose-binding lectin status is associated with risk of major infection following myeloablative sibling allogeneic hematopoietic stem cell transplantation. Blood. 2008;112(5):2120–8.

319. Bochud PY, Chien JW, Marr KA, Leisenring WM, Upton A, Janer M, et al. Toll-like receptor 4 polymorphisms and aspergillosis in stem-cell transplantation. N Engl J Med. 2008;359(17):1766–77.

320. Zaia JA, Sun JY, Gallez-Hawkins GM, Thao L, Oki A, Lacey SF, et al. The effect of single and combined activating killer immunoglobulin-like receptor genotypes on cytomegalovirus infection and immunity after hematopoietic cell transplantation. Biol Blood Marrow Transplant. 2009;15(3):315–25.

Infections in Solid Organ Transplant Recipients

12

Shahid Husain and Coleman Rotstein

Introduction

Solid organ transplant (SOT) recipients are unique among immunocompromised hosts. Similar to other immunocompromised patients, they are susceptible to infections caused by endogenous organisms through reactivation of pre-existing or latent infections but also infections caused by exogenous organisms acquired from the environment or other personnel. However, what is unique to SOT recipients is that they are also predisposed to infections that may be transmitted from the donor themselves [1]. Thus, one can approach infections in SOT recipients according to a timeline of infection. This timeline correlates with the host's immunity to infection counterbalanced by the host's susceptibility to infection due to the superimposed immunosuppression produced by the immunosuppressive agents used to prevent rejection of the transplanted organ. An additional issue regarding infections in SOT recipients is that the typical signs and symptoms of infection are often absent or blunted due to the presence of this immunosuppression.

S. Husain (✉) · C. Rotstein (✉)
Division of Infectious Diseases, Department of
Medicine, University of Toronto, and Multi-organ
Transplant Program, University Health Network,
Toronto, ON, Canada
e-mail: Shahid.Husain@uhn.ca; Coleman.Rotstein@
uhn.ca

Overview of Infections in SOT

SOT recipients are at a higher risk for both common and opportunistic infections compared to immunocompetent individuals. Among the SOT recipients, small bowel transplant recipients have the highest risk of infections at any time point after transplant followed by lung transplant recipients. In the absence of allograft rejection, kidney transplantation probably has the lowest risk of infections.

The type of infection that a transplant recipient gets depends on several factors. Most important is perhaps the "net state of immunosuppression" which is an abstract concept, and none of the known surrogate markers, such as immunosuppressive drug levels or T cell functional assays, predict the risk with certainty. As immunosuppression is highest during the early period of transplant, the risk of infection is highest during that period.

Timeline of Infection in SOT Recipients

Traditionally, three risk periods have been defined, an initial one during the 1st month after transplantation, a second period between 1 and 6 months, and a third period that extends beyond 6 months (Fig. 12.1) [1]. However, it is to be noted that these designations are arbitrary and

© Springer International Publishing AG, part of Springer Nature 2018
B. H. Segal (ed.), *Management of Infections in the Immunocompromised Host*,
https://doi.org/10.1007/978-3-319-77674-3_12

Fig. 12.1 Relative distribution of pathogens posttransplantation

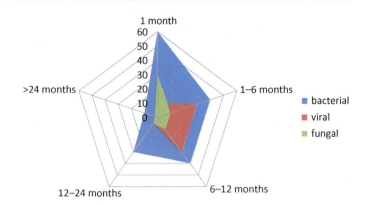

modified by the net state of immunosuppression and the use of various prophylactic strategies to prevent infection.

Infections Occurring in the 1st Month

This period can also be called the period of nosocomial infection or period of donor-derived infections. Bacterial infections associated with the surgical procedure or donor-derived infections are predominant during this period. Most clinical syndromes noted during this period are the result of surgery, such as surgical site infection, mediastinitis, empyema, subdiaphragmatic abscesses, or retroperitoneal abscesses [2]. The etiology of these bacterial organisms depends on the origin of the bacteria producing the infection such as those infections arising from intra-abdominal surgery (superficial epidermal origin versus organ/space infections arising from gastrointestinal organs), and their susceptibility will be determined by previous exposure to antibiotics along with the pattern prevalent in the community.

Another common source of infection during this period is donor-derived infections. With the increased use of high-risk donors who may be infected at the time of organ procurement, the rate of donor-derived infections in transplant recipients is rising. The most common donor-derived infections are bacterial infections. Every organ procurement organization has standardized procedures to detect these infections. As a general rule, bacteremia in the donor increases the risk in all organs retrieved; positive BAL cultures from the donor are significant risks only for lung transplant recipients, while a positive urine culture from the donor may cause urinary tract infection in renal transplant recipients. Among the fungi, *Candida* species are the most common; *Cryptococcus neoformans*, *Histoplasma capsulatum*, and *Coccidioides immitis* have been identified as causes of donor-derived infection, and inadvertent transmissions have been noted for *Aspergillus* species as well. Similarly, among the viruses, rabies, lymphocytic choriomeningitis virus (LCMV), HIV, hepatitis C virus (HCV), and West Nile virus (WNV) have also been reported to cause donor-derived infection, albeit rarely. Prior colonization with *Aspergillus* or *Pseudomonas* species in lung transplant recipients and *Candida* colonization in liver transplant recipients may also cause severe disease [3–9].

Infections from 1 to 6 Months

This period is also called the period of reactivation of latent infection or opportunistic infections. Bacterial infections are not the major infections during this period. Herpes virus reactivation, especially Cytomegalovirus infections, is noted during this period in the absence of antiviral prophylaxis. Similarly, BK virus infections in kidney transplant recipients [10] and HCV infection in the liver transplant recipients are the major concerns. Among the opportunistic infections, *Pneumocystis jirovecii* infection in the absence of prophylaxis or cryptococcal and *Aspergillus* infection also occur during this period. Infections with *Listeria*, *Nocardia*, *Toxoplasma*, *Strongyloides*, *Leishmania*, and *Trypanosoma cruzi* may also be found during this period. Prophylaxis with trimethoprim-sulfamethoxazole and antifungal and antiviral agents may either abort the risk or shift the timeline of these opportunistic infections [11, 12].

Infections After 6 Months

This period is also called community-acquired infection period. *Aspergillus* or other mold infections are more common in transplant recipients during this period. In the winter season, the transplant recipients are more likely to get influenza or community-acquired respiratory virus infection than reactivation of latent viral infections. Latent viral infection presentation in the later months may be with a more severe form of disease (e.g., cytomegalovirus (CMV) colitis, herpes simplex virus (HSV) encephalitis, or Epstein-Barr virus (EBV) posttransplant lymphoproliferative disorder) as the prophylaxis or surveillance use wanes after 1 year of transplant. However, these events are not very common [13]. However, allograft rejection requiring intensive immunosuppressive therapy increases the risk of common bacterial and viral infections as well as opportunistic pathogens regardless of the time after transplantation.

Approach to Infections in SOT Recipients

The transplant recipients are very complex, and only a consistent methodological approach can unravel the mysteries of the diagnosis. A list of key questions in history is shown in Table 12.1.

Bacterial Infections in SOT

Infections may occur in up to 80% of SOT recipients [14]. Bacterial infections predominate over other types of infection, occurring in 43–60% of lung transplant recipients [15] and up to 71% in

Table 12.1 List of essential questions to be asked in a transplant recipient suspected of infection

When was the transplant performed? (timeline of infections)
Transplantation history
Transplant serology
Increase risk of CMV in D+/R- transplants
History of rejection episodes
Augmented or change in immunosuppression
Type of transplant
Lung → Pneumonia
Kidney/pancreas → UTI
Liver → GI
Heart→ Mediastinitis
Travel history
Endemic mycoses
Pets
Toxoplasmosis
History of ill contact
Viruses
Respiratory, Parvovirus, HSV, etc.
Compliance with prophylactic drugs, e.g., PJP prophylaxis

liver transplant recipients [16, 17]. In fact, bloodstream infections caused by bacteria are a major cause of morbidity and mortality posttransplant [18–20]. In renal transplant recipients, urinary tract infections appear to be the main source of these bacteremias [21]. This fact relates to manipulation of the urinary tract at the time of surgery, the presence of ureteric stents posttransplant, and preexistent reflux in these recipients. This is underscored in the aforementioned surveillance study of SOT recipients from Spain where 39% of the bacteremias in 1400 renal transplant recipients were identified as being of urinary tract origin and as a result were due to Gram-negative bacteria (62–70%) [18, 21]. In contrast, among liver transplant recipients, bacterial bloodstream infection is most often intravascular catheter-related and may be produced almost equally by Gram-negative and Gram-positive bacteria [18, 22]. However, one must be cognizant that surgical site infections mainly caused by bacteria may be present in up to 41.3% of living donor liver transplants [23]. Palmer and colleagues reported that 25% of 176 consecutive lung transplant recipients developed bloodstream infections of which *Staphylococcus aureus* and

Pseudomonas aeruginosa were most common [24]. The origin of bacteremias in lung transplant recipients appears to be the lungs (46% of the time and particularly during the first 30 days posttransplant) and vascular catheter-related infection (41% of the time and most common after 30 days posttransplant) based on a multicenter study of 305 patients with bacteremias [19]. Once more, the Spanish SOT cohort study found that 11% of heart transplant recipients developed bloodstream infections, with coagulase-negative staphylococci predominating as a cause of bacteremia (27%) followed by *S. aureus* accounting for 21% with central intravascular devices (44%), far exceeding pulmonary (9%) and surgical site infection (9%) as the foci of infection for the bacteremias [18]. Pancreatic transplant recipients develop bacterial and in particular bloodstream infections most commonly in the first 3 months posttransplant related to surgical site infections (organ/space surgical site infections) [25]. Similarly, in intestinal transplant recipients, bacterial infections are predominately related to surgical site infections due to surgical technical complications [26].

Clinical manifestations of bacteremias in SOT recipients may range from an insidious presentation without major symptoms or signs such as fever or hypotension but rather subtle symptoms or findings such as merely having a chill or an elevated white blood cell count, to overt findings of septic shock. Appropriate diagnostic testing should be undertaken to include blood cultures (from each lumen of a central venous catheter and a peripheral vein), sputum culture, and urine cultures. Often in the case of lung transplant recipients because of the range of potential pathogens to be considered, bronchoscopy to obtain diagnostic cultures may be necessary. Empiric antibiotic therapy should take into account a number of important factors such as previous colonizing organisms, recent duration of hospitalization predisposing them to more resistant organisms, receipt of antibiotics in the past 90 days [27], travel history to destinations where resistant organisms may be harbored, and possible origins of the infection. Specific therapy should ensure adequate coverage of potential pathogens including Gram-positive and Gram-negative pathogens.

Viral Infections in SOT

Viral infections are the second most frequent infections encountered in SOT recipients. In lung transplant recipients, 23–31% of all infections experienced were of viral origin of which CMV was the most common [15]. The greatest risk of CMV infection occurred in those recipients seronegative for CMV who received an organ from a seropositive donor (D+R-), whereas CMV-seropositive recipients have an intermediate risk of developing CMV infection after transplantation [28]. EBV, another DNA virus in the *Herpesviridae* family, may produce a primary infection in seronegative recipients receiving seropositive donor organs and subsequently be associated with posttransplant lymphoproliferative disorder (PTLD) [29]. In fact, PTLD may develop in 3–12% of lung transplant recipients [29]. Reactivation of herpes simplex virus (HSV 1 and 2) in the orolabial or genital locations is fairly common after transplantation as seroprevalence of antibody reaches >80% by the age of 60 in North America [30, 31]. Nevertheless, local spread and dissemination may occur in lung and other SOT recipients due to their immunosuppressive therapy [32]. Similarly, herpes zoster has an incidence of 8–11% in the first 4 years after transplantation and often may be disseminated at presentation in lung transplant recipients [33, 34]. Viral infections occurred in 19.3% of a consecutive liver transplant cohort in Colombia [17]. CMV infections accounted for the majority of these infections (62.5%) followed by herpes virus infections. Once again the risk for CMV infection in liver transplant recipients was highest in D+R- transplants [28]. The risk of EBV-related PTLD is considered to be in the moderate range [29]. Herpes simplex infection may cause devastating outcomes such as fulminant hepatitis after liver transplantation. Surprisingly, human herpes virus 6 may also be prevalent in 14–82% of liver transplant recipients [35].

The most common clinical presentation of HSV is orolabial, genital, or perianal disease and is manifested by vesicular lesions and/or ulcerations [36, 37]. However, HSV may produce disseminated disease involving the skin, esophagus (usually upper two-thirds), liver, and lungs [32]. Herpes keratitis is another form of HSV infection involving the eye. Rapid diagnosis may be achieved by means of PCR testing of open lesions [38]. Oral therapy with acyclovir, famciclovir, or valacyclovir may be employed for localized infection, but for more extensive visceral or disseminated disease, acyclovir 10 mg/kg every 8 h (dose based on adults with normal renal function) intravenously should be initiated [38]. Similarly, herpes zoster may present as a localized dermatomal vesicular eruption but can readily disseminate [33]. Therapy varies from oral medication (acyclovir, famciclovir, or valacyclovir) for mild dermatomal eruptions to intravenous acyclovir 10 mg/kg every 8 h intravenously for disseminated disease [39].

In contrast, CMV infection may present in three ways: CMV replicating in the bloodstream (CMV viremia), CMV syndrome when fever and/or malaise are accompanied by leucopenia or thrombocytopenia, and CMV disease where tissue invasion occurs with visceral involvement [28]. Diagnosis is made by an assessment of CMV viral load and its presence in tissues. Similarly, response to therapy is reflected in a reduction in CMV viral load. Treatment with oral valganciclovir may be adequate for CMV infection, but for CMV disease with or without organ involvement, intravenous ganciclovir is preferred [28]. EBV may produce infectious mononucleosis symptoms (fever, pharyngitis, lymphadenopathy, hepatosplenomegaly, and atypical lymphocytosis) in addition to organ involvement with hepatitis, pneumonitis, and hematological abnormalities (leukopenia, hemolytic anemia, thrombocytopenia, and hemophagocytosis) [29]. Far more devastating manifestations include the development of EBV-linked PTLD that may be manifested by the same aforementioned signs and symptoms noted with EBV infectious mononucleosis [29]. The first line of therapy for treatment of PTLD involves reduction in immunosuppression. Other modalities of therapy that may be required for the treatment of PTLD are rituximab and antineoplastic chemotherapy [29]. Antiviral therapy is not of value for PTLD. Once more response to therapy is gauged by following the EBV viral load.

Fungal Infections in SOT

Invasive fungal infections (IFI) in SOT recipients are often unrecognized and thus underestimated. The cumulative incidence of IFI in the SOT patients (16,808 patients) included in the Transplant-Associated Surveillance Network (TRANSNET) was 3.1% [40]. However, within the TRANSNET multicenter study, the incidence varied considerably among the transplanted organs: small bowel 11.6%, lung and heart–lung 8.6%, liver 4.7%, pancreas and kidney pancreas 4.0%, heart 3.4%, and kidney 1.3% [40]. Variation in incidence of IFI was also noted among the transplant center sites (ranging from 1.2% to 6.1%) [40]. The prevalence of IFI solely in lung transplant recipients has been observed to be 9.1% in a retrospective review single center [41] and 10–14% in a review of data from a number of centers [15]. *Aspergillus* was the predominant fungus producing IFIs in lung transplant recipients (44%) followed by *Candida* (23%) and then other molds (19.8%) according to the TRANSNET database [40]. In contrast, Neofytos and colleagues assessed IFIs at 17 transplant centers including 108 lung transplant recipients and demonstrated that aspergillosis accounted for 63% of the 134 IFIs in these recipients, while *Candida* accounted for 23.9% and other molds 9.7% [42].

Although another study in a single center reflected a higher rate of IFI in liver transplant recipients (8.4%) [17] compared to the TRANSNET data, there was concurrence in both studies that *Candida* spp. produced the bulk of the IFIs observed (approximately 70%). The next most common pathogen producing IFIs in liver transplant recipients was *Aspergillus* spp. [17, 40, 42]. Similarly, in renal, pancreas, and heart transplant recipients, *Candida* spp. were demonstrated to be the most common fungal pathogen inciting IFIs and was usually followed by *Aspergillus* spp. except in renal transplant recipients where *Cryptococcus* spp. superseded *Aspergillus* as a cause of IFIs [40, 42].

Invasive candidiasis predominantly presents as candidemia that may be vascular catheter-related or arising from the gastrointestinal tract. In contrast, in liver transplant recipients, an intra-abdominal focus may be more frequent. Thus, invasive candidiasis may present as a clinical spectrum of symptoms and signs from asymptomatic disease to septic shock. Diagnosis of this entity is based on the isolation of *Candida* spp. from blood or a sterile body site. Surrogate markers such as the 1–3 beta-D-glucan assay have been used as ancillary aids in the diagnosis of invasive candidiasis, but their availability is limited [43, 44]. Treatment of invasive candidiasis has been updated recently by the Infectious Diseases Society of America who calls for the use of echinocandins intravenously (anidulafungin, caspofungin, or micafungin) at least initially with subsequent streamlining based on organism identification and susceptibilities [45].

As stated above invasive aspergillosis (IA) of the lung is the predominant IFI noted in lung transplant recipients but plays a less prominent role in producing IFIs in liver and heart transplant recipients [46]. Since *Aspergillus* conidia are ubiquitous in the environment, they easily reach the lung, and thus pulmonary IA is the major manifestation of infection. The diagnosis of this infection most commonly involves CT scan of the chest findings (nodules with or without a halo sign, cavitation, or air crescent sign) with a positive culture for *Aspergillus* spp. in respiratory secretions or a positive serological marker (serum or bronchoalveolar lavage galactomannan) [47]. The use of bronchoalveolar lavage fluid galactomannan testing as a surrogate marker of IA has greatly enhanced the diagnosis of this entity. Once again, the Infectious Diseases Society of America has recently produced updated treatment guidelines for IA [48], and voriconazole is recommended as the mainstay of therapy.

Cryptococcal disease usually manifests as meningitis or pulmonary disease. Lung involvement solely may occur in 33% of recipients with cryptococcal infection but extrapulmonary involvement may be present in 50–75% of SOT recipients with cryptococcal disease [49]. Symptoms may be subtle such as a persistent headache in the case of cryptococcal meningitis or progress to sepsis. Similarly, pulmonary lesions may present as asymptomatic colonization and nodules on chest imaging or produce respiratory distress [49]. Therapy for these infections has been outlined in the guidance provided by the Infectious Diseases Society of America and usually involves fluconazole for mild infection, and for moderate to severe infection, an amphotericin B formulation with flucytosine initially followed by fluconazole for a prolonged period of time [50]. Simultaneous reduction in immunosuppression is also beneficial.

Mycobacterial, Pneumocystis, and Nocardia Infections in SOT

The incidence of other infections produced by a variety of other pathogens in SOT recipients is far less frequent than those infections discussed above. Specifically, infections produced by mycobacteria, *Pneumocystis jirovecii*, and *Nocardia* spp. were less frequent in lung transplant recipients accounting for only 4–10% of all the infections in this patient group [15]. Mycobacterial infection may be subdivided into *M. tuberculosis* infection and those infections caused by nontuberculous mycobacteria (NTM). The prevalence of tuberculosis (TB) in SOT recipients ranges from 1.2% to 6.4% in developed nations but can be as high as 15% in endemic locales [51]. The majority of active TB cases developed in the 1st year posttransplant (median 11.2 months) when immunosuppression is at its height and was most common among renal transplant recipients in a retrospective study undertaken at Columbia University Medical Center [52]. NTM infections have been reported in 0.16–0.38% of renal transplant recipients, 0.24–2.8% of heart transplant patients, 0.46–8.0% of lung transplant recipients, and 0.04% of liver transplants [53]. However, other investigators have determined that NTM infections occur more frequently in lung transplant recipients (53 of 237, 23%) [54]. NTM are a heterogeneous group of organisms, with varying potential to cause invasive disease. Some species such as *M. abscessus* may produce aggressive and disseminated infection in SOT recipients (particularly lung transplant recipients [54, 55]), whereas *M. gordonae* rarely causes invasive disease [56].

In lung transplant recipients, *M. avium* complex is isolated most frequently (69.8%), followed by *M. abscessus* (9.4%) and *M. gordonae* (7.5%) [54]. In the TRANSNET database, *P. jirovecii* was demonstrated in only 1% of the incidence cohort [40]. There is a paucity of incidence data otherwise [57]. Similarly, nocardiosis has been identified in 0.7–3.5% based in recent reviews [58]. Peleg and coworkers identified *Nocardia* infection in 0.6% of 5126 SOT recipients from 1995 to 2005 [59]. The highest frequency was noted in lung transplants (3.5%) followed by heart (2.5%), small bowel (1.3%), kidney (0.2%), and liver transplants (0.1%). The lung was the sole organ affected in 77% of those infected. In contrast, others have demonstrated a lower rate of nocardiosis (0.4%) with a higher rate of lung involvement (89%) and skin manifestations in 26% [60].

Most cases of TB in SOT recipients arise from reactivation of latent infection. As such, symptoms may not be as overt as expected [61], although fever, night sweats, and weight loss do occur in recipients who are subsequently diagnosed with TB. The diagnosis may be delayed until a specimen from a potentially infected body site is culture positive or histopathological verification of infection is documented. The standard four-drug regimen (isoniazid, rifampin, pyrazinamide, and ethambutol) for 2 months followed by isoniazid and rifampin for additional 4 months is preferred for the treatment of tuberculosis [61]. Rifampin can accelerate the metabolism of several drugs, e.g., calcineurin inhibitors, and serum levels and dose modifications are necessary.

Pulmonary and skin involvement are the most common presentations of NTM infection particularly in lung transplant recipients [62]. *M. abscessus* is particularly prone to dissemination with both lung and skin involvement [54, 55]. Lung findings may range from nodules to infiltrates and also cavitation. The diagnosis of these infections should have the diagnostic principles previously established [56]. Therapy of these infections may require two, three, or even four drugs depending on the organism's susceptibility for a prolonged period of time [63].

Pneumocystis jirovecii presents with a more abrupt onset in SOT recipients manifested by fever, shortness of breath, and a nonproductive cough with interstitial pulmonary infiltrates [57]. Bronchoscopy with bronchoalveolar lavage or transbronchial biopsy is the preferred method of diagnosis. Trimethoprim-sulfamethoxazole is still the mainstay of therapy. Nocardiosis primarily involves the lung in SOT recipients, but central nervous system involvement may be present in one third of the cases [59]. Radiologically, nocardiosis produces nodular lesions that may cavitate [58, 60]. Diagnosis of this infection requires sampling an infected site with culture-based or histologic proof of the organism. Therapy with an appropriate antimicrobial agent is predicated on identification of the organism and susceptibility testing [33]. Preferred agents have included trimethoprim-sulfamethoxazole, ceftriaxone, imipenem/meropenem, amikacin, and linezolid [58].

Parasitic Infections in SOT

Parasitic infections are increasing in number in SOT recipients. This trend relates to increased leisure travel in transplant recipients, the expansion of transplant programs to endemic areas within Latin America and the potential of patients receiving their transplants from previously infected asymptomatic donors, immigration of both recipients and potential donors with asymptomatic or latent infection from endemic areas, and the use of newer immunosuppressive agents in lieu of cyclosporine-based immunosuppression that possesses antiparasitic activity [64]. As an example, seronegative cardiac transplant recipients are at greatest risk of developing toxoplasmosis if the transplanted organ is from a seropositive donor as might be the case if the donor is from an endemic area (Latin America or sub-Saharan Africa) and latent infection is present in the donor myocardium when no prophylaxis for toxoplasmosis is provided [65]. Among non-cardiac transplant recipients, the origin of toxoplasmosis is more varied [64]. Another parasitic infection of considerable import in Latin

America is Chagas disease. This disease caused by *Trypanosoma cruzi* may affect transplant recipient in three distinct fashions: (a) heart transplant recipients with chronic infection and thus are at risk of reactivation posttransplant; (b) non-cardiac transplant recipients with chronic *T. cruzi* infection who are at risk of reactivation posttransplant; and (c) uninfected SOT recipient who may receive an organ or blood products from an infected donor [64]. Chagasic cardiomyopathy is the third leading cause for heart transplantation in Brazil accounting for 21.9% of all heart transplants [66]. Moreover, reactivation of past infection after transplantation is relatively common and occurs in 27–43% [66, 67].

Leishmaniasis is transmitted by the bite of a female sand fly and has its peak prevalence in tropical and subtropical areas of Asia, the Middle East, Africa, Southern Europe, Central America, and South America [68]. Similar to Chagas disease, infection in transplant patients may be acquired from (a) a new infection, (b) reactivation of a previous infection, and (c) transmission in the transplanted organ [64].

The parasitic infections are a varied group with varied clinical manifestations. In particular, toxoplasmosis may cause lymphadenopathy, hepatosplenomegaly, brain abscesses, and pancytopenia. The definitive diagnosis rests on demonstrating tachyzoites in histopathological specimens of infected tissue [64]. Primary therapy involves sulfadiazine, pyrimethamine, and leucovorin; high-dose trimethoprim-sulfamethoxazole is an alternative. Leishmaniasis produces fever, hepatosplenomegaly, and pancytopenia. Once more the diagnosis is made by the demonstration of the parasite histopathologically from affected tissue. Liposomal amphotericin B is an effective therapy for this infection [68].

Donor-Derived Infections

Infections acquired by the organ transplant recipient from the donor may be classified as those that are expected such as CMV or hepatitis B where a priori knowledge of the donor's infected status is known and the recipient can then be monitored for signs of infection. In contrast, unexpected infections originating in the donor may arise in the recipient such as *Mycobacterium tuberculosis*, lymphocytic choriomeningitis, or fungal pathogens such as *Histoplasma capsulatum*. It is these unexpected infections that are of greatest concern. Definitions for donor-derived infections have been promulgated and have gained acceptance in many jurisdictions [69]. This framework includes proven (definitive proof of infectious disease found in both the donor and recipient), probable, possible, unlikely, excluded (clear evidence of an alternative origin of infection), intervention without documented transmission (presumptive infection without proof), positive assay without disease transmission and not assessable [69]. Donor-derived infections accounted for 0.2% of all deceased organ donation transplants according to the Organ Procurement and Transplant Network survey between 2005 and 2011 [4]. Donor-derived viral infections predominated with bacterial, fungal, and parasitic infections following in descending order in the organ recipients [4]. However a recent update from 2013 on donor-derived transmission events has highlighted the increase in potential reportable events [70]. It was demonstrated that 203 of the 284 potential donor-derived transmission events were due to infection (71.4%) with 24 (11.8%) proven/probable infections noted [70]. Donor-derived bacterial infections were most frequent among the proven/probable infections (11/24, 46%) including two methicillin-resistant *Staphylococcus aureus* infections followed by viral (8/24, 33%) and fungal plus parasitic accounting for five infections (21%).

The impact of donor-derived infection may be enhanced in the future with the impetus to utilize increased infection risk donors to meet organ transplantation needs. In fact, a guidance has been created by the Canadian Society of Transplantation and the Canadian National Transplant Research Program concerning this issue to address the expanding utilization of such organs [71].

Future Considerations

As discussed above, infections posttransplant arise from the effect of immunosuppressive medication on the immune system increasing the recipient's susceptibility to infection. One approach to reduce the impact and incidence of infection in the post-transplant period has been the practice of antimicrobial prophylaxis. Antimicrobial prophylaxis has been employed for potential donor-derived bacterial infection through perioperative prophylaxis [3], CMV infection via antiviral prophylaxis for varying durations of time according to the type of transplant of individuals at higher risk for CMV infection (CMV mismatch transplants where the virus is acquired from the donor, or recipient positive individuals where there may be reactivation of latent infection) [28], antifungal prophylaxis particularly for lung and liver transplant recipients where fungal infection may be endogenous or exogenous [72, 73], prophylaxis for *Pneumocystis jirovecii* [57], or prophylaxis for potential parasitic infections such as toxoplasmosis [64]. These efforts have reduced morbidity and mortality but are not uniformly successful.

However, it may be possible to obviate the need for immunosuppressive therapy by novel means. Some investigators have attempted to use non-myeloablative conditioning regimens or the infusion of donor stem cells to create chimerism in SOT recipients and thus induce immune tolerance of the transplanted organ [74]. By resetting the immune system to induce tolerance, immunosuppression to prevent rejection is unnecessary thus reducing the potential risk for infections. Another strategy being explored is the isolation of regulatory T cells for subsequent infusion to suppress rejection produced by T cell responsiveness [75]. Again, this strategy may achieve the goal of immune tolerance thus precluding the need for immunosuppressive medications and thus reducing the risk of post-transplant infections.

Others have sought to identify those individuals predisposed to infectious complications posttransplant by assessing genetic polymorphisms. For example, after liver transplantation, the adaptive immune response is blunted through the use of immunosuppressive agents, and it is the innate immune response that is the primarily involved in controlling infectious pathogens [14]. Molecules operative in the innate immune response such as toll-like receptors and the lectin pathway of complement

activation are directed to defend against bacteria [76]. Single nucleotide polymorphisms (SNP) or genetic mutations in the aforementioned genes may contribute to poor performance by the recipient in controlling bacterial infection. Specifically, perturbations in toll-like receptor 2, a receptor for Gram-positive bacterial cell wall peptidoglycan, and impaired cytokine via a SNP (e.g., the R753Q SNP in toll-like receptor 2) produce defective intracellular signaling and impaired cytokine secretion. This mutation has been associated with more frequent bacterial and viral infections, particularly CMV and hepatitis C infection after liver transplantation [77–79]. Specifically, hepatitis C virus recurrence after liver transplantation was associated with single nucleotide polymorphisms resulting in high producers of TNF-alpha [80]. Furthermore, polymorphisms in the lectin pathway of the complement system activation may be an important risk factor for bacterial infection after transplantation [81, 82]. Further elucidation of the genetic profiles of both donor and recipients may portend alterations in the innate immune system and the predilection to infection. Such novel strategies may help devise a personalized approach to infection preventive measures in the future for SOT recipients.

In conclusion, SOT recipients are predisposed to infections due to endogenous latent infection or reactivated microorganisms, exogenous ones acquired from the environment or other personnel, as well as those that may be derived from the donor because of the immunosuppressive agents administered to reduce the risk of rejection. Bacteria, viruses, fungi, and parasites all contribute to this heightened susceptibility to infection. Efforts to reverse this propensity to infection by utilizing antimicrobial prophylaxis, reducing immunosuppression when necessary, and obviating the need for immunosuppression all together have met with varied success. In addition, manipulation of the immune system to induce tolerance through non-myeloablative transplantation or infusion of donor stem cells or genetic alterations to correct immune deficiencies may yet meet this need; however, these modalities require further investigation.

References

1. Fishman JA. Infection in solid-organ transplant recipients. N Engl J Med. 2007;357(25):2601–14.
2. Dorschner P, McElroy LM, Ison MG. Nosocomial infections within the first month of solid organ transplantation. Transplant Infect Dis: Off J Transplant Soc. 2014;16(2):171–87.
3. Ison MG, Grossi P. Donor-derived infections in solid organ transplantation. Am J Transplant: Off J Am Soc Transplant Am Soc Transplant Surg. 2013;13(Suppl 4):22–30.
4. Ison MG, Nalesnik MA. An update on donor-derived disease transmission in organ transplantation. Am J Transplant: Off J Am Soc Transplant Am Soc Transplant Surg. 2011;11(6):1123–30.
5. Wan Q, Luo A, Ye Q, Liu S, Zhou J. Predictors of shock and mortality in solid organ transplant recipients with bacteremia caused by non-lactose-fermenting gram-negative bacilli. Infect Dis (London, England). 2016;48(1):32–9.
6. Wan QQ, Ye QF, Yuan H. Multidrug-resistant Gram-negative bacteria in solid organ transplant recipients with bacteremias. Eur J Clin Microbiol Infect Dis: Off Publ Eur Soc Clin Microbiol. 2015;34(3):431–7.
7. Lanini S, Costa AN, Puro V, et al. Incidence of carbapenem-resistant gram negatives in Italian transplant recipients: a nationwide surveillance study. PLoS One. 2015;10(4):e0123706.
8. Shields RK, Clancy CJ, Gillis LM, et al. Epidemiology, clinical characteristics and outcomes of extensively drug-resistant Acinetobacter baumannii infections among solid organ transplant recipients. PLoS One. 2012;7(12):e52349.
9. Ruiz I, Gavalda J, Monforte V, et al. Donor-to-host transmission of bacterial and fungal infections in lung transplantation. Am J Transplant: Off J Am Soc Transplant Am Soc Transplant Surg. 2006;6(1):178–82.
10. Hirsch HH. BK virus: opportunity makes a pathogen. Clin Infect Dis. 2005;41(3):354–60.
11. Kotton CN, Kumar D, Caliendo AM, et al. International consensus guidelines on the management of cytomegalovirus in solid organ transplantation. Transplantation. 2010;89(7):779–95.
12. Tong CY, Bakran A, Peiris JS, Muir P, Herrington CS. The association of viral infection and chronic allograft nephropathy with graft dysfunction after renal transplantation. Transplantation. 2002;74(4):576–8.
13. Cervera C, Fernandez-Ruiz M, Valledor A, et al. Epidemiology and risk factors for late infection in solid organ transplant recipients. Transplant Infect Dis: Off J Transplant Soc. 2011;13(6):598–607.
14. Pedersen M, Seetharam A. Infections after orthotopic liver transplantation. J Clin Exp Hepatol. 2014;4(4):347–60.
15. Alexander BD, Tapson VF. Infectious complications of lung transplantation. Transplant Infect Dis: Off J Transplant Soc. 2001;3(3):128–37.
16. Romero FA, Razonable RR. Infections in liver transplant recipients. World J Hepatol. 2011;3(4):83–92.
17. Vera A, Contreras F, Guevara F. Incidence and risk factors for infections after liver transplant: single-center experience at the University Hospital Fundacion Santa Fe de Bogota, Colombia. Transplant Infect Dis: Off J Transplant Soc. 2011;13(6):608–15.
18. Moreno A, Cervera C, Gavalda J, et al. Bloodstream infections among transplant recipients: results of a nationwide surveillance in Spain. Am J Transplant: Off J Am Soc Transplant Am Soc Transplant Surg. 2007;7(11):2579–86.
19. Husain S, Chan KM, Palmer SM, et al. Bacteremia in lung transplant recipients in the current era. Am J Transplant Off: J Am Soc Transplant Am Soc Transplant Surg. 2006;6(12):3000–7.
20. Kritikos A, Manuel O. Bloodstream infections after solid-organ transplantation. Virulence. 2016;7(3):329–40.
21. Chuang P, Parikh CR, Langone A. Urinary tract infections after renal transplantation: a retrospective review at two US transplant centers. Clin Transpl. 2005;19(2):230–5.
22. Bert F, Larroque B, Paugam-Burtz C, et al. Microbial epidemiology and outcome of bloodstream infections in liver transplant recipients: an analysis of 259 episodes. Liver Transplant: Off Publ Am Assoc Study Liver Dis Int Liver Transplant Soc. 2010;16(3):393–401.
23. Yamamoto M, Takakura S, Iinuma Y, et al. Changes in surgical site infections after living donor liver transplantation. PLoS One. 2015;10(8):e0136559.
24. Palmer SM, Alexander BD, Sanders LL, et al. Significance of blood stream infection after lung transplantation: analysis in 176 consecutive patients. Transplantation. 2000;69(11):2360–6.
25. Singh RP, Farney AC, Rogers J, et al. Analysis of bacteremia after pancreatic transplantation with enteric drainage. Transplant Proc. 2008;40(2):506–9.
26. Guaraldi G, Cocchi S, Codeluppi M, et al. Outcome, incidence, and timing of infectious complications in small bowel and multivisceral organ transplantation patients. Transplantation. 2005;80(12):1742–8.
27. Safdar N, Maki DG. The commonality of risk factors for nosocomial colonization and infection with antimicrobial-resistant Staphylococcus aureus, enterococcus, gram-negative bacilli, Clostridium difficile, and Candida. Ann Intern Med. 2002;136(11):834–44.
28. Razonable RR, Humar A. Cytomegalovirus in solid organ transplantation. Am J Transplant: Off J Am Soc Transplant Am Soc Transplant Surg. 2013;13(Suppl 4):93–106.
29. Allen UD, Preiksaitis JK. Epstein-Barr virus and posttransplant lymphoproliferative disorder in solid organ transplantation. Am J Transplant: Off J Am Soc Transplant Am Soc Transplant Surg. 2013;13(Suppl 4):107–20.
30. Schillinger JA, Xu F, Sternberg MR, et al. National seroprevalence and trends in herpes simplex virus type 1 in the United States, 1976–1994. Sex Transm Dis. 2004;31(12):753–60.

31. Xu F, Sternberg MR, Kottiri BJ, et al. Trends in herpes simplex virus type 1 and type 2 seroprevalence in the United States. JAMA. 2006;296(8):964–73.

32. Smyth RL, Higenbottam TW, Scott JP, et al. Herpes simplex virus infection in heart-lung transplant recipients. Transplantation. 1990;49(4):735–9.

33. Gourishankar S, McDermid JC, Jhangri GS, Preiksaitis JK. Herpes zoster infection following solid organ transplantation: incidence, risk factors and outcomes in the current immunosuppressive era. Am J Transplant: Off J Am Soc Transplant Am Soc Transplant Surg. 2004;4(1):108–15.

34. Pergam SA, Forsberg CW, Boeckh MJ, et al. Herpes zoster incidence in a multicenter cohort of solid organ transplant recipients. Transplant Infect Dis: Off J Transplant Soc. 2011;13(1):15–23.

35. Razonable RR, Rivero A, Brown RA, et al. Detection of simultaneous beta-herpesvirus infections in clinical syndromes due to defined cytomegalovirus infection. Clin Transpl. 2003;17(2):114–20.

36. Pettersson E, Hovi T, Ahonen J, et al. Prophylactic oral acyclovir after renal transplantation. Transplantation. 1985;39(3):279–81.

37. Seale L, Jones CJ, Kathpalia S, et al. Prevention of herpesvirus infections in renal allograft recipients by low-dose oral acyclovir. JAMA. 1985;254(24):3435–8.

38. Wilck MB, Zuckerman RA. Herpes simplex virus in solid organ transplantation. Am J Transplant: Off J Am Soc Transplant Am Soc Transplant Surg. 2013;13(Suppl 4):121–7.

39. Pergam SA, Limaye AP. Varicella zoster virus in solid organ transplantation. Am J Transplant: Off J Am Soc Transplant Am Soc Transplant Surg. 2013;13(Suppl 4):138–46.

40. Pappas PG, Alexander BD, Andes DR, et al. Invasive fungal infections among organ transplant recipients: results of the Transplant-Associated Infection Surveillance Network (TRANSNET). Clin Infect Dis: Off Publ Infect Dis Soc Am. 2010;50(8):1101–11.

41. Pinney MF, Rosenberg AF, Hampp C, Schain D, Akindipe O, Baz M. Invasive fungal infections in lung transplant recipients not receiving routine systemic antifungal prophylaxis: 12-year experience at a university lung transplant center. Pharmacotherapy. 2011;31(6):537–45.

42. Neofytos D, Fishman JA, Horn D, et al. Epidemiology and outcome of invasive fungal infections in solid organ transplant recipients. Transplant Infect Dis: Off J Transplant Soc. 2010;12(3):220–9.

43. Silveira FP, Kusne S. Candida infections in solid organ transplantation. Am J Transplant: Off J Am Soc Transplant Am Soc Transplant Surg. 2013;13(Suppl 4):220–7.

44. Ostrosky-Zeichner L, Alexander BD, Kett DH, et al. Multicenter clinical evaluation of the (1-->3) beta-D-glucan assay as an aid to diagnosis of fungal infections in humans. Clin Infect Dis: Off Publ Infect Dis Soc Am. 2005;41(5):654–9.

45. Pappas PG, Kauffman CA, Andes DR, et al. Clinical Practice Guideline for the Management of Candidiasis: 2016 update by the Infectious Diseases Society of America. Clin Infect Dis: Off Publ Infect Dis Soc Am. 2016;62(4):e1–50.

46. Singh N, Husain S. Aspergillosis in solid organ transplantation. Am J Transplant: Off J Am Soc Transplant Am Soc Transplant Surg. 2013;13(Suppl 4):228–41.

47. De Pauw B, Walsh TJ, Donnelly JP, et al. Revised definitions of invasive fungal disease from the European Organization for Research and Treatment of Cancer/ Invasive Fungal Infections Cooperative Group and the National Institute of Allergy and Infectious Diseases Mycoses Study Group (EORTC/MSG) Consensus Group. Clin Infect Dis: Off Publ Infect Dis Soc Am. 2008;46(12):1813–21.

48. Patterson TF, Thompson GR 3rd, Denning DW, et al. Practice guidelines for the diagnosis and management of aspergillosis: 2016 update by the Infectious Diseases Society of America. Clin Infect Dis: Off Publ Infect Dis Soc Am. 2016;63(4):e1–e60.

49. Baddley JW, Forrest GN. Cryptococcosis in solid organ transplantation. Am J Transplant: Off J Am Soc Transplant Am Soc Transplant Surg. 2013;13(Suppl 4):242–9.

50. Perfect JR, Dismukes WE, Dromer F, et al. Clinical practice guidelines for the management of cryptococcal disease: 2010 update by the Infectious Diseases Society of America. Clin Infect Dis: Off Publ Infect Dis Soc Am. 2010;50(3):291–322.

51. Munoz P, Rodriguez C, Bouza E. Mycobacterium tuberculosis infection in recipients of solid organ transplants. Clin Infect Dis: Off Publ Infect Dis Soc Am. 2005;40(4):581–7.

52. Lopez de Castilla D, Schluger NW. Tuberculosis following solid organ transplantation. Transplant Infect Dis: Off J Transplant Soc. 2010;12(2):106–12.

53. Piersimoni C. Nontuberculous mycobacteria infection in solid organ transplant recipients. Eur J Clin Microbiol Infect Dis: Off Publ Eur Soc Clin Microbiol. 2012;31(4):397–403.

54. Knoll BM, Kappagoda S, Gill RR, et al. Nontuberculous mycobacterial infection among lung transplant recipients: a 15-year cohort study. Transplant Infect Dis: Off J Transplant Soc. 2012;14(5):452–60.

55. Morales P, Gil A, Santos M. Mycobacterium abscessus infection in transplant recipients. Transplant Proc. 2010;42(8):3058–60.

56. Griffith DE, Aksamit T, Brown-Elliott BA, et al. An official ATS/IDSA statement: diagnosis, treatment, and prevention of nontuberculous mycobacterial diseases. Am J Respir Crit Care Med. 2007;175(4):367–416.

57. Martin SI, Fishman JA. Pneumocystis pneumonia in solid organ transplantation. Am J Transplant: Off J Am Soc Transplant Am Soc Transplant Surg. 2013;13(Suppl 4):272–9.

58. Clark NM, Reid GE. Nocardia infections in solid organ transplantation. Am J Transplant: Off J Am Soc Transplant Am Soc Transplant Surg. 2013;13(Suppl 4):83–92.

59. Peleg AY, Husain S, Qureshi ZA, et al. Risk factors, clinical characteristics, and outcome of Nocardia infection in organ transplant recipients: a matched

case-control study. Clin Infect Dis: Off Publ Infect Dis Soc Am. 2007;44(10):1307–14.

60. Santos M, Gil-Brusola A, Morales P. Infection by Nocardia in solid organ transplantation: thirty years of experience. Transplant Proc. 2011;43(6):2141–4.

61. Subramanian AK, Morris MI. Mycobacterium tuberculosis infections in solid organ transplantation. Am J Transplant: Off J Am Soc Transplant Am Soc Transplant Surg. 2013;13(Suppl 4):68–76.

62. Doucette K, Fishman JA. Nontuberculous mycobacterial infection in hematopoietic stem cell and solid organ transplant recipients. Clin Infect Dis: Off Publ Infect Dis Soc Am. 2004;38(10):1428–39.

63. Keating MR, Daly JS. Nontuberculous mycobacterial infections in solid organ transplantation. Am J Transplant: Off J Am Soc Transplant Am Soc Transplant Surg. 2013;13(Suppl 4):77–82.

64. Schwartz BS, Mawhorter SD. Parasitic infections in solid organ transplantation. Am J Transplant: Off J Am Soc Transplant Am Soc Transplant Surg. 2013;13(Suppl 4):280–303.

65. Fernandez-Sabe N, Cervera C, Farinas MC, et al. Risk factors, clinical features, and outcomes of toxoplasmosis in solid-organ transplant recipients: a matched case-control study. Clin Infect Dis: Off Publ Infect Dis Soc Am. 2012;54(3):355–61.

66. Campos SV, Strabelli TM, Amato Neto V, et al. Risk factors for Chagas' disease reactivation after heart transplantation. J Heart Lung Transplant: Off Publ Int Soc Heart Transplant. 2008;27(6):597–602.

67. Diez M, Favaloro L, Bertolotti A, et al. Usefulness of PCR strategies for early diagnosis of Chagas' disease reactivation and treatment follow-up in heart transplantation. Am J Transplant: Off J Am Soc Transplant Am Soc Transplant Surg. 2007;7(6):1633–40.

68. Prevention CfDCa. Parasites – Leishmaniasis. Last updated: January 10, 2013.

69. Garzoni C, Ison MG. Uniform definitions for donor-derived infectious disease transmissions in solid organ transplantation. Transplantation. 2011;92(12):1297–300.

70. Green M, Covington S, Taranto S, et al. Donor-derived transmission events in 2013: a report of the Organ Procurement Transplant Network Ad Hoc Disease Transmission Advisory Committee. Transplantation. 2015;99(2):282–7.

71. Guidance on the use of increased infectious risk donors for organ transplantation. Transplantation. 2014;98(4):365–9.

72. Luong ML, Chaparro C, Stephenson A, et al. Pretransplant Aspergillus colonization of cystic fibrosis patients and the incidence of post-lung transplant invasive aspergillosis. Transplantation. 2014;97(3):351–7.

73. Evans JD, Morris PJ, Knight SR. Antifungal prophylaxis in liver transplantation: a systematic review and network meta-analysis. Am J Transplant: Off J Am Soc Transplant Am Soc Transplant Surg. 2014;14(12):2765–76.

74. Granados JM, Benichou G, Kawai T. Hematopoietic stem cell infusion/transplantation for induction of allograft tolerance. Curr Opin Organ Transplant. 2015;20(1):49–56.

75. Muller YD, Seebach JD, Buhler LH, Pascual M, Golshayan D. Transplantation tolerance: clinical potential of regulatory T cells. Self Nonself. 2011;2(1):26–34.

76. van Hoek B, de Rooij BJ, Verspaget HW. Risk factors for infection after liver transplantation. Best practice & research. Clin Gastroenterol. 2012;26(1):61–72.

77. Brown RA, Gralewski JH, Eid AJ, Knoll BM, Finberg RW, Razonable RR. R753Q single-nucleotide polymorphism impairs toll-like receptor 2 recognition of hepatitis C virus core and nonstructural 3 proteins. Transplantation. 2010;89(7):811–5.

78. Brown RA, Gralewski JH, Razonable RR. The R753Q polymorphism abrogates toll-like receptor 2 signaling in response to human cytomegalovirus. Clin Infect Dis: Off Publ Infect Dis Soc Am. 2009;49(9):e96–9.

79. Eid AJ, Brown RA, Paya CV, Razonable RR. Association between toll-like receptor polymorphisms and the outcome of liver transplantation for chronic hepatitis C virus. Transplantation. 2007;84(4):511–6.

80. Mas VR, Fisher RA, Maluf DG, et al. Polymorphisms in cytokines and growth factor genes and their association with acute rejection and recurrence of hepatitis C virus disease in liver transplantation. Clin Genet. 2004;65(3):191–201.

81. Cervera C, Balderramo D, Suarez B, et al. Donor mannose-binding lectin gene polymorphisms influence the outcome of liver transplantation. Liver Transplant: Off Publ Am Assoc Study Liver Dis Int Liver Transplant Soc. 2009;15(10):1217–24.

82. Worthley DL, Johnson DF, Eisen DP, et al. Donor mannose-binding lectin deficiency increases the likelihood of clinically significant infection after liver transplantation. Clin Infect Dis: Off Publ Infect Dis Soc Am. 2009;48(4):410–7.

Onyema Ogbuagu and R. Douglas Bruce

Introduction

The acquired immunodeficiency syndrome (AIDS) was first recognized three and a half decades ago with the harbinger being the discovery of opportunistic infections initially in a cluster of young homosexual males in the United States who were, at the time, not known to have any known immune-compromising condition [1]. Subsequently, other risk groups for the syndrome were identified, other than homosexual or bisexual men, including hemophiliacs, heroin users, and Haitian immigrants [2]. The identification of AIDS among female partners of homosexual men drew attention to sexual transmission of the disease [3]. It took 2 years after the report on the first cluster of cases in 1981, primarily occurring in San Francisco and New York City [4], that the definitive link between the clinical syndrome and the etiologic virus, lymphadenopathy-associated virus (LAV) or human T-lymphotropic virus III (HTLV III), later termed the human immunodeficiency virus (HIV), was definitively isolated and described by French scientists, Francoise Barre-Sinoussi and Luc Montagnier, both of whom

were eventually awarded Nobel prizes for their work 25 years later [5–7].

In the ensuing decades, there were reports from across the globe of confirmed cases of HIV/AIDS impacting millions of people [8]. As of 2014, 36.9 million people are living with HIV/AIDS (PLWHA) with approximately two million new infections occurring annually [9]. It is estimated that since 2000, 25 million died because of AIDS-related illnesses with 1.2 million in 2014 alone [9, 10]. A majority of PLWHA are in middle- and low-income countries with 66% of new adult and greater than 90% of pediatric cases occurring in sub-Saharan Africa – one of the hardest hit regions in the world [10].

The drivers of the epidemic remain sexual transmission primarily among men who have sex with men (MSM) and heterosexual sex, infected sexual partners who are either not aware of their infection or not receiving antiretroviral drug treatment, and sharing of unsterile syringes or paraphernalia among people who inject drugs [11]. Vertical transmission from infected mothers to their babies continues to occur primarily in low-resource settings where interventions to prevent mother-to-child transmission are lacking or insufficient [12, 13]. The risk of HIV transmission through blood transfusion or organ transplantation is very low due to improved screening of donors.

Since 1981, significant advances have occurred in the knowledge and understanding of HIV viral

O. Ogbuagu
Section of Infectious Diseases, Yale University School of Medicine, New Haven, CT, USA

R. D. Bruce (✉)
Yale University School of Medicine, Cornell Scott-Hill Health Center, New Haven, CT, USA
e-mail: robert.bruce@yale.edu

© Springer International Publishing AG, part of Springer Nature 2018
B. H. Segal (ed.), *Management of Infections in the Immunocompromised Host*,
https://doi.org/10.1007/978-3-319-77674-3_13

structure and pathogenesis, natural history, disease manifestation, treatment, and prevention. Highly effective, tolerable, and simplified treatment regimens have led to improved life expectancy among PLWHA though access and affordability remain barriers to optimal coverage globally [14]. In spite of these improvements, high rates of morbidity and mortality continue, especially among individuals in low-resource settings or globally among vulnerable populations including ethnic minorities, MSM and transgendered individuals, women, people with substance use disorders, sex workers, prisoners, the poor, children, and adolescents [15, 16].

The morbidity and mortality from HIV are a direct result of opportunistic infections, which take advantage of a weakened immune system and/or may occur as a consequence of off-target end-organ injury from an activated immune system's efforts to control the virus. These include a wide array of clinical conditions including infections caused by a broad range of pathogens – bacterial, fungal, viral, and parasitic – which occur at a higher frequency than in immune-competent individuals, occur in unusual sites or may be disseminated, and/or are associated with neurologic disorders or cancers. Furthermore, with the aging of the HIV population, it is now appreciated that other conditions including renal disease, neurocognitive disorders, cancers, and cardiovascular and cerebrovascular disease may occur as long-term complications and are also contributing to morbidity and mortality [17, 18].

This chapter will focus specifically on infections that occur in HIV-infected individuals with an emphasis on the spectrum, epidemiology, pathogenesis, clinical presentation, management, and prevention of the infections.

Immune Defects in HIV-Infected Individuals

While CD4 T-cell depletion is the hallmark and a reliable measure of the degree of immune dysfunction in HIV-infected individuals, HIV broadly impacts multiple components of the immune system [19]. This was recognized early in the AIDS epidemic where studies showed that there were diminished CD4 and CD8 T-cell proliferation following exposure to antigens and anti-CD3 monoclonal antibody as well as decreased CD4 T helper cell activity in individuals with AIDS compared to those without HIV [20, 21]. Diminished immunoglobulin production by B-cells was observed in vitro following mitogen stimulation, in spite of the observed hyperproduction of immunoglobulins (specifically IgG) in vivo that occurs in specimens from patients with AIDS [20]. Similarly, decreased functioning of antigen-presenting cells (monocytes and dendritic cells) and natural killer cells has also been described [22, 23]. Some of these effects may occur prior to significant CD4 T-cell depletion but may become more prominent in individuals with long-term infection and/or who have developed AIDS [20, 24].

These studies have demonstrated the negative or altering impact of HIV infection on both innate and adaptive arms of the immune system. Together, the maladaptive responses underscore the increased risks for opportunistic infections that are not entirely reflected by and may occur independent of the decreased CD4 T-cell counts.

Natural History of HIV Infection and AIDS

Clinically, HIV infection progresses through three stages. First, a local is established at the site of inoculation, with subsequent regional spread and systemic dissemination, all of which occur during the acute phase of infection. Some individuals will develop signs and symptoms of an acute illness at the time of systemic viral dissemination (median time following infection 3–4 weeks) which auto-resolves even without any specific therapy. Subsequently, there is a variable period of clinical latency during which many individuals remain asymptomatic, followed by progression to AIDS.

The early events in HIV infection have been well elucidated. Following inoculation of the virus at vulnerable sites where infection may be promoted by certain host and local factors such as mucosal ulceration in the setting of a sexually transmitted disease (STD) [25], there is local replication of the virus and then regional spread to adjacent tissue and draining lymph nodes, after which there is widespread dissemination of the virus when it enters the blood stream. This phase of infection typically occurs within 2 weeks of infection at which time the virus can be detected in plasma by commercially available viral load assays. Coincident with this rise in viral load is a massive depletion of organ-specific (primarily in the gut) and peripheral blood lymphocytes, and this may be measured as a depletion of CD4 T-cells in the peripheral blood. During this period of disseminated infection, there is a concurrent establishment of organ-specific reservoirs in sites such as the central nervous system (CNS) and genitourinary system.

Following this acute rise in viremia, immune-mediated control of the virus occurs, which is driven principally by CD8 T-cell-mediated cytotoxicity and cytolysis directed against infected CD4-expressing cells. This may result in suppression of viral replication and establishment of a viral "set point" that is tightly regulated until late stages of the infection coincident with the development of AIDS. This viral set point determines the rate of CD4 decline over time.

Certain individuals do not experience a CD4 decline in spite of long-term infection with HIV. These are individuals typically with robust CD8 T-cell immune responses to viral infection or express certain immune phenotypes that confer an increased ability to suppress viral replication. These comprise elite controllers and long-term nonprogressors (viremic controllers) who suppress HIV viral loads to levels that are either undetectable by commercial viral load assays or to low levels, typically <10,000 copies, respectively. An understanding of how these individuals exert immune control of the virus has not been fully elucidated but remains a subject of keen interest as it might inform current and future strategies to cure, control, and/or prevent HIV.

It was established early on in the HIV epidemic that certain opportunistic infections (OIs) tend to occur below specific CD4 thresholds such that the susceptibility to and occurrence of certain OIs can be reliably predicted based on measured CD4 T-cell counts in people with HIV, assuming no other coexistent immune compromising conditions [26]. In the absence of effective combination antiretroviral therapy (cART), individuals with CD4 count <200 cells/mm^3 and/or CD4% <14 will develop an opportunistic infection at a median duration of 12–18 months from the time of dropping below that threshold. Based on epidemiologic observations, these laboratory criteria comprise the surveillance definition of AIDS. Furthermore, individuals with advanced HIV infection, i.e., CD4 count <50cells/mm^3, are susceptible to a broad range of opportunistic pathogens, which confer a poor prognosis. For these individuals, the median survival in the absence of cART is 12–18 months. Even when treated, these individuals experience higher rates of immunologic failure than those initiating therapy at higher CD4 counts (>50 cells/mm^3), lending credence to the World Health Organization (WHO) and US Department of Health and Human Services (DHHS) guidelines that support initiation of cART as soon as possible from the time of diagnosis for all individuals with HIV.

Viral Infections in HIV Infection

Human Herpesviruses

Introduction

Herpesviruses (HHVs) are a family of double-stranded DNA viruses, which, like HIV, have the unique ability to persist for the life of the human host. They do so by evading human immune responses and establishing latency in either neural tissue or tissues of the monocyte-macrophage system [27]. Human herpesvirus (HHVs 1–3), also referred to as alphaherpesviruses, establish latency in neural tissue, while HHVs 4–8 are lymphotropic, establishing latency in cells of the monocyte-macrophage system. The seroprevalence of HHVs among patients with HIV infection far exceeds seroprevalence rates among individuals without HIV. One study demonstrated that Epstein-Barr virus (EBV), HHV-8, cytomegalovirus (CMV), and herpes simplex virus-1 (HSV-1) were detected by polymerase chain reaction (PCR) in the saliva of people with HIV at a higher frequency (90%, 57%, 31%, and 16%, respectively) than controls without HIV (48%, 24%, 2%, and 2%, respectively) [28].

Herpesviruses carry epidemiologic and clinical significance in patients with HIV infection. Certain herpesviruses such as HSV-1 and HSV-2 can cause ulcerations or "cold sores" thereby disrupting mucosal integrity at vulnerable site such as male and female genitalia and, therefore, increase risk of HIV transmission during sexual intercourse [29]. Also, the presence of herpesvirus infections such as HSV-2, EBV, and cytomegalovirus (CMV) has been associated with increased HIV plasma viremia and is recognized as risk factors for faster HIV disease progression with morbidity and mortality implications [29–31]. Furthermore, the presence of CMV and EBV viremia has been associated with slower decay of HIV viral loads on ART [30]. Some positive interactions, however, have been reported such as the observation that HHV-6 and HHV-7 may decrease replication of HIV virus that exclusively utilize the chemokine co-receptor, CCR5, for entry into target cells and down-regulate CD4 receptors on T-cells thereby slowing disease progression [32].

HIV, by virtue of its negative effect on the immune system, interacts synergistically with HHVs resulting in increased risk of viral reactivation and development of end-organ or disseminated disease and malignancies associated with the HHVs [27, 33]. While HHV infections in the healthy host may be benign or result in mild self-limited illnesses, the same infections may carry serious consequences in immune-compromised hosts (see Table 13.1). The epidemiology, clinical presentation, diagnosis, and management of these consequential HHV infections in HIV-infected individuals will be discussed below.

Herpes Simplex Virus (HSV)

The two types of viruses that make up this group are HSV-1, which predominantly causes orolabial ulcers and typically acquired early in life, and HSV-2, which primarily causes anogenital disease and is typically acquired following onset of sexual activity [34]. However, either virus can cause similar disease syndromes at either location, may involve visceral organs, or cause disseminated disease. Both viruses are similar with 70% of their genome being identical [35].

Epidemiology

The prevalence of seropositivity to HSV-2 among individuals with HIV disease ranges from 30% to 90% depending on the type of population studied [36, 37]. An incidence rate of 4.4/10 person-years (pys) was reported among participants of a US military HIV natural history study (NHS) and was higher among African Americans (6.45/100pys) compared to Caucasians (3.46/100pys) [36]. HSV-2 seroprevalence increases with age and occurs at relatively higher frequencies among MSM and female sex workers, as well as ethnic minorities in the United States (African American and Latino) [37]. Individuals of lower socioeconomic status and those with more sexual partners and pregnancies also have higher infection rates [38, 39]. Some studies have found higher HSV-2 prevalence among women with HIV compared to men [40]. HSV-1 infection is generally more prevalent than HSV-2, with rates ranging from 30% to 78% [37, 40]. HSV-1 seropositivity may protect against HSV-2 acquisition and vice versa, but this has not been uniformly shown across studies [40, 41].

The epidemiologic links between HIV and HSV are significant. HSV-2 infection is associated with a two to four times increased risk of HIV disease acquisition likely through the breakdown of a natural skin barrier [36, 42–44]. Similarly, as HSV-2 seropositivity is associated with increased plasma HIV viral loads, it may potentially increase disease transmission risk [45]. However, a study showed no effect of HSV-2 seropositivity or viral shedding on HIV viremia in seminal and cervico-vaginal secretions, thereby challenging the contribution of HSV-2 to HIV disease transmission [46]. Incident HSV-2 infections also serve as a marker of sexual risk behaviors that place an individual at increased risk of HIV acquisition. Herpes simplex virus is transmitted through direct contact with oral and

Table 13.1 Clinical syndromes associated with herpesviruses in HIV patients

Herpesvirus	Nomenclature	Associated clinical syndromes
HHV-1	HSV-1	Orolabial and genital ulcers, aseptic meningitis, cranial nerve (CN) VII paralysis, transverse myelitis, disseminated cutaneous disease, keratitis, retinitis, esophagitis, bronchitis, pneumonitis, hepatitis, proctitis, herpetic whitlow
HHV-2	HSV-2	Genital and orolabial ulcers, meningoencephalitis, transverse myelitis, disseminated cutaneous disease, proctitis
HHV-3	VZV	Meningoencephalitis, CN VII paralysis, transverse myelitis, disseminated cutaneous disease, keratitis, retinitis, pneumonitis, hepatitis
HHV-4	EBV	Burkitt Lymphoma, primary CNS lymphoma (PCNSL), hepatitis, oral hairy leukoplakia
HHV-5	CMV	Meningoencephalitis, polyradiculopathy, transverse myelitis, retinitis, pneumonitis, esophagitis, colitis, hepatitis, cholangiopathy
HHV-6	HHV-6	Meningitis, encephalitis
HHV-7	HHV-7	Hepatitis, myeloradiculoneuropathy
HHV-8	HHV-8/ KSHV	Multicentric Castleman disease (MCD), Kaposi sarcoma (KS), primary effusion lymphoma

genital secretions including from individuals with active lesions or who shed the virus during asymptomatic periods. The incubation period is approximately 2–13 days (average 3–6 days).

Pathogenesis

Following inoculation of the virus into epithelial surfaces (skin or mucous membranes), the virus is able to evade immune responses, accesses axon terminals, and establishes latency in sensory ganglia – trigeminal or sacral ganglia for oral or genital HSV infections, respectively. Viral replication is typically limited to the epidermis or epithelial surface of mucous membranes [47]. Initial human innate (toll-like receptors [TLRs] and cytokine products) and later adaptive immune responses (CD8 T-cells, antibodies directed against viral proteins) aim to control viral replication and subsequent reactivation [47]. Subclinical reactivation and shedding of viruses may occur with varying frequencies depending on multiple factors including host immune status and environmental factors including stress and concurrent illnesses, malnutrition, and pregnancy [47].

Clinical Presentation

The clinical spectrum of HSV disease ranges from asymptomatic to severe and prolonged illness predominantly occurring in individuals who are immunocompromised and are experiencing a first episode of HSV illness. Genital lesions in particular, beyond discomfort, can be stigmatizing for individuals who experience outbreaks. Oropharyngeal lesions may cause severe oral pain and interfere with swallowing and feeding. Visceral HSV disease is uncommon and occurs predominantly in individuals who are older, receiving steroids or other immunocompromising medications including those undergoing cancer chemotherapy or transplant recipients, and other immunocompromised patients such as individuals with HIV disease. HSV hepatitis and meningitis, which can be recurrent however, can occur in immunocompetent hosts. Mollaret's meningitis, which is recurrent aseptic meningitis, most commonly results from recurrent HSV-2.

A typical HSV lesion is localized and progresses through multiple stages – a prodrome of burning or tingling, followed by development of papular lesions that progress to vesicles, which subsequently ulcerate. Regional lymph nodes may be enlarged. In immunocompromised patients, lesions may coalesce forming large superficial ulcers, which can persist for prolonged periods and may be mistaken for other lesions, such as decubitus ulcers in the perianal region. Lesions may become superinfected, but otherwise are not pustular. Resolution of the lesions is heralded by crusting and typically leaves no scarring.

HSV esophagitis typically presents as odynophagia, which can be frequently disabling and interfere with eating. HSV hepatitis may present with "anicteric hepatitis" syndrome, characterized by rapid rise in liver transaminases initially without hyperbilirubinemia or clinical jaundice, and may result in serious consequences including fulminant hepatic failure if unrecognized and untreated early. Ocular disease may present as keratitis with patients complaining of foreign body sensation, redness of eye, and pain. Acute retinal necrosis (ARN) and progressive outer retinal necrosis (PORN) are feared complications of HSV ocular infection. Central nervous system disorders associated with HSV include Bell's palsy, transverse myelitis, meningitis that could be recurrent (Mollaret's meningitis), and a severe meningoencephalitis [35], the latter occurring in both adults and infants from vertical transmission. Rare clinical syndromes include pneumonitis and herpetic paronychia or "whitlow."

Diagnosis

Genital herpes may be diagnosed clinically based on the characteristic appearance of the lesions. Unlike VZV, HSV lesions do not take on a dermatomal distribution but are more regional in distribution (e.g., orolabial or perianal). Other diseases may mimic HSV, and therefore definitive diagnosis requires laboratory testing. Swabs of active lesions (typically with a cotton tip or Dacron) can be sent for detection of HSV DNA by nucleic acid amplification/PCR, antigen detection, or culture [48]. Cytologic examination of smears of lesions or biopsy specimens with Tzanck or Papanicolaou stains, though inexpensive, has poor sensitivity and specificity. However, detection of antigens by immunofluorescence has improved detection rates with sensitivity ranging from 70% to 90% for smears of genital ulcers [48]. While viral culture remains the gold standard, HSV DNA detection by nucleic acid amplification testing (NAAT) or PCR remains the most sensitive and specific detection method (98% and up to 100%, respectively) and is the preferred method of testing [48]. As type-specific antibodies are usually absent in early HSV disease, antibody testing is best reserved to confirm prior exposure or past infections and has the advantage of distinguishing between HSV-1 and HSV-2.

Treatment/Management

Acyclovir, available in oral and intravenous formulations, is the first-line medication for treatment of HSV. Oral valacyclovir and famciclovir are alternatives with greater oral bioavailability and less frequent dosing than acyclovir. All require dosage adjustment for patients with renal insufficiency. IV acyclovir is used for more serious infections. Penciclovir has poor oral bioavailability; thus its use is limited to topical application to active lesions [49]. Prolonged duration of therapy may be required for immunocompromised patients with extensive mucocutaneous lesions to achieve a cure. Of the clinical syndromes caused by HSV, encephalitis is a medical emergency [35]. Intravenous acyclovir is the mainstay of therapy, and steroids may be used for individuals who develop severe brain edema. Mortality rates are high, and survivors have high frequencies of neurologic deficits.

Mutations in viral thymidine kinase may render HSV resistant to acyclovir and may be found in 5–25% of immunocompromised patients receiving acyclovir prophylaxis or treatment [50]. In these cases, foscarnet or cidofovir, the latter administered with probenecid to prevent nephrotoxicity, are alternative treatment options [50]. Medications in early phase clinical trials that have shown some promise include pritelivir and amenamevir, which belong to a new class of antivirals that are helicase-primase inhibitors [49].

Prevention

There are no available vaccines against HSV, but some candidates are in development [49]. Individuals at risk for recurrent disease reactivation can be maintained on antiviral prophylaxis, which may also serve to prevent disease transmission. Avoiding contact with active lesions and use of condoms during sexual intercourse are also effective ways of preventing disease transmission. HSV transmission, however, can result from asymptomatic viral shedding.

Varicella Zoster Virus
Introduction

Varicella zoster virus (VZV), a DNA virus, is distributed worldwide. While primary varicella zoster virus infection (chickenpox) can occur in any host (healthy or immune compromised), reactivation herpes zoster disease (shingles) typically occurs in the elderly and other immunocompromised hosts. In people with HIV, herpes zoster episodes are a harbinger of the development of AIDS. VZV can be potentially life-threatening in individuals with HIV, particularly individuals with low CD4 counts where it may present as prolonged or disseminated cutaneous or visceral disease typically associated with higher morbidity and mortality, especially when manifesting as a neurologic syndrome [51].

Epidemiology

Primary VZV infection typically occurs in childhood but can occasionally present in unvaccinated adolescents and adults [52]. In settings where varicella vaccines are not offered routinely, seroprevalence rates of 50% by age 3 and 94% by age 7 have been reported [53]. VZV is shed in oral secretions, but, unlike HSV, asymptomatic shedding is rare [54]. VZV is extremely contagious and may be transmitted by contact from individuals with active cutaneous lesions that have not undergone crusting. Respiratory droplets, however, are thought to be the primary mode of transmission [55]. Herpes zoster infection occurs more frequently among people with HIV than HIV-negative persons. A study of MSM showed that the incidence rate of herpes zoster was much higher among men with HIV (29.4 cases/100 person-years) versus 2.0 cases per 100 person-years among seronegative men [56]. While the risk of VZV reactivation in HIV-infected individuals in the cART era has decreased, there remains an increased risk of three times higher than that of the general population [57, 58]. Not unexpected is the observation in cohorts of people with HIV that low CD4 counts and not being on cART are identified risk factors for herpes zoster [59].

Pathogenesis

Following inhalational exposure to VZV, the virus invades the epithelial and immune cells of lymphoid tissue of the respiratory tract as well as the tonsils [47]. Thereafter, infected T-cells are thought to traffic the virus systemically and may initiate primary infection in the dermal tissue.

Innate immune responses including toll-like receptor-mediated processes as well as humoral responses are then able to abort or control the primary infection; however the virus is able to evade complete eradication by, among other things, modulating interferon signaling [47]. The mechanism of VZV reactivation is poorly understood, but it is generally thought that cellular immunity plays a significant role in maintaining latency of VZV primarily in sensory neural tissue, and thus factors which impair those responses can lead to reactivation of infection.

Clinical Presentation

Primary varicella infection typically presents as a generalized rash that progresses from macular to papular and to vesicular lesions, which are occasionally intensely pruritic and spread in a centrifugal pattern. Lesions may appear over 4–5 days and therefore may be at different stages of evolution at the time of presentation [60]. Superinfection of the lesions may occur with scratching, with bacterial organisms like *Staphylococcus aureus* and beta-hemolytic streptococci predominating and, although uncommon, may lead to deeper soft tissue infections and septic shock [61]. Bullous or hemorrhagic lesions may occur in immunocompromised hosts [61].

Herpes zoster lesions, on the other hand, frequently involve multiple dermatomes in HIV-infected patients, coalesce to form large lesions, last for prolonged periods on the order of weeks, and take longer to heal with reepithelization. Disseminated herpes zoster infection may also occur in immunocompromised hosts and may be indistinguishable from varicella zoster or disseminated herpes simplex infection. A rare syndrome of herpes zoster reactivation manifesting as dermatomal or radicular pain without a rash referred to as *zoster sine herpete* has been described.

Pneumonitis is rare but presents as cough, dyspnea, and hemoptysis typically occurring after the rash has erupted [52]. Chest radiograph may reveal diffuse interstitial infiltrates, and mortality without treatment is approximately 30% [52]. Neurologic syndromes associated with VZV include encephalitis, cerebellar ataxia syndrome, aseptic meningitis, Bell's palsy, Ramsay

Hunt syndrome (Bell's palsy plus herpes zoster oticus), transverse myelitis, and Guillain Barre syndrome. A post-infectious granulomatous angiitis may result in ischemic injury or hemorrhage. Ocular disease may involve multiple structures including necrotizing retinal syndromes – acute retinal necrosis (ARN) and progressive outer retinal necrosis (PORN). Headache, fever, and altered mentation are typical symptoms of VZV encephalitis, which is the most feared of the neurologic syndromes with up to 20% of survivors having residual neurologic sequelae [52]. Focal neurologic signs include cranial nerve palsies and seizures [62]. Other visceral diseases, such as hepatitis, are rare.

Diagnosis

It is possible to diagnose primary VZV infection on clinical grounds based on the characteristic appearance and spread of its rash, sometimes described as "dew drops on a rose petal" that reflects vesicular lesions on an erythematous base. Otherwise, lesions may be unroofed, and a VZV monoclonal antibody test or viral culture may identify and/or isolate the virus, respectively [60]. PCR is the most sensitive test and can be used on a wide range of biologic specimens including cerebrospinal fluid, blood, amniotic fluid, tissue, and bronchoalveolar lavage specimens [60]. For patients with VZV meningoencephalitis, cerebrospinal fluid analysis typically reveals a mononuclear pleocytosis, frequently with red blood cells, and an elevated protein [63]. Detection of VZV antibodies has limited diagnostic utility for active infection except when isolated in the CSF. IgM antibodies may not be detectable early in infection and have suboptimal sensitivity, and false-positive tests occur [60]. In general, testing for VZV-specific IgG should be limited to the identification of which susceptible individuals require active and/or passive immunization to prevent infection.

Treatment/Management

The nucleoside analogue acyclovir and prodrugs valacyclovir (acyclovir) and famciclovir (penciclovir) are treatment options for VZV [60]. The latter two drugs have better oral bioavailability, but all drugs may decrease the severity and duration and reduce the risk of complications associated with VZV infection. They may also be used for prophylaxis against herpes zoster in people with HIV [64]. Intravenous acyclovir is the formulation of choice for CNS disease. Acyclovir is generally well tolerated, but gastrointestinal, hepatic, and renal toxicities may occur. Similar to HSV, mutations in viral thymidine kinase may render VZV resistant to acyclovir, and in those instances, intravenous foscarnet may be used [60]. Antiviral resistance is rare and typically occurs in immunocompromised patients, such as those with AIDS, and prolonged antiviral agent exposure allowing for the selection of resistant viral mutants.

Prognosis/Prevention

Varicella infection may be prevented by receipt of two doses of a live attenuated vaccine (Varivax), which is universally recommended for all children beginning at age 12–15 months with a protective efficacy of about 90% [65]. Adolescents and adults may receive catch-up vaccinations at any time; however, being a live vaccine, it is contraindicated in immunocompromised individuals and pregnant women. For people with HIV, the vaccine may be safely administered at CD4 counts >200 cells/uL. On the other hand, vaccination against herpes zoster is recommended for individuals aged 50 years and older. Similar to the VZV vaccine, it may be administered cautiously in patients with CD4 count >200 cells/uL [66]. A herpes zoster vaccine, Zostavax, has been shown in the short term (<7 years post receipt), to decrease reactivation episodes by about 40–70% and the complication of postherpetic neuralgia by 60–83% [67]. A newer non-live adjuvanted subunit vaccine, Shingrix, was approved by the US FDA in October 2017 and has replaced Zostavax as the recommended vaccine to prevent herpes zoster (efficacy of >90%) and postherpetic neuralgia (efficacy of 91%) [68]. As with many vaccines, protective effectiveness may decline over time.

In the hospital, HIV-positive patients with VZV infection should be placed on both airborne and contact isolation until lesions have crusted [69].

Epstein-Barr Virus

Introduction

Human herpesvirus 4, Epstein-Barr virus (EBV), is one of the most common viral infections in the world. Among people with HIV, chronic EBV infection is associated with a wide spectrum of clinical disorders including benign conditions such as oral hairy leukoplakia and more serious life-threatening conditions including primary CNS lymphoma and Burkitt's and other non-Hodgkin's lymphomas (NHL). The epidemiology, pathogenesis, clinical presentation, and management of EBV infection are discussed below.

Epidemiology

EBV is very common worldwide with seroprevalence of >90% in adults. In a review of participants of the US NHANES, among children aged 6–19 years, non-Hispanic blacks had a higher prevalence than non-Hispanic whites, and risk factors include older age, low household income, and absence of health insurance coverage [70]. The primary route of transmission is saliva; therefore shared utensils or drinking cups and toothbrushes may be vectors. Other means of acquisition of the virus include sexual contact, organ transplant, and blood transfusion. Incubation is approximately 6 weeks [71].

Pathogenesis

Following introduction into the oral cavity, EBV infects epithelial cells wherein it replicates and then spreads to involve the lymphoid tissue of the Waldeyer's ring from where it disseminates hematogenously. Primarily, CD8 T-cell lymphocytes exert immune control over EBV replication. Dendritic cells and other antigen-presenting cells promote T-cell activity [72].

Clinical Presentation

Primary EBV infection is usually asymptomatic. It can cause a mononucleosis syndrome with cardinal symptoms including fever, myalgias, pharyngitis, swollen lymph glands particularly of posterior cervical chain, rash, and hepatosplenomegaly. The splenomegaly may occasionally be massive and leaves the individual prone to life-threatening splenic rupture with abdominal trauma. Classically, use of ampicillin may provoke a rash. Symptoms typically last for about 2 weeks, but prolonged fatigue lasting months is common. Oral hairy leukoplakia typically manifests as white coloration on the lateral aspect of the tongue in patients with immunodeficiency and may be misdiagnosed as oral candidiasis.

EBV-associated malignancies commonly present with "B symptoms" of fevers, weight loss, night sweats, and lymphadenopathy; and in HIV-infected patients, the diagnosis may be delayed as providers may attribute the symptoms to and pursue an evaluation for a chronic infection. Primary CNS lymphoma typically manifests as a solitary space-occupying lesion on brain imaging, which may be accompanied by edema with neurologic symptoms reflecting the location of the tumor. Seizures may complicate the syndrome and may frequently be the presenting symptom.

Diagnosis

While atypical lymphocytes may be noted on a peripheral blood smear, it is not pathognomonic for EBV infection. The heterophile or monospot antibody test is useful to diagnose primary EBV infection but has suboptimal sensitivity but with greater specificity depending on the assay used ranging from 70% to 92% and 96–100%, respectively [73]. The monospot test is also prone to false negative very early in infection. Acute EBV infection may be diagnosed by detection of IgM or rise in IgG antibodies to EBV capsid antigen. While not used routinely for diagnostic purposes, an EBV viral load assay will be positive in patients with infectious mononucleosis but has the limitation of being unable to differentiate reactivation from primary infection. The role of viral load assays for the diagnosis of primary CNS lymphoma is limited but may be useful as the specificity of detection of the virus in CSF is upward of 79% [74]; the sensitivity of CSF cytology is very poor (15%), but flow cytometry for clonal B-cells may improve case detection [75]. The definitive diagnosis of primary CNS lymphoma may require biopsy where other modalities fail. Burkitt's lymphoma and other NHL may be diagnosed by lymph node or bone marrow biopsies.

Treatment/Management

The antiviral acyclovir has activity against EBV; however treatment of the primary infection is limited to symptomatic therapy including antipyretics and anti-inflammatory agents as the antiviral drug has been shown to have no effect on the disease course. Oral hairy leukoplakia typically resolves with immune reconstitution in patients with HIV, but treatment with acyclovir and topical podophyllin or retinoic acid will lead to faster resolution but with high rates of recurrence.

The mainstay of treatment for primary CNS lymphoma is brain irradiation and chemotherapy [76]. For other HIV-associated lymphomas, outcomes improve with both targeted chemotherapy for the malignancy and immune reconstitution with antiretroviral therapy [77]. Therapy of lymphomas depends on the histologic type with varying chemotherapeutic regimens used such as R-EPOCH (rituximab, etoposide + prednisone + vincristine + cyclophosphamide + doxorubicin) used for the treatment of diffuse large B-cell lymphoma and Burkitt's lymphoma. High-dose chemotherapy with hematopoietic stem cell transplant is an attractive option that carries a high risk of complications but with high cure rates [77].

Prognosis/Prevention

The prognosis of EBV-associated infectious mononucleosis is excellent. Very rarely, individuals with primary infection develop an encephalitis which may be fatal. Splenomegaly associated with EBV may last for a month after the infection, so during that time individuals may wish to avoid contact sports or other conditions that may predispose to abdominal trauma. Among individuals with HIV, the prognosis of EBV-associated lymphomas is historically poor, but outcomes have improved with cART-mediated immune reconstitution and chemotherapy with 2-year survival rates for diffuse large cell B lymphomas and Burkitt's lymphoma at 67% and 75%, respectively. There is no preventative vaccine for EBV infection.

Cytomegalovirus (CMV)

Introduction

Cytomegalovirus, a lymphotropic beta-herpesvirus, is the largest of the human herpes viruses. It is also referred to as human herpes virus 5. At the time that the AIDS syndrome was first recognized, CMV disease was identified as a frequent opportunistic infection that contributed significantly to morbidity among patients with the syndrome, typically manifesting as a sight-threatening retinitis. With the availability of cART, however, the contribution of CMV to morbidity among people with HIV has decreased significantly.

Epidemiology

CMV is a common infection worldwide, in part owing to its transmissibility in a wide range of bodily fluids, including saliva, breast milk, urine, and seminal and cervicovaginal secretions. CMV can be transmitted transplacentally from mother to child, by blood transfusion and transplanted organs. In the United States, the CDC estimates that 50–80% of adults are infected with the virus by the age of 40. Risk factors for CMV infection include infection with other herpes viruses, poor nutritional status, and living in crowded dwellings [78]. Individuals caring for young children and babies are at particularly high risk. Among cohorts of people with HIV, MSM have higher seropositivity rates compared to other risk groups. Seroprevalence rates are also higher in developing compared to developed countries [78].

Pathogenesis

CMV, like other herpes viruses, establishes latency in the human host. Patients with advanced HIV infection (AIDS) are at risk for CMV reactivation and organ disease. Studies suggest that both humoral- and cellular-mediated immune responses are involved with the control of CMV replication. The virus is able to avoid full eradication by evasive mechanisms including elaboration of proteins, which protect infected cells against lysis by natural killer cells [79].

There have been various reported interactions between HIV and CMV, which impact the pathogenesis of HIV disease. CMV infection may increase infection of CD4 T-cells by HIV, promote T-cell depletion by apoptotic mechanisms, and may promote reactivation of latent virus and HIV viral replication [78].

Clinical Presentation

The majority of individuals with primary CMV infection are asymptomatic. Similarly, an overwhelming majority of individuals with reactivation viremia show no signs or symptoms of end-organ involvement. Symptomatic individuals are likely to be those with compromised immune systems such as people with HIV, transplant recipients, and individuals undergoing intensive chemotherapy. Symptomatic primary CMV infection is rarely life-threatening and typically manifests, after an incubation period of 28–60 days, as a mild "flu-like" illness with symptoms and signs such as fever, fatigue, lymphadenopathy, sore throat, and splenomegaly. An erythematous rash and hepatomegaly may also be noted on physical examination. The clinical syndrome is frequently accompanied by hallmark laboratory abnormalities including leukopenia, lymphopenia, or lymphocytosis with atypical cells, thrombocytopenia, and elevated serum transaminases (aspartate > alanine aminotransferase).

Women who acquire CMV during pregnancy, especially during the first half, are at risk of fetal infection complicated by adverse events including severe neurologic disease and disability. The majority (80%) of infants with vertical CMV infection, however, never develop symptoms. Congenital CMV disease may manifest as microcephaly, sensorineural hearing loss, mental retardation, neuromuscular disorders, and ocular disease including optic atrophy and chorioretinitis [80].

Individuals with high levels of CMV reactivation viremia are more likely to have end-organ disease. CMV can infect almost every organ and may manifest as meningitis, encephalitis, myelitis, polyradiculopathy, retinitis, pneumonitis, esophagitis, hepatitis, cholangiopathy, and colitis. In patients with advanced HIV infection, CMV retinitis is a common manifestation, and regular symptom screening for ocular symptoms and ophthalmologic exams should be performed in patients with AIDS and CD4 count <50/ul.

Diagnosis

CMV viremia may be detected using nucleic acid assays in plasma specimens. The diagnosis of end-organ disease requires a compatible clinical syndrome and confirmation of the presence of the virus either by its detection in tissue (e.g., ulcerative lesions or tissue biopsy specimens) by antigen or nucleic acid testing or evidence of its characteristic cytopathic effect on tissue specimens on microcopy. CMV retinitis is diagnosed through funduscopic visualization of pathognomonic retinal changes including white exudates with or without hemorrhage and/or areas of retinal necrosis in a susceptible symptomatic host. A definitive diagnosis of encephalitis or radiculopathy may be made if CMV is detected in cerebrospinal fluid in patients with neurologic symptoms matching the syndrome and with brain imaging showing periventricular or meningeal enhancement and spine imaging with thickened nerve roots, respectively [81].

Treatment/Management

Antivirals with activity against CMV include ganciclovir, valganciclovir, foscarnet, and cidofovir. Ganciclovir and its prodrug valganciclovir are typically first-line drugs used for treatment of CMV disease. Mutation in CMV's phosphotransferase -gene (UL97) confers resistance to ganciclovir, while mutations in the polymerase gene (UL54) make virus resistant to foscarnet, cidofovir, and ganciclovir [82]. In such cases, maribavir and brincidofovir are other antiviral agents that have activity against CMV [83]. A pyrimidine synthesis inhibitor, leflunomide, has also been used successfully to treat multidrug-resistant CMV infection [84].

Prognosis/Prevention

Studies have shown that CMV reactivation is a predictor of both end-organ disease and mortality in patients with AIDS [85, 86]. While CMV infection causes severe morbidity, it is likely that the increased mortality observed is a reflection of vulnerable hosts succumbing to other life-threatening infections associated with severe immune deficiency. Certainly, central nervous system end-organ diseases carry a worse prognosis than others. There is mixed data on the efficacy of preemptive anti-CMV treatment for patients with AIDS to mitigate this mortality risk [85, 86]. Furthermore, anti-CMV treatment is frequently associating with severe toxicities.

Individuals at risk for CMV infection include those who work with young children and babies. Pregnant women are advised to wash hands with soap and water after contact with bodily fluids including urine and saliva to prevent primary infection. Healthcare workers who adhere to standard infection control precautions do not appear to have higher rates of primary CMV infection compared to that of the general population.

There is no effective vaccine for the prevention of CMV infection or reactivation.

Human Herpesviruses 6 and 7 (HHV-6 and HHV-7)

Introduction

The relevance of human herpes virus 6 (HHV-6) infection in patients with HIV infection is unclear. The viral infection has been associated with a lymphadenopathy syndrome in patients, but its role in the development of lymphoproliferative disorders is still speculative at best as the detection of HHV-6 in tumor cells does not prove a causal role [87]. Observations suggest that HHV-6 coinfection in HIV individuals may lead to higher viral replication and thereby promote progression to AIDS [87]. HHV-7 is not thought to cause any significant clinical syndrome in people with HIV, so this section will include information on HHV-6 alone.

Epidemiology

HHV-6 infection is more common in people with HIV compared to those without [88]. PCR tests performed on gastric and colon biopsy specimens to detect HHV-6 DNA showed that 50% and 70% of HIV-infected individuals harbored the virus at these sites, respectively [88]. Seropositivity as high as 100% has also been reported [89]. Infection in immunocompromised patients may be caused by either variant A or B HHV-6. the former causing disease more frequently in immunocompromised individuals. HHV-6 is thought to be transmitted primarily by oral secretions.

Pathogenesis

HHV-6 has a trophism for certain host cells including monocytes, macrophages, T- and B-cells, NK cells, glial cells, and megakaryocytes. It establishes latency in peripheral blood mononuclear cells (PBMCs) and other sites including the oropharynx, salivary glands, female genital tract, and brain tissue [90]. Clinical disease in HIV-infected persons typically results from reactivation of latent infection. Some studies have demonstrated excess seropositivity of HHV-6 and detected HHV-6 sequences in patients with Hodgkin's disease and non-Hodgkin's lymphoma [90].

Clinical Presentation

HHV-6 infection can cause hepatitis or a mononucleosis syndrome indistinguishable from primary infection associated with other herpes viruses or HIV infection [90]. Fever and maculopapular rash that occur few days after fever are most common with primary infection. Gastrointestinal, respiratory, and central nervous symptoms may also occur. On exam, there may be hepatosplenomegaly. Hepatitis and encephalitis are clinical syndromes suggesting end-organ involvement. A prolonged benign lymphadenopathy syndrome may also occur subsequently in people with HIV.

Diagnosis

The diagnosis of HHV-6 infection is made by positive serologic tests (antibodies) or by detection of HHV-6 DNA by PCR testing or culture on body fluid specimens (blood, saliva, stool, or urine) or tissue specimens. The virus can also be detected by immunohistochemical staining of tissue or culture of body fluids and tissue. As "benign" reactivation of HHV-6 can occur without causing any end-organ disease, positive tests have to be interpreted in light of the patient's presenting syndrome to support a causal relationship.

Treatment/Management

There is no specific treatment for HHV-6 infection other than supportive measure, although the antivirals, ganciclovir and foscarnet, have been used in some cases.

Prognosis/Prevention

HHV-6 infections typically have an excellent prognosis in immunocompetent individuals; however, in people with AIDS, disseminated infection can result in death.

Human Herpesvirus 8 (HHV-8)

Introduction

Human herpes virus 8 (HHV-8) is responsible for three distinct clinical syndromes in people with HIV: Kaposi sarcoma, primary effusion lymphoma (also known as body cavity lymphoma), and multicentric Castleman disease (angiofollicular lymph node hyperplasia), all of which are neoplastic disorders. Kaposi sarcoma is the most common of the three and can occur in people with HIV regardless of CD4 count. A newer clinical syndrome yet to fully elucidated is an inflammatory cytokine condition with high mortality which lacks abnormal pathologic findings on lymph node histology [91]. A brief overview of the epidemiology, clinical presentation, and management of the syndromes is discussed below.

Epidemiology

Multicentric Castleman disease (MCD), a more aggressive form of angiofollicular lymph node hyperplasia, tends to occur predominantly in men and presents in the fifth to sixth decade of life [92]. The disease frequently coexists with Kaposi sarcoma (KS). AIDS-related KS (the epidemic form) differs from endemic KS in that it affects a younger population and has a more aggressive clinical course [93]. Primary effusion lymphoma (PEL), like MCD, frequently coexists with KS, and patients with the disease share the same clinico-demographic profiles.

Pathogenesis

Human herpesvirus 8 (HHV-8) infects a variety of host cells including monocytes and endothelial and B-cells in which it is able to establish latency by evading host immune processes and can induce proliferation and prevent apoptosis. Multiple viral proteins encoded by HHV-8 have been implicated in angiogenesis and oncogenesis [94]. Also encoded is a viral interleukin 6, and together with dysregulated human interleukin 6, they play a role in the pathogenesis of the HHV-8-associated clinical syndromes. Infection of activated lymphocytes by HHV-8 has been implicated in MCD.

Clinical Presentation

KS commonly presents as nodules or macules on skin or mucous membranes, which are often violaceous and with a range of colors including purple, red, or brown [93]. Lesions may be painful and can ulcerate and bleed. Lymphadenopathy is a common feature and may represent reactive or involved lymph nodes or may represent a separate opportunistic infection or neoplasm. Lesions in the bowel and lungs are only visible with invasive procedures with risk of bleeding with biopsy attempts. Other viscera that may rarely be affected include the liver, spleen, and bones.

Patients with MCD typically present with fever, lymphadenopathy, hepatosplenomegaly, and, less commonly, pulmonary symptoms, edema and ascites [92]. Patient with PEL may have lymphocytic effusions in the pleura, peritoneum, or pericardium. Extracavitary disease is rare.

Diagnosis

KS lesions show characteristic spindle-shaped cells in which HHV-8 can be detected by immunostaining. MCD is diagnosed by biopsy of affected lymph nodes for histology. For MCD, the plasma cell variant tends to predominate over the hyaline vascular variant (80–90% of cases), or there may be cases with mixed histology [92]. For PEL, the virus may be detected in malignant B-cells (which may be coinfected with EBV).

Treatment/Management

Mucocutaneous KS may respond to initiation of ART with immune recovery alone. The addition of chemotherapy to its management may lead to faster resolution of lesions but does not impact overall survival [95]. However, for visceral disease and extensive or complicated mucocutaneous disease, chemotherapy should be included in management of those forms of KS.

ART with immune reconstitution is insufficient to control MCD. Rituximab alone, CHOP, and a combination of the two are the most popular chemotherapeutic regimens. Due to the few cases of the disorder, trials to compare regimens are lacking, and there is no data on the comparative effectiveness of these regimens. Patients with copresenting KS and MCD may have a flare of KS with the use of rituximab alone; therefore concurrent treatment with liposomal doxorubicin or other chemotherapeutic agent with activity against KS is advocated [94]. Steroid use has also been associated with a flare in KS lesions [93]. Stem cell transplantation may be attempted in relapsed MCD after second remission with chemotherapy [92].

PEL is treated with R-EPOCH (cyclophosphamide, doxorubicin, etoposide, vincristine, and prednisone) or CHOP (cyclophosphamide, doxorubicin, vincristine, and prednisone). Other agents under investigation include pomalidomide or lenalidomide [94].

Prognosis/Prevention

The mortality rate of MCD in HIV-infected patients appears to be better than that of noninfected patients (44% vs 65%) [92]. Patients with PEL have a 2-year survival of 30–40% even following chemotherapy. Mortality from all three disease syndromes appears to have improved in the cART era supporting a beneficial role of cART. No preventive vaccines exist for HHV-8 to prevent HHV-8-associated diseases.

Polyoma Viruses (JC Virus)

Introduction

The polyoma viruses, JC and BK viruses, were first recognized in 1965 and 1971, respectively. Both viruses were named after the individuals from whom the viruses were first identified, John Cunningham virus (JCV) and BK virus (BKV). Both viruses cause unique clinical syndromes in immunocompromised patients. JCV is associated primarily with a severe demyelinating neurologic syndrome called progressive multifocal leukoencephalopathy (PML). BKV is associated with hemorrhagic cystitis and allograft loss in patients who have renal transplants. While BK viremia and viruria may be identified in people with HIV, it is not clear that there are clinical consequences of the infection.

Epidemiology

While infections with JCV occur rarely in people with AIDS (mean CD4 at diagnosis 84–104 cells/mm^3) [96], clinical disease from BKV in HIV-

positive patients occurs in the context of other conditions and/or treatments, e.g., renal transplantation and hematopoietic stem cell transplantation. Polymerase chain reaction (PCR)-based surveys of HIV patients reveal that 8–33% have been exposed to BK virus [97, 98] and 16–50% have evidence of JCV [99–101]. Prior to the availability of cART, 5–10% of AIDS patient developed PML. The mode of transmission is unclear, but the tonsils, GI tract, and kidneys may be reservoirs of the virus [101].

Pathogenesis

PML results from cytolysis and demyelination associated with JCV replication within astrocytes and oligodendrocytes. With declining T-cell immunity, loss of immune control allows for reactivation of latent virus from tissue reservoirs particularly the kidneys [101]. Interestingly, it has been demonstrated that for patients with BK virus coinfection, antibodies against BKV capsid protect against the development of PML [102].

Clinical Presentation

JCV results in four distinct clinical syndromes. It can cause PML, a fulminant variant of encephalopathy involving cortical pyramidal neurons [103], meningitis, and a granule cell neuronopathy which preferentially affects the cerebellum with clinical symptoms of ataxia, nystagmus, and tremor. Because PML can affect any area of the brain, typically with multisite involvement, symptoms differ widely between patients. In people with HIV, motor symptoms predominate over cognitive and language deficits [101]. Common symptoms include weakness, gait changes, sensory symptoms, cognitive impairment, visual symptoms, headache, behavioral abnormalities, and seizures. Fever is unusual and should prompt a search for a concurrent or an alternative diagnosis.

Diagnosis

Radiologically, PML presents as multifocal demyelination involving white matter of the brain with parieto-occipital and frontal lobes of the brain most commonly involved, and occasionally deep gray matter structures are involved [101]. Brain MRI is more sensitive than CT scans and the lesions, which are frequently coalescent and measure up to a few centimeters and are hypointense on T1 and hyperintense on T2 and flair sequences. Occasionally PML lesions show gadolinium enhancement. There is typically no edema associated with PML lesions. Detection of JCV DNA by PCR in the CSF is 92% sensitive [104]. The use of PCR may prevent the need for tissue biopsy to confirm or differentiate the diagnosis of PML from other diseases like multiple sclerosis. If a biopsy is performed, however, a classic triad of "bizarre astrocytes," demyelination, and enlarged oligodendroglial nuclei is pathognomonic of PML [96].

Treatment/Management

PML and other clinical syndromes associated with JCV represent an antiretroviral treatment emergency as immune reconstitution is the only means of controlling disease progression. Following initiation of cART, immune reconstitution inflammatory syndrome (IRIS) may develop and can mimic disease progression. Treatments which have shown some promise for JCV virus-associated disease, but that have not been rigorously evaluated in clinical trials, include mirtazapine, cidofovir, mefloquine, and dimethyl fumarate [105].

Prognosis

Mortality in patients with PML ranges from 20% to 80%, and survivors typically suffer persistent neurologic deficits [106].

Chronic Hepatitis B and C

Introduction

Hepatitis B and C contribute disproportionately to morbidity and mortality among people with HIV. These infections are particularly prevalent among HIV cohorts as they share similar routes of transmissions – sexual and vertical transmission as well as by exposure to blood or infected bodily fluids. Complications caused by these infections, including liver fibrosis with progression to cirrhosis and the development of hepatocellular carcinoma, may be accelerated in people with HIV. Because of this, liver-related mortality has surpassed AIDS and its complications as the leading cause of death in people with HIV [107]. Chronic viral hepatitis, however, is both preventable and treatable (and curable for HCV).

Epidemiology

The prevalence of HCV infection among cohorts of people with HIV ranges from 2.4% to 82.4%, with most regions averaging around 30% coinfection rates [107, 108]. Hepatitis B virus infection is much less common with prevalence rates ranging from 6% to 20% with highest coinfection rates reported in Asia and Africa where vertical transmission is the most common mode of infection [109]. Risk factors for HBV infection include intravenous drug and cocaine use and low educational level. There are ten genotypes for hepatitis B and six main viral genotypes for hepatitis C that are distributed worldwide.

Pathogenesis

HIV-infected patients have lower rates of spontaneous clearance of HCV infection compared to uninfected counterparts, although increased clearance has been reported with initiation of ART [107, 110]. For those with chronic HCV and HBV infection, HIV infection accelerates progression to cirrhosis and hepatic decompensation presumably through multiple mechanisms including its effect on pro-fibrosis mediators, induction of hepatocyte apoptosis, and HIV-associated immune dysregulation [109]. Unlike patients with HCV, individuals with HBV may frequently develop hepatocellular carcinoma in the absence of liver cirrhosis [109].

Clinical Presentation

While symptoms with acute infection may occur in patients with HBV infection after an incubation period of 1–6 months, it is very rare in patients with HCV infection. In HBV, prodromal phases of symptoms including fever, anorexia, malaise, nausea, vomiting, abdominal pain, and jaundice are frequently reported symptoms. Jaundice, hepatomegaly, and splenomegaly may also be present. HBV flares may occur and resemble symptoms of acute infection. HBV has been linked to polyarteritis nodosa (PAN). People with HCV are mostly asymptomatic, but pruritus, fatigue, arthralgia, paresthesia, myalgias, and sicca syndrome are potential extrahepatic manifestations. HCV has been linked to porphyria cutanea tarda and mixed cryoglobulinemia. Epidemiologically, HCV is associated with type 2 diabetes. Fulminant acute hepatitis is rare for both HBV and HCV infections.

Diagnosis

A positive hepatitis B surface antigen (HBsAg) suggests the presence of replicating virus. Detection of IgM antibodies to hepatitis B core antigen suggests acute infection. Persistence of HBsAg for 6 months confirms the diagnosis of chronic infection. These tests examine the host response to HBV, while quantitation of serum HBV DNA is used to assess active viral infection. Hepatitis C infection is diagnosed based on the detection of antibodies to hepatitis C; however, the test does not discriminate between cleared, cured, and active infection. A reflex HCV RNA assay is recommended to determine the presence of the virus. Assessment of response to therapy for both chronic HBV and HCV infections is based on serial assessment of viral load detection.

Treatment/Management

The treatment of HCV has been revolutionized since the approval of the first ever direct-acting antiviral drugs (DAAs) in 2011. The DAAs provide shorter treatment durations, higher cure rates, and greater regimen tolerability than previous interferon- and ribavirin-based regimens. HCV-HIV coinfected patients should have priority for treatment given the synergy of both viral infections, which results in higher rates of liver-related morbidity. The currently approved treatment regimens for HCV disease in HIV-infected patients are listed below (see Table 13.2). Reports of HBV flares in untreated HBV patients undergoing HCV therapy have prompted recommendation that HBV screening be performed routinely in patients for whom HCV therapy is being considered [111].

The mainstay of HBV treatment is nucleoside analogues: tenofovir, emtricitabine, lamivudine, and entecavir [112]. While lamivudine monotherapy has been used for HBV treatment, its low barrier to resistance limits the therapeutic length of this medication. Compared with other nucleoside analogues, tenofovir has the advantage of a high resistance barrier, retains activity against lamivudine resistant virus, and, like lamivudine and emtricitabine, has activity against HIV [113]. Oral adefovir and subcutaneously administered interferon monotherapy have largely been abandoned due to toxicity profiles and/or low resistance barrier. In general, patients with HIV and HBV coinfection should be treated for both concurrently given the availability of antiviral drugs with activity against both viruses. HBV viral load (DNA) measurements are useful for monitoring response to HBV treatment and also to assess for antiviral resistance for chronically treated patients. A viral load, however, is not predictive for a treatment endpoint and sustained response once medications are discontinued. For HBeAg-positive patients, treatment endpoints include loss and seroconversion of HBeAg, loss of HBsAg, and, the most elusive endpoint, development of hepatitis B surface antibody (HBsAb) [113]. The latter two treatment endpoints also apply to HBeAb-negative patients.

Prognosis/Prevention

The liver-related complications of HBV and HCV can be prevented with early diagnosis and treatment. Recent studies have shown, however, that patients with cirrhosis may experience regression of their fibrosis (up to 50% of individuals); however, in spite of successful treatment, a minority of patients may still develop hepatocellular cancer (HCC). Extrahepatic manifestations can occur with both viral infections and contribute significantly to morbidity and mortality including renal complications. Hepatitis B may be prevented by vaccination. Unvaccinated persons who are exposed to HBV may be administered with hepatitis B immune globulin (HBIG) to

Table 13.2 Recommended initial HCV treatment regimens for HIV-infected patients by genotype and significant antiretroviral (ARV) drug interactions (American Association for the Study of Liver Diseases [AASLD] and endorsed by the Infectious Diseases Society of America [IDSA], October 2016)

	Recommended treatment regimens	Contraindicated ARVs
HCV genotypes 1a and 1b	Elbasvir/grazoprevir × 12 weeks[a, b, c]	Cobicistat, efavirenz, etravirine, nevirapine, any protease inhibitor
	Ledipasvir/sofosbuvir × 12 weeks[b, c]	Tipranavir. Risk of increased tenofovir levels with boosted regimens (cobicistat or ritonavir)
	Paritaprevir/ritonavir/ombitasvir/dasabuvir × 12 weeks[c, f]	Darunavir, efavirenz, ritonavir boosted lopinavir and tipranavir, etravirine, nevirapine, cobicistat or rilpivirine
	Simeprevir/sofosbuvir × 12 weeks	Cobicistat, efavirenz, etravirine, nevirapine, any protease inhibitor, tipranavir
	Sofosbuvir/velpatasvir × 12 weeks[b, c]	Efavirenz, etravirine, nevirapine or tipranavir
	Sofosbuvir/daclatasvir × 12 weeks	Tipranavir
HCV genotype 2	Sofosbuvir/velpatasvir × 12 weeks[d]	As above
HCV genotype 3	Sofosbuvir/velpatasvir × 12 weeks[d]	As above
	Sofosbuvir/daclatasvir × 12 weeks[e]	As above
HCV genotype 4	Paritaprevir/ritonavir/ombitasvir + ribavirin × 12 weeks[d, f]	Darunavir, efavirenz, ritonavir boosted lopinavir and tipranavir, etravirine, nevirapine, cobicistat, rilpivirine, didanosine, stavudine, or zidovudine
	Sofosbuvir/velpatasvir × 12 weeks[d]	As above
	Elbasvir/grazoprevir × 12 weeks[d]	As above
	Sofosbuvir/ ledipasvir × 12 weeks[d]	As above
HCV genotypes 5 and 6	Sofosbuvir/velpatasvir × 12 weeks[d]	As above
	Sofosbuvir/ledipasvir × 12 weeks[d]	As above

[a]For patients with no baseline resistance-associated variants (RAVs), 16 weeks of treatment is recommended when RAVs are present
[b]Treatment regimens may also be used for patients with genotype 1a with compensated liver cirrhosis
[c]Treatment regimens may also be used for patients with genotype 1b with compensated liver cirrhosis
[d]Can be used for patients with no liver cirrhosis and compensated liver cirrhosis
[e]Should be extended to 24 weeks for patients with compensated liver cirrhosis (with or without ribavirin)
[f]This regimen containing ritonavir should only be used in patients on antiretroviral therapy

prevent infection. Antiviral agents and administration of HBIG post-delivery may be used to prevent vertical transmission of HBV infection. There is no vaccine against HCV.

Human Papilloma Virus (HPV)

Introduction

As in the general population, HPV seroprevalence is high among HIV-infected individuals. There is a recognized interaction between HPV and HIV, as development of HPV-associated cancers occurs at a much higher frequency in people with HIV, particularly anal cancer among MSM and cervical cancer in women,

the second most common cancer worldwide for that demographic. Routine screening for these cancers allows for early detection and improved patient outcomes.

Epidemiology

HPV is transmitted between individuals through skin-to-skin contact and via bodily fluids and is implicated in the pathogenesis of cervical, anal, penile, and certain head and neck cancers [114]. High-risk genotypes that predispose to these cancers include 16, 18, 31, 33, 35, 95, 45, 51, 52, 56, 58, 59, 68, 73, and 82 [115]. The prevalence of these high-risk genotypes varies in population studies. In women with HIV, surveillance studies have shown that 33–64% harbor at least one high-risk genotype and up to 12% have more than one [116–118]. The prevalence may be higher in young women (<20 years), women with indicators of high-risk sexual behavior (history of STDs and number of sexual partners), and women with HIV infection who have low CD4 counts and use oral contraceptives [115, 116, 119]. While higher sexual activity indices are associated with higher prevalence of HPV infection in men, it is not clear that circumcision is protective [120]. Anal HPV infection is associated with receptive anal intercourse, and in MSM with HIV, prevalence rates may be up to 93%, with 73.5% having high-risk genotypes [121]. Unlike HIV, female-to-male transmission of HPV is thought to be higher than male-to-male transmission [122].

Pathogenesis

The HPV genome encodes 8 early and late genes which encode 6 early proteins and 2 late proteins. Much of their roles have been elucidated. For example, early proteins 6 and 7 (E6 and E7, respectively) are both involved in cell-cycle entry and cell proliferation, as well as degrading the tumor suppressors p53 and pRb, respectively [123]. When HPV infects epithelial cells, its genome is integrated into the host cell where expression of its oncoproteins results in cellular transformation [123, 124]. High-risk HPV genotypes are able to drive proliferation of the cells typically in the basal layer of the epithelium, while low-risk HPV genotypes do not appear to cause abnormal proliferation of the cells they infect [123].

Clinical Presentation

HPV disease is asymptomatic in most individuals. Certain HPV strains cause warts that may be present on the penis, scrotum, perineum, cervix, vagina, urethra, vulva, and anus. HPV lesions may appear as keratotic lesions (less common) or the typical cauliflower-like lesions which may be smooth, flat, or dome shaped [120]. Among people with HIV, particularly people with AIDS, these lesions may grow very large in size creating unsightly and disfiguring lesions with resultant complications (e.g., urethral HPV causing outflow obstruction). HPV-associated cancers are the most severe manifestation [120].

Diagnosis

HPV disease (warts) may be diagnosed clinically based on the appearance of its characteristic skin lesions. Biopsies may be performed if they appear atypical and/or there is concern for a malignancy. Abnormal cervical or anal bleeding should prompt evaluation for cancerous lesions.

Treatment/Management

Topical imiquimod is effective for the treatment of anogenital warts with clearance rates of up to 29% after 16 weeks of application [121, 122]. Podofilox, sinecatechins, bichloracetic acid, and trichloroacetic acid are topical alternatives. Cryotherapy is also used with varying degrees of success; surgical removal may be indicated for complicated warts such as those causing penile meatal obstruction or that are refractory to medical therapy [122]. The treatment arsenal for HPV-associated malignancies include surgery, radiotherapy, chemotherapy, and anti-angiogenic agents, and treatment modalities are tailored to the type of cancer, stage, and patient characteristics [124].

Prognosis/Prevention

Regression of HPV disease does occur frequently after infection; one study found that 60% of women with HIV had regression of genital warts without treatment in the 1st year of their diagnosis and up to 82% when followed further out (13 years) [121]. Cervical cancer screening should begin at age 21, with cervical cytology performed every 3 years. Women older than 30 should have cervical cytology and HPV testing every 5 years or using the same strategy outlined for younger women up to age 65 [125]. Women with HIV should have three negative annual cervical cytology screens prior to initiating screenings every 3 years [125]. There is no data on the optimal screening strategy and frequency for anal cancers in men in spite of the recognition that HPV disease constitutes a significant disease burden to men with HIV. Most clinics caring for this patient population perform annual screening for MSM with referrals for high-resolution anoscopy with any abnormal cytology result.

Bivalent, quadrivalent, and nanovalent vaccines exist for the prevention of HPV disease and may be administered to children up to the age of

26. These vaccines all protect against the major genotypes that cause HPV-associated cancers (HPV 16 and 18) and decrease dysplasia [114, 121]. Importantly, condoms do not offer complete protection against HPV disease [120].

Bacterial Infections in HIV Infections

Clinical Bacterial Syndromes

It was recognized early in the HIV epidemic that people with HIV were particularly vulnerable not just to opportunistic pathogens but that they also experience recurrent bacterial infections such as pneumonia, sinusitis, meningitis, skin and soft tissue infections, and other pyogenic processes. In recognition of this occurrence, the US CDC incorporated recurrent bacterial pneumonia in the list of AIDS-defining conditions. With some infections, such as enteritis caused by non-typhoidal salmonella, *Shigella*, and *Campylobacter*, secondary bloodstream infections may occur [126]. With the introduction and widespread use of effective cART as well as trimethoprim-sulfamethoxazole prophylaxis in patients with AIDS, the burden of bacterial infections in HIV-infected patients has decreased but remains above the risk for individuals without HIV. Therefore, surveillance for specific bacterial infections (e.g., screening for sexually transmitted diseases and tuberculosis) and institution of preventative measures where possible are important parts of the management of someone living with HIV.

Spectrum of Infection

The spectrum of bacterial infections in HIV-infected patients includes common infections such as pneumonia, bloodstream and urinary tract infections, as well as skin and soft tissue infection which are typically the most frequent presentations but also includes bacterial infections that are sexually transmitted such as syphilis, gonorrhea, and chlamydia [127, 128]. In addition to STDs, MSM can acquire proctocolitis with bacteria including Shigella, non-typhoidal salmonella and Clostridium difficile. People who inject drugs (a common comorbidity among HIV-infected cohorts) may present with skin and soft tissue infections, vascular infection (septic thrombophlebitis), and bacterial endocarditis.

Epidemiology

One study showed that bacterial infections are responsible for up to 15% of mortality among people with HIV in an urban setting [129]. The common bacterial pathogens isolated in the bloodstream of patients who present with community-acquired infections vary by region, but the most commonly reported include *Streptococcus pneumoniae*, the *Enterobacteriaceae*, *Staphylococcus aureus*, and coagulase-negative staphylococci (usually associated with intravascular devices) [126].

Pathogenesis

In HIV infection, there is a paradoxical B-cell hyperactivation and hyporesponsiveness [130]. This is evidenced by diminished responses to vaccines which also reflects diminished T-cell function. Similarly, cells of the innate immune system including monocyte-macrophage, natural killer cells, and dendritic cells also show some dysfunction [131, 132]. Together, this immune dysregulation increases the susceptibility of people with HIV to bacterial infections.

Clinical Presentation

The clinical presentation of bacterial infections depends on the type, but certain considerations must be included for people with HIV. Patients with AIDS may have muted or no constitutional symptoms even when they have serious infections due to immunosuppression. Leukocytosis may not be present although high normal white blood cell counts, with neutrophilia and/or bandemia, should raise concern for an infectious process. Similarly, the degree of cellular pleocytosis in bodily fluids may underrepresent the degree of inflammation in the compartment. Sweats may be a reasonable surrogate for fevers which patients may not always recognize or report, and high normal temperature should be taken seriously in the setting of immunosuppression.

Diagnosis

Diagnostic tests should be performed targeting the suspected clinical syndrome as would typically be performed in an immunocompetent host. Inflammatory markers such as ESR may be challenging to interpret as baseline levels may be elevated in people with HIV compared to healthy controls [133]. On the other hand, discriminatory tests like procalcitonin, which can help distinguish bacterial from nonbacterial infectious processes, perform well in this patient population [134, 135]. Every effort should be made to obtain relevant cultures or other diagnostic tests preferably before initiation of antibiotic therapy.

As with the clinical presentation, radiologic findings may be absent or lack prominence in patients with low CD4 counts such as a "normal-appearing" chest radiograph which may occur in a patient with pneumonia. Where clinical suspicion is high, it is advisable to obtain more sensitive imaging modalities such as a chest CT scan for a pulmonary process. Because of a typically broad differential diagnosis factoring in the host immunity, invasive diagnostic testing may be indicated so as to establish a timely diagnosis to guide appropriate management.

Treatment/Management

There are several key management principles, first of which is to maintain a high index of suspicion for infection based on clinical symptoms, derangements in vital signs, and laboratory abnormalities. Secondly, it is paramount to obtain appropriate cultures prior to initiating antibiotics, including draining accessible abscesses if present. Thirdly, initiating appropriate and timely empiric antibiotics, triaging the patient to the appropriate level of care, and considering host factors when deciding on the duration of therapy for the infection are important management principles.

Prognosis and Prevention

Because of a higher risk of secondary blood stream infections and impaired host immune responses, and occasional late recognition of sepsis by providers due to subtle presentations, bacterial infections remain a significant cause of mortality among people with HIV, especially those with AIDS [136]. Endovascular and CNS infections typically carry a worse prognosis. Pneumococcal vaccination, oral care, and medication-assisted therapy or syringe exchange programs for people who inject drugs can significantly prevent bacterial infections.

Bartonella Infections (Bacillary Angiomatosis)

Introduction

There are many *Bartonella* species that cause various diseases in humans, but bacillary angiomatosis in people with HIV is typically caused by *Bartonella henselae* and *Bartonella quintana*. Disseminated disease may occur, but the mortality is low.

Epidemiology

Bartonella infections have multiple modes of transmission including contact with infected animals or by arthropod vectors including cat fleas which are transmitted occasionally by a scratch by infested cat claws (*B. henselae*). Poor personal and environmental hygiene promotes the habitat of the human body louse, *Pediculus humanus*, the vector for *B. quintana*. As a result, homelessness and poor socioeconomic status are risk factors for infection [137]. Surprisingly, high rates of occult Bartonella bacteremia have been reported in people with HIV, with one study reporting a prevalence of 10% based on PCR surveys suggesting that it is an underrecognized disease [138].

Pathogenesis

Following inoculation in to the blood, *B. henselae* and *B. quintana* adhere to and penetrate into endothelial cells where they replicate ultimately resulting in the development of reactive vasoproliferative lesions.

Clinical Presentation

Fever, skin lesions resembling Kaposi sarcoma, and lymphadenopathy are the prominent symptoms of bacillary angiomatosis. The skin lesions may take the form of angiomatous nodules, papules, or plaques, which may be red, purple, or skin colored, of different sizes with smooth or eroded surfaces [139–141]. Visceral disease involving the respiratory and GI tracts, brain, bone, and lymph nodes has been described, and symptoms referable to sites may be present. Disease caused by *B. quintana* tends to present with more neurologic features including cranial nerve deficits and seizures, while lymphadenopathy predominates for *B. henselae* [137, 140]. Endocarditis may result from Bartonella infections (a leading cause of culture-negative endocarditis), but this has been rarely reported in individuals with HIV infection [142].

Diagnosis

While rare, the diagnosis of bacillary angiomatosis should be considered in a person with HIV with multiple vascular-appearing skin papules or nodules. Serology is the mainstay of diagnosis with a rise in titers over time essentially confirming the diagnosis. Histopathology of affected organs (lymph node, liver, bone marrow) may reveal the organism with specialized staining (Warthin-Starry) or by detection of the organism using PCR [137]. *Bartonella* species are Gram-negative bacteria, and in patients with disseminated disease, blood cultures may be positive; however, the organisms are fastidious and slow-growing, so they are not always recovered in cultures. PCR tests on blood may be more sensitive for bacteremia [143].

Treatment/Management

Doxycycline and erythromycin are the mainstay of treatment for bacillary angiomatosis, and a duration of 3 months is recommended [141, 144].

Prognosis/Prevention

With appropriate management, complete resolution of skin lesions occurs; however, relapses are common. There is no preventative vaccine.

Mycobacterial Infections (TB and MAC)

Introduction

The cellular immune defects associated with HIV create particularly vulnerability for mycobacterial infections. In areas endemic for tuberculosis (TB), it contributes significantly to morbidity and is a leading cause of mortality. Mycobacterial infections are a frequent cause of immune reconstitution inflammatory syndrome (IRIS) . In non-endemic areas, *Mycobacterium tuberculosis* and *Mycobacterium avium complex* (MAC) are frequent opportunistic infections, the latter being more common in patients with advanced HIV disease.

Mycobacterium Tuberculosis (M.Tb)

Epidemiology

TB frequently coexists in people with HIV. In certain endemic countries, up to 70% of all TB cases occur in people with HIV. Reactivation of latent tuberculosis is very high in people with HIV, occurring at an annual rate of 1 in 10. This rate approximates the lifetime risk in an immunocompetent individual. Risk factors include male gender, low socioeconomic status, and poor living conditions [145]. People who inject drugs are a subpopulation that is also disproportionally impacted. Concurrent immunosuppressive medications or conditions further increase the risk of tuberculosis infection or reactivation.

Pathogenesis

Diminished T-cell-mediated immunity underlies the predisposition to mycobacterial infections. While pulmonary tuberculosis can occur at any CD4 count, disseminated and extrapulmonary forms of the disease occur at lower CD4 counts. The macrophage dysfunction which occurs in people with HIV is believed to contribute to the inability to confine the organism to the site of infection, allowing dissemination.

Clinical Presentation

The presentation of TB in people with HIV is similar in most respects to that of immunocompetent hosts. A chronic syndrome of fevers, malaise, night sweats, weight loss, and cough with or without hemoptysis should prompt a diagnostic evaluation for pulmonary TB. Of note, a cough of short duration (0–14 days) should not preclude a consideration of TB as studies have shown that cases may be detected in patients who report shorter cough periods [146]. In endemic areas, extrapulmonary disease occurs more frequently in people with HIV than in the general population, and clinical manifestations are typically referent to the organ system involved. More importantly, the clinician must bear in mind that TB can affect almost any organ system and that a high index of suspicion is warranted. Patients with unexplained pleural or pericardial effusions and ascites should have these serosal effusions sampled and tested for infectious etiologies including mycobacteria and for malignancy.

Diagnosis

Findings of chest radiography in people with HIV with pulmonary TB range from normal to grossly abnormal with focal or multilobar infiltrates, nodular or cavitary lesions with intrathoracic adenopathy, and pleural effusions being the most frequent disease patterns. A miliary pattern of pulmonary infiltrates suggests disseminated disease.

The diagnosis of TB typically requires isolation of the organism from tissue specimens and to differentiate it from other mimicking conditions including other mycobacterial infections. Sputum collection for acid-fast bacilli (AFB) smears for the evaluation of pulmonary disease are best collected in the morning for optimal yield, and multiple specimens may be sent to improve testing yield. "Sterile pyuria" in the setting of an epidemiologic risk for TB should prompt an evaluation for genitourinary disease. For patients with disseminated disease, bone marrow, lymph node, or liver biopsy specimens may be obtained for testing. Improved diagnostics including the GeneXpert MTB-RIF test which allow for both rapid detection of TB and rifampicin resistance, as well as liquid culture techniques such as the Mycobacterium growth indicator tube (MGIT), have led to significant shortening of the laboratory time required to diagnose TB. Furthermore, these diagnostic tests can be utilized for non-pulmonary specimens for the diagnosis of extrapulmonary disease. Genotyping of smear-positive specimens, where available, may provide useful preliminary information on the isolate's susceptibility profile to first- and second-line medications. One important caveat patient with HIV and AFB smear-negative sputa can have culture-positive sputa and retain the potential to transmit TB to others. Where possible, all sputa should be held for culture to rule out this possibility.

The role of tuberculin skin tests and interferon gamma release assays in the diagnosis of active tuberculosis is limited as they do not differentiate latent from active disease. Furthermore, in people with HIV with severe CD4 depletion, or who are anergic from malnutrition or other causes, the tests may be falsely negative.

Treatment/Management

The treatment of TB depends on the site or sites of involvement and susceptibility profile of the tuberculosis isolate (see Table 13.3). CNS and osteoarticular tuberculosis and multidrug-resistant isolates require modification of the choice and duration of treatment. Adjunctive steroids may be used in patients with meningitis and pericarditis and those experiencing TB-IRIS. Drug interactions complicate the management of TB in people with HIV. The non-nucleoside reverse transcriptase inhibitor, efavirenz, and integrase inhibitors are the preferred base medications to be used in combination with rifampicin. Protease inhibitors are best avoided, and rifampicin increases their metabolism and results in subtherapeutic drug levels. Rifampicin may be substituted with rifabutin to further decrease the interaction potential [145]. Also overlapping side effects such as hepatotoxicity must be considered.

Following diagnosis, local health departments or other appropriate authorities should be notified of diagnosed cases to arrange for medication

Table 13.3 Recommended treatment duration recommendations for drug-susceptible pulmonary and extrapulmonary tuberculosis (TB) (WHO guidelines 2010)

Form of tuberculosis	Recommended antitubercular drug treatment duration
Pulmonary and extrapulmonary tuberculosis[a]	6 months (2 months RHZE, 4 months RH)
Tuberculous meningitis	9–12 months (2 months RHZE, 7–10 months RH)
Bone and joint tuberculosis	9 months (2 months RHZE, 7 months RH)

E ethambutol, *H* isoniazid, *R* rifampicin, *Z* pyrazinamide
[a]Except central nervous system and bone and joint tuberculosis

supervision, often referred to as directly observed therapy (DOTs), and for contact tracing as applicable.

The timing of initiation of cART following a diagnosis of TB was explored in the SAPIT trial. The study showed a mortality benefit for patients with CD4 count <50 cell/mm^3 who were initiated on cART within 2 weeks of TB diagnosis and treatment compared to a group for whom cART was deferred. There was more IRIS in the early cART initiators; therefore, deferred cART for at least 4 weeks following initiation of antimycobacterial therapy may be advisable for those with CD4 count >50 cells/mm^3 [147].

Infection control considerations are critical to reduce the spread of TB. Patients with suspected pulmonary TB should be immediately placed on airborne isolation to decrease risk of transmission to both healthcare workers and other hospitalized patients. Because patients with extrapulmonary disease frequently have pulmonary foci, precautions should be extended to these patients until pulmonary disease is ruled out. Isolation precautions may be lifted with documented sputum conversion and after 1–2 weeks of treatment. One important caveat is that HIV-positive patients with AFB smear-negative sputa can have culture-positive sputa and retain the potential to transmit TB to others.

Prognosis

The patient's prognosis depends on prompt recognition of the infection, type of organ involvement, and institution of appropriate therapy with good adherence. Pleural and pericardial TB may result in long-term sequelae including trapped lung and constrictive pericarditis. Individuals with TB meningitis may have residual neurologic disability. Severe bony destruction by Pott's disease may require surgical stabilization.

TB can be prevented by intensive case finding (to address community-based transmission), isoniazid prevention therapy (for individuals with latent infection), and observance of infection control precautions. The BCG vaccine reduces the incidence of tuberculosis in infants and children.

Mycobacterium Avium Complex (MAC)
Introduction

Mycobacterium avium complex is a ubiquitous organism that is a common cause of infection in people with AIDS, typically manifesting as disseminated disease and is a frequent cause of IRIS.

Epidemiology

In the pre-cART era, the prevalence of MAC among AIDS patients was as high as 40% and is a marker of mortality [148]. *Mycobacterium avium* is the principal disease-causing species. The organism is acquired primarily by inhalation, but ingestion is also a significant means of infection. Risk factors for disease include CD4 count <50 cells/mm^3 and previous colonization with MAC.

Pathogenesis

As described for TB, diminished cellular immunity, as well as impairment in macrophage function, is the immunologic basis for increased susceptibility to MAC infection in people with HIV. Certain primary immune deficiencies have been also implicated in increased susceptibility to mycobacterial infections [149].

Clinical Presentation

With cART, isolated organ involvement has been reported including isolated pulmonary disease and may reflect the impact of cART on host immunologic status [150]. The clinical presentation of disseminated MAC (dMAC) is nonspecific; however, in patients with advanced HIV infection (e.g., CD4 <50/mm^3), constitutional symptoms of weight loss, fatigue, intermittent fevers, night sweats, as well as organ-centered symptoms, such as diarrhea, lymphadenitis, and/or abdominal pain, should prompt the clinician to include a workup for MAC. Hepatosplenomegaly and lymphadenopathy may also be present.

Diagnosis

The diagnosis of MAC can be made by isolating the organism in blood (by culture) or by a biopsy of affected tissue including the bone marrow and/or liver in disseminated disease. While blood culture has reasonable sensitivity, the results do not return quickly enough, typically taking 2–4 weeks to grow in culture. If there is pulmonary involvement, multiple sputa may be sent for AFB smear and culture but interpreted with caution as MAC is an occasional contaminant of respiratory specimens. When AFB are identified in clinical specimens, rapid PCR tests may detect MAC shortening the time-specific species identification, which, in the past, had to be identified only after growth in culture. Certain laboratory abnormalities such as cytopenias (suggesting bone marrow involvement) and elevated liver transaminase or alkaline phosphatase (suggesting liver involvement) in the context of a compatible syndrome favor MAC as the etiology.

Treatment/Management

The anchor for the treatment of MAC is the macrolides: clarithromycin or azithromycin. These have excellent penetration into the intracellular compartment which makes them ideal for treating MAC, an intracellular pathogen. Combination therapy is the norm for the dual benefit of synergistic bactericidal activity and to prevent the emergence of drug resistance. Clarithromycin appears to be superior to azithromycin with regard to microbiologic clearance of the organism. Rifabutin and ethambutol are typically used in addition to a macrolide offering the advantage in clinical trials of improving clinical cure rates with less relapse. Aminoglycosides can be added for severe disease although long-term use carries the risk of renal and hearing complications. As with the treatment of TB, the use of rifabutin and clarithromycin raises risk of drug-drug interactions including with cART. Treatment for dMAC should be continued for at least 1 year and/or for 3–6 months after CD4 stays above 100 cells/mm^3, whichever is longer.

Prognosis

To the extent that MAC in patients with AIDS reflects severely impaired immune status, it has been shown in multiple studies to correlate with an increased risk of mortality. Prevention may take the form of primary prophylaxis with intermittent azithromycin for HIV patients at risk for dMAC. For individuals with a past episode, secondary prophylaxis with azithromycin or clarithromycin should be given until sufficient immune recovery (>100 cells/mm^3).

Parasitic Infection

Toxoplasmosis

Introduction

Toxoplasmosis is a common protozoal infection that afflicts people with AIDS who have more advanced HIV infection (i.e., CD4 <50 cells/mm^3), typically occurring as reactivation of prior infection in the setting of being severely immunocompromised.

Epidemiology

Toxoplasma gondii, an obligate intracellular protozoan and the causative organism of toxoplasmosis, is acquired via ingestion of raw/undercooked meats or contact with cats and their feces containing oocysts. Vertical transmission of tachyzoites can occur and is the only form of person-to-person transmission known to occur. The incubation period is 10–23 days. Seroprevalence rates of 10–90% have been reported, with higher rates observed in certain European and developing countries [151].

Pathogenesis

When *Toxoplasma* cysts or oocysts are ingested, bradyzoites or sporozoites are released, respectively, and penetrate the lining of the gastrointestinal tract where they are transported via lymphatics and are subsequently disseminated through the bloodstream. At the tissue level, the organism proliferates, producing necrotic foci. In severely immunodeficient individuals, this process can progress without disruption, leading to clinically overt disease.

Clinical Presentation

In people with AIDS, the most common presentation of toxoplasmosis is cerebral disease which typically manifests as multiple ring-enhancing lesions on CT scan and MRI brain imaging [152]. Seizures, fevers, altered mentation, and focal neurologic deficits are frequent findings. Rarely, dissemination may occur with rash. Ocular, cardiac, and pulmonary disease can occur but are also uncommon.

Diagnosis

Exposure to *Toxoplasma gondii* can be determined by the detection of IgG antibodies; however, the test does not distinguish active infection from past exposure. A negative IgG test makes toxoplasmosis unlikely. *Toxoplasma* PCR may be assessed in various body fluids or tissue specimens but has suboptimal sensitivity. Biopsies may be attempted on involved organs to enable detection of the organism; however, for the brain, risks may outweigh benefits. As such, a therapeutic trial of agents known to be active against the protozoan may first be attempted, and, if there is no improvement in 1–2 weeks, invasive diagnostic testing will then be justified. This usually results in the diagnosis of an alternate etiology of the brain lesion.

Treatment/Management
The standard of care for toxoplasmosis is combination treatment with pyrimethamine with leucovorin and sulfadiazine. High-dose trimethoprim-sulfamethoxazole is an alternative. A combination of pyrimethamine and leucovorin with clindamycin or atovaquone is appropriate for patients with allergies to sulfa-containing medications. Steroids may be used for severe brain swelling with mass effect. A 6-week treatment course is recommended followed by secondary prophylaxis in people with HIV until the CD4 count remains above 200 cells/mm^3 for 3–6 months. Antiepileptic medications may be required if the patient presents with seizures.

Prognosis
With prompt and appropriate treatment, toxoplasmosis usually responds to appropriate therapy; however, neurologic deficits may persist.

Fungal Infections

General Introduction
Certain fungal infections are particularly common in people with HIV: these include cutaneous infections, *Pneumocystis jirovecii* pneumonia, endemic mycoses, cryptococcal disease, and mucocutaneous candidiasis. Filamentous fungal infections such as aspergillosis and mucormycoses are less common, for unclear reasons, unless related to other immunocompromising conditions such as receipt of cancer chemotherapy,

posttransplant, steroid use, or poorly controlled diabetes mellitus. This section will discuss common fungal infections in people living with HIV.

Oropharyngeal Candidiasis

Introduction
Candidiasis is the most frequent opportunistic fungal infection observed in people with HIV. Oral candidiasis is a reliable marker of severe immune deficiency and heralds the susceptibility to other opportunistic infections if the individual remains untreated. Esophageal candidiasis and candidiasis of the upper airway tract are designated as AIDS-defining conditions.

Epidemiology
Colonization with *Candida* occurs in up to 65% of adults [153]. There are no differences in colonization rates between people with and without HIV. Risk factors for clinical disease include smoking, dentures, use of inhaled or systemic steroids or other immunosuppressant medications, xerostomia, and exposure to broad spectrum antibiotics [153]. The most common species causing disease in people with HIV is *Candida albicans*. Other species that cause disease include *C. glabrata* and *C. krusei*, which may be the predominant species in patients receiving fluconazole. *C. glabrata* is variably fluconazole-sensitive, while *C. krusei* is fluconazole-resistant. Invasive visceral candidiasis and bloodstream infections may occur in people with HIV with other comorbidities, such as cancer chemotherapy-associated mucositis and neutropenia and indwelling vascular devices.

Pathogenesis
Candida species are common commensals of the human gastrointestinal tract. *Candida* species possess enzymes known as secreted aspartyl proteases (SAPs), which facilitate adherence and damage to epithelial surfaces [154]. These SAPs degrade host epithelial cell-mediated anticandidal immune responses which play a role in suppressing the development of clinical disease. On the other hand, protease inhibitors used in the treatment of HIV may impede adherence

mechanisms of *Candida* as HIV protease has homology with Candida SAPs [153, 154]. CD4 cells, through expression of TH-17 cytokines, also participate in the defense against *Candida* infection [154].

Clinical Presentation
Oropharyngeal candidiasis in HIV patients manifests as three forms: (1) white dense plaques, semi-adherent to the buccal mucosa, palate, gingivae, tongue, or throat, (2) erythematous patches at the same sites, and (3) hyperplastic firmly adherent plaques on the buccal mucosa, palate, and tongue that may mimic oral hairy leukoplakia [153]. Dysphagia in the setting of oral candidiasis usually implies esophageal involvement. Odynophagia is unusual and should raise concern for ulcerative disease, most frequently caused by HSV or CMV. Severe disease can impair taste sensation and, in patients with dysphagia, impair nutrition and the ability to take oral medications.

Diagnosis
The diagnosis can be made by its characteristic clinical appearance and confirmed by resolution with antifungal therapy. Oral swabs for fungal stains and culture are indicated in patients who do not respond to treatment and may reveal species that are resistant to the chosen therapy, for example, *Candida krusei* in patient who is treated with fluconazole. Esophageal candidiasis is easily visualized and identified by upper endoscopy; however, the invasive test is not warranted in all cases.

Treatment/Management
Spontaneous resolution of candidiasis is uncommon in adults with HIV, and treatment is generally indicated. Topical therapies with clotrimazole or nystatin are effective treatments. Gentian violet has been shown to be a lower-cost and equally effective alternative to oral nystatin for the treatment of oropharyngeal candidiasis [155]. Oral azoles allow for systemic treatment with higher efficacy than nystatin [156]. Azole-resistant *Candida* species, however, will require treatment with an intravenous echinocandin or an amphotericin B formulation. Treatment duration of 14 days is recommended and relapses are common.

Prognosis/Prevention
Candidiasis responds quickly to antifungal drugs and typically resolves within a week. *Candida* vaccines are in early phase development [157].

Pneumocystis jirovecii Pneumonia (PJP)

Introduction
Pneumocystis jirovecii pneumonia (PJP) was one of the opportunistic infections that drew attention to the AIDS epidemic. It remains one of the most common opportunistic infections, irrespective of setting, reflecting the global distribution of the causative organism. An improved understanding of the natural history and pathogenesis of disease caused by the organism has led to advancements in its management, which has translated into improved treatment outcomes for patients.

Epidemiology
Pneumocystis jirovecii (formerly *P. carinii*) is acquired via inhalation. The organism has a predilection for the lungs where the trophic form predominates over the cystic stage of the fungus. Colonization without clinical disease is well described, and human-to-human transmission can occur [158]. Before cART, up to 80% of people with AIDS developed disease associated with the organism. Since cART and widespread use of antimicrobial prophylaxis, the incidence has dramatically declined.

Pathogenesis
Alveolar macrophages are thought to be the primary host defense against *Pneumocystis* [159]. Immunoglobulins (IgG) and other opsonins are also involved with the macrocytic phagocytosis of invading organisms. CD4 T-cells produce cytokines in response to *Pneumocystis*, which facilitate recruitment of neutrophils and macrophages to the lung but also mediate tissue damage [159]. Thereby, tissue damage occurs from the immune response to the organism rather than the organism itself.

Clinical Presentation

Patients with PJP typically report a subacute syndrome of dyspnea that is worse on exertion, dry cough, low-grade fever, and malaise. While tachypnea and exertional hypoxia are common, cyanosis is rare. Lung exam may be normal or demonstrate diffuse dry crackles. There is usually no wheezing. Extrapulmonary pneumocytosis (liver, spleen, brain, retina, or kidney) is rare.

Diagnosis

The typical radiographic appearance of PJP is that of bilateral ground-glass opacities more easily identified on a high-resolution chest CT than X-ray. In patients who received inhaled pentamidine for prophylaxis, upper lobe disease alone may occur. Focal consolidation, pleural effusions, or intrathoracic adenopathy is unusual and should prompt search for an alternate primary or concurrent etiology. Granulomatous disease manifesting as nodular opacities on chest imaging has also been reported in a minority of patients with PJP [160]. The definitive diagnosis of PJP requires visualization of the teacup-shaped fungal forms in respiratory secretions including induced sputum or bronchoalveolar lavage, the latter specimen being more sensitive. While transbronchial biopsies are very helpful from a diagnostic standpoint, the risk of pneumothorax is high and may not justify the invasive procedure. A surrogate marker of the fungus, $1 \rightarrow 3$ beta-D-glucan, may be useful where bronchoscopy is not available and has a sensitivity of 92% and a specificity of 65% [161, 162]. The low specificity, however, reflects the cross-reaction with other fungi such as *Candida*, *Aspergillus*, and *Histoplasma* which is a significant limitation. Although frequently used historically, the utility of an elevated LDH as a screening test to assess the likelihood of PJP is problematic as it has suboptimal sensitivity and specificity [163].

Treatment/Management

Trimethoprim/sulfamethoxazole (15–20/75–100 mg/kg/day) [Bactrim] is the mainstay of therapy. This may be given orally in mild to moderate disease, while IV is used for severe disease. Individuals unable to tolerate Bactrim can take atovaquone for mild to moderate disease. In severe disease, IV pentamidine or IV clindamycin + primaquine are reasonable options, although with significant toxicities. A 21-day treatment duration is recommended and is usually successful for the vast majority of patients. For individuals with a paO2 <70 mmHg or A-a gradient >35 mmHg, the use of a tapering course of adjunctive steroids confers a mortality benefit and decreases the probability of requiring mechanical ventilator support. After treatment is completed, people with HIV should be placed on prophylaxis until the CD4 count recovers to above 200 cell/mm^3 for at least 3 months.

Prognosis

The mortality rate from PJP is about 10–20% in people with HIV [159].

Histoplasmosis

Introduction

Histoplasmosis is a significant cause of morbidity and mortality among people with HIV, especially individuals living in areas endemic to the fungus. Its presentation may mimic mycobacterial disease and limited diagnostics, especially in resource-limited settings, and may lead to delayed recognition of the disease. A synopsis of the epidemiology, clinical presentation, management, and prevention is presented below.

Epidemiology

The causative organism of histoplasmosis, *Histoplasma capsulatum*, has a worldwide distribution and may be isolated in soil, bird, and bat droppings [164]. Three varieties of the fungus have been described with regional differences in distribution: *H. capsulatum* var. *duboisii* being found in Africa (African histoplasmosis), *H. capsulatum* var. *capsulatum* in the Americas, and *H. capsulatum* var. *farciminosum*, which causes disease in animals in Africa and the Middle East [164]. African histoplasmosis is reported to occur very rarely in people with HIV [165]. In the United States, the Ohio and Mississippi valley regions are endemic for histoplasmosis. Two to

25% of people with HIV living in endemic areas develop clinical disease [164]. Exposure to birds including chickens and low baseline CD4 counts (<150 cells/mm^3) have been identified as risk factors for the disease [166].

Pathogenesis

Histoplasma, a dimorphic fungus, exists in its yeast form at body temperature and as a mold at cooler temperatures. Humans become infected through inhalation of its micronidia or hyphal forms, and in the lungs, the organism is ingested by phagocytic cells of the innate immune system (macrophages, neutrophils, and dendritic cells), which also facilitate its dissemination to mediastinal and hilar lymph nodes and organs of the reticuloendothelial system [164]. When cell mediated immunity is depressed, clinical disease is more likely; otherwise, a latent, asymptomatic infection typically results following exposure.

Clinical Presentation

In people with HIV, clinical disease may result from acute infection or reactivation of latent foci. Clinical syndromes of histoplasmosis include acute and chronic pulmonary infection. Disseminated disease is the most common presentation in people living with AIDS. Less common presentations include pericardial, cutaneous, gastrointestinal, ocular, musculoskeletal, central nervous system, and rheumatologic disease [167]. Disseminated histoplasmosis may involve any organ.

Patients with histoplasmosis typically present with nonspecific chronic symptoms of fatigue, fever, headache, and weight loss. Those with pulmonary disease may report cough and dyspnea and may be found to be hypoxic. Individuals with esophageal disease may report dysphagia or odynophagia, and diarrhea may be a marker of bowel involvement. Examination may reveal hepatic or splenic enlargement, peripheral lymphadenopathy, and a skin rash particularly in patients with disseminated infection [164]. Patients with CNS disease may present with neurologic symptoms including deficits attributable to a space-occupying lesion (histoplasmoma).

Diagnosis

Patients with pulmonary disease may have a myriad of findings: diffuse interstitial infiltrates and miliary and cavitary lung disease associated with mediastinal or hilar adenopathy. The presence of calcified granulomata may signify past exposure. An elevated LDH level is frequently observed, and pancytopenia suggests bone marrow involvement. Histoplasma antigen detection tests are a useful diagnostic marker with variable sensitivity (42–100%), depending on the test and specimen used. Serum and urine antigen testing is a very useful test for detection of systemic histoplasmosis. The test cross-reacts with other fungal infections such as blastomycosis, coccidioidomycosis, and aspergillosis [168]. Blood cultures may be useful in patients with disseminated disease. Fungal stains and cultures should be performed on all tissue specimens with bone marrow specimens offering the highest yield, but cultures may take up to 6 weeks to yield positive results. PCR tests are a helpful adjunct test that may be performed on tissue specimens with the advantage of more rapid diagnosis, though sensitivity remains suboptimal [168]. Seroconversion following exposure to *Histoplasma capsulatum* typically occurs 4 weeks following exposure. Antibodies do not distinguish latent from active infection, though a negative test makes chronic infection less likely. In addition, antibody testing has a limitation of lower sensitivity in people with HIV (90%) [167].

Treatment/Management

For patients with severe or disseminated histoplasmosis, intravenous liposomal amphotericin B as induction therapy for at least 2 weeks (or 4–6 weeks for patients with CNS disease) followed by oral itraconazole for 1 year is the recommended treatment [169]. As there are significant drug interactions between itraconazole and antiretroviral drugs including efavirenz and protease inhibitors, adjustments may have to be made to HIV therapy. Fluconazole is less effective than itraconazole for the treatment of histoplasmosis [164].

Prognosis/Prevention

Severe fatal forms of histoplasmosis have been described that present as severe sepsis with multi-organ failure and may occur in 10–20% of people with HIV with mortality rates as high as 70% [164]. People with HIV living in endemic areas should be considered for itraconazole prophylaxis (200 mg/day) when CD4 counts fall below 150 cell/mm^3. Secondary prophylaxis should be continued until CD4 counts >150 cells/mm^3 for 6 months on cART and after they have received at least 12 months of antifungal therapy with negative fungal blood cultures and with a serum *Histoplasma* antigen <2 ng/mL [169].

Cryptococcal Infection

Introduction

Central nervous system (CNS) disease associated with cryptococcal infection is a major cause of morbidity in people with HIV/AIDS with a significant mortality rate in spite of optimal management. As with other opportunistic infections, the availability of cART has led to decreased incidence of this serious condition.

Epidemiology

Cryptococcal disease in HIV-infected patients is primarily caused by two species of *Cryptococcus*, *Cryptococcus neoformans* and *Cryptococcus gattii*. The latter organism has a predilection for forming cryptococcomas in the CNS, causing disease in immunocompetent individuals, and some strains have a high fluconazole minimum inhibitory concentration [170]. *C. neoformans* is globally distributed, although with significant variation in the prevalence of species and molecular types. The yeast has been isolated from tree hollows, soil, and bird droppings [170, 171]. The prevalence of cryptococcal infection among people with HIV ranges from 5% to 8% in developed countries but is higher in developing countries. The portal of entry is likely inhalation of yeasts. In people with HIV, the most common presentation of cryptococcal infection is meningitis; however, pulmonary, lymph node, and musculoskeletal can occur. Skin disease is often a marker of dissemination [171]. The incubation period is not well defined and ranges from 1 to 110 months [170].

Pathogenesis

Following inhalation, cryptococcal organisms invade lung tissue and subsequently disseminate through the blood stream. The polysaccharide capsule of the yeast enables it to evade or suppress host immune responses, and enzymes like urease promote its ability to penetrate human tissue. Defective neutrophil, natural killer (NK), dendritic cell, and monocyte-macrophage function have been shown, primarily in animal models, to be associated with susceptibility to cryptococcal disease [172–175]. In humans, impaired cellular immunity is the major risk factor for *C. neoformans* meningitis. In cryptococcal meningitis, the organism can obstruct CSF drainage through the arachnoid granulations, commonly leading to hydrocephalus which is a life-threatening complication of the disease [176].

Clinical Presentation

Generalized and nonspecific symptoms of cryptococcal disease include fevers with chills and/or sweats and weight loss. Individuals with CNS disease may have a headache as their solitary symptom, nuchal rigidity, photophobia, and other classical signs of meningismus are frequently absent. Abnormal mentation, blurring of vision, focal neurologic deficits with cranial nerve VI involvement being the most common, and seizures may occur especially if there are concurrent brain space-occupying lesions (cryptococcomas). Cognitive impairment, gait ataxia, urinary incontinence, and/or vomiting should raise concerns for raised intracranial pressure associated with CNS disease [177]. Cryptococcal pneumonia typically manifests with cough with or without hemoptysis, dyspnea, and pleuritic chest pain. Skin lesions of *Cryptococcus* may be nodular or exhibit the characteristic central umbilication resembling *Molluscum contagiosum* lesions; however, cryptococcal lesions are typically larger. Biopsies are required to establish the diagnosis.

Diagnosis

In patients with cryptococcal meningitis, head imaging may reveal ventriculitis with or without ventricular dilatation, and focal nodules or cystic lesions may be demonstrated [171]. CSF analysis typically reveals a lymphocytic predominance of white blood cells, with high protein and low glucose. Characteristically, opening pressures are elevated in patients with cryptococcal meningitis. Organisms may be rapidly identified by the use of India ink stain (sensitivity of 70–90%). Otherwise cultures of CSF or other specimens (e.g., blood or tissue) are very sensitive and typically yield growth of the organism within 2–5 days. Cryptococcus will grow on most standard blood culture media and fungal media including Sabouraud Dextrose Agar. Cryptococcal antigen tests have the advantage of rapid diagnosis with a titer of >1:4 having >90% sensitivity for detection of disease [177]. Chest imaging may reveal focal infiltrates, nodules, and/or cavitary disease. Large lesions mimicking malignancy may occur. Biopsies of the skin, lymph node, bone marrow, lungs, and brain or other tissue specimens, when performed, allow for direct visualization of the organisms in tissue with specialized stains.

Treatment/Management

Treatment of CNS cryptococcosis occurs in three phases: induction, consolidation, and maintenance. There is robust evidence showing that induction treatment with amphotericin B and flucytosine confers a morbidity and mortality benefit [178]. Liposomal amphotericin offers the advantage of better CNS penetration and less nephrotoxicity than conventional amphotericin B. In areas where flucytosine is unavailable, fluconazole may be used as a substitute in combination with amphotericin, but studies have shown lack of a mortality benefit compared to amphotericin alone [178]. Induction phase of treatment should be for 2 weeks or until CSF cultures are negative, whichever comes last. In patients with cryptococcomas, prolonged induction phases up to 6 weeks are recommended by the Infectious Diseases Society of America (IDSA) [179]. Consolidation phase consists of fluconazole 400–800 mg once

daily for an 8-week period and then maintenance therapy (or secondary prophylaxis) with fluconazole 200 mg once daily until CD4 counts are above 100 cells/mm^3 for >3 months. The use of adjunctive steroids has not been shown to impact mortality and leads to higher adverse effects and disability in patients with AIDS-associated cryptococcal meningitis [180]. Recent clinical trials have shown that sertraline may be a reasonable substitute for fluconazole for the treatment of cryptococcal meningitis [181, 182].

An important component of managing cryptococcal meningitis is the monitoring of electrolytes. Amphotericin B causes electrolyte wasting, and hypokalemia and hypomagnesemia are serious risks during treatment, as well as acute kidney injury, and significant renal impairment can increase flucytosine levels, leading to marrow and gastrointestinal toxicity. Also, ongoing monitoring of intracranial pressure is critical with changes in clinical status such as worsening headache, vomiting, and new or evolving neurologic deficits. Spinal taps may be required daily until pressure normalizes. In a minority of patients, an external ventricular drain or a ventriculoperitoneal shunt may be placed to provide relief of spinal fluid pressure. Patients with seizures in the setting of CNS lesions require antiepileptics.

Another important consideration in patients with cryptococcal meningitis is the timing of antiretroviral therapy for patients who are cART naïve. Studies show higher mortality in patients who receive cART within 2 weeks of the diagnosis and treatment compared to deferred therapy (after 4–5 weeks) [183]. Initiation of cART at four or more weeks into treatment of cryptococcal meningitis is recommended.

In isolated pulmonary, lymph node, or skin disease, fluconazole alone may be an adequate treatment.

Prognosis

Mortality from cryptococcal meningitis ranges from 5.5% to 25% with survivors also experiencing residual neurologic and intellectual disability. Outcomes are worse in resource-limited settings. Predictors of mortality include a low CSF WBC count (<20 cells per high-power field), altered mental status, high fungal burden, and older age (>50 years), and slow rate of clearance of CSF infection have been associated with increased mortality [184]. The development of immune reconstitution inflammatory syndrome (IRIS) with introduction of cART may mimic disease progression or relapse and can pose a great challenge to the clinician to differentiate them. IRIS can lead to increased morbidity and mortality.

The best way to prevent cryptococcal meningitis is the maintenance of a robust CD4 count with cART. Studies do support the use of fluconazole prophylaxis for patients with asymptomatic cryptococcal antigenemia for the prevention of end-organ disease [185].

Immune Reconstitution Inflammatory Syndrome (IRIS)

HIV-infected patients initiated on cART and who achieve viral suppression typically experience improvements in immune responses demonstrated by a rise in CD4 counts. This phenomenon may result in inflammatory responses to an existing opportunistic pathogen manifesting as a new manifestation of a previously undiagnosed subclinical infection (unmasking IRIS) or worsening of an already diagnosed infection (paradoxical IRIS) typically occurring 3–6 months following initiation of cART [186]. However, shorter periods of occurrence of IRIS of under a week or longer period of months to years have been reported. Patients on the integrase strand transfer inhibitor class of antiretrovirals, which cause steep virologic decay, experience disproportionately higher rates of IRIS compared to other classes of antiretrovirals [186]. Other risk factors for IRIS include a low CD4 count and high HIV viral load at treatment initiation [187].

The presentation of IRIS is nonspecific but is attributable to an inflammatory response to the infecting pathogen, and symptoms or signs are manifest at sites where the organism is present. For example, a patient with *Pneumocystis jirovecii* pneumonia may develop adult respiratory distress syndrome with worsening hypoxia, or a patient with cerebral toxoplasmosis may have worsening brain edema around a focal brain lesion and/or manifest new (previously undetected) lesions on imaging with worsening neurologic signs. For patients with CNS OIs, development of IRIS may be catastrophic and lead to mortality.

While IRIS is a clinical diagnosis, a thorough diagnostic evaluation targeted at the patient's signs and symptoms is prudent and may include a thorough physical exam (such as eye exams for CMV retinitis); blood tests including cultures for bacteria, acid-fast bacilli, and fungi; cerebrospinal fluid examination; imaging; and tissue biopsies. As IRIS may mimic disease progression, consideration should be given to possible resistance of the pathogen to the therapy administered prior to the event.

As a rule, the management of IRIS should not include discontinuation of antiretroviral except in very extreme cases that are life-threatening. Anti-inflammatory medications such as aspirin and nonsteroidal anti-inflammatory drugs may be used to provide symptom relief. The use of steroids should be done very judiciously as it may cause more harm than benefit except for well-defined syndromes such as TB-IRIS where it has been shown to decrease length of hospitalization and improve patients' quality of life [188].

Due to concerns for paradoxical IRIS, delaying initiation of cART for no more than a 2-week period from the initiation of treatment of most OIs may prevent its occurrence, but delayed cART initiation beyond the 2-week timeframe may also result in adverse consequences [189]. One OI for which this recommendation does not apply is cryptococcal meningitis where early cART initiation (<4 weeks) may lead to increased mortality [183].

Future Directions

For the HIV-infected patient, improving rates of early diagnosis as well as access to and utilization of effective cART is the most important factor that has and will continue to lead to a decline in the incidence of OIs [11, 190]. However, achieving those goals is particularly difficult for low-resource settings, such as sub-Saharan Africa that have been disproportionately impacted by the HIV epidemic. In recent years, better diagnostics have led to faster and more accurate identification of OIs, and these are expected to continue to evolve positively. For treatment of OIs, it is hoped that future studies will inform better ways to utilize or administer existing treatments or evaluate new treatments that should result in improved management and outcomes of patients with HIV-associated OIs.

References

1. (CDC) CfDC. Kaposi's sarcoma and Pneumocystis pneumonia among homosexual men – New York City and California. MMWR Morb Mortal Wkly Rep. 1981;30(25):305–8.
2. Jaffe HW, Bregman DJ, Selik RM. Acquired immune deficiency syndrome in the United States: the first 1,000 cases. J Infect Dis. 1983;148(2):339–45.
3. Harris C, Small CB, Klein RS, Friedland GH, Moll B, Emeson EE, et al. Immunodeficiency in female sexual partners of men with the acquired immunodeficiency syndrome. N Engl J Med. 1983;308(20):1181–4.
4. (CDC) Cfdc. A cluster of Kaposi's sarcoma and Pneumocystis carinii pneumonia among homosexual male residents of Los Angeles and Orange Counties, California. MMWR Morb Mortal Wkly Rep. 1982;31(23):305–7.
5. Barre-Sinoussi F, Chermann JC, Rey F, Nugeyre MT, Chamaret S, Gruest J, et al. Isolation of a T-lymphotropic retrovirus from a patient at risk for acquired immune deficiency syndrome (AIDS). Science (New York, NY). 1983;220(4599):868–71.
6. Gallo RC, Sarin PS, Gelmann EP, Robert-Guroff M, Richardson E, Kalyanaraman VS, et al. Isolation of human T-cell leukemia virus in acquired immune deficiency syndrome (AIDS). Science (New York, NY). 1983;220(4599):865–7.
7. Editors. Francoise Barre-Sinoussi and Luc Montagnier share the 2008 Nobel Prize for Physiology and Medicine for their discovery of the human immunodeficiency virus (HIV). AIDS (London, England). 2009;23(1):1.
8. Kilmarx PH. Global epidemiology of HIV. Curr Opin HIV AIDS. 2009;4(4):240–6.
9. (WHO) WHO. Global summary of the AIDS epidemic 2014. 2015.
10. UNAIDS. 2030: ending the AIDS epidemic. Fact Sheet 2015. 2015.
11. Frieden TR, Foti KE, Mermin J. Applying public health principles to the HIV epidemic – how are we doing? N Engl J Med. 2015;373(23):2281–7.
12. Luzuriaga K, Mofenson LM. Challenges in the elimination of pediatric HIV-1 infection. N Engl J Med. 2016;374(8):761–70.
13. Liotta G, Marazzi MC, Mothibi KE, Zimba I, Amangoua EE, Bonje EK, et al. Elimination of mother-to-child transmission of HIV infection: the drug resource enhancement against AIDS and malnutrition model. Int J Environ Res Public Health. 2015;12(10):13224–39.
14. Hoos D, El-Sadr WM, Dehne KL. Getting the balance right: scaling-up treatment and prevention. Glob Publ Health. 2017 Apr;12(4):483-497.
15. Althoff KN, Rebeiro P, Brooks JT, Buchacz K, Gebo K, Martin J, et al. Disparities in the quality of HIV care when using US department of health and human services indicators. Clin Infect Dis: Off Publ Infect Dis Soc Am. 2014;58(8):1185–9.
16. Ogbuagu O, Bruce RD. Reaching the unreached: treatment as prevention as a workable strategy to mitigate HIV and its consequences in high-risk groups. Curr HIV/AIDS Rep. 2014;11(4):505–12.
17. Palella FJ Jr, Baker RK, Moorman AC, Chmiel JS, Wood KC, Brooks JT, et al. Mortality in the highly active antiretroviral therapy era: changing causes of death and disease in the HIV outpatient study. J Acquir Immune Defic Syndr. 2006;43(1):27–34.
18. Smith CJ, Ryom L, Weber R, Morlat P, Pradier C, Reiss P, et al. Trends in underlying causes of death in people with HIV from 1999 to 2011 (D:A:D): a multicohort collaboration. Lancet (London, England). 2014;384(9939):241–8.
19. Bowen DL, Lane HC, Fauci AS. Immunopathogenesis of the acquired immunodeficiency syndrome. Ann Intern Med. 1985;103(5):704–9.
20. Miedema F, Petit AJ, Terpstra FG, Schattenkerk JK, de Wolf F, Al BJ, et al. Immunological abnormalities in human immunodeficiency virus (HIV)-infected asymptomatic homosexual men. HIV affects the immune system before CD4+ T helper cell depletion occurs. J Clin Invest. 1988;82(6):1908–14.
21. Ciobanu N, Welte K, Kruger G, Venuta S, Gold J, Feldman SP, et al. Defective T-cell response to PHA and mitogenic monoclonal antibodies in male homosexuals with acquired immunodeficiency syndrome and its in vitro correction by interleukin 2. J Clin Immunol. 1983;3(4):332–40.
22. Miedema F. Immunological abnormalities in the natural history of HIV infection: mechanisms and clinical relevance. Immunodefic Rev. 1992;3(3):173–93.
23. Katz JD, Mitsuyasu R, Gottlieb MS, Lebow LT, Bonavida B. Mechanism of defective NK cell activity in patients with acquired immunodeficiency syndrome (AIDS) and AIDS-related complex. II. Normal antibody-dependent cellular cytotoxicity (ADCC) mediated by effector cells defective in natural killer (NK) cytotoxicity. J Immunol (Baltimore, Md: 1950). 1987;139(1):55–60.

24. Schroff RW, Gottlieb MS, Prince HE, Chai LL, Fahey JL. Immunological studies of homosexual men with immunodeficiency and Kaposi's sarcoma. Clin Immunol Immunopathol. 1983;27(3):300–14.

25. Wu L. Biology of HIV mucosal transmission. Curr Opin HIV AIDS. 2008;3(5):534–40.

26. Moore RD, Chaisson RE. Natural history of opportunistic disease in an HIV-infected urban clinical cohort. Ann Intern Med. 1996;124(7):633–42.

27. Gianella S, Massanella M, Wertheim JO, Smith DM. The sordid affair between human herpesvirus and HIV. J Infect Dis. 2015;212(6):845–52.

28. Miller CS, Berger JR, Mootoor Y, Avdiushko SA, Zhu H, Kryscio RJ. High prevalence of multiple human herpesviruses in saliva from human immunodeficiency virus-infected persons in the era of highly active antiretroviral therapy. J Clin Microbiol. 2006;44(7):2409–15.

29. Munawwar A, Singh S. Human herpesviruses as Copathogens of HIV infection, their role in HIV transmission, and disease progression. J Lab Phys. 2016;8(1):5–18.

30. Gianella S, Anderson CM, Var SR, Oliveira MF, Lada SM, Vargas MV, et al. Replication of human herpesviruses is associated with higher HIV DNA levels during antiretroviral therapy started at early phases of HIV infection. J Virol. 2016;90(8):3944–52.

31. Griffiths PD. CMV as a cofactor enhancing progression of AIDS. J Clin Virol: Off Publ Pan Am Soc Clin Virol. 2006;35(4):489–92.

32. Lisco A, Vanpouille C, Margolis L. Coinfecting viruses as determinants of HIV disease. Curr HIV/AIDS Rep. 2009;6(1):5–12.

33. Pinzone MR, Berretta M, Cacopardo B, Nunnari G. Epstein-barr virus- and Kaposi sarcoma-associated herpesvirus-related malignancies in the setting of human immunodeficiency virus infection. Semin Oncol. 2015;42(2):258–71.

34. Nahmias AJ, Lee FK, Beckman-Nahmias S. Seroepidemiological and -sociological patterns of herpes simplex virus infection in the world. Scand J Infect Dis Suppl. 1990;69:19–36.

35. Steiner I, Kennedy PG, Pachner AR. The neurotropic herpes viruses: herpes simplex and varicella-zoster. Lancet Neurol. 2007;6(11):1015–28.

36. Koren M, Wang X, Blaylock JM, Okulicz JF, Whitman TJ, Deiss RG, et al. Brief report: the epidemiology of herpes simplex virus type 2 infections in a large cohort of HIV-infected patients, 2006–2014. Med Surveill Mon Rep. 2016;23(3):11–5.

37. Cohen JA, Sellers A, Sunil TS, Matthews PE, Okulicz JF. Herpes simplex virus seroprevalence and seroconversion among active duty US air force members with HIV infection. J Clin Virol: Off Publ Pan Am Soc Clin Virol. 2016;74:4–7.

38. Mertz GJ. Epidemiology of genital herpes infections. Infect Dis Clin N Am. 1993;7(4):825–39.

39. Da Rosa-Santos OL, Goncalves da Silva A, Pereira AC Jr. Herpes simplex virus type 2 in Brazil: seroepidemiologic survey. Int J Dermatol. 1996;35(11):794–6.

40. Smith JS, Robinson NJ. Age-specific prevalence of infection with herpes simplex virus types 2 and 1: a global review. J Infect Dis. 2002;186(Suppl 1):S3–28.

41. Looker KJ, Garnett GP. A systematic review of the epidemiology and interaction of herpes simplex virus types 1 and 2. Sex Transm Infect. 2005;81(2):103–7.

42. Freeman EE, Weiss HA, Glynn JR, Cross PL, Whitworth JA, Hayes RJ. Herpes simplex virus 2 infection increases HIV acquisition in men and women: systematic review and meta-analysis of longitudinal studies. AIDS (London, England). 2006;20(1):73–83.

43. Brown JM, Wald A, Hubbard A, Rungruengthanakit K, Chipato T, Rugpao S, et al. Incident and prevalent herpes simplex virus type 2 infection increases risk of HIV acquisition among women in Uganda and Zimbabwe. AIDS (London, England). 2007;21(12):1515–23.

44. Freedman E, Mindel A. Epidemiology of herpes and HIV co-infection. J HIV Ther. 2004;9(1):4–8.

45. Tan DH, Murphy K, Shah P, Walmsley SL. Herpes simplex virus type 2 and HIV disease progression: a systematic review of observational studies. BMC Infect Dis. 2013;13:502.

46. Chu K, Jiamton S, Pepin J, Cowan F, Mahakkanukrauh B, Suttent R, et al. Association between HSV-2 and HIV-1 viral load in semen, cervico-vaginal secretions and genital ulcers of Thai men and women. Int J STD AIDS. 2006;17(10):681–6.

47. Kinchington PR, Leger AJ, Guedon JM, Hendricks RL. Herpes simplex virus and varicella zoster virus, the house guests who never leave. Herpesviridae. 2012;3(1):5.

48. LeGoff J, Pere H, Belec L. Diagnosis of genital herpes simplex virus infection in the clinical laboratory. Virol J. 2014;11:83.

49. Birkmann A, Zimmermann H. HSV antivirals – current and future treatment options. Curr Opin Virol. 2016;18:9–13.

50. Chen Y, Scieux C, Garrait V, Socie G, Rocha V, Molina JM, et al. Resistant herpes simplex virus type 1 infection: an emerging concern after allogeneic stem cell transplantation. Clin Infect Dis: Off Publ Infect Dis Soc Am. 2000;31(4):927–35.

51. Brown M, Scarborough M, Brink N, Manji H, Miller R. Varicella zoster virus-associated neurological disease in HIV-infected patients. Int J STD AIDS. 2001;12(2):79–83.

52. Gnann JW Jr. Varicella-zoster virus: atypical presentations and unusual complications. J Infect Dis. 2002;186(Suppl 1):S91–8.

53. Davidovici BB, Balicer RD, Klement E, Green MS, Mendelson E, Smetana Z, et al. Comparison of the dynamics and correlates of transmission of Herpes Simplex Virus-1 (HSV-1) and Varicella-Zoster Virus

(VZV) in a sample of the Israeli population. Eur J Epidemiol. 2007;22(9):641–6.

54. van Velzen M, Ouwendijk WJ, Selke S, Pas SD, van Loenen FB, Osterhaus AD, et al. Longitudinal study on oral shedding of herpes simplex virus 1 and varicella-zoster virus in individuals infected with HIV. J Med Virol. 2013;85(9):1669–77.

55. Wharton M. The epidemiology of varicella-zoster virus infections. Infect Dis Clin N Am. 1996;10(3):571–81.

56. Buchbinder SP, Katz MH, Hessol NA, Liu JY, O'Malley PM, Underwood R, et al. Herpes zoster and human immunodeficiency virus infection. J Infect Dis. 1992;166(5):1153–6.

57. Grabar S, Tattevin P, Selinger-Leneman H, de La Blanchardiere A, de Truchis P, Rabaud C, et al. Incidence of herpes zoster in HIV-infected adults in the combined antiretroviral therapy era: results from the FHDH-ANRS CO4 cohort. Clin Infect Dis: Off Publ Infect Dis Soc Am. 2015;60(8):1269–77.

58. Blank LJ, Polydefkis MJ, Moore RD, Gebo KA. Herpes zoster among persons living with HIV in the current antiretroviral therapy era. J Acquir Immune Defic Syndr. 2012;61(2):203–7.

59. Jansen K, Haastert B, Michalik C, Guignard A, Esser S, Dupke S, et al. Incidence and risk factors of herpes zoster among hiv-positive patients in the german competence network for HIV/AIDS (KompNet): a cohort study analysis. BMC Infect Dis. 2013;13:372.

60. Sauerbrei A. Diagnosis, antiviral therapy, and prophylaxis of varicella-zoster virus infections. Eur J Clin Microbiol Infect Dis: Off Publ Eur Soc Clin Microbiol. 2016;35(5):723–34.

61. Aebi C, Ahmed A, Ramilo O. Bacterial complications of primary varicella in children. Clin Infect Dis: Off Publ Infect Dis Soc Am. 1996;23(4):698–705.

62. De Broucker T, Mailles A, Chabrier S, Morand P, Stahl JP. Acute varicella zoster encephalitis without evidence of primary vasculopathy in a case-series of 20 patients. Clin Microbiol Infect. 2012;18(8):808–19.

63. Gilden D, Cohrs RJ, Mahalingam R, Nagel MA. Varicella zoster virus vasculopathies: diverse clinical manifestations, laboratory features, pathogenesis, and treatment. Lancet Neurol. 2009;8(8):731–40.

64. Barnabas RV, Baeten JM, Lingappa JR, Thomas KK, Hughes JP, Mugo NR, et al. Acyclovir prophylaxis reduces the incidence of herpes zoster among HIV-infected individuals: results of a randomized clinical trial. J Infect Dis. 2016;213(4):551–5.

65. Chaves SS, Lopez AS, Watson TL, Civen R, Watson B, Mascola L, et al. Varicella in infants after implementation of the US varicella vaccination program. Pediatrics. 2011;128(6):1071–7.

66. Aberg JA, Gallant JE, Ghanem KG, Emmanuel P, Zingman BS, Horberg MA. Primary care guidelines for the management of persons infected with HIV: 2013 update by the HIV Medicine Association of the

Infectious Diseases Society of America. Clin Infect Dis: Off Publ Infect Dis Soc Am. 2014;58(1):1–10.

67. Hales CM, Harpaz R, Ortega-Sanchez I, Bialek SR, Control CfD, Prevention. Update on recommendations for use of herpes zoster vaccine. MMWR Morb Mortal Wkly Rep. 2014;63(33):729–31.

68. Lal H, Cunningham AL, Godeaux O, Chlibek R, Diez-Domingo J, Hwang SJ, et al. Efficacy of an adjuvanted herpes zoster subunit vaccine in older adults. N Engl J Med. 2015;372(22):2087–96.

69. Siegel JD, Rhinehart E, Jackson M, Chiarello L. 2007 Guideline for isolation precautions: preventing transmission of infectious agents in health care settings. Am J Infect Control. 2007;35(10 Suppl 2):S65–164.

70. Balfour HH Jr, Sifakis F, Sliman JA, Knight JA, Schmeling DO, Thomas W. Age-specific prevalence of Epstein-Barr virus infection among individuals aged 6–19 years in the United States and factors affecting its acquisition. J Infect Dis. 2013;208(8):1286–93.

71. Dunmire SK, Grimm JM, Schmeling DO, Balfour HH Jr, Hogquist KA. The incubation period of primary Epstein-Barr virus infection: viral dynamics and immunologic events. PLoS Pathog. 2015;11(12):e1005286.

72. Dunmire SK, Hogquist KA, Balfour HH. Infectious mononucleosis. Curr Top Microbiol Immunol. 2015;390(Pt 1):211–40.

73. Elgh F, Linderholm M. Evaluation of six commercially available kits using purified heterophile antigen for the rapid diagnosis of infectious mononucleosis compared with Epstein-Barr virus-specific serology. Clin Diagn Virol. 1996;7(1):17–21.

74. Ivers LC, Kim AY, Sax PE. Predictive value of polymerase chain reaction of cerebrospinal fluid for detection of Epstein-Barr virus to establish the diagnosis of HIV-related primary central nervous system lymphoma. Clin Infect Dis. 2004;38(11):1629–32.

75. Patrick LB, Mohile NA. Advances in primary central nervous system lymphoma. Curr Oncol Rep. 2015;17(12):60.

76. Abrey LE, Yahalom J, DeAngelis LM. Treatment for primary CNS lymphoma: the next step. J Clin Oncol: Off J Am Soc Clin Oncol. 2000;18(17):3144–50.

77. Krishnan A, Zaia JA. HIV-associated non-Hodgkin lymphoma: viral origins and therapeutic options. Hematol Educ Prog Am Soc Hematol Am Soc Hematol Educ Prog. 2014;2014(1):584–9.

78. Adland E, Klenerman P, Goulder P, Matthews PC. Ongoing burden of disease and mortality from HIV/CMV coinfection in Africa in the antiretroviral therapy era. Front Microbiol. 2015;6:1016.

79. Reyburn HT, Mandelboim O, Vales-Gomez M, Davis DM, Pazmany L, Strominger JL. The class I MHC homologue of human cytomegalovirus inhibits attack by natural killer cells. Nature. 1997;386(6624):514–7.

80. Stagno S, Pass RF, Cloud G, Britt WJ, Henderson RE, Walton PD, et al. Primary cytomegalovirus infection

in pregnancy: incidence, transmission to fetus, and clinical outcome. JAMA. 1986;256(14):1904–8.

81. Erice A, Tierney C, Hirsch M, Caliendo AM, Weinberg A, Kendall MA, et al. Cytomegalovirus (CMV) and human immunodeficiency virus (HIV) burden, CMV end-organ disease, and survival in subjects with advanced HIV infection (AIDS Clinical Trials Group Protocol 360). Clin Infect Dis: Off Publ Infect Dis Soc Am. 2003;37(4):567–78.

82. Gohring K, Hamprecht K, Jahn G. Antiviral drug- and multidrug resistance in cytomegalovirus infected SCT patients. Comput Struct Biotechnol J. 2015;13:153–9.

83. Griffiths P, Lumley S. Cytomegalovirus. Curr Opin Infect Dis. 2014;27(6):554–9.

84. Verkaik NJ, Hoek RA, van Bergeijk H, van Hal PT, Schipper ME, Pas SD, et al. Leflunomide as part of the treatment for multidrug-resistant cytomegalo-virus disease after lung transplantation: case report and review of the literature. Transplant Infect Dis: Off J Transplant Soc. 2013;15(6):E243–9.

85. Mayaphi SH, Brauer M, Morobadi DM, Mazanderani AH, Mafuyeka RT, Olorunju SA, et al. Cytomegalovirus viral load kinetics in patients with HIV/AIDS admitted to a medical intensive care unit: a case for pre-emptive therapy. PLoS One. 2014;9(4):e93702.

86. Mattioni S, Pavie J, Porcher R, Scieux C, Denis B, De Castro N, et al. Assessment of the efficacy and safety of pre-emptive anti-cytomegalovirus (CMV) therapy in HIV-infected patients with CMV virae-mia. Int J STD AIDS. 2015;26(5):306–12.

87. Dolcetti R, Di Luca D, Carbone A, Mirandola P, De Vita S, Vaccher E, et al. Human herpesvirus 6 in human immunodeficiency virus-infected indi-viduals: association with early histologic phases of lymphadenopathy syndrome but not with malig-nant lymphoproliferative disorders. J Med Virol. 1996;48(4):344–53.

88. Falasca F, Maida P, Gaeta A, Verzaro S, Mezzaroma I, Fantauzzi A, et al. Detection and quantification of EBV, HHV-6 and CMV DNA in the gastroin-testinal tract of HIV-positive patients. Infection. 2014;42(6):1033–7.

89. Campadelli-Fiume G, Mirandola P, Menotti L. Human herpesvirus 6: an emerging pathogen. Emerg Infect Dis. 1999;5(3):353–66.

90. Luppi M, Torelli G. The new lymphotropic herpes-viruses (HHV-6, HHV-7, HHV-8) and hepatitis C virus (HCV) in human lymphoproliferative diseases: an overview. Haematologica. 1996;81(3):265–81.

91. Uldrick TS, Wang V, O'Mahony D, Aleman K, Wyvill KM, Marshall V, et al. An interleukin-6-related systemic inflammatory syndrome in patients co-infected with Kaposi sarcoma-associated herpes-virus and HIV but without Multicentric Castleman disease. Clin Infect Dis: Off Publ Infect Dis Soc Am. 2010;51(3):350–8.

92. Mylona EE, Baraboutis IG, Lekakis LJ, Georgiou O, Papastamopoulos V, Skoutelis A. Multicentric

Castleman's disease in HIV infection: a systematic review of the literature. AIDS Rev. 2008;10(1):25–35.

93. Chabria S, Barakat L, Ogbuagu O. Steroid-exacerbated HIV-associated cutaneous Kaposi's sarcoma immune reconstitution inflammatory syn-drome: 'Where a good intention turns bad'. Int J STD AIDS. 2016;27(11):1026–9.

94. Goncalves PH, Ziegelbauer J, Uldrick TS, Yarchoan R. Kaposi sarcoma herpesvirus-associated disor-ders and related diseases. Curr Opin HIV AIDS. 2016;12:47.

95. Mosam A, Shaik F, Uldrick TS, Esterhuizen T, Friedland GH, Scadden DT, et al. A randomized controlled trial of highly active antiretroviral ther-apy versus highly active antiretroviral therapy and chemotherapy in therapy-naive patients with HIV-associated Kaposi sarcoma in South Africa. J Acquir Immune Defic Syndr. 2012;60(2):150–7.

96. Berger JR, Aksamit AJ, Clifford DB, Davis L, Koralnik IJ, Sejvar JJ, et al. PML diagnostic criteria: consensus statement from the AAN Neuroinfectious Disease Section. Neurology. 2013;80(15):1430–8.

97. Martinez MJ, Moreno C, Levican J, Pena M, Gaggero A, Chnaiderman J. BK and JC polyoma-virus detection in leukocyte extracts of peripheral blood samples of HIV+ patients from the north area of Santiago. Rev Chilena Infectol: organo oficial Soc Chil Infectol. 2016;33(3):298–302.

98. Akhgari S, Mohraz M, Azadmanesh K, Vahabpour R, Kazemimanesh M, Aghakhani A, et al. Frequency and subtype of BK virus infection in Iranian patients infected with HIV. Med Microbiol Immunol. 2016;205(1):57–62.

99. Sundsfjord A, Flaegstad T, Flo R, Spein AR, Pedersen M, Permin H, et al. BK and JC viruses in human immunodeficiency virus type 1-infected per-sons: prevalence, excretion, viremia, and viral regu-latory regions. J Infect Dis. 1994;169(3):485–90.

100. Behzad-Behbahani A, Klapper PE, Vallely PJ, Cleator GM, Khoo SH. Detection of BK virus and JC virus DNA in urine samples from immunocom-promised (HIV-infected) and immunocompetent (HIV-non-infected) patients using polymerase chain reaction and microplate hybridisation. J Clin Virol: Off Publ Pan Am Soc Clin Virol. 2004;29(4):224–9.

101. Adang L, Berger J. Progressive multifocal leukoen-cephalopathy. F1000Research. 2015;4.

102. Rossi F, Li X, Jacobson L, Levine AJ, Chen Y, Palella FJ, et al. BK virus capsid antibodies are asso-ciated with protection against subsequent develop-ment of PML in HIV-infected patients. Virology. 2015;485:467–72.

103. Wuthrich C, Dang X, Westmoreland S, McKay J, Maheshwari A, Anderson MP, et al. Fulminant JC virus encephalopathy with productive infec-tion of cortical pyramidal neurons. Ann Neurol. 2009;65(6):742–8.

104. McGuire D, Barhite S, Hollander H, Miles M. JC virus DNA in cerebrospinal fluid of human immuno-deficiency virus-infected patients: predictive value

for progressive multifocal leukoencephalopathy. Ann Neurol. 1995;37(3):395–9.

105. Baharnoori M, Lyons J, Dastagir A, Koralnik I, Stankiewicz JM. Nonfatal PML in a patient with multiple sclerosis treated with dimethyl fumarate. Neurol (R) Neuroimmunol Neuroinflammation. 2016;3(5):e274.

106. Casado JL, Corral I, Garcia J, Martinez-San Millan J, Navas E, Moreno A, et al. Continued declining incidence and improved survival of progressive multifocal leukoencephalopathy in HIV/AIDS patients in the current era. Eur J Clin Microbiol Infect Dis: Off Publ Eur Soc Clin Microbiol. 2014;33(2):179–87.

107. Klein MB, Rockstroh JK, Wittkop L. Effect of coinfection with hepatitis C virus on survival of individuals with HIV-1 infection. Curr Opin HIV AIDS. 2016;11(5):521–6.

108. Platt L, Easterbrook P, Gower E, McDonald B, Sabin K, McGowan C, et al. Prevalence and burden of HCV co-infection in people living with HIV: a global systematic review and meta-analysis. Lancet Infect Dis. 2016;16(7):797–808.

109. Taddei TH, Lo Re V 3rd, Justice AC. HIV, aging, and viral coinfections: taking the long view. Curr HIV/AIDS Rep. 2016;13(5):269–78.

110. Stenkvist J, Nystrom J, Falconer K, Sonnerborg A, Weiland O. Occasional spontaneous clearance of chronic hepatitis C virus in HIV-infected individuals. J Hepatol. 2014;61(4):957–61.

111. Wahle RC, Perez RM, Pereira PF, Oliveira EM, Emori CT, Uehara SN, et al. Hepatitis B virus reactivation after treatment for hepatitis C in hemodialysis patients with HBV/HCV coinfection. Brazilian J Infect Dis: Off Publ Braz Soc Infect Dis. 2015;19(5):533–7.

112. Soriano V, Labarga P, de Mendoza C, Pena JM, Fernandez-Montero JV, Benitez L, et al. Emerging challenges in managing hepatitis B in HIV patients. Curr HIV/AIDS Rep. 2015;12(3):344–52.

113. Fung S, Kwan P, Fabri M, Horban A, Pelemis M, Hann HW, et al. Tenofovir disoproxil fumarate (TDF) vs. emtricitabine (FTC)/TDF in lamivudine resistant hepatitis B: a 5-year randomised study. J Hepatol. 2017 Jan;66(1):11-18.

114. Cox JT. Epidemiology and natural history of HPV. J Fam Pract. 2006;Suppl:3–9.

115. Moore RA, Ogilvie G, Fornika D, Moravan V, Brisson M, Amirabbasi-Beik M, et al. Prevalence and type distribution of human papillomavirus in 5,000 British Columbia women – implications for vaccination. Cancer Causes Control : CCC. 2009;20(8):1387–96.

116. Mujuni F, Mirambo MM, Rambau P, Klaus K, Andreas M, Matovelo D, et al. Variability of high risk HPV genotypes among HIV infected women in Mwanza, Tanzania- the need for evaluation of current vaccine effectiveness in developing countries. Infect Agents Cancer. 2016;11:49.

117. Macleod IJ, O'Donnell B, Moyo S, Lockman S, Shapiro RL, Kayembe M, et al. Prevalence of human papillomavirus genotypes and associated cervical squamous intraepithelial lesions in HIV-infected women in Botswana. J Med Virol. 2011;83(10):1689–95.

118. Stuardo V, Agusti C, Godinez JM, Montoliu A, Torne A, Tarrats A, et al. Human papillomavirus infection in HIV-1 infected women in Catalonia (Spain): implications for prevention of cervical cancer. PLoS One. 2012;7(10):e47755.

119. Temmerman M, Tyndall MW, Kidula N, Claeys P, Muchiri L, Quint W. Risk factors for human papillomavirus and cervical precancerous lesions, and the role of concurrent HIV-1 infection. Int J Gynaecol Obstet: Off Organ Int Fed Gynaecol Obstet. 1999;65(2):171–81.

120. Weaver BA. Epidemiology and natural history of genital human papillomavirus infection. J Am Osteopath Assoc. 2006;106(3 Suppl 1):S2–8.

121. Massad LS, Xie X, Darragh T, Minkoff H, Levine AM, Watts DH, et al. Genital warts and vulvar intraepithelial neoplasia: natural history and effects of treatment and human immunodeficiency virus infection. Obstet Gynecol. 2011;118(4):831–9.

122. Park IU, Introcaso C, Dunne EF. Human papillomavirus and genital warts: a review of the evidence for the 2015 centers for disease control and prevention sexually transmitted diseases treatment guidelines. Clin Infect Dis: Off Publ Infect Dis Soc Am. 2015;61(Suppl 8):S849–55.

123. Doorbar J. Model systems of human papillomavirus-associated disease. J Pathol. 2016;238(2):166–79.

124. Lee SJ, Yang A, Wu TC, Hung CF. Immunotherapy for human papillomavirus-associated disease and cervical cancer: review of clinical and translational research. J Gynecol Oncol. 2016;27(5):e51.

125. Committee on Practice Bulletins—Gynecology. Practice Bulletin No. 168: cervical cancer screening and prevention. Obstet Gynecol. 2016;128(4):e111–30.

126. Huson MA, Stolp SM, van der Poll T, Grobusch MP. Community-acquired bacterial bloodstream infections in HIV-infected patients: a systematic review. Clin Infect Dis: Off Publ Infect Dis Soc Am. 2014;58(1):79–92.

127. Flagg EW, Weinstock HS, Frazier EL, Valverde EE, Heffelfinger JD, Skarbinski J. Bacterial sexually transmitted infections among HIV-infected patients in the United States: estimates from the Medical Monitoring Project. Sex Transm Dis. 2015;42(4):171–9.

128. Sogaard OS, Reekie J, Ristola M, Jevtovic D, Karpov I, Beniowski M, et al. Severe bacterial non-aids infections in HIV-positive persons: incidence rates and risk factors. J Infect. 2013;66(5):439–46.

129. Uhlenkott MC, Buskin SE, Kahle EM, Barash E, Aboulafia DM. Causes of death in the era of highly active antiretroviral therapy: a retrospective analysis of a hybrid hematology-oncology and HIV practice and the Seattle/King county adult/adolescent spec-

trum of HIV-related diseases project. Am J Med Sci. 2008;336(3):217–23.

130. Moir S, Malaspina A, Ogwaro KM, Donoghue ET, Hallahan CW, Ehler LA, et al. HIV-1 induces phenotypic and functional perturbations of B cells in chronically infected individuals. Proc Natl Acad Sci U S A. 2001;98(18):10362–7.

131. Rook AH, Masur H, Lane HC, Frederick W, Kasahara T, Macher AM, et al. Interleukin-2 enhances the depressed natural killer and cytomegalovirus-specific cytotoxic activities of lymphocytes from patients with the acquired immune deficiency syndrome. J Clin Invest. 1983;72(1):398–403.

132. Grassi F, Hosmalin A, McIlroy D, Calvez V, Debre P, Autran B. Depletion in blood CD11c-positive dendritic cells from HIV-infected patients. AIDS (London, England). 1999;13(7):759–66.

133. Ndakotsu MA, Salawu L, Durosinmi MA. Relation between erythrocyte sedimentation rate, clinical and immune status in HIV-infected patients. Niger J Med: J Natl Assoc Res Doctors Niger. 2008;17(4):420–2.

134. Phatlhane DV, Ipp H, Erasmus RT, Zemlin AE. Evaluating the use of procalcitonin in an asymptomatic, HIV-infected antiretroviral therapy-naive, South African cohort. Clin Chem Lab Med. 2016;54(3):501–8.

135. Schleicher GK, Herbert V, Brink A, Martin S, Maraj R, Galpin JS, et al. Procalcitonin and C-reactive protein levels in HIV-positive subjects with tuberculosis and pneumonia. Eur Respir J. 2005;25(4):688–92.

136. Berger BJ, Hussain F, Roistacher K. Bacterial infections in HIV-infected patients. Infect Dis Clin N Am. 1994;8(2):449–65.

137. Gasquet S, Maurin M, Brouqui P, Lepidi H, Raoult D. Bacillary angiomatosis in immuno-compromised patients. AIDS (London, England). 1998;12(14):1793–803.

138. Frean J, Arndt S, Spencer D. High rate of Bartonella henselae infection in HIV-positive outpatients in Johannesburg, South Africa. Trans R Soc Trop Med Hyg. 2002;96(5):549–50.

139. Justa RF, Carneiro AB, Rodrigues JL, Cavalcante A, Girao ES, Silva PS, et al. Bacillary angiomatosis in HIV-positive patient from Northeastern Brazil: a case report. Rev Soc Bras Med Trop. 2011;44(5):641–3.

140. Koehler JE, Tappero JW. Bacillary angiomatosis and bacillary peliosis in patients infected with human immunodeficiency virus. Clin Infect Dis: Off Publ Infect Dis Soc Am. 1993;17(4):612–24.

141. Forrestel AK, Naujokas A, Martin JN, Maurer TA, McCalmont TH, Laker-Opwonya MO, et al. Bacillary angiomatosis masquerading as Kaposi's sarcoma in East Africa. J Int Assoc Providers AIDS Care. 2015;14(1):21–5.

142. Spach DH, Callis KP, Paauw DS, Houze YB, Schoenknecht FD, Welch DF, et al. Endocarditis caused by Rochalimaea quintana in a patient infected with human immunodeficiency virus. J Clin Microbiol. 1993;31(3):692–4.

143. Sander A, Penno S. Semiquantitative species-specific detection of Bartonella henselae and Bartonella quintana by PCR-enzyme immunoassay. J Clin Microbiol. 1999;37(10):3097–101.

144. Koehler JE, Sanchez MA, Tye S, Garrido-Rowland CS, Chen FM, Maurer T, et al. Prevalence of Bartonella infection among human immunodeficiency virus-infected patients with fever. Clin Infect Dis: Off Publ Infect Dis Soc Am. 2003;37(4):559–66.

145. Montales MT, Chaudhury A, Beebe A, Patil S, Patil N. HIV-associated TB syndemic: a growing clinical challenge worldwide. Front Public Health. 2015;3:281.

146. Otero L, Ugaz R, Dieltiens G, Gonzalez E, Verdonck K, Seas C, et al. Duration of cough, TB suspects' characteristics and service factors determine the yield of smear microscopy. Trop Med Int Health: TM & IH. 2010;15(12):1475–80.

147. Abdool Karim SS, Naidoo K, Grobler A, Padayatchi N, Baxter C, Gray AL, et al. Integration of antiretroviral therapy with tuberculosis treatment. N Engl J Med. 2011;365(16):1492–501.

148. Corti M, Palmero D. Mycobacterium avium complex infection in HIV/AIDS patients. Expert Rev Anti-Infect Ther. 2008;6(3):351–63.

149. Casanova JL, Abel L. Genetic dissection of immunity to mycobacteria: the human model. Annu Rev Immunol. 2002;20:581–620.

150. Salama C, Policar M, Venkataraman M. Isolated pulmonary Mycobacterium avium complex infection in patients with human immunodeficiency virus infection: case reports and literature review. Clin Infect Dis: Off Publ Infect Dis Soc Am. 2003;37(3):e35–40.

151. Walle F, Kebede N, Tsegaye A, Kassa T. Seroprevalence and risk factors for Toxoplasmosis in HIV infected and non-infected individuals in Bahir Dar, Northwest Ethiopia. Parasit Vectors. 2013;6(1):15.

152. Le LT, Spudich SS. HIV-associated neurologic disorders and central nervous system opportunistic infections in HIV. Semin Neurol. 2016;36(4):373–81.

153. Pankhurst CL. Candidiasis (oropharyngeal). BMJ Clin Evid. 2013;2013:1304.

154. Cassone A, Cauda R. Candida and candidiasis in HIV-infected patients: where commensalism, opportunistic behavior and frank pathogenicity lose their borders. AIDS (London, England). 2012;26(12):1457–72.

155. Mukherjee PK, Chen H, Patton LL, Evans S, Lee A, Kumwenda J, et al. Topical gentian violet compared to nystatin oral suspension for the treatment of oropharyngeal candidiasis in HIV-1 Infected participants. AIDS. 2017 Jan 2;31(1):81-88.

156. Pienaar ED, Young T, Holmes H. Interventions for the prevention and management of oropharyngeal candidiasis associated with HIV infection in adults and children. Cochrane Database Syst Rev. 2010;11(11):Cd003940.

157. Cassone A. Vulvovaginal *Candida albicans* infections: pathogenesis, immunity and vaccine prospects. BJOG: Int J Obstet Gynaecol. 2015;122(6):785–94.
158. Morris A, Beard CB, Huang L. Update on the epidemiology and transmission of Pneumocystis carinii. Microbes Infect/Inst Pasteur. 2002;4(1):95–103.
159. Tasaka S. Pneumocystis pneumonia in human immunodeficiency virus-infected adults and adolescents: current concepts and future directions. Clin Med Insights Circ Respir Pulm Med. 2015;9(Suppl 1):19–28.
160. Kim HW, Heo JY, Lee YM, Kim SJ, Jeong HW. Unmasking granulomatous pneumocystis jirovecii pneumonia with nodular opacity in an HIV-infected patient after initiation of antiretroviral therapy. Yonsei Med J. 2016;57(4):1042–6.
161. Sax PE, Komarow L, Finkelman MA, Grant PM, Andersen J, Scully E, et al. Blood (1->3)-beta-D-glucan as a diagnostic test for HIV-related Pneumocystis jirovecii pneumonia. Clin Infect Dis: Off Publ Infect Dis Soc Am. 2011;53(2):197–202.
162. Kamada T, Furuta K, Tomioka H. Pneumocystis pneumonia associated with human immunodeficiency virus infection without elevated (1 --> 3)-beta-D glucan: a case report. Respir Med Case Rep. 2016;18:73–5.
163. Esteves F, Cale SS, Badura R, de Boer MG, Maltez F, Calderon EJ, et al. Diagnosis of Pneumocystis pneumonia: evaluation of four serologic biomarkers. Clin Microbiol Infect. 2015;21(4):379. e1–10.
164. Adenis AA, Aznar C, Couppie P. Histoplasmosis in HIV-infected patients: a review of new developments and remaining gaps. Curr Trop Med Rep. 2014;1:119–28.
165. Loulergue P, Bastides F, Baudouin V, Chandenier J, Mariani-Kurkdjian P, Dupont B, et al. Literature review and case histories of Histoplasma capsulatum var. duboisii infections in HIV-infected patients. Emerg Infect Dis. 2007;13(11):1647–52.
166. McKinsey DS, Spiegel RA, Hutwagner L, Stanford J, Driks MR, Brewer J, et al. Prospective study of histoplasmosis in patients infected with human immunodeficiency virus: incidence, risk factors, and pathophysiology. Clin Infect Dis: Off Publ Infect Dis Soc Am. 1997;24(6):1195–203.
167. Wheat LJ. Laboratory diagnosis of histoplasmosis: update 2000. Semin Respir Infect. 2001;16(2):131–40.
168. Wheat LJ. Improvements in diagnosis of histoplasmosis. Expert Opin Biol Ther. 2006;6(11):1207–21.
169. Panel on Opportunistic Infections in HIV-Infected Adults and Adolescents. Guidelines for the prevention and treatment of opportunistic infections in HIV-infected adults and adolescents: recommendations from the Centers for Disease Control and Prevention, the National Institutes of Health, and the HIV Medicine Association of the Infectious Diseases Society of America. Available at http://aidsinfo.nih.gov/contentfiles/lvguidelines/adult_oi.pdf. Accessed 10 Oct 2016.
170. Chen SC, Meyer W, Sorrell TC. Cryptococcus gattii infections. Clin Microbiol Rev. 2014;27(4):980–1024.
171. Ogbuagu O, Villanueva M. Extensive central nervous system Cryptococcal disease presenting as immune reconstitution syndrome in a patient with advanced HIV: report of a case and review of management dilemmas and strategies. Infect Dis Rep. 2014;6(4):5576.
172. Wright L, Bubb W, Davidson J, Santangelo R, Krockenberger M, Himmelreich U, et al. Metabolites released by *Cryptococcus neoformans* var. neoformans and var. gattii differentially affect human neutrophil function. Microbes Infect/Inst Pasteur. 2002;4(14):1427–38.
173. Islam A, Li SS, Oykhman P, Timm-McCann M, Huston SM, Stack D, et al. An acidic microenvironment increases NK cell killing of *Cryptococcus neoformans* and Cryptococcus gattii by enhancing perforin degranulation. PLoS Pathog. 2013;9(7):e1003439.
174. Charlier C, Nielsen K, Daou S, Brigitte M, Chretien F, Dromer F. Evidence of a role for monocytes in dissemination and brain invasion by *Cryptococcus neoformans*. Infect Immun. 2009;77(1):120–7.
175. Huston SM, Li SS, Stack D, Timm-McCann M, Jones GJ, Islam A, et al. Cryptococcus gattii is killed by dendritic cells, but evades adaptive immunity by failing to induce dendritic cell maturation. J Immunol (Baltimore, Md: 1950). 2013;191(1):249–61.
176. Loyse A, Wainwright H, Jarvis JN, Bicanic T, Rebe K, Meintjes G, et al. Histopathology of the arachnoid granulations and brain in HIV-associated cryptococcal meningitis: correlation with cerebrospinal fluid pressure. AIDS (London, England). 2010;24(3):405–10.
177. Bicanic T, Harrison TS. Cryptococcal meningitis. Br Med Bull. 2004;72(1):99–118.
178. Day JN, Chau TT, Wolbers M, Mai PP, Dung NT, Mai NH, et al. Combination antifungal therapy for cryptococcal meningitis. N Engl J Med. 2013;368(14):1291–302.
179. van der Horst CM, Saag MS, Cloud GA, Hamill RJ, Graybill JR, Sobel JD, et al. Treatment of cryptococcal meningitis associated with the acquired immunodeficiency syndrome. National Institute of Allergy and Infectious Diseases Mycoses Study Group and AIDS Clinical Trials Group. N Engl J Med. 1997;337(1):15–21.
180. Beardsley J, Wolbers M, Kibengo FM, Ggayi AB, Kamali A, Cuc NT, et al. Adjunctive dexamethasone in HIV-associated cryptococcal meningitis. N Engl J Med. 2016;374(6):542–54.
181. Smith KD, Achan B, Hullsiek KH, McDonald TR, Okagaki LH, Alhadab AA, et al. Increased antifungal drug resistance in clinical isolates of *Cryptococcus neoformans* in Uganda. Antimicrob Agents Chemother. 2015;59(12):7197–204.
182. Rhein J, Morawski BM, Hullsiek KH, Nabeta HW, Kiggundu R, Tugume L, et al. Efficacy of adjunc-

tive sertraline for the treatment of HIV-associated cryptococcal meningitis: an open-label dose-ranging study. Lancet Infect Dis. 2016;16(7):809–18.

183. Boulware DR, Meya DB, Muzoora C, Rolfes MA, Huppler Hullsiek K, Musubire A, et al. Timing of antiretroviral therapy after diagnosis of cryptococcal meningitis. N Engl J Med. 2014;370(26):2487–98.

184. Jarvis JN, Bicanic T, Loyse A, Namarika D, Jackson A, Nussbaum JC, et al. Determinants of mortality in a combined cohort of 501 patients with HIV-associated Cryptococcal meningitis: implications for improving outcomes. Clin Infect Dis: Off Publ Infect Dis Soc Am. 2014;58(5):736–45.

185. Kaplan JE, Vallabhaneni S, Smith RM, Chideya-Chihota S, Chehab J, Park B. Cryptococcal antigen screening and early antifungal treatment to prevent cryptococcal meningitis: a review of the literature. J Acquir Immune Defic Syndr. 2015;68(Suppl 3):S331–9.

186. Dutertre M, Cuzin L, Demonchy E, Pugliese P, Joly V, Valantin MA, et al. Initiation of antiretroviral therapy containing integrase inhibitors increases the risk of IRIS requiring hospitalization. J Acquir Immune Defic Syndr. 2017;76(1):e23–e6.

187. Manzardo C, Guardo AC, Letang E, Plana M, Gatell JM, Miro JM. Opportunistic infections and immune reconstitution inflammatory syndrome in HIV-1-infected adults in the combined antiretroviral therapy era: a comprehensive review. Expert Rev Anti-Infect Ther. 2015;13(6):751–67.

188. Meintjes G, Wilkinson RJ, Morroni C, Pepper DJ, Rebe K, Rangaka MX, et al. Randomized placebo-controlled trial of prednisone for para-doxical TB-associated immune reconstitution inflammatory syndrome. AIDS (London, England). 2010;24(15):2381–90.

189. Zolopa A, Andersen J, Powderly W, Sanchez A, Sanne I, Suckow C, et al. Early antiretroviral therapy reduces AIDS progression/death in individuals with acute opportunistic infections: a multicenter randomized strategy trial. PLoS One. 2009;4(5):e5575.

190. Brooks JT, Kaplan JE, Holmes KK, Benson C, Pau A, Masur H. HIV-associated opportunistic infections – going, going, but not gone: the continued need for prevention and treatment guidelines. Clin Infect Dis: Off Publ Infect Dis Soc Am. 2009;48(5):609–11.

Infections in Patients with Autoimmune Diseases

14

Neil U. Parikh, Mark F. Sands, and Stanley A. Schwartz

Introduction

The relationship between autoimmunity and infections is complex and bi-directional. Infections have been associated with the induction of autoimmunity as well as protection from autoimmune diseases [1–6]. Infectious agents may play both a causative and protective role in the pathogenesis of some autoimmune disorders like Sjogren's syndrome [7]. Infections are a common cause of morbidity and mortality in patients with systemic autoimmune diseases [8]. Considerable evidence has emerged regarding the greater susceptibility of patients with autoimmune disorders to infections due to predisposition from autoimmunity itself as well as the use of immunosuppressive therapy [9].

Infections Leading to Autoimmunity

Rheumatic fever is a classic example of Group A *Streptococcus* infection inducing autoimmunity. Molecular mimicry between host and bacterial proteins seems to be a major pathogenic mechanism. In rheumatic fever, a large group of bacterial proteins, M proteins, intercalated within the cell walls of Group A streptococci, bear structural similarities with various human heart proteins resulting in both cell-mediated and humoral autoimmune reactions to cardiac structures, including valves, myosin, and endothelium [10].

Molecular mimicry is due to common or shared immunologic epitopes between a microorganism and its host. Other proposed pathogenic mechanisms include the release of cryptic (hidden) or sequestered antigens, epitope spreading, anti-idiotype antibodies, antigenic complementarity, the bystander effect, or the infection itself [11, 12]. The theory of cryptic antigens is based on the concept that tissue damage can release cryptic self-antigens that activate host T cells that were not deleted or tolerized during thymic education. Epitope spreading as a basis for the pathogenesis of autoimmune reactions is similar to cryptic antigens in that sequestered self-antigens may be released from tissues initially damaged by an inflammatory response or infection. Subdominant epitopes of the released self-antigen may then be recognized and differentiated from the initial

N. U. Parikh
University of Central Florida, Orlando, FL, USA

M. F. Sands · S. A. Schwartz (✉)
Division of Allergy, Immunology & Rheumatology, Department of Medicine, University at Buffalo, Buffalo General Medical Center, Buffalo, NY, USA
e-mail: mfsands@buffalo.edu; sasimmun@buffalo.edu

© Springer International Publishing AG, part of Springer Nature 2018
B. H. Segal (ed.), *Management of Infections in the Immunocompromised Host*, https://doi.org/10.1007/978-3-319-77674-3_14

epitope [13, 14]. The anti-idiotype theory derives from the idea that an antibody directed at a viral antigen used by the virus to bind to a host cell could also bind to the host cell potentially injuring the cell as a form of autoimmunity [11] (the same concept applies to antigens from non-viral pathogens). The theory of antigenic complementarity proposes that pairs of molecularly complementary antigens induce pairs of complementary antibodies or T-cell receptors such that each antibody or T-cell receptor mimics one of the antigens, resulting in loss of the self-nonself distinction [15]. The bystander effect theory states that viral infections cause activation of antigen-presenting cells that in turn activate autoreactive T cells that can then initiate autoimmune disease (bystander activation of autoreactive immune T cells). Additionally, virus-specific T cells also might initiate immunological responses to kill infected cells, and the inflammatory mediators produced lead to bystander killing of uninfected neighboring cells [12].

Among viruses predisposing to autoimmunity, cytomegalovirus (CMV), Epstein–Barr virus

(EBV), and parvovirus B19 are the most frequently implicated [16–18]. Chronic antigenic stimulation by hepatitis C virus is considered a key mechanism sustaining the proliferation of rheumatoid factor-secreting B-cell clones [19] that may predispose to autoimmune complications, such as mixed cryoglobulinemia. Inflammatory bowel disease (IBD) is an example of interplay between commensal and pathogenic bacteria leading to autoimmune disease [20, 21]. Gut microbiota by themselves are known to drive autoimmune arthritis by promoting differentiation and migration of Peyer's patch T follicular helper cells [22]. Figure 14.1, adapted from Maddur et al. [9], summarizes the interplay between infections, immune system effector cells, and autoantibodies that neutralize the key immune system components.

Autoimmunity Leading to Infections

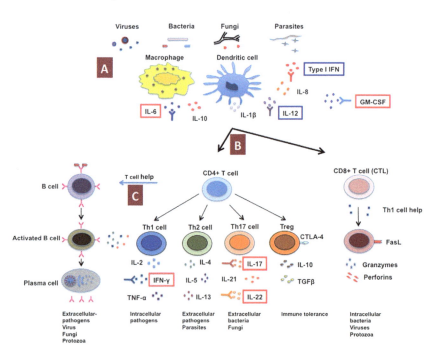

Fig. 14.1 Antigens from infecting pathogens are recognized and presented by innate immune cells (**a**) such as macrophages and dendritic cells to CD4+ and CD8+ T cells (**b**). CD8+ cytotoxic T cells (CTL) recognize endogenous antigens presented by MHC class I molecules and express cytotoxic functions upon activation. CD4+ T cells recognize antigens presented in the context of MHC class II molecules, and under the influence of innate cells and the cytokine milieu, CD4+ T cells can be differentiated into subsets such as Th1, Th2, Th17, and regulatory

Disease-Specific Immune Dysregulation

Systemic Lupus Erythematosus (SLE)

There is a complex interplay between infection, autoimmunity, and immunosuppression in SLE. Deficiencies in the early components of the classical complement pathway (C1q, C1r, C1s, C2, and C4) predispose patients to developing SLE. More than 90% of C1q-deficient individuals develop SLE. Factors that lead to increased risk of infections include mannose-binding lectin deficiency, C1q deficiency, hypocomplementemia secondary to consumption, defects in autophagy, dysfunctional B- and T-cell responses, and functional asplenia [23]. Most infections are caused by common bacterial pathogens, followed by opportunistic fungi. Moreover, immunosuppressive therapies commonly used for SLE further increase the incidence of opportunistic infections. C2 deficiency is known to predispose individuals, particularly children, to infections with encapsulated bacteria such as *Streptococcus pneumonia*, *Haemophilus influenzae* type B, and *Neisseria meningitidis* [24]. Patients with multiple serious infections have increased joint damage by radiography and more physical dysfunction [25]. Table 14.1 highlights the various mechanisms of immunological dysfunction in SLE.

Rheumatoid Arthritis (RA)

Immunological dysregulation including altered cytokine profile and defects in cellular and humoral immunity associated with a chronic inflammatory state increases the risk of infections [26]. Table 14.1 summarizes the immunological dysfunctions associated with rheumatoid arthritis. The use of steroids, disease-modifying antirheumatic drugs (DMARDs), and biologics all contribute to a predisposition to infections. The types of infections associated with the use of immunosuppressive agents are listed in Table 14.2.

Sjogren's Syndrome

Sjogren's syndrome is an autoimmune disease primarily involving the exocrine glands. The risk of lymphoproliferative disorders associated with *Helicobacter pylori*, human herpesvirus 6, human T-lymphotropic virus type I, and Epstein–Barr virus has been described in case reports [27]. Cytopenias and monoclonal gammopathies are commonly seen. Low C4 levels and CD4$^+$ lymphocytopenia contribute to increased risk of infections [28, 29]. These mechanisms are summarized in Table 14.1.

Miscellaneous Disorders

Common Variable Immunodeficiency (CVID)

CVID is a primary immunodeficiency disorder characterized by impaired B-cell differentiation with defective immunoglobulin production and T-cell dysfunction in some subgroups. CVID affects about 1 in 25,000 Caucasians [30]. Although CVID is classified as a primary immune deficiency disorder, patients with CVID have

---

Fig. 14.1 (continued) T cells (Tregs) that secrete distinct cytokines. CD4+ T cells provide help to B cells to produce antigen-specific antibodies (**c**). However, neutralizing autoantibodies may be produced against any of these key components of the immune system critical for mounting antimicrobial responses and might either predispose the host to an increased risk of bacterial, viral, and fungal opportunistic infections or exacerbate ongoing infections. Indeed, in patients with infections, the occurrence of neutralizing autoantibodies against several key cytokines such as IFN-γ, IL-6, GM-CSF, IL-17, and IL-22 (highlighted in *red boxes*) that interfere with the host immune response to pathogens has been demonstrated. Autoantibodies against type I IFNs and IL-12 also have been reported and may play a role in predisposition to infections (highlighted in *blue boxes*). Abbreviations: CTLA-4 cytotoxic T lymphocyte antigen-4, CTL cytotoxic T lymphocyte, FasL Fas ligand, GM-CSF granulocyte/macrophage colony-stimulating factor, IFN interferon (Adapted with permission from Maddur et al. [9])

Table 14.1 Mechanisms of immunological dysfunction in rheumatic diseases

Disease	Associated mechanism(s) of immunological dysfunction
Rheumatoid Arthritis (RA)	Defects in cellular immunity
	Hyperproduction of IL-17 cells and IL-23 with perpetuation of local inflammation, induction of angiogenesis, osteoclastogenesis, and, ultimately, destruction of cartilage and bone
	Altered regulatory T cells: these cells express TNF-receptor II, which make them susceptible to the immunomodulatory effects of TNF-α
	Defects in humoral immunity
	Hyperproduction of inflammatory cytokines TNF-α and IL-6, contributing to perpetuation of inflammation and autoactivation of B cells
	Antibodies against the formation of immune complexes from responses to debris of dead cells in RA synovium
	Formation of tertiary lymphoid structures in synovium by hyperstimulation of B cells by factors secreted by synovium such as B-cell-activating factor (BAFF)
	Altered regulatory B cells: these cells overproduce IL-10, probably downregulating immune responses to tolerizing T cells
	Chronic hyperinflammatory state
	Excess production of pro-inflammatory cytokines such as TNF-α
Systemic Lupus Erythematosus (SLE)	Dysfunction of the phagocytic activity of monocytes
	Decreased production of TNF-α; deficit in the generation of superoxide
	Dysfunction of B lymphocytes
	Hypogammaglobulinemia
	Antibodies against neutrophil cytoplasmic components
	Antibodies against the Fc-γ receptor
	Defects in cellular immunity, quantitative and functional alternations in T lymphocytes and subtypes
	Lymphocytopenia
	Decreased CD4$^+$ T-cell counts
	Reduced IL-2 and INF-γ production
	Decreased and altered regulatory T-cell populations
	Functional asplenia
	Impaired reticuloendothelial system, with defect in the removal of circulating immune complexes and elimination of microorganisms
	Low levels and dysfunction of complement
	Depletion of C1q and C1r/C1s and other complement components, e.g., C3, C5–C9
	Deficit of mannose-binding lectin
	Dysfunction of opsonization (formation of anti-C1q antibodies)
	Alteration of Fc-γ RIIa
	Decreased synthesis of immunoglobulins
Sjogren's syndrome	CD4$^+$ T-cell lymphocytopenia
	Low levels of complement, especially C4 (either genetically determined decreased production or secondary to consumption)

Adapted with permission from infection and autoimmunity, 2e: *Yehuda Shoenfeld, Nancy Agmon-Levin and Noel Rose*

Table 14.2 Mechanisms of immunological dysfunction and their relationship with pharmacological agents and infectious pathogens in autoimmune diseases

Immunological abnormality	Pharmacologic agents	Bacteria	Fungi	Viruses	Protozoal
Dysfunction of cellular immunity	Corticosteroids Methotrexate Azathioprine Cyclosporine A	Tuberculous and non-tuberculous mycobacteria, *Mycoplasma* spp., *Listeria monocytogenes*, *Nocardia* spp., *Salmonella* spp.	*Pneumocystis jiroveci*, *Cryptococcus neoformans*, dimorphic fungi, e.g., *Histoplasma capsulatum*, *Blastomyces dermatitidis*, and *Coccidioides immitis*	Cytomegalovirus, *Epstein—Barr* virus, Varicella Zoster virus	*Toxoplasma gondii*, *Strongyloides stercoralis*
Dysfunction of humoral immunity	Corticosteroids (high dose), Azathioprine, Cyclophosphamide, and other alkylating agents	*Streptococcus pneumonia*, *Haemophilus influenzae*, *Neisseria meningitidis*			
Quantitative or functional neutropenia and/or qualitative defects of phagocytic function	Corticosteroids, Azathioprine, Methotrexate, Cyclophosphamide, and other alkylating agents	*Staphylococcus aureus* *Streptococcus* spp. *Nocardia* spp. *Escherichia coli* *Pseudomonas aeruginosa* *Klebsiella* spp. Other *Enterobactericeae*	*Candida* spp., *Aspergillus* spp.		
Blockade of tumor necrosis factor (TNF)	Infliximab, adalimumab, etanercept, golimumab	Tuberculosis and non-tuberculous mycobacteria, *Mycoplasma* spp., *Listeria monocytogenes*	Dimorphic fungi		

Adapted with permission from infection and autoimmunity, 2e: *Yehuda Shoenfeld, Nancy Agmon-Levin and Noel Rose*

evidence of immune dysregulation leading to autoimmunity and a variety of inflammatory disorders. Nearly all patients who do not receive replacement IgG therapy develop bacterial infections resulting in pneumonia, rhinosinusitis, conjunctivitis, otitis media, septic arthritis, and sepsis due to encapsulated organisms. Other common infections include giardiasis and *Mycoplasma* infections [31, 32]. Autoimmune hematologic disorders such as idiopathic thrombocytopenia purpura are the most common autoimmune conditions in these patients.

Selective IgA Deficiency (sIgAD)

sIgAD is the most common primary immunodeficiency disorder in humans. Its worldwide incidence varies depending on the ethnic background. In the United States, the frequency is estimated to be from 1 in 223 to 1 in 1000 individuals in community studies and from 1 in 333 to 1 in 3000 persons among healthy blood donors [33]. sIgAD is defined as the isolated deficiency of serum immunoglobulin (Ig) A in the setting of normal serum levels of Ig G and Ig M in an individual older than 4 years of age in whom other causes of hypogammaglobulinemia have been excluded [34]. The majority of individuals with sIgAD are asymptomatic. Others manifest recurrent sinopulmonary infections, autoimmune disorders, gastrointestinal infections, allergies, or, less commonly, anaphylaxis when transfused with blood products from donors with IgA. SLE, Graves' disease, Type 1 diabetes, vitiligo, rheumatoid arthritis, immune thrombocytopenia, and myasthenia gravis are associated with sIgAD [35, 36].

Human Immunodeficiency Virus (HIV) Infection

The list of reported autoimmune diseases in HIV-infected individuals includes SLE, antiphospholipid antibody syndrome, vasculitis, primary biliary cirrhosis, polymyositis, Graves' disease, and idiopathic thrombocytopenic purpura. Among mechanisms leading to autoimmunity, several hypotheses exist: direct role of virus replication within the blood vessel wall [37], immune complex-mediated disease, dysregulation of the B-/T-lymphocyte interaction, molecular mimicry, and polyclonal B-lymphocyte activation that might favor the synthesis of autoantibodies [38, 39]. Also, HIV-infected patients manifest an array of autoantibodies including anticardiolipin, anti-β2 glycoprotein, anti-DNA, anti-small nuclear ribonucleoproteins (snRNP), anti-thyroglobulin, anti-thyroid peroxidase, anti-myosin, and anti-erythropoietin antibodies. These are present in up to 23% of HIV-infected patients usually without any clinical manifestation [40, 41].

Reactive Arthritis

Reactive arthritis is a form of arthritis that is associated with enteric and genitourinary pathogens such as *Chlamydia trachomatis*, *Chlamydia pneumoniae*, *Yersinia*, *Salmonella*, *Clostridium difficile*, and *Shigella* and *Campylobacter* species. Antibiotic therapy is aimed at treating the underlying infection that triggered the arthritis.

Idiopathic CD4 Lymphocytopenia (ICL)

ICL is a rare disorder that is poorly understood and associated with autoimmune diseases. Autoimmune disorders were reported in 14.2% patients with ICL. Cryptococcal infections were most prevalent in ICL patients (26.6%), followed by *Mycobacteria* (17%), *Candida* (16.2%), and VZV infections (13.1%) [42, 43].

Drugs Commonly Used to Treat Autoimmune Disorders

Corticosteroids

Corticosteroids are broad-spectrum immunosuppressants that affect the immune system by multiple actions [44, 45]. They induce increased transcription of genes coding for anti-inflammatory proteins, inhibit the expression of multiple inflammatory genes, impair phagocyte and T-cell functions, and induce T-cell apoptosis predisposing to bacterial, fungal, viral, and protozoal infections. Patients with newly diagnosed autoimmune diseases are at high risk of developing intracellular infection during initial treatment with glucocorticoids (GCs). The presence of diabetes, lymphocytopenia, increased age, and male gender are independent predictors for serious intracellular infections in patients with newly diagnosed autoimmune diseases initially treated with high-dose (>30 mg/day) GCs [46]. Interestingly, the use of the lowest possible GC dose at night during peak production of TNF and other inflammatory cytokines could dramatically decrease the risk of infections in patients with autoimmune disorders [8, 46–48].

Conventional Disease-Modifying Antirheumatic Drugs (DMARDs)

Methotrexate (MTX)

MTX inhibits purine and pyrimidine synthesis and suppresses methyltransferase activity with accumulation of polyamines, reduction of antigen-dependent T-cell proliferation, and promotion of adenosine release [49]. These mechanisms contribute to the toxicity of MTX and may increase the risk of infections, but its overall positive effect on the activity of autoimmune diseases results in a reduction of risk factors for infections. Evidence of an increased prevalence of pneumonia or reactivation of latent infections with MTX therapy remains controversial [50]. Common opportunistic infections include *Pneumocystis jiroveci* pneumonia and herpes zoster infection. Accelerated nodulosis is a well-known complication of methotrexate therapy in rheumatoid arthritis patients, characterized by the rapid appearance of subcutaneous nodules (2 mm to several cm) on the hands, elbows, and feet [51]. In case of mild viral infections, MTX therapy can be continued. With bacterial infections that require antibiotic therapy, MTX should be discontinued until the antibiotic course has been completed, inflammatory markers have returned to baseline levels, and clinical symptoms are resolved. If opportunistic infections occur during MTX treatment, they can be severe and sometimes life threatening [52, 53].

Azathioprine

Azathioprine halts DNA replication and blocks the purine synthesis pathway. The 6-thioguanine metabolites of azathioprine mediate its immunosuppressive effects. Chronic immunosuppression with azathioprine increases the risk of malignancy as well as common and opportunistic infections. Leukopenia associated with its use can sometimes lead to severe infections.

Cyclosporine

Cyclosporine complexes with cyclophilin and inhibits the phosphatase activity of calcineurin which is required for the transcription and translation of cytokine genes such as IL-2. IL-2 is necessary for the activation of resting T lymphocytes. Infections reported with cyclosporine use are commonly viral, but bacterial and fungal infections can also occur. These are summarized in Table 14.2.

Other Non-immunosuppressive DMARDs

Several DMARDs including hydroxychloroquine and dapsone (both antimalarials), parenteral gold, sulfasalazine, tetracyclines, and bucillamine are not associated with an increased risk for infections. Contrary to common perception, it is important for clinicians to recognize that DMARDs are less immunosuppressive than corticosteroids. Clinical trials have not shown a higher incidence of infection in patients receiving leflunomide, a pyrimidine synthesis inhibitor, compared to patients receiving placebo. However, leflunomide is not recommended for patients with immunodeficiency or serious infections. Disseminated fungal or viral infections or opportunistic infections have not been reported during clinical trials with leflunomide.

Cyclophosphamide

Cyclophosphamide and chlorambucil are the only two pharmacological agents currently available that can modulate the population of memory

B cells. The introduction of cyclophosphamide led to a dramatic increase in survival of patients with Wegener's granulomatosis [54]. Reversible myelosuppression is common with the use of cyclophosphamide, and the degree of leucopenia and neutropenia is proportional to the dose used. Also, its prolonged use can lead to bone marrow suppression. Studies have demonstrated that severe infection occurred in 15% of patients treated with cyclophosphamide. Community-acquired pneumonia was the most frequent infection followed by herpes zoster [55, 56]. Targeting a minimal white blood cell (WBC) count of 3000–4000/microliter as a safe range, a reduction of the dose of cyclophosphamide when the white count falls below this level will prevent serious infections in patients receiving this drug.

Biologics

Anti-TNF-α Agents

Numerous studies have reported an increased rate of infections with anti-TNF-α therapies, especially reactivation of mycobacterial and dimorphic fungal infections. EBV-associated lymphoma is an additional risk of this class of agents. A Cochrane analysis found infliximab and certolizumab to be associated with an elevated risk for serious infections in comparison to placebo [57]. Standard-dose and high-dose biological drugs (with or without traditional DMARDs) are associated with an increase in serious infections in rheumatoid arthritis compared with traditional DMARDs alone; low-dose biological drugs are not associated with an increased rate of infections [58]. Particular caution should be exercised when using anti-TNFα therapy in patients with latent tuberculosis infection, and screening should be implemented to identify such patients prior to initiation of therapy [59]. Cyclosporine A and anti-TNF-α agents seem to be safe, in terms of viral load and liver toxicity, in the treatment of HIV- or HCV-infected patients with systemic autoimmune diseases [60, 61].

Anakinra (Anti IL-1)

Anakinra, an antagonist of the IL-1 receptor, is FDA approved for the treatment of rheumatoid arthritis and neonatal-onset multisystem inflammatory disease (NOMID). Anakinra in combination with other antirheumatic DMARDs is safe, with a rate of serious infections slightly higher in the anakinra group than in the placebo group (2.1% vs. 0.4%) [62].

Rituximab (RTX)

Rituximab is a monoclonal antibody directed against the CD20 antigen on B lymphocytes and is indicated for the treatment of rheumatoid arthritis, granulomatosis with polyangiitis (Wegener's granulomatosis), and microscopic polyangiitis. Most infections after RTX therapy are minor and involve the upper respiratory or urinary tracts. A slight increase in serious infections (5.2 versus 3.7 per 100 patient-years) over placebo in a large multicenter trial was reported [63]. The risk factors for severe infections include chronic lung and/or cardiac disease, extra-articular involvement, and low IgG before RTX treatment. This suggests that serum IgG should be checked and the risk–benefit ratio of RTX discussed for patients found to have low levels of IgG [64]. Given reports of humoral immunosuppression after RTX use, it is prudent to enumerate B-cell counts before initiating treatment [65, 66].

Abatacept

Abatacept inhibits T-cell activation by binding to CD80 and CD86 on antigen presenting cells and is used for the treatment of RA unresponsive to DMARDs or biologics. Infections were more common in abatacept-treated patients than in placebo-treated patients (37.6% vs. 32.3%, respectively). The majority of infections were mild to moderate. The rate of serious infections was the same in abatacept-treated patients (2.3%) and placebo-treated patients (2.3%). The Orencia and Rheumatoid Arthritis (ORA) data registry indicated that patients treated with abatacept had more comorbidities in clinical trials, and serious infections were slightly more frequent. In the ORA registry, predictive risk factors of serious infections include age and history of serious infections [67, 68].

Natalizumab

Natalizumab is a monoclonal antibody against the alpha-4 subunit of integrin molecules that prevents the adhesion and transmigration of leucocytes from vasculature to inflamed tissues. Natalizumab is used for the treatment of relapsing multiple sclerosis and Crohn's disease. Progressive multifocal leukoencephalopathy (PML) due to the reactivation of the polyoma JC virus is a rare and frequently fatal opportunistic infection that has been well reported in patients with rheumatic diseases. The contributions of predisposing factors such as underlying disease and immunosuppressive drugs are not completely understood. Natalizumab has the clearest pattern of a small but definite risk for PML [69].

Differentiating Infections from Autoimmunity

It is well known that a higher degree of immunosuppression puts patients with autoimmune disorders at greater risk of infections. When patients with underlying autoimmune disorders have a deterioration of their health, it is often challenging to differentiate between a newly acquired infection, reactivation of an existing infection, and worsening of the underlying autoimmune disease. As an example, granulomatosis with polyangiitis (formerly known as Wegener's granulomatosis) is a small-vessel vasculitis characterized by granulomatous and necrotizing inflammation that affects the respiratory tract and/or kidneys. New-onset fever, cough, and dyspnea in a patient with granulomatosis with microscopic polyangiitis in remission could arise due to many reasons. Cytomegalovirus infection and reactivation are common causes of pneumonitis. Cyclophosphamide and azathioprine used for the treatment of vasculitis have been proposed as causes of hypersensitivity pneumonitis [70]. Worsening of underlying disease is always a concern and the Birmingham Vasculitis Activity Score (BVAS) is a valid, disease-specific activity index for patients with granulomatosis with polyangiitis that can be used as tool [71]. These patients warrant careful evaluation with serology, imaging, and bronchoalveolar lavage with culture to rule out potential infectious complications.

Therapeutic Options for Autoimmunity-Associated Infectious Diseases

Therapeutic strategies should be directed at controlling the infection as well as inhibiting the autoimmune response. A common approach is the use of antimicrobial agents and immunosuppressive treatments simultaneously. Another approach is using plasmapheresis to remove temporarily autoantibodies triggering the disease flare. Since plasmapheresis does not eliminate autoantibody-producing plasma cells, B-cell-targeted therapies using monoclonal antibodies have become mainstream therapy. However, suppression of B-cell function can result in hypogammaglobulinemia and antibody deficiencies that can predispose to recurring infections. Immunoglobulin (Ig) G replacement therapy, both intravenous (IV) and subcutaneous (SC), has been used to treat secondary humoral immunodeficiencies associated with B-cell-directed monoclonal antibody therapies [65, 66]. High-dose (1–2 g/kg) intravenous immunoglobulin (IVIG) has a long history as immunomodulatory therapy for a wide range of autoimmune disorders [72]. IVIG targets both cellular and soluble mediators of autoimmunity and inhibits disease by multimodal, mutually nonexclusive mechanisms such as anti-idiotypic antibodies to autoantibodies, induction of B-cell tolerance, regulation of the immunoglobulin repertoire, suppression of innate antigen-presenting cells, inhibition of T-cell help to B cells, and expansion of CD4$^+$CD25$^+$ regulatory T cells. The latter are critical for maintaining immune tolerance to prevent autoimmunity. A combination of antimicrobial agents, immunosuppression, B-cell-targeted therapies, and immunomodulation by IVIG is a reasonable approach to treat autoimmunity and associated infections [9, 73–75].

Several new recommendations for the vaccination of adults with autoimmune inflammatory diseases represent an important step forward in the prevention of infections in these high-risk patients [76]. The lay literature is rife with reports that vaccination against infectious diseases preceded the onset of rheumatologic disorders. However, a causal relationship has not been definitively established. Interestingly, influenza and pneumococcal vaccines have been found to be safe and, generally, protective in patients with systemic lupus erythematosus and rheumatoid arthritis [77]. Many patients with autoimmune disease are relatively poor responders to vaccine antigens and may require high-dose vaccines, additional boosters, and/or adjuvants. The protective value of vaccines in patients with autoimmune disease is well-established based on sound epidemiologic data, while the possibility that vaccines may induce or exacerbate autoimmune disease remains speculative [78]. Guidelines for vaccination of patients with autoimmune, inflammatory, and rheumatologic diseases should be followed to prevent infections [79]. Live vaccines such as measles, mumps, and rubella (MMR), varicella, Bacille Calmette-Guérin (BCG), and oral polio vaccine (OPV) are contraindicated in SLE patients with active disease or on high-dose immunosuppressive therapy as they can result in vaccine-acquired infection.

Toll-like receptor (TLR) antagonists, including quinine-derived antimalarial drugs such as hydroxychloroquine and quinacrine, reduce mortality in SLE and reduce the incidence of infections. Antimalarials exert their therapeutic effects through inhibition of TLR7 and TLR9

activation by blocking endosomal acidification; they should be used if not otherwise contraindicated [80, 81].

Future Directions

Strategies for suppressing the inflammatory response using anti-cytokine and monoclonal antibody-based therapies could pave the way for avoiding pathogenic autoimmunity without inhibiting protective immunity. Developing vaccines against pathogens inciting autoimmunity is an arduous task but could have tremendous preventive benefits. Using specific monoclonal antibodies to block the immune response to shared epitopes might be a strategy to prevent autoimmunity with molecular mimicry as its basis.

Research on the microbiome of the gut has significantly increased in recent years, and its role in the etiology of intestinal and extraintestinal autoimmune diseases is now recognized. Development of therapies aimed at altering the behavior of the microbiome or understanding the metabolites generated that affect immunity is a fascinating new avenue in medicine that could prevent autoimmunity.

Summary

Patients with autoimmune disorders become susceptible to common as well as opportunistic infections by various mechanisms. This susceptibility may arise from the disease itself and/or from the use of immunosuppressive medications. While treatment-associated infections are possible, it is challenging to distinguish a flare up of the underlying autoimmune disease from an infection. There is increased morbidity and mortality from infections in patients with autoimmune diseases; hence, it is important to recognize and treat any infections early. Greater efforts should be taken to prevent infections in these patients.

References

1. Doria A, Canova M, Tonon M, Zen M, Rampudda E, Bassi N, et al. Infections as triggers and complications of systemic lupus erythematosus. Autoimmun Rev. 2008;8(1):24–8.
2. Kallenberg CG, Tadema H. Vasculitis and infections: contribution to the issue of autoimmunity reviews devoted to "autoimmunity and infection". Autoimmun Rev. 2008;8(1):29–32.
3. Randone SB, Guiducci S, Cerinic MM. Systemic sclerosis and infections. Autoimmun Rev. 2008;8(1):36–40.
4. Sotgiu S, Angius A, Embry A, Rosati G, Musumeci S. Hygiene hypothesis: innate immunity, malaria and multiple sclerosis. Med Hypotheses. 2008;70(4):819–25.
5. Zandman-Goddard G, Shoenfeld Y. Parasitic infection and autoimmunity. Lupus. 2009;18(13):1144–8.
6. Sheikh KA, Nachamkin I, Ho TW, Willison HJ, Veitch J, Ung H, et al. Campylobacter jejuni lipopolysaccharides in Guillain-Barre syndrome: molecular mimicry and host susceptibility. Neurology. 1998;51(2):371–8.
7. Kivity S, Arango MT, Ehrenfeld M, Tehori O, Shoenfeld Y, Anaya JM, et al. Infection and autoimmunity in Sjogren's syndrome: a clinical study and comprehensive review. J Autoimmun. 2014;51:17–22.
8. Cutolo M, Seriolo B, Pizzorni C, Secchi ME, Soldano S, Paolino S, et al. Use of glucocorticoids and risk of infections. Autoimmun Rev. 2008;8(2):153–5.
9. Maddur MS, Vani J, Lacroix-Desmazes S, Kaveri S, Bayry J. Autoimmunity as a predisposition for infectious diseases. PLoS Pathog. 2010;6(11):e1001077.
10. Cunningham MW. Rheumatic fever, autoimmunity, and molecular mimicry: the streptococcal connection. Int Rev Immunol. 2014;33(4):314–29.
11. Root-Bernstein R, Fairweather D. Complexities in the relationship between infection and autoimmunity. Curr Allergy Asthma Rep. 2014;14(1):407.
12. Fujinami RS, von Herrath MG, Christen U, Whitton JL. Molecular mimicry, bystander activation, or viral persistence: infections and autoimmune disease. Clin Microbiol Rev. 2006;19(1):80–94.
13. Vanderlugt CJ, Miller SD. Epitope spreading. Curr Opin Immunol. 1996;8(6):831–6.
14. Lehmann PV, Sercarz EE, Forsthuber T, Dayan CM, Gammon G. Determinant spreading and the dynamics of the autoimmune T-cell repertoire. Immunol Today. 1993;14(5):203–8.
15. Root-Bernstein R. Antigenic complementarity in the induction of autoimmunity: a general theory and review. Autoimmun Rev. 2007;6(5):272–7.
16. Doria A, Zampieri S, Sarzi-Puttini P. Exploring the complex relationships between infections and autoimmunity. Autoimmun Rev. 2008;8(2):89–91.
17. Lunardi C, Tinazzi E, Bason C, Dolcino M, Corrocher R, Puccetti A. Human parvovirus B19 infection and autoimmunity. Autoimmun Rev. 2008;8(2):116–20.
18. Ryan KR, Patel SD, Stephens LA, Anderton SM. Death, adaptation and regulation: the three pillars of immune tolerance restrict the risk of autoimmune disease caused by molecular mimicry. J Autoimmun. 2007;29(4):262–71.
19. Zignego AL, Piluso A, Giannini C. HBV and HCV chronic infection: autoimmune manifestations and lymphoproliferation. Autoimmun Rev. 2008;8(2):107–11.
20. Hansen R, Thomson JM, El-Omar EM, Hold GL. The role of infection in the aetiology of inflammatory bowel disease. J Gastroenterol. 2010;45(3):266–76.
21. Packey CD, Sartor RB. Interplay of commensal and pathogenic bacteria, genetic mutations, and immunoregulatory defects in the pathogenesis of inflammatory bowel diseases. J Intern Med. 2008;263(6):597–606.
22. Teng F, Klinger CN, Felix KM, Bradley CP, Wu E, Tran NL, et al. Gut microbiota drive autoimmune arthritis by promoting differentiation and migration of Peyer's patch T follicular helper cells. Immunity. 2016;44(4):875–88.
23. Caza T, Oaks Z, Perl A. Interplay of infections, autoimmunity, and immunosuppression in systemic lupus erythematosus. Int Rev Immunol. 2014;33(4):330–63.
24. Jonsson G, Truedsson L, Sturfelt G, Oxelius VA, Braconier JH, Sjoholm AG. Hereditary C2 deficiency in Sweden. Medicine (Baltimore). 2005;84(1):23–34.
25. Iguchi-Hashimoto M, Hashimoto M, Fujii T, Hamaguchi M, Furu M, Ishikawa M, et al. The association between serious infection and disease outcome in patients with rheumatoid arthritis. Clin Rheumatol. 2016;35(1):213–8.
26. al-Janadi M, al-Balla S, al-Dalaan A, Raziuddin S. Cytokine profile in systemic lupus erythematosus, rheumatoid arthritis, and other rheumatic diseases. J Clin Immunol. 1993;13(1):58–67.
27. Fox RI. Sjogren's syndrome. Lancet. 2005;366(9482):321–31.
28. Mandl T, Bredberg A, Jacobsson LT, Manthorpe R, Henriksson G. CD4+ T-lymphocytopenia – a frequent finding in anti-SSA antibody seropositive patients with primary Sjogren's syndrome. J Rheumatol. 2004;31(4):726–8.
29. Hersey P, Lawrence S, Prendergast D, Bindon C, Benson W, Valk P. Association of Sjögren's syndrome with C4 deficiency, defective reticuloendothelial function and circulating immune complexes. Clin Exp Immunol. 1983;52(3):551–60.
30. Hammarström L, Vorechovsky I, Webster D. Selective IgA deficiency (SIgAD) and common variable immunodeficiency (CVID). Clin Exp Immunol. 2000;120(2):225–31.
31. Bloom KA, Chung D, Cunningham-Rundles C. Osteoarticular infectious complications in patients with primary immunodeficiencies. Curr Opin Rheumatol. 2008;20(4):480–5.
32. Cunningham-Rundles C, Bodian C. Common variable immunodeficiency: clinical and immunological features of 248 patients. Clin Immunol (Orlando, Fla). 1999;92(1):34–48.

33. Cunningham-Rundles C. Physiology of IgA and IgA deficiency. J Clin Immunol. 2001;21(5):303–9.

34. Yel L. Selective IgA deficiency. J Clin Immunol. 2010;30(1):10–6.

35. Jorgensen GH, Gardulf A, Sigurdsson MI, Sigurdardottir ST, Thorsteinsdottir I, Gudmundsson S, et al. Clinical symptoms in adults with selective IgA deficiency: a case-control study. J Clin Immunol. 2013;33(4):742–7.

36. Wang N, Shen N, Vyse TJ, Anand V, Gunnarson I, Sturfelt G, et al. Selective IgA deficiency in autoimmune diseases. Mol Med. 2011;17(11–12):1383–96.

37. Matsumoto R, Nakamizo S, Tanioka M, Miyachi Y, Kabashima K. Leukocytoclastic vasculitis with eosinophilic infiltration in an HIV-positive patient. Eur J Dermatol: EJD. 2011;21(1):103–4.

38. Iordache L, Launay O, Bouchaud O, Jeantils V, Goujard C, Boue F, et al. Autoimmune diseases in HIV-infected patients: 52 cases and literature review. Autoimmun Rev. 2014;13(8):850–7.

39. Zandman-Goddard G, Shoenfeld Y. HIV and autoimmunity. Autoimmun Rev. 2002;1(6):329–37.

40. Martinez V, Diemert MC, Braibant M, Potard V, Charuel JL, Barin F, et al. Anticardiolipin antibodies in HIV infection are independently associated with antibodies to the membrane proximal external region of gp41 and with cell-associated HIV DNA and immune activation. Clin Infect Dis: Off Publ Infect Dis Soc Am. 2009;48(1):123–32.

41. Savige JA, Chang L, Horn S, Crowe SM. Anti-nuclear, anti-neutrophil cytoplasmic and anti-glomerular basement membrane antibodies in HIV-infected individuals. Autoimmunity. 1994;18(3):205–11.

42. Ahmad DS, Esmadi M, Steinmann WC. Idiopathic CD4 Lymphocytopenia: spectrum of opportunistic infections, malignancies, and autoimmune diseases. Avicenna J Med. 2013;3(2):37–47.

43. Regent A, Autran B, Carcelain G, Cheynier R, Terrier B, Charmeteau-De Muylder B, et al. Idiopathic CD4 lymphocytopenia: clinical and immunologic characteristics and follow-up of 40 patients. Medicine (Baltimore). 2014;93(2):61–72.

44. Rhen T, Cidlowski JA. Anti-inflammatory action of glucocorticoids – new mechanisms for old drugs. N Engl J Med. 2005;353(16):1711–23.

45. Barnes PJ. Anti-inflammatory actions of glucocorticoids: molecular mechanisms. Clin Sci (Lond). 1998;94(6):557–72.

46. Migita K, Arai T, Ishizuka N, Jiuchi Y, Sasaki Y, Izumi Y, et al. Rates of serious intracellular infections in autoimmune disease patients receiving initial glucocorticoid therapy. PLoS One. 2013;8(11):e78699.

47. Cutolo M, Otsa K, Aakre O, Sulli A. Nocturnal hormones and clinical rhythms in rheumatoid arthritis. Ann N Y Acad Sci. 2005;1051:372–81.

48. Atzeni F, Bendtzen K, Bobbio-Pallavicini F, Conti F, Cutolo M, Montecucco C, et al. Infections and treatment of patients with rheumatic diseases. Clin Exp Rheumatol. 2008;26(1 Suppl 48):S67–73.

49. Tian H, Cronstein BN. Understanding the mechanisms of action of methotrexate: implications for the treatment of rheumatoid arthritis. Bull NYU Hosp Jt Dis. 2007;65(3):168–73.

50. Caporali R, Caprioli M, Bobbio-Pallavicini F, Montecucco C. DMARDS and infections in rheumatoid arthritis. Autoimmun Rev. 2008;8(2):139–43.

51. Patatanian E, Thompson DF. A review of methotrexate-induced accelerated nodulosis. Pharmacotherapy. 2002;22(9):1157–62.

52. Albrecht K, Muller-Ladner U. Side effects and management of side effects of methotrexate in rheumatoid arthritis. Clin Exp Rheumatol. 2010;28(5 Suppl 61):S95–101.

53. McLean-Tooke A, Aldridge C, Waugh S, Spickett GP, Kay L. Methotrexate, rheumatoid arthritis and infection risk: what is the evidence? Rheumatology (Oxford). 2009;48(8):867–71.

54. Hoffman GS, Kerr GS, Leavitt RY, Hallahan CW, Lebovics RS, Travis WD, et al. Wegener granulomatosis: an analysis of 158 patients. Ann Intern Med. 1992;116(6):488–98.

55. Cavallasca JA, Costa CA, Maliandi MDR, Contini LE, Fernandez de Carrera E, Musuruana JL. Severe infections in patients with autoimmune diseases treated with cyclophosphamide. Reumatol Clín (Engl Ed). 2015;11(4):221–3.

56. Singh JA, Cameron C, Noorbaloochi S, Cullis T, Tucker M, Christensen R, et al. Risk of serious infection in biological treatment of patients with rheumatoid arthritis: a systematic review and meta-analysis. Lancet. 2015;386(9990):258–65.

57. Singh JA, Wells GA, Christensen R, Tanjong Ghogomu E, Maxwell L, Macdonald JK, et al. Adverse effects of biologics: a network meta-analysis and Cochrane overview. Cochrane Database Syst Rev. 2011;2:CD008794.

58. de Assis MR, Heymann RE. Care against infections in rheumatic autoimmune diseases. Rev Bras Reumatol. 2015;55(4):317.

59. Lalvani A, Millington KA. Screening for tuberculosis infection prior to initiation of anti-TNF therapy. Autoimmun Rev. 2008;8(2):147–52.

60. Galeazzi M, Giannitti C, Manganelli S, Benucci M, Scarpato S, Bazzani C, et al. Treatment of rheumatic diseases in patients with HCV and HIV infection. Autoimmun Rev. 2008;8(2):100–3.

61. Cavazzana I, Ceribelli A, Cattaneo R, Franceschini F. Treatment with etanercept in six patients with chronic hepatitis C infection and systemic autoimmune diseases. Autoimmun Rev. 2008;8(2):104–6.

62. Fleischmann RM, Schechtman J, Bennett R, Handel ML, Burmester G-R, Tesser J, et al. Anakinra, a recombinant human interleukin-1 receptor antagonist (r-metHuIL-1ra), in patients with rheumatoid arthritis: a large, international, multicenter, placebo-controlled trial. Arthritis Rheum. 2003;48(4):927–34.

63. Cohen SB, Emery P, Greenwald MW, Dougados M, Furie RA, Genovese MC, et al. Rituximab for rheu-

matoid arthritis refractory to anti–tumor necrosis factor therapy: results of a multicenter, randomized, double-blind, placebo-controlled, phase III trial evaluating primary efficacy and safety at twenty-four weeks. Arthritis Rheum. 2006;54(9):2793–806.

64. Gottenberg JE, Ravaud P, Bardin T, Cacoub P, Cantagrel A, Combe B, et al. Risk factors for severe infections in patients with rheumatoid arthritis treated with rituximab in the autoimmunity and rituximab registry. Arthritis Rheum. 2010;62(9):2625–32.

65. Barmettler S, Price C. Continuing IgG replacement therapy for hypogammaglobulinemia after rituximab – for how long? J Allergy Clin Immunol. 2015;136(5):1407–9.

66. Kaplan B, Kopyltsova Y, Khokhar A, Lam F, Bonagura V. Rituximab and immune deficiency: case series and review of the literature. J Allergy Clin Immunol Pract. 2014;2(5):594–600.

67. Genovese MC, Becker J-C, Schiff M, Luggen M, Sherrer Y, Kremer J, et al. Abatacept for rheumatoid arthritis refractory to tumor necrosis factor α inhibition. N Engl J Med. 2005;353(11):1114–23.

68. Salmon JH, Gottenberg JE, Ravaud P, Cantagrel A, Combe B, Flipo RM, et al. Predictive risk factors of serious infections in patients with rheumatoid arthritis treated with abatacept in common practice: results from the Orencia and Rheumatoid Arthritis (ORA) registry. Ann Rheum Dis. 2016;75:1108–13.

69. Boren EJ, Cheema GS, Naguwa SM, Ansari AA, Gershwin ME. The emergence of progressive multifocal leukoencephalopathy (PML) in rheumatic diseases. J Autoimmun. 2008;30(1–2):90–8.

70. Lee IH, Kang GW, Kim KC. Hypersensitivity pneumonitis associated with azathioprine therapy in a patient with granulomatosis with polyangiitis. Rheumatol Int. 2016 Jul;36(7):1027–32.

71. Stone JH, Hoffman GS, Merkel PA, Min YI, Uhlfelder ML, Hellmann DB, Specks U, Allen NB, Davis JC, Spiera RF, Calabrese LH, Wigley FM, Maiden N, Valente RM, Niles JL, Fye KH, McCune JW, St Clair EW, Luqmani RA. International Network for the Study of the Systemic Vasculitides (INSSYS). A

disease-specific activity index for Wegener's granulomatosis: modification of the Birmingham Vasculitis Activity Score. International Network for the Study of the Systemic Vasculitides (INSSYS). Arthritis Rheum. 2001 Apr;44(4):912–20.

72. Schwartz SA. Intravenous immunoglobulin (IVIG) for the therapy of autoimmune disorders. J Clin Immunol. 1990;10(2):81–9.

73. Ahmed AR, Spigelman Z, Cavacini LA, Posner MR. Treatment of pemphigus vulgaris with rituximab and intravenous immune globulin. N Engl J Med. 2006;355(17):1772–9.

74. Dorner T, Radbruch A, Burmester GR. B-cell-directed therapies for autoimmune disease. Nat Rev Rheumatol. 2009;5(8):433–41.

75. Elluru SR, Vani J, Delignat S, Bloch MF, Lacroix-Desmazes S, Kazatchkine MD, et al. Modulation of human dendritic cell maturation and function by natural IgG antibodies. Autoimmun Rev. 2008;7(6):487–90.

76. Meyer-Olson D, Witte T. Immunology: prevention of infections in patients with autoimmune diseases. Nat Rev Rheumatol. 2011;7(4):198–200.

77. Conti F, Rezai S, Valesini G. Vaccination and autoimmune rheumatic diseases. Autoimmun Rev. 2008;8(2):124–8.

78. Murdaca G, Orsi A, Spano F, Puppo F, Durando P, Icardi G, et al. Influenza and pneumococcal vaccinations of patients with systemic lupus erythematosus: current views upon safety and immunogenicity. Autoimmun Rev. 2014;13(2):75–84.

79. Westra J, Rondaan C, van Assen S, Bijl M. Vaccination of patients with autoimmune inflammatory rheumatic diseases. Nat Rev Rheumatol. 2015;11(3):135–45.

80. Ruiz-Irastorza G, Ramos-Casals M, Brito-Zeron P, Khamashta MA. Clinical efficacy and side effects of antimalarials in systemic lupus erythematosus: a systematic review. Ann Rheum Dis. 2010;69(1):20–8.

81. Kuznik A, Bencina M, Svajger U, Jeras M, Rozman B, Jerala R. Mechanism of endosomal TLR inhibition by antimalarial drugs and imidazoquinolines. J Immunol. 2011;186(8):4794–804.

Antibacterial and Antifungal Agents: The Challenges of Antimicrobial-Resistant Infections in Immunocompromised Hosts

Matthew W. McCarthy, Thomas Baker,
Michael J. Satlin, and Thomas J. Walsh

Introduction

Antimicrobial resistance may be intrinsic or acquired and is associated with poor clinical outcomes and breakthrough infections during treatment and prophylaxis. Given their frequent healthcare exposure, the immunocompromised are at higher risk for infection attributed to multidrug-resistant organisms. This increased risk, combined with identification through culturing techniques that can take several days, may lead to immunocompromised patients being placed empirically on antibiotics and antifungal agents that are not active against resistant organisms. Thus, patients with resistant infections may experience significant delays in receiving appropriate antimicrobial therapy. Understanding the underlying mechanisms of antibiotic resistance is critical to both choosing appropriate active therapy and developing new antimicrobial agents. Resistance mechanisms, which will be reviewed below, are extensive and vary across species. The most common mechanisms include alteration of drug target site, enzymatic drug inactivation, decreased bacterial membrane permeability, and drug efflux.

M. W. McCarthy (✉) · T. Baker · M. J. Satlin
T. J. Walsh
Department of Infectious Diseases, Weill Cornell Medicine, New York, NY, USA
e-mail: mwm9004@med.cornell.edu

For each major drug class, this section will describe these common resistance mechanisms and organisms frequently harboring them, examples of resistance emerging in immunocompromised patients, and alternative agents available for treatment of these resistant organisms (Table 15.1).

β-Lactam Agents (Penicillins, Cephalosporins, and Monobactams)

Mechanisms of Resistance

Drug Inactivation

Resistance to β-lactam agents is frequently mediated through bacterial production of β-lactamase enzymes. These enzymes are capable of hydrolyzing the β-lactam ring, leading to drug inactivation. Initially isolated from *E. coli* in 1940, the first β-lactamase was dubbed penicillinase for its ability to inactivate the then newly discovered penicillin (Abraham). In the 1940s, plasmid-mediated penicillin resistance quickly spread among *Staphylococcus aureus* and is now exceedingly common (Barber). In the 1960s and 1970s, the world saw the emergence and expansion of TEM- and SHV-type β-lactamases capable of inactivating penicillins and narrow-spectrum cephalosporins (Datta, Hawkey). Then, after the

© Springer International Publishing AG, part of Springer Nature 2018
B. H. Segal (ed.), *Management of Infections in the Immunocompromised Host*,
https://doi.org/10.1007/978-3-319-77674-3_15

Table 15.1 Antibiotic classes with common mechanisms of resistance, organism expressing resistance, and available alternative agents

Agent class	Mechanism of resistance	Organism	Alternative agents
β-Lactams	β-Lactamases (non-carbapenemase)	Enterobacteriaceae	Carbapenems
		P. aeruginosa	Fluoroquinolones
		S. maltophilia	Aminoglycosides
		A. baumannii	
	PBPs	MRSA	Vancomycin
			Daptomycin
		S. pneumoniae	Levofloxacin
			Macrolides
Carbapenems	Carbapenemases	Enterobacteriaceae	Polymyxin-based combination therapy
		P. aeruginosa	Ceftazidime-avibactam (if KPC-mediated resistance)
	Drug permeability	A. baumannii	
	Drug efflux	S. maltophilia (chromosomal)	+/− high-dose, prolonged infusion carbapenem if MIC ≤8 μg/mL
Fluoroquinolones	DNA gyrase modification	Enterobacteriaceae	β-lactams
		P. aeruginosa	Aztreonam
			Aminoglycosides
	Topoisomerase IV modification	MRSA	Macrolides (not MRSA)
		S. pneumoniae	β-lactams
			Daptomycin
			Linezolid
Aminoglycosides	Aminoglycoside-modifying enzymes	Enterobacteriaceae	
		P. aeruginosa	
		S. maltophilia	β-lactams
		A. baumannii	Aztreonam
	16S rRNA methylation	Enterococcus spp.	Fluoroquinolones
		S. aureus	
Glycopeptides/ lipopeptides	D-Ala-D-Ala modification	Enterococcus spp.	
		S. aureus (rare)	Linezolid
			Ceftaroline
	D-Ala-D-Ala overproduction	S. aureus (rare)	Telavancin

development of third-generation cephalosporins, TEM- and SHV-type extended-spectrum β-lactamases (ESBLs) with the ability to hydrolyze extended-spectrum β-lactams were described in the 1980s (Kitzis). In the early 1990s, CTX-M-derived β-lactamases, also capable of extended-spectrum hydrolysis, were first recognized. This family of plasmid-mediated resistance spread rapidly worldwide, and CTX-M enzymes are now the world's most prevalent ESBLs (Canton).

AmpC β-lactamases, like ESBLs, are capable of inactivating penicillins and most cephalosporins, but not carbapenems. Unlike ESBLs, they are not effectively inhibited by β-lactamase inhibitors, like clavulanate and tazobactam.

AmpC β-lactamase genes can be located both chromosomally and on plasmids and are often expressed at only a low level. However, the expression of these enzymes can be markedly upregulated upon exposure to β-lactam antibiotics (Jacoby). Thus, organisms possessing AmpC β-lactamase genes may initially test susceptible to third-generation cephalosporins, like ceftriaxone or ceftazidime, but subsequently develop resistance to these antibiotics during therapy due to the inducible expression of these enzymes (Choi, Chow).

β-Lactamases also play an important role in carbapenem resistance, but this will be discussed in the next section.

Alteration of Drug Target

If they avoid hydrolysis by β-lactamases, β-lactam antibiotics bind covalently to penicillin-binding proteins (PBPs) in the bacterial cytoplasmic membrane, leading to inhibition of cell wall synthesis and eventual cell lysis. Certain Gram-positive bacteria, however, develop resistance by producing PBPs with low affinity for β-lactam antibiotics. Without the ability to adequately bind its intended target, the β-lactam can no longer effectively inhibit bacterial growth (Zapun).

Bacteria Expressing This Form of Resistance

Drug Inactivation

Among Gram-negative bacteria, β-lactamases are widespread and are commonly encountered in *Enterobacteriaceae*, *Pseudomonas aeruginosa*, *Acinetobacter baumannii*, and *Stenotrophomonas maltophilia*. Enterobacteriaceae are an important family of bacteria that inhabit the gastrointestinal tract and are a common cause of Gram-negative bacteremia in immunocompromised hosts (Trecarichi). Prominent pathogens in this family include *E. coli*, *Klebsiella pneumoniae*, and *Enterobacter* species. ESBLs, like CTX-M, are most commonly identified in *E. coli* and *Klebsiella* species [12]. Enterobacteriaceae that most commonly harbor AmpC β-lactamases are often referred to as the SPICE organisms (*Serratia marcescens*, **P**rovidencia, **i**ndole-positive *Proteus*, *Citrobacter*, and *Enterobacter* species) (Jacoby).

Alteration of Drug Target

Arguably the most clinically relevant bacterial alteration of a β-lactam drug target is seen in methicillin-resistant *Staphylococcus aureus* (MRSA). This resistance is most commonly mediated through the expression of the mecA gene. This gene encodes PBP2a, a penicillin-binding protein with low affinity for β-lactam antibiotics. This allows for resistance to methicillin, nafcillin, oxacillin, cephalosporins (with the exception of some newer generation cephalosporins), and carbapenems. Ceftaroline and some newer cephalosporins retain activity against MRSA. The mecA gene is located on a staphylococcal chromosome cassette (SCCmec), a mobile genetic element, and was likely originally acquired from a coagulase-negative staphylococcal species (Gutmann).

Examples in the Immunocompromised

Drug Inactivation

There are numerous reports documenting the emergence of ESBL-producing *Enterobacteriaceae* (ESBL-E) bacteremia in patients with hematologic malignancies. These reports suggest that in some regions, ESBL-E comprises 17–37% of all bacteremias due to *Enterobacteriaceae* in this population and that this incidence is increasing (Cornejo, Montassier, Mihu). Risk factors for ESBL-E bacteremia in immunosuppressed patients include recent hospitalizations or antibiotic exposure, intensive care unit (ICU) admissions, and prolonged durations of hospitalization and neutropenia (Cornejo, Gudiol, Kang, Kim, Oliviea, Ha). Mortality rates following ESBL-E bacteremia in patients with hematologic malignancies range from 13% to 45% and are higher when compared to non-ESBL-E bacteremias (Cornejo, Trecharichi, Gudiol, Kang, Kim, Ha, Metan, Yemisen). Inappropriate initial antibiotic therapy in ESBL infection has repeatedly been shown to be a risk factor for increased mortality (Cornejo, Gudiol, Kang, Hyle).

Data regarding the incidence of AmpC β-lactamase-producing *Enterobacteriaceae* (AmpC-E) infections in immunocompromised patients are limited; most clinical microbiology laboratories do not perform phenotypic or genotypic testing to detect AmpC β-lactamases. Some studies show that *Enterobacter* spp. (which typically harbor AmpC β-lactamases) cause 5–8% of Gram-negative bacteremias in patients with hematologic malignancies, making them the fourth most common cause of Gram-negative bacteremia in this population (Gudiol 2013; Trecarichi, Metan, Kara).

Alteration of Drug Target

Although *S. aureus* has been shown to be disproportionately prevalent among patients with hematological malignancy, the impact of MRSA in the immunocompromised has not been well defined (Skov). One study examining 494 patients with MRSA and 505 patients with methicillin-sensitive *S. aureus* (MSSA) infections found that MRSA infection was more prevalent in patients with cancer. In that same study, patients with MRSA infection were 50% more likely to die in hospital (Hanberger). One study of 223 patients with cancer and MRSA bacteremia treated with vancomycin found a treatment failure rate of 54%. Hematologic malignancy and hematopoietic stem cell transplantation (HSCT) were both found to be risk factors for MRSA-associated mortality (Mahajan). As vancomycin is widely used in this population, clinically overt MRSA infections may be thwarted from developing.

Alternative Agents

Drug Inactivation

Even when ESBL-E test susceptible to cefepime or piperacillin-tazobactam (PTZ), clinical data suggest that infections due to ESBL-E may not respond as well to these agents as compared to carbapenems. A propensity score-matched, observational study of ESBL-E bacteremias found that patients treated with cefepime were more likely to have a clinical or microbiological failure and had higher 30-day mortality than those who received carbapenem therapy (Lee). Additionally, a recent observational study of patients with ESBL-E bacteremia found that risk of death doubled when PTZ was used empirically instead of a carbapenem, despite all isolates being susceptible to both PTZ and carbapenems (Tamma).

The increase in mortality seen with cefepime and PTZ therapy may be because the minimum concentrations of these antibiotics required to inhibit growth of ESBL-E increases when the number of organisms inoculated is increased (Thomson). This "inoculum effect" is not seen with carbapenems. Based on current data,

carbapenems remain the preferred agents for the treatment of ESBL-E bacteremias, regardless of cefepime or PTZ susceptibility results.

Carbapenems are also generally considered the first-line treatment for serious infections due to AmpC-E, given that they are stable to hydrolysis by most AmpC enzymes and do not exhibit an inoculum effect [60]. However, no randomized trials have been conducted to definitively determine the optimal therapy. Penicillins and third-generation cephalosporins, such as ceftriaxone and ceftazidime, should not be used as these organisms may upregulate AmpC expression and develop resistance on therapy. Cefepime, however, has relative stability against AmpC β-lactamases compared to other cephalosporins and may have a role in the treatment of AmpC-E infections. Two observational studies of AmpC-E infections showed no differences in outcomes between patients treated with either carbapenems or cefepime ([109], Lee). Limited observational data suggest that PTZ has similar effectiveness to carbapenems when AmpC-E test susceptible to PTZ (Marcos, Harris). Fluoroquinolones are another option in treating AmpC-E infections, and a recent meta-analysis demonstrated favorable outcomes with fluoroquinolones for this indication (Harris).

Alteration of Drug Target

Numerous parenteral agents are currently available for invasive MRSA infections. These include vancomycin, daptomycin, linezolid, and ceftaroline. Each of these agents, however, has unique advantages and limitations; providers should consider patient factors, infection location, and susceptibility data when selecting an agent. For MRSA bacteremia, the Infectious Diseases Society of America (IDSA) currently recommends the first-line use of either vancomycin or daptomycin (Liu). Daptomycin should be avoided in lung infections, however, given its inactivation by pulmonary surfactant. Ceftaroline, a fifth-generation cephalosporin, has been approved for the treatment of complicated skin and soft tissue infection and community-acquired pneumonia, but not yet MRSA bacteremia. Also of note, in a randomized control trial, high-dose trimethoprim-sulfamethoxazole failed to achieve non-inferiority to vancomycin for treatment of severe MRSA infections (Bashara).

Carbapenems

Mechanism of Resistance

Drug Inactivation
In areas with high rates of carbapenem-resistant *Enterobacteriaceae* (CRE), the most common resistance mechanism is the presence of a carbapenemase. This is a β-lactamase enzyme capable of hydrolyzing and inactivating carbapenems and all other β-lactam agents. These enzymes are also stable against commonly used β-lactamase inhibitors. Although occasionally chromosomally encoded, genes that encode for carbapenemases are typically located on plasmids, and these genes can be transferred both within bacterial species and across different species and genera. To date, a number of carbapenemases have been described, including *K. pneumoniae* carbapenemase (KPC), New Delhi metallo-β-lactamase (NDM), OXA-48-type, Verona integron-encoded metallo-β-lactamase (VIM), and IMP-type enzymes. These different carbapenemases predominate in different geographical areas. KPC is common in the United States, South America, Italy, Greece, Israel, and China, whereas NDMs predominate in India and Pakistan, and OXA-48-type carbapenemases predominate in Mediterranean Europe, North Africa, and Turkey.

Decreased Bacterial Membrane Permeability
A decrease in bacterial cellular membrane permeability can be accomplished through the downregulation or total absence of porins. Porins are proteins that cross the cellular membrane, forming a pore through which various molecules, including carbapenems, can diffuse. This decrease in permeability to carbapenems, usually combined with background β-lactamase production or other resistance mechanisms, can lead to clinical carbapenem resistance (Trias).

Bacteria Expressing This Form of Resistance

Drug Inactivation
Carbapenemases are most commonly encountered in Gram-negative organisms. The naturally occurring, chromosomally encoded carbapenemases are typically seen in *S. maltophilia* and *Elizabethkingia meningoseptica*. Carbapenemases acquired through plasmid transfer are more common in *Enterobacteriaceae* (including *K. pneumoniae* and *E. coli*), *P. aeruginosa*, and *A. baumannii*. These plasmids also frequently carry genes conferring resistance to other antibiotic classes, such as fluoroquinolones and aminoglycosides, leaving few treatment options (Satlin).

Decreased Bacterial Membrane Permeability
P. aeruginosa is also capable of achieving carbapenem resistance through the downregulation of the porin OprD. When working in concert with underlying AmpC β-lactamase production and potentially other efflux modifications, these isolates can become fully carbapenem resistant (Trias). Porins also play a role in carbapenem resistance seen in *Enterobacteriaceae*, specifically *K. pneumoniae* and *Enterobacter* species (Doumith).

Examples in the Immunocompromised

The epidemiology of CRE infections in immunocompromised hosts is unclear and has only recently been investigated. In a study of neutropenic patients with hematologic malignancies, exposures to β-lactam-β-lactamase inhibitors, trimethoprim-sulfamethoxazole, glucocorticoids, and having a prior culture that grew CRE were independent risk factors for the development of CRE bacteremia (Satlin).

The overall reported mortality rates after CRE infections in patients with hematologic malignancies are high, ranging from 44% to 72%. Two factors likely contribute to these high mortality rates. First, detection of CRE from blood cultures using traditional microbiologic methods typically takes

2–3 days, and most patients do not receive CRE-active therapy during this time. Second, the treatment options for CRE infections are limited due to their extensive resistance profiles.

Alternative Agents

The optimal therapeutic regimen for CRE infections has yet to be identified; no large randomized clinical trials comparing treatment options have been completed. Observational studies of CRE bacteremia in the general population suggest that combination therapy with at least two antibiotics to which the infecting organism tests susceptible is more effective than monotherapy [119]. These studies also suggest that despite the presence of carbapenemases, adjunctive therapy with a carbapenem, in combination with active agents, may be associated with decreased mortality. It is important to note that these improved outcomes were observed when high doses and prolonged infusions of carbapenems were used (e.g., 2 gm. of meropenem infused over 3 h, every 8 h) and when the minimum inhibitory concentration of the carbapenem was ≤ 8 mg/L.

Ceftazidime-avibactam is a new agent with potent in vitro activity against KPC-producing, but not NDM-producing, *Enterobacteriaceae*. This compound was recently approved in the United States for complicated intra-abdominal and urinary tract infections. It represents the first approved β-lactam/β-lactamase inhibitor showing activity against KPC-producing CRE (Castanheira). However, clinical trials that led to approval of this agent enrolled very few patients with CRE infection or immunocompromised patients (Liscio).

Fluoroquinolones

Mechanism of Resistance

Alteration of Drug Target Site
The primary mechanism underlying fluoroquinolone resistance is spontaneously occurring mutations in chromosomal genes leading to alteration of drug target site. In Gram-negative organisms,

this occurs in DNA gyrase (topoisomerase II), while in Gram-positive bacteria, topoisomerase IV is altered. These enzymes are important in the formation of both positive and negative supercoils in DNA or, in other words, the winding and unwinding of bacterial DNA strands. The enzymes' structures consist of A and B subunits encoded by the *gyrA* and *gyrB*, respectively, for DNA gyrase and *parC* and *parE*, respectively, for topoisomerase IV. The most common forms of resistance are due to mutations to the A subunit, although B subunit mutations have also been described (Wolfson). These structural changes to DNA gyrase and topoisomerase IV lead to a decrease in fluoroquinolone binding affinity and reduce their efficacy.

Interestingly, plasmid-mediated quinolone resistance (*qnr*) genes have recently been identified in *Enterobacteriaceae*. These *qnr* gene products protect DNA gyrase and topoisomerase IV from fluoroquinolone binding. *Qnr* genes are, by themselves, not sufficient for clinical resistance, but they enable prolonged survival during drug exposure and widen the available window for selection of chromosomal mutations (Tran).

Bacteria Expressing This Form of Resistance

Alteration of Drug Target
Rates of fluoroquinolone resistance are rising across Gram-negative species and have been linked to the frequent and widespread use of these agents. Among Gram-negative bacteria, the *Enterobacteriaceae* and *P. aeruginosa* are particularly problematic (Lautenbach, Polk, Neuhauser). Indeed, one US cancer center saw a rise in fluoroquinolone-resistant *E. coli* bacteremia from 28% in 1999 to 60% in 2008 (Mihu). Regarding Gram-positive species, MRSA (more commonly than MSSA) frequently harbors fluoroquinolone resistance [113]. Although the rate of fluoroquinolone resistance among *Streptococcus pneumoniae* has remained relativity low in the United States, it appears to be increasing worldwide (Chen, Hooper).

Examples in the Immunocompromised

Fluoroquinolone used as antimicrobial prophylaxis during prolonged chemotherapy-induced neutropenia is a common practice. Current IDSA guidelines recommend fluoro-quinolone prophylaxis with levofloxacin or ciprofloxacin in high-risk patients with expected durations of prolonged and profound neutropenia (ANC ≤ 100 cells/mm^3 for >7 days) (Freifeld). This regimen importantly targets both *P. aeruginosa* and other Gram-negative organisms, like the *Enterobacteriaceae*, which are frequent causes of life-threatening infections in this patient population.

The ultimate impact of fluoroquinolone prophy-laxis, however, is not entirely clear. A meta-analysis completed in 2005 showed a significant survival benefit for neutropenic patients placed on prophy-laxis [37]. That being said, there is growing concern surrounding bacterial resistance and fluoroquino-lone prophylaxis. The use of fluoroquinolones in patients with cancer has been well linked to increas-ing rates of resistance at individual cancer centers (Leibovici, Reuter, Kern, Martino, Mihu). Indeed, two of these centers found that bacterial resistance rates fell after discontinuing routine fluoroquino-lone prophylaxis without finding a significant impact on patient morbidity (Kern, Martino). More recently, a single center study found that fluoroqui-nolone prophylaxis in patients with cancer was also significantly associated with the emergence of MRSA, multidrug-resistant *E. coli*, and multidrug resistance *P. aeruginosa* infections (Rangaraj 2010). Given these concerns, some advocate that preva-lence monitoring of fluoroquinolone resistance among Gram-negative organisms should be per-formed at institutions where routine fluoroquino-lone prophylaxis is employed.

Alternative Agents

For Gram-negative infections resistant to fluo-roquinolones, multiple alternative agents are available for therapy. For patients with a severe β-lactam allergy, monobactams (aztreonam) and aminoglycosides can be considered as these agents provide broad Gram-negative and anti-pseudomonal coverage. The aminoglycosides, however, are limited by nephrotoxicity, otoves-tibular toxicity, and historical data suggest that aminoglycoside monotherapy is associated with comparatively poor outcomes after Gram-negative bacteremia in neutropenic patients (Bodey). If there is no concern for β-lactam allergy, and depending on the organism and type of infection, β-lactams, β-lactam-β-lactamase inhibitor (BL-BLI) combinations, cephalosporins, and carbapenems are other potential alternatives.

Fluoroquinolones are generally most reliable for certain Gram-positive infections like *S. pneu-monia* or *Enterococcus* species. This is due to cur-rent rates of resistance, limited potency against these organisms, and their propensity for rapid development of resistance while on therapy. For suspected or confirmed *S. pneumoniae* infections, β-lactams and macrolides are both potential alter-natives. However, treatment regimens should take into account location and severity of the infection.

Aminoglycosides

Mechanism of Resistance

Enzymatic Drug Inactivation
The prominent mechanism of aminoglycoside resistance is mediated through the action of aminoglycoside-modifying enzymes. The genes for these proteins can be present chromosomally or spread through plasmids or transposons. This modification and inactivation is achieved through drug phosphorylation, acetylation, or nucleoti-dylation and generally occurs during the transport of aminoglycosides across the cytoplasmic mem-brane. Once modified, the drug cannot no longer effectively bind its intended target site (Smith).

Alteration of Drug Target Site
It is increasingly recognized that aminoglycoside resistance can also be mediated through target site alteration. Aminoglycosides act by binding the

bacterial 16S rRNA and subsequently inhibiting protein synthesis. Methylation of this 16S rRNA, however, can interfere with aminoglycoside binding and greatly diminish drug efficacy. There are numerous identified methyltransferases responsible for 16S rRNA methylation, including the Rmt/Arm families (Zhou). This alteration confers high-level resistance to all currently available parenteral aminoglycosides. Unfortunately, this mechanism appears to be increasingly encountered worldwide (Fritsche, Yamane, Dhoi).

A variety of other mechanisms not discussed here, including a decrease in bacterial cellular membrane permeability and drug efflux, also have roles in aminoglycoside resistance. These generally provide low-level resistance, but can work together in concert to produce fully resistant clinical isolates (Houghton).

Bacteria Expressing This Form of Resistance

Enzymatic Drug Inactivation

Aminoglycoside-modifying enzymes have been identified in a range of in Gram-negative bacteria, like *Enterobacteriaceae*, *P. aeruginosa*, *S. maltophilia*, and *A. baumannii*. Resistance is more likely to be seen in multidrug-resistant organisms, such as CRE or ESBL-E (Haidar). This is likely because these modifying genes are commonly present on plasmids also carrying genes conferring resistance to other antibiotic classes. Importantly, aminoglycoside-modifying enzymes are also seen in Gram-positive bacteria, such as *Staphylococcus* and *Enterococcus* species (Ardia, Leclercq, Niu, Feizaba). Although the use of aminoglycosides for *Staphylococcal* infections has fallen out of favor, the propensity of these genes to also accompany β-lactamases results in a loss of synergistic combination therapy for serious enterococcal infections.

Alteration of Drug Target Site

P. aeruginosa and *K. pneumoniae* isolates producing 16S rRNA methyltransferase were first reported in 2003 (Galimand, Yokoyama). Since that time, they have been increasingly detected in *Enterobacteriaceae*, *P. aeruginosa*, and other Gram-negative organisms, including *Acinetobacter* species (Fritsche, Zhou, Doi, Yamane). Given the ability of these genes to spread through both horizontal transfer and clonal expansion, the prevalence of this resistance is expected to rise.

Examples in the Immunocompromised

As described before, CRE are an expanding threat to the immunocompromised. Given the horizontal transfer of plasmids carrying multiple antibiotic resistance genes, these multidrug-resistant organisms are frequently resistant to aminoglycosides in addition to carbapenems. Indeed, aminoglycosides are not reliably active against CRE, as almost all are resistant to tobramycin and approximately one-half are resistant to gentamicin and amikacin (Marquez, Sanchez). However, aminoglycosides remain viable options for treatment of multidrug-resistant *P. aeruginosa*. A study completed in Turkey found that in patients with high-risk hematologic malignancy, roughly 10% of *P. aeruginosa* bloodstream isolates were resistant to amikacin (Kara). Aminoglycosides, unfortunately, have high toxicity rates and are associated with poor outcomes in oncology patients with *P. aeruginosa* bacteremia compared to the use of β-lactam agents (Bodey).

Alternative Agents

Aminoglycosides are generally used only synergistically in Gram-positive infections but have a primary role in combination with beta-lactams against a broad range of aerobic Gram-negative organisms, including *Enterobacteriaceae*, *P. aeruginosa*, and *Acinetobacter* species. If aminoglycoside resistance is suspected or confirmed, then providers may be able to choose from fluoroquinolones, β-lactams, BL-BLI combinations, cephalosporins, and carbapenems as potential alternatives. As stated previously, however, frequently aminoglycoside resistance will coincide with multiple other antibiotic resistance mechanisms. In the setting of CRE infections, last resort regimens include polymyxins (colistin and polymyxin B), tigecycline, and fosfomycin. Unfortunately, each of these treatment options has major limitations.

Glycopeptides and Lipopeptides

Mechanism of Resistance

Alteration of Drug Target Site

Glycopeptides (vancomycin and teicoplanin) function by binding the C-terminal D-Alanine–D-Alanine (D-Ala-D-Ala) site of late peptidoglycan precursors, ultimately preventing cross-linking and inhibiting proper cell wall synthesis. Resistance can occur through modification of the binding site D-Ala-D-Ala. Most commonly, the *vanA* gene encodes for peptidoglycan precursors with a D-alanine-D-lactate terminus (D-Ala-D-Lac), diminishing glycopeptide binding affinity and drug efficacy. The vanA gene can be either chromosomally or plasmid encoded, with the latter allowing for gene transfer to other species and genera through conjugation. Although encountered less frequently, *vanB*, *vanC*, *vanD*, *vanE*, and *vanG* genes have also been described conferring vancomycin resistance (Reynolds).

Daptomycin, a lipopeptide, inserts into the bacterial cell membrane and combines with other drug molecules to form aggregates. This aggregation leads to the development of ion channels, causing subsequent rapid bacterial cell depolarization and ultimate cell death. Resistance of Gram-positive bacteria to daptomycin remains rare. A clear resistance mechanism has yet to be elucidated but likely involves interfering with the ability of daptomycin to bind and interact with the bacterial cell wall. For example, a gain-of-function mutation in the *mprF* gene leads to an increased ratio of lysyl-phosphatidylglycerol to phosphatidylglycerol present in the cell wall. This decrease in phosphatidylglycerol limits both drug interaction with the cell membrane and formation of functional aggregates (Friedman).

Reduced Drug Availability

Reduced susceptibility to glycopeptides can also be achieved through overproduction of the drug's target site. In vancomycin-intermediate *S. aureus* (VISA) isolates, reduced susceptibility to vancomycin is achieved by the formation of an unusually thick bacterial cell wall. This increase in D-Ala-D-Ala binding sites decreases the overall availability of vancomycin and increases its minimum inhibitory concentration (Hiramatsu). The underlying genetic changes responsible for this thickened cell wall are not well understood. However, mutations in several different genes, including vraR, graRS, and walRK, have all been identified as potential mechanisms (Howden).

Bacteria Expressing This Form of Resistance

Alteration of Drug Target Site

Glycopeptide resistance is most often encountered in *Enterococcus* spp., like *E. faecalis* and *E. faecium*. Vancomycin-resistant *Enterococcus* (VRE) is increasingly encountered, with 2006–2007 surveillance data revealing vancomycin resistance in 33% of pathogenic *Enterococcus* species (Hidron NHSN). Data from the UK, Europe, and Middle East suggest a lower percentage of VRE when compared to the US, closer to 10% (Brown, Werner, Fontana, Emanaini).

In 2002, the first vancomycin-resistant *S. aureus* (VRSA) isolate was reported in the United States. Subsequent DNA sequencing of this isolate revealed the presence of the *vanA* gene, likely transferred from an accompanying VRE infection. Since 2002 there have been at least 13 additional cases of VRSA identified, with a majority of cases from patients where VRE was also isolated (Sievert). Gene transfer of *vanA* from VRE to *S. aureus* has since been recreated in vitro (de Niederhäusern).

Although lipopeptide resistance is rare, it appears to occur more frequently in *Enterococcus* spp. compared to *S. aureus*. Descriptions of overt daptomycin-resistant *Enterococcus* infections are limited to case reports (Kanafani, Long, Hidron). In *S. aureus*, treatment failures and non-susceptible daptomycin minimum inhibitory concentrations have been reported (Fowler, Hayden, Marty).

Reduced Drug Availability

The first *S. aureus* isolate with intermediate susceptibility to vancomycin was reported in 1997. There has subsequently been numerous published clinical infections with VISA (Fridkin). Common factors in these cases include ongoing or recent hemodialysis and prolonged vancomycin exposure in the months preceding infection. The burden of these isolates, however, remains low. Surveillance data from the US and Europe in 2007 found *S. aureus* isolates with vancomycin MICs ≥4 mcg/mL represented less than 0.3% of all MIC values (Tenover).

Examples in the Immunocompromised

VRE are more frequently encountered in the immunocompromised population. A retrospective study at one cancer institution found that VRE was responsible for 54% of all bacteremias in the first 30 days following HSCT (Kamboj). Another center found that VRE colonization was common among HSCT patients, occurring in 40% of cases. Of those patients colonized, 34% subsequently developed VRE bloodstream infections (Weinstock). In the immunocompromised, VRE Infection has been associated with prolonged hospital stays and increased morbidity and mortality (Vydra). Mortality following VRE infection is high, approaching 40% in some studies, but attributable mortality due to VRE infection is unclear (Peel, Vydra). It may be that infection with VRE is more a marker of disease severity in high-risk, critically ill patients (Avery).

Alternative Agents

Glycopeptides

Over the last two decades, alternative therapies for glycopeptide-resistant organisms have expanded. For invasive VRE infections, granted the isolate is not ampicillin-sensitive, both linezolid and daptomycin are the mainstays of therapy. There is limited clinical trial data, however,

establishing efficacy of these agents. Data surrounding the use of linezolid are primarily in compassionate use settings, where outcomes were generally favorable (Birmingham, El-Khoury). However, significant adverse effects to linezolid can occur, especially during prolonged therapy, including thrombocytopenia, anemia, lactic acidosis, and peripheral neuropathy. Given the potential to induce serotonin syndrome, care must also be taken when administered with selective serotonin reuptake inhibitors. Ceftaroline has no activity against *Enterococcus* species and should not be used as primary therapy for VRE infections. There may be some data, however, for its use synergistically with daptomycin (Sakoulas).

Lipopeptides

Alternatives to daptomycin may need to be considered based on the infecting organism, site of infection, patient allergy, or drug side effects (including elevations in serum creatine kinase levels). Similarly to glycopeptides, linezolid and ceftaroline are possible alternative therapies. Additionally, the lipoglycopeptides, including telavancin, are newer agents available for Gram-positive infections. These agents share similar mechanisms to the glycopeptides. The bactericidal potency of telavancin is higher, however, and thus retains activity against VISA, VRSA, and some VRE isolates (Leuthner). However, telavancin has only received approval for acute bacterial skin and soft tissue infections due to Gram-positive pathogens and hospital-acquired pneumonia when other alternatives are not suitable.

Antifungal Agents

There are three major classes of antifungal agents: triazoles (fluconazole, itraconazole, voriconazole, posaconazole, isavuconazole), polyenes (nystatin, various formulations of amphotericin B), and echinocandins (caspofungin, micafungin, anidulafungin) (McCarthy). Below, we review what is known about the resistance mechanisms associated with these agents, examine the challenges associated with treating these organisms, and explore how novel diagnostic platforms may aid in the selection of appropriate antimicrobial therapy.

Triazole Resistance

The triazole drugs are the largest class of antifungals used in the clinical practice and as agricultural fungicides. These agents, which include ketoconazole, fluconazole, voriconazole, itraconazole, posaconazole, and isavuconazole, are becoming less effective in treating some medical mycoses due to the emergence of less susceptible fungal isolates (Snelders). Resistance to azoles used in medicine has arisen, in part, because of the use of prophylaxis in susceptible patients and prolonged treatment courses in those with known infection.

Triazole resistance can arise due to single mutations in the drug target lanosterol 14α-demethylase (Erg11p/CYP51) (Warrilow). The CLSI M27-A3 methodology requires reading MIC endpoints for triazoles visually in order to identify the lowest concentration with a prominent reduction in growth as compared with the control. This method is robust and reproducible but may be time-consuming and labor-intensive. In this setting, other platforms have recently emerged to aid in the detection of triazole resistance. *Aspergillus fumigatus* is the most common cause of invasive mold infection in immunocompromised patients. The commercially developed PathoNostics AsperGenius® species assay is a multiplex real-time PCR capable of detecting aspergillosis and genetic markers associated with azole resistance that is validated for testing bronchoalveolar lavage (BAL) fluids, replacing the requirement for culture to differentiate susceptible from resistant *A. fumigatus* strains (White).

The assay detects TR34, L98H, T289A, and Y121F mutations, known as resistance associated mutations (RAMs), in CYP51A, a gene that encodes cytochrome p450 sterol 14α-demethylase, the target of azoles. A large retrospective, multicenter study evaluated the diagnostic performance of the AsperGenius® on BAL fluid and correlated the presence of these RAMs with azole treatment failure and mortality in patients with hematologic disease and suspected invasive aspergillosis (Chong). Two hundred and one patients contributed one BAL sample, 88 served as positive controls, and 113 were negative controls. PCR was positive in 74 of 88 positive controls, and azole treatment failure was observed in 6 of 8 patients with a RAM compared with 12 of 45 patients without RAMs ($P = 0.01$). The sensitivity, specificity, positive predictive value, and negative predictive value were 84%, 80%, 76% and 87%, respectively. A 6-week mortality was nearly three times higher in patients with RAMs (50.0% versus 18.6%; $P = 0.07$) suggesting that assay had a good diagnostic performance on BAL fluid and that detection of RAMs was associated with poor prognosis.

This promising platform has distinct limitations. Although more than 15 *Cyp51A* RAMs have been described, only four appear in the current iteration of the assay and these mutations tend to originate from the environment, not from prolonged azole treatment. Other non-genotype mechanisms of resistance include increased copy number of CYP51A, efflux, and mutation of components of mitochondrial complex I. Given the potentially profound impact on patient care— early detection of RAMs can lead to prompt adaptation of the antifungal regimen—further development of this real-time multiplex PCR assay and others are needed to incorporate additional RAMs, including non-*Cyp51A* mechanisms that also confer acquired azole resistance to *A. fumigatus* and other filamentous fungi [20–22]. Other platforms, including matrix-assisted laser desorption ionization–time of flight mass spectrometry (MALDI-TOF MS), which relies on the generation of a microorganism's "protein fingerprint," are currently being evaluated as a tool for triazole susceptibility testing (Becker).

Polyene Resistance

Polyenes represent a class of biologically active fungal metabolites isolated from the genus *Streptomyces*, an aerobic actinomycete obtained from soil (Donovick). While more than 100 polyene agents have been described, formulations of amphotericin B are the most commonly used drugs to treat fungal infections in humans. Resistance to amphotericin B is uncommon, but it is increasing in the context of emerging pathogens, such as *Candida lusitaniae* and *Candida guilliermondii*, as well as species of *Aspergillus*, *Fusarium*, *Scedosporium*, and *Trichosporon*.

Amphotericin B acts mainly at the plasma membrane and impairs membrane barrier function (Broughton). Susceptibility to polyenes depends on membrane structure, including sterols and other components such as phospholipids. Sterols are essential components of eukaryotic cells, and ergosterol is the principal sterol in the fungal cell membrane. Similar to mammalian cholesterol, ergosterol serves as a bio-regulator of membrane fluidity and of membrane integrity and permeability. Amphotericin B has toxic effects on mammalian cells. It has been shown that in the presence of serum, amphotericin B binding is not limited to membrane-binding, but also to binding with low density lipoprotein (LDL) receptors. These toxic effects may be due to its capacity to modify or weaken the structure of LDLs by an oxidative process.

Intrinsic resistance to amphotericin B is rare among pathogenic fungi infecting humans, and acquired resistance during therapy is even less common. However, resistant strains have been identified. Identification of a particular pathogen to the species level helps to predict possible polyene resistance and can be extremely important to help guide the choice of antifungal therapy. For example, most isolates of *Aspergillus terreus* are resistant to amphotericin B in vitro (Blum). Clinical resistance, i.e., failure of antifungal therapy, is multifactorial and depends on a variety of factors, such as the immune status of the host, pharmacokinetics of the antifungal agent, and the species of infecting fungus. In many instances, resistance to amphotericin B may not be related to the MIC but to failure of the antifungal agent to penetrate into infected tissue.

The MIC of amphotericin B can vary depending upon the test format, type of media, and the fungal species being evaluated. The CLSI has developed a standardized broth dilution methodology for in vitro susceptibility testing of *Candida* species against amphotericin B, but this method cannot always distinguish between amphotericin B-susceptible and amphotericin B-resistant isolates due to the narrow range of MIC values that is generated.

There is a narrow range of MIC values (0.06–2 μg/mL) for amphotericin B against *Candida* species; therefore, a one-dilution shift in a breakpoint can greatly alter how susceptibility or resistance is reported. *Candida* spp. with MIC >1 μg/mL are considered resistant to amphotericin B. Limitations with the current methodologies have precluded the establishment of interpretative MIC breakpoints for amphotericin B for yeasts and molds.

Echinocandin Resistance

Echinocandins inhibit the synthesis of glucan in the fungal cell wall via noncompetitive inhibition of the enzyme 1,3-β glucan synthase and are often the treatment of choice for invasive candidiasis. Acquired resistance of *Candida* species to echinocandins is typically mediated via acquisition of point mutations in the FKS genes encoding the major subunit of its target enzyme and MICs against *Candida* isolates occasionally exceed the breakpoints for resistance (Perlin). This observation has led to concerns about the sensitivity of the CLSI-recommended methodology in identifying resistant isolates and led to a revision in echinocandin interpretive breakpoints by considering factors such as relative differences in susceptibility among *Candida* spp., epidemiological MIC cutoff values (ECVs), molecular mechanisms of resistance, β-1,3-D-glucan synthase enzyme kinetics, pharmacokinetic (PK) and pharmacodynamic (PD) data, and published clinical data linking MICs with therapeutic outcomes (Pfaller).

Although the echinocandins have been in clinical use since 2001, there have been numerous reports of echinocandin resistance in patients with invasive candidiasis. In almost all cases, the echinocandin resistance mechanism implicates the drug target, Fks, particularly in highly conserved hot spots regions (Pham). However, more resistance mechanisms may remain to be described given that Fks mutations have not been identified in some echinocandin-resistant isolates.

A novel and highly accurate diagnostic platform has recently been developed for rapid identification of FKS mutations associated with echinocandin resistance (Zhao). The assay uses allele-specific molecular beacon probes and DNA melt analysis and has the potential to overcome the deficiencies of existing in vitro susceptibility based assays to identify echinocandin resistance. Susceptibility testing is warranted in immunocompromised patients as well as those with prior exposure to these agents.

Emergence of Multidrug-Resistant Organisms

Candida auris is a novel ascomycetous yeast species first isolated from the external ear canal of a patient in a Japanese hospital in 2008 (Clancy). The organism has since become the first globally emerging fungal pathogen that exhibits multidrug resistance as well as a strong potential for nosocomial transmission. The rapid spread across four continents may be indicative of increasing selection pressures from the widespread use of antifungal agents, and molecular typing suggests that the clinical isolates are highly related within each country but distinct between continents (Lockhart). In some cases, *C. auris* is resistant to all existing antifungal agents; in other cases, it may demonstrate high-grade triazole resistance coupled with echinocandin susceptibility. However, there are reports of rapid acquisition of echinocandin resistance while on therapy.

The emergence of antifungal resistance to the most commonly used classes of drugs—triazoles, polyenes, and echinocandins—is an expanding public health threat, underscored by the paucity of novel antifungal compounds in preclinical or clinical development (Srinivasan). Successfully confronting antifungal resistance will require strategic investment in novel diagnostic platforms, therapeutics, and public health education, as well as enhanced approaches to chemoprophylaxis.

Conclusions and Future Directions

The immunocompromised are an incredibly vulnerable population, who are at risk for a number of bacterial and fungal infections with both complicated resistance patterns and mechanisms. This chapter reviewed some of the most relied upon classes of antimicrobial agents with an emphasis on common bacteria and fungi expressing resistance, examples of emergence in the immunocompromised, and alternative antimicrobial therapies. Resistance may be encountered in the drug-exposed or drug-naïve patients and is particularly challenging when it concerns infection with acquired resistance that cannot be predicted from the species identification itself. Due to the expanding spectrum of causative agents, fast and accurate pathogen detection systems are necessary to identify resistant organisms to confront the expanding threat of drug-resistant infections in patients with immune impairment.

Early recognition of resistant pathogens is essential in the initiation of antimicrobial therapy targeted against these organisms. Screening by surveillance cultures or by PCR swabs of patients undergoing cancer chemotherapy or HSCT may identify patients who are colonized with resistant organisms allowing targeted empirical therapy. Advances in T2 technology and rapid multiplexed molecular systems applied to blood, urine, and BAL fluid may detect resistant pathogens to guide preemptive therapy of documented infections.

A new generation of antibacterial and antifungal agents is being developed against resistant pathogens. Novel beta-lactamase inhibitors, tetracyclines, cephalosporins, pleuromutilins, peptides, and other molecules offer potentially new options for treatment of MDR Gram-negative bacillary pathogens, while tri-terpene $(1{\rightarrow}3)$-β-D-glucan synthase cell wall biosynthesis inhibitors, glycosylphosphatidylinositol inhibitors, and orotomides are new antifungal agents designed for treatment of resistant pathogenic fungi. Carefully conducted predictive preclinical studies and thoughtfully designed clinical trials in immunocompromised hosts are being pursued to meet the challenges of these organisms.

While the technical and regulatory hurdles associated with antimicrobial drug development are well-documented, several new developments are cause for optimism. On August 29, 2017, the US Food and Drug Administration (FDA) approved meropenem/vaborbactam fixed combination for the treatment adults with complicated urinary tract infections (cUTI). The decision was based on substantial preclinical and clinical data, including two recent trials involving hundreds of adults with cUTI. Meropenem/vaborbactam represents a powerful new treatment option to address antibiotic-resistant pathogens, including *Klebsiella pneumoniae* carbapenemase (KPC)-producing bacteria that exhibit resistance to most antimicrobial agents. Vaborbactam is a new boron-based inhibitor of several classes of β-lactamases that has been developed in combination with meropenem for the treatment of resistant bacterial pathogens, and recent work suggests this combination may one day be used to address other forms of infection, including bacteremia and lower respiratory tract infection.

This is but one of many new compounds in development. Another new agent, cefiderocol (formerly known as S-649266), is a novel siderophore cephalosporin that has significant antimicrobial activity against a variety of MDR bacteria, including strains that produce carbapenemases such as *Klebsiella pneumoniae* carbapenemase (KPC) and New Delhi metallo-β-lactamase (NDM)-1. Siderophores are small, high-affinity, iron-chelating compounds that are produced by a variety of bacteria and fungi and are among the strongest soluble Fe^{3+}-binding agents known. One potentially powerful application is to use the iron transport abilities of siderophores to carry drugs into cells by preparation of conjugates between siderophores and antimicrobial agents, which has sometimes been referred to as the "Trojan Horse" approach. We are encouraged by this ingenious strategy for the development of anti-infective therapies and believe it will serve as a model for other drugs in development. Circumventing bacterial mechanisms of resistance will require creativity as well as sustained investment to meet the needs of the expanding population of patients who are susceptible to these potentially deadly infections.

References

1. Abraham EP, Chain E. An enzyme from bacteria able to destroy penicillin. Nature. 1940;1446:837.
2. Ardia N, Sareyyupoglu B, Ozyurt M, et al. Investigation of aminoglycoside modifying enzyme genes in methicillin-resistant staphylococci. Microbiol Res. 2006;161:49–56.
3. Avery R, Kalaycio M, Pohlman B, Sobecks R, Kuczkowski E, Andresen S, Mossad S, Shamp J, Curtis J, Kosar J, Sands K, Serafin M, Bolwell B. Early vancomycin resistant enterococcus (VRE) bacteraemia after allogenic bone marrow transplantation is associated with a rapidly deteriorating clinical course. Bone Marrow Transplant. 2005;35:497–9.
4. Balkan II, Aygun G, Aydın S, et al. Blood stream infections due to OXA-48-like carbapenemase-producing Enterobacteriaceae: treatment and survival. Int J Infect Dis. 2014;26:51–6.
5. Barber M, Rozwadowska-Dowzenko M. Infection by penicillin-resistant staphylococci. Lancet. 1948;2:641–4.
6. Becker PT, de Bel A, Martiny D, Ranque S, Piarroux R, Cassagne C, et al. Identification of filamentous fungi isolates by MALDI-TOF mass spectrometry: clinical evaluation of an extended reference spectra library. Med Mycol. 2014;52(8):826–34.
7. Blum G, Perkofer S, Haas H, et al. Potential basis for amphotericin B resistance in *Aspergillus terreus*. Antimicrob Agents Chemother. 2008;52(4):1553–5.
8. Bodey GP, Jadeja L, Elting L. Pseudomonas bacteremia. Retrospective analysis of 410 episodes. Arch Intern Med. 1985;145:1621–9.
9. Bow, Bow EJ. Fluoroquinolones, antimicrobial resistance and neutropenic cancer patients. Curr Opin Infect Dis. 2011;24(6):–545.
10. Broughton MC, Bard M, Lees ND. Polyene resistance in ergosterol producing strains of *Candida albicans*. Mycoses. 1991;34:75–83.
11. Brown DF, Hope R, Livermore DM, Brick G, Broughton K, George RC, et al. Non-susceptibility trends among enterococci and non-pneumococcal streptococci from bacteraemias in the UK and Ireland, 2001–06. J Antimicrob Chemother. 2008;62(Suppl 2):ii75–85.
12. Canton. CTX-M enzymes: origin and diffusion. Front Microbiol. 2012;3:110.
13. Canton R, Coque TM. The CTX-M beta-lactamase pandemic. Curr Opin Microbiol. 2006;9:466–75.
14. Castanheira M, Mills JC, Costello SE, et al. Ceftazidime-avibactam activity tested against Enterobacteriaceae isolates from U.S. hospitals (2011–2013) and characterization of b-lactamase-producing strains. Antimicrob Agents Chemother. 2015;59:3509–17.
15. Chen DK, McGeer A, de Azavedo JC, Low DE. Decreased susceptibility of Streptococcus pneumoniae to fluoroquinolones in Canada. Canadian

Bacterial Surveillance Network. N Engl J Med. 1999;341:233–9.

16. Choi S-H, Lee JE, Park SJ, et al. Emergence of antibiotic resistance during therapy for infections caused by Enterobacteriaceae producing AmpC beta-lactamase: implications for antibiotic use. Antimicrob Agents Chemother. 2008;52:995–1000.

17. Chong GM, van der Beek MT, von dem Borne PA, Boelens J, Steel E, Kampinga GA, et al. PCR-based detection of Aspergillus fumigatus Cyp51A mutations on bronchoalveolar lavage: a multicentre validation of the AsperGenius assay® in 201 patients with haematological disease suspected for invasive aspergillosis. J Antimicrob Chemother. 2016;71:3528–35.

18. Chow JW, Fine MJ, Shlaes DM, et al. Enterobacter bacteremia: clinical features and emergence of antibiotic resistance during therapy. Ann Intern Med. 1991;115:585–90.

19. Clancy CJ, Nguyen MH. Emergence of Candida auris: an international call to arms. Clin Infect Dis. 2017;64(2):141–3.

20. Cornejo-Juarez P, Perez-Jimenez C, Silva-Sanchez J, et al. Molecular analysis and risk factors for *Escherichia coli* producing extended-spectrum b-lactamase bloodstream infection in hematological malignancies. PLoS One. 2012;7:e35780.

21. Daikos GL, Tsaousi S, Tzouvelekis LS, et al. Carbapenemase-producing *Klebsiella pneumoniae* bloodstream infections: lowering mortality by antibiotic combination schemes and the role of carbapenems. Antimicrob Agents Chemother. 2014;58:2322–8.

22. Datta N, Kontomichalou P. Penicillinase synthesis controlled by infectious R factors in Enterobacteriaceae. Nature. 1965;208:239–41.

23. Nidehhausern D, de Niederhäusern S, Bondi M, Messi P, Iseppi R, Sabia C, Manicardi G, Anacarso I. Vancomycin-resistance transferability from VanA enterococci to *Staphylococcus aureus*. Curr Microbiol. 2011;62(5):1363–7. https://doi.org/10.1007/s00284-011-9868-6. Epub 2011 Jan 15.

24. Doi Y, Arakawa Y. 16S ribosomal RNA methylation: emerging resistance mechanism against aminoglycosides. Clin Infect Dis. 2007;45:88–94.

25. Donovick R, Gold W, Pagano JF, Stout HA. Amphotericins A and B, antifungal antibiotics produced by a streptomycete. I. In vitro studies. Antibiot Annu. 1955;3:579–86.

26. Doumith M, Ellington MJ, Livermore DM, Woodford N. Molecular mechanisms disrupting porin expression in ertapenem-resistant Klebsiella and Enterobacter spp. clinical isolates from the UK. J Antimicrob Chemother. 2009;63:659–67.

27. El-Khoury J, Fishman JA. Linezolid in the treatment of vancomycin-resistant Enterococcus faecium in solid organ transplant recipients: report of a multicenter compassionate-use trial. Transpl Infect Dis. 2003;5:121.

28. Emanaini. Prevalence of vancomycin-resistant Enterococcus in Iran: a systematic review and meta-analysis.

29. Feizabadi MM, Shokrzadeh L, Sayady S, Asadi S. Transposon Tn5281 is the main distributor of the aminoglycoside modifying enzyme gene among isolates of Enterococcus faecalis in Tehran hospitals. Can J Microbiol. 2008;54:887–90.

30. Fontana R, Ligozzi M, Mazzariol A, Veneri G, Cornaglia G. Resistance of enterococci to ampicillin and glycopeptide antibiotics in Italy. The Italian Surveillance Group for Antimicrobial Resistance. Clin Infect Dis. 1998;27(Suppl 1):S84–6.

31. Fowler VG Jr, Boucher HW, Corey GR, Abrutyn E, Karchmer AW, Rupp ME, Levine DP, Chambers HF, Tally FP, Vigliani GA, et al. Daptomycin versus standard therapy for bacteremia and endocarditis caused by *Staphylococcus aureus*. N Engl J Med. 2006;355:653–65.

32. Freifeld, Freifeld AG, Bow EJ, Sepkowitz KA, Boeckh MJ, Ito JI, Mullen CA, Raad II, Rolston KV, Young JA, Wingard JR. Clinical practice guideline for the use of antimicrobial agents in neutropenic patients with cancer: 2010 update by the infectious diseases society of America. Infectious Diseases Society of America. Clin Infect Dis. 2011;52(4):e56–93. https://doi.org/10.1093/cid/cir073.

33. Freire MP, Pierrotti LC, Filho HHC, et al. Infection with *Klebsiella pneumoniae* carbapenemase (KPC)-producing *Klebsiella pneumoniae* in cancer patients. Eur J Clin Microbiol Infect Dis. 2015;34:277–86.

34. Fridkin, Fridkin SK. Vancomycin-intermediate and -resistant *Staphylococcus aureus*: what the infectious disease specialist needs to know. Clin Infect Dis. 2001;32(1):108.

35. Friedman L, Alder JD, Silverman JA. Genetic changes that correlate with reduced susceptibility to daptomycin in *Staphylococcus aureus*. Antimicrob Agents Chemother. 2006;50:2137–45.

36. Fritsche TR, Castanheira M, Miller GH, et al. Detection of methyltransferases conferring high-level resistance to aminoglycosides in Enterobacteriaceae from Europe, North America and Latin America. Antimicrob Agents Chemother. 2008;52:1843–5.

37. Gafter-Gvili A, Fraser A, Paul M, et al. Meta-analysis: antibiotic prophylaxis reduces mortality in neutropenic patients. Ann Intern Med. 2005;142:979–95.

38. Galimand M, Courvalin P, Lambert T. Plasmid-mediated high-level resistance to aminoglycosides in Enterobacteriaceae due to 16S rRNA methylation. Antimicrob Agents Chemother. 2003;47:2565–71.

39. Girmenia C, Rossolini GM, Piciocchi A, et al. Infections by carbapenem-resistant *Klebsiella pneumoniae* in SCT recipients: a nationwide retrospective survey from Italy. Bone Marrow Transplant. 2015;50:282–8.

40. Gudiol C, Bodro M, Simonetti A, et al. Changing aetiology, clinical features, antimicrobial resistance, and outcomes of bloodstream infection in neutropenic cancer patients. Clin Microbiol Infect. 2013;19:474–9.

41. Gudiol C, Calatayud L, Garcia-Vidal C, et al. Bacteraemia due to extended-spectrum beta-lactamase-producing Escherichia coli (ESBL-EC) in cancer patients: clinical features, risk factors, molecular epidemiology and outcome. J Antimicrob Chemother. 2010;65:333–41.

42. Gutmann, Michel M, Gutmann L. Methicillin-resistant Staphylococcus aureus and vancomycin-resistant enterococci: therapeutic realities and possibilities. Lancet. 1997;349(9069):1901.

43. Ha YE, Kang C-I, Cha MK, et al. Epidemiology and clinical outcomes of bloodstream infections caused by extended-spectrum b-lactamase-producing Escherichia coli in patients with cancer. Int J Antimicrob Agents. 2013;42:403–9.

44. Haidar G, Haidar G, Alkroud A, Cheng S, Churilla TM, Churilla BM, Shields RK, Doi Y, Clancy CJ, Nguyen. Association between presence of aminoglycoside modifying enzymes and in vitro activity of gentamicin, tobramycin, amikacin and plazomicin against KPC and ESBL-producing Enterobacter spp. Antimicrob Agents Chemother. 2016;60:5208–14.

45. Hanberger. Increased mortality associated with meticillin-resistant Staphylococcus aureus (MRSA) infection in the Intensive Care Unit: results from the EPIC II study.

46. Harris PNA, Wei JY, Shen AW, et al. Carbapenems versus alternative antibiotics for the treatment of bloodstream infections caused by Enterobacter, Citrobacter or Serratia species: a systematic review with metaanalysis. J Antimicrob Chemother. 2016;71:296–306.

47. Hawkey PM. Molecular epidemiology of clinically significant antibiotic resistance genes. Br J Pharmacol. 2008;153:S406–13.

48. Hayden MK, Rezai K, Hayes RA, Lolans K, Quinn JP, Weinstein RA. Development of Daptomycin resistance in vivo in methicillin-resistant Staphylococcus aureus. J Clin Microbiol. 2005;43:5285–7. PMID:16207998.

49. Hidron AI, Schuetz AN, Nolte FS, Gould CV, Osborn MK. Daptomycin resistance in Enterococcus faecalis prosthetic valve endocarditis. J Antimicrob Chemother. 2008;61:1394–6.

50. Hindron, Hidron AI, Edwards JR, Patel J, Horan TC, Sievert DM, Pollock DA, Fridkin SK, National Healthcare Safety Network Team, Participating National Healthcare Safety Network Facilities. NHSN annual update: antimicrobial-resistant pathogens associated with healthcare-associated infections: annual summary of data reported to the National Healthcare Safety Network at the Centers for Disease Control and Prevention, 2006–2007. Infect Control Hosp Epidemiol. 2008;29(11):996.

51. Hiramatsu K. Vancomycin-resistant Staphylococcus aureus: a new model of antibiotic resistance. Lancet Infect Dis. 2001;1:147–55.

52. Hooper DC. Fluoroquinolone resistance among Gram-positive cocci.

53. Houghton JL, Green KD, Chen W, et al. The future of aminoglycosides: the end or the renaissance? ChemBioChem. 2010;11(7):880–902.

54. Howden. Evolution of multidrug resistance during Staphylococcus aureus infection involves mutation of the essential two component regulator WalKR.

55. Hyle EP, Lipworth AD, Zaoutis TE, et al. Impact of inadequate initial antimicrobial therapy on mortality in infections due to extended-spectrum beta-lactamase-producing enterobacteriaceae: variability by site of infection. Arch Intern Med. 2005;165:1375–80.

56. Jacoby GA. AmpC beta-lactamases. Clin Microbiol Rev. 2009;22:161–82.

57. Kamboj M, Chung D, Seo SK, Pamer EG, Sepkowitz KA, Jakubowski AA, Papanicolaou G. The changing epidemiology of vancomycin-resistant Enterococcus (VRE) bacteraemia in allogenic hematopoietic stem cell transplant (HSCT) recipients. Biol Blood Marrow Transplant. 2010;16:1576–81.

58. Kanafani ZA, Federspiel JJ, Fowler VG Jr. Infective endocarditis caused by daptomycin-resistant Enterococcus faecalis: a case report. Scand J Infect Dis. 2007;39:75–7.

59. Kang C-I, Chung DR, Ko KS, et al. Risk factors for infection and treatment outcome of extended-spectrum b-lactamase-producing Escherichia coli and Klebsiella pneumoniae bacteremia in patients with hematologic malignancy. Ann Hematol. 2012;91:115–21.

60. Kang C-I, Pai H, Kim S-H, et al. Cefepime and the inoculum effect in tests with Klebsiella pneumoniae producing plasmid-mediated AmpC-type beta-lactamase. J Antimicrob Chemother. 2004;54:1130–3.

61. Kara Ö, Zarakolu P, Aşçioğlu S, Etgül S, Uz B, Büyükaşik Y, Akova M. Epidemiology and emerging resistance in bacterial bloodstream infections in patients with hematologic malignancies. Infect Dis (Lond). 2015;47:686–93.

62. Kern WV, Klose K, Jellen-Ritter AS, et al. Fluoroquinolone resistance of Escherichia coli at a cancer center: epidemiologic evolution effects of discontinuing prophylactic fluoroquinolone use in neutropenic patients with leukemia. Eur J Clin Microbiol Infect Dis. 2005;24:111–8.

63. Kim S-H, Kwon J-C, Choi S-M, et al. Escherichia coli and Klebsiella pneumoniae bacteremia in patients with neutropenic fever: factors associated with extended-spectrum b-lactamase production and its impact on outcome. Ann Hematol. 2013;92:533–41.

64. Kitzis MD, Billot-Klein D, Goldstein FW, Williamson R, Tran VN, Carlet J, et al. Dissemination of the novel plasmid-mediated

beta-lactamase CTX-1, which confers resistance to broad-spectrum cephalosporins, and its inhibition by beta-lactamase inhibitors. Antimicrob Agents Chemother. 1988;32:9–14.

65. Lautenbach E, Fishman NO, Bilker WB, Castiglioni A, Metlay JP, Edelstein PH, Strom BL. Risk factors for fluoroquinolone resistance in nosocomial *Escherichia coli* and *Klebsiella pneumoniae* infections. Arch Intern Med. 2002;162:2469–77.

66. Leclercq R. Enterococci aquire new kinds of resistance. Clin Infect Dis. 1997;24(suppl 1):880–4.

67. Lee N-Y, Lee C-C, Huang W-H, et al. Cefepime therapy for monomicrobial bacteremia caused by cefepime susceptible extended-spectrum beta-lactamase-producing Enterobacteriaceae: MIC matters. Clin Infect Dis. 2013;56:488–95.

68. Lee N-Y, Lee C-C, Li C-W, et al. Cefepime therapy for monomicrobial *enterobacter cloacae* bacteremia: unfavorable outcomes in patients infected by cefepime-susceptible dose-dependent isolates. Antimicrob Agents Chemother. 2015;59:7558–63.

69. Leibovici L, Paul M, Cullen M, et al. Antibiotic prophylaxis in neutropenic patients: new evidence, practical decisions. Cancer. 2006;107:1743–51.

70. Leuthner KD, Cheung CM, Rybak MJ. Comparative activity of the new lipoglycopeptide telavancin in the presence and absence of serum against 50 glycopeptide non-susceptible staphylococci and three vancomycin-resistant *Staphylococcus aureus*. J Antimicrob Chemother. 2006;58:338–43.

71. Birmingham MC, Rayner CR, Meagher AK, Flavin SM, Batts DH, Schentag JJ. Linezolid for the treatment of multidrug-resistant, gram-positive infections: experience from a compassionate-use program. Clin Infect Dis. 2003;36(2):159–68.

72. Liscio JL, Mahoney MV, Hirsch EB. Ceftolozane/tazobactam and ceftazidime/avibactam: two novel b-lactam/b-lactamase inhibitor combination agents for the treatment of resistant Gram-negative bacterial infections. Int J Antimicrob Agents. 2015;46:266–71.

73. Liu, Liu C, Bayer A, Cosgrove SE, Daum RS, Fridkin SK, Gorwitz RJ, Kaplan SL, Karchmer AW, Levine DP, Murray BE, Rybak M J, Talan DA, Chambers HF, Infectious Diseases Society of America. Clinical practice guidelines by the infectious diseases society of America for the treatment of methicillin-resistant *Staphylococcus aureus* infections in adults and children. Clin Infect Dis. 2011;52(3):e18–55.

74. Lockhart SR, Etienne KA, Vallabhaneni S, Farooqi J, Chowdhary A, Govender NP, et al. Simultaneous emergence of multidrug-resistant Candida auris on 3 continents confirmed by whole-genome sequencing and epidemiological analyses. Clin Infect Dis. 2017;64(2):134–40.

75. Long JK, Choueiri TK, Hall GS, Avery RK, Sekeres MA. Daptomycin-resistant Enterococcus faecium in a patient with acute myeloid leukemia. Mayo Clin Proc. 2005;80:1215–6.

76. Mahajan, Mahajan SN, Shah JN, Hachem R, Tverdek F, Adachi JA, Mulanovich V, Rolston KV, Raad II, Chemaly RF. Characteristics and outcomes of methicillin-resistant *staphylococcus aureus* bloodstream infections in patients with cancer treated with vancomycin: 9-year experience at a comprehensive cancer center. Oncologist. 2012;17(10):1329–36.

77. Marcos M, Inurrieta A, Soriano A, et al. Effect of anti- ~ microbial therapy on mortality in 377 episodes of Enterobacter spp. bacteraemia. J Antimicrob Chemother. 2008;62:397–403.

78. Marquez P, Terashita D, Dassey D, et al. Population based incidence of carbapenem-resistant *Klebsiella pneumoniae* along the continuum of care, Los Angeles County. Infect Control Hosp Epidemiol. 2013;34:144–50. [49]

79. Martino R, Subira M, Altes A, et al. Effect of discontinuing prophylaxis with norfloxacin in patients with hematologic malignancies and severe neutropenia. A matched case-control study of the effect on infectious morbidity. Acta Haematol. 1998;99:206–11.

80. Marty FM, Yeh WW, Wennersten CB, Venkataraman L, Albano E, Alyea EP, Gold HS, Baden LR, Pillai SK. Emergence of a clinical daptomycin-resistant *Staphylococcus aureus* isolate during treatment of methicillin-resistant *Staphylococcus aureus* bacteremia and osteomyelitis. J Clin Microbiol. 2006;44:595–7.

81. McCarthy M, Rosengart A, Schuetz AN, Kontoyiannis DP, Walsh TJ. Mold infections of the central nervous system. N Engl J Med. 2014;371(2):150–60.

82. Metan G, Demiraslan H, Kaynar LG, et al. Factors influencing the early mortality in haematological malignancy patients with nosocomial Gram negative bacilli bacteraemia: a retrospective analysis of 154 cases. Braz J Infect Dis. 2013;17:143–9.

83. Mihu CN, Rhomberg PR, Jones RN, et al. *Escherichia coli* resistance to quinolones at a comprehensive cancer center. Diagn Microbiol Infect Dis. 2010;67:266–9.

84. Miles-Jay. Evaluation of routine pre-transplant screening for methicillin-resistant *Staphylococcus aureus* in hematopoietic cell transplant recipients.

85. Montassier E, Batard E, Gastinne T, et al. Recent changes in bacteremia in patients with cancer: a systematic review of epidemiology and antibiotic resistance. Eur J Clin Microbiol Infect Dis. 2013;32:841–50.

86. Muto CA, Pokrywka M, Shutt K, et al. A large outbreak of Clostridium difficile-associated disease with an unexpected proportion of deaths and colectomies at a teaching hospital following increased fluoroquinolone use. Infect Control Hosp Epidemiol. 2005;26:273–80. 187. Pepin J

87. Neuhauser MM, Weinstein RA, Rydman R, et al. Antibiotic resistance among gram-negative bacilli in US intensive care units: implications for fluoroquinolone use. JAMA. 2003;289:885.

88. Niu, Niu H, Yu H, Hu T, Tian G, Zhang L, Guo X, Hu H, Wang Z. The prevalence of aminoglycoside-modifying enzyme and virulence genes among enterococci with high-level aminoglycoside resistance in Inner Mongolia, China. Braz J Microbiol. 2016;47(3):691–6.

89. Oliveira AL, de Souza M, Carvalho-Dias VMH, et al. Epidemiology of bacteremia and factors associated with multi-drug-resistant Gram-negative bacteremia in hematopoietic stem cell transplant recipients. Bone Marrow Transplant. 2007;39:775–81.

90. Pagano L, Caira M, Trecarichi EM, et al. Carbapenemase-producing *Klebsiella pneumoniae* and hematologic malignancies. Emerg Infect Dis. 2014;20:1235–6.

91. Peel T, Cheng AC, Spelman T, Huysmans M, Spelman D. Differing risk factors for vancomycin-resistant and vancomcyin-sensitive enterococcal bacteraemia. Clin Microbiol Infect. 2012;18:388–94.

92. Perlin DS. Echinocandin resistance in Candida. Clin Infect Dis. 2015;61(Suppl 6):S612–7.

93. Pfaller MA, et al. Clinical breakpoints for the echinocandins and Candida revisited: integration of molecular, clinical, and microbiological data to arrive at species-specific interpretive criteria. Drug Resist Updat. 2011;14:164–76.

94. Pham CD, Iqbal N, Bolden CB, Kuykendall RJ, Harrison LH, Farley MM, et al. Role of FKS mutations in Candida glabrata: MIC values, echinocandin resistance, and multidrug resistance. Antimicrob Agents Chemother. 2014;58(8):4690–6.

95. Polk RE, Johnson CK, McClish D, et al. Predicting hospital rates of fluoroquinolone-resistant Pseudomonas aeruginosa from fluoroquinolone use in US hospitals and their surrounding communities. Clin Infect Dis. 2004;39:497.

96. Qureshi ZA, Paterson DL, Potoski BA, et al. Treatment outcome of bacteremia due to KPC-producing *Klebsiella pneumoniae*: superiority of combination antimicrobial regimens. Antimicrob Agents Chemother. 2012;56:2108–13.

97. Rangaraj G, Granwehr BP, Jiang Y, et al. Perils of quinolone exposure in cancer patients: breakthrough bacteremia with multidrug-resistant organisms. Cancer. 2010;116:967–73.

98. Reuter S, Kern WV, Sigge A, et al. Impact of fluoroquinolone prophylaxis on reduced infection-related mortality among patients with neutropenia and hematologic malignancies. Clin Infect Dis. 2005;40:1087–93.

99. Reynolds, Reynolds PE. Structure, biochemistry and mechanism of action of glycopeptide antibiotics. Eur J Clin Microbiol Infect Dis. 1989;8(11):943.

100. Saheb N, Coulombe MA, et al. Emergence of fluoroquinolones as the predominant risk factor for Clostridium difficileassociated diarrhea: a cohort study during an epidemic in Quebec. Clin Infect Dis. 2005;41:1254–60.

101. Sakoulas, Sakoulas G, Rose W, Nonejuie P, Olson J, Pogliano J, Humphries R, Nizet V. Ceftaroline restores daptomycin activity against daptomycin-nonsusceptible vancomycin-resistant Enterococcus faecium. Antimicrob Agents Chemother. 2014;58(3):1494–500. Epub 2013 Dec 23.

102. Sanchez GV, Master RN, Clark RB, et al. *Klebsiella pneumoniae* antimicrobial drug resistance, United States, 1998–2010. Emerg Infect Dis. 2013;19:133–6.

103. Satlin MJ, Jenkins SG, Walsh TJ. The global challenge of carbapenem-resistant Enterobacteriaceae in transplant recipients and patients with hematologic malignancies. Clin Infect Dis. 2014;58:1274–83.

104. Sievert DM, Rudrik JT, Patel JB, et al. Vancomycin-resistant *Staphylococcus aureus* in the United States, 2002–2006. Clin Infect Dis. 2008;46(5):668–74.

105. Skov, Skov R, et al. *Staphylococcus aureus* bacteremia: a 14-year nationwide study in hematological patients withmalignant disease or agranulocytosis. Scand J Infect Dis. 1995;27:563–8.

106. Smith CA, Baker EN. Aminoglycoside antibiotic resistance by enzymatic deactivation. Curr Drug Targets Infect Disord. 2002;2(2):143–60.

107. Snelders E, Huis In 't Veld RA, Rijs AJ, Kema GH, Melchers WJ, Verweij PE. Possible environmental origin of resistance of Aspergillus fumigatus to medical triazoles. Appl Environ Microbiol. 2009;75(12):4053–7.

108. Srinivasan A, Lopez-Ribot JL, Ramasubramanian AK. Overcoming antifungal resistance. Drug Discov Today Technol. 2014;11:65–71.

109. Tamma PD, Girdwood SCT, Gopaul R, et al. The use of cefepime for treating AmpC b-lactamase-producing Enterobacteriaceae. Clin Infect Dis. 2013;57:781–8.

110. Tamma PD, Han JH, Rock C, et al. Carbapenem therapy is associated with improved survival compared with piperacillin-tazobactam for patients with extended-spectrum b-lactamase bacteremia. Clin Infect Dis. 2015;60:1319–25.

111. Tenover, Tenover FC, Moellering RC Jr. The rationale for revising the clinical and laboratory standards institute vancomycin minimal inhibitory concentration interpretive criteria for *Staphylococcus aureus*. Clin Infect Dis. 2007;44(9):1208.

112. Thomson KS, Moland ES. Cefepime, piperacillin-tazobactam, and the inoculum effect in tests with extended-spectrum beta-lactamase-producing Enterobacteriaceae. Antimicrob Agents Chemother. 2001;45:3548–54.

113. Tillotson GS, Draghi DC, Sahm DF, et al. Susceptibility of *Staphylococcus aureus* isolated from skin and wound infections in the United States 2005–07: laboratory-based surveillance study. J Antimicrob Chemother. 2008;62:109–15.

114. Tran JH, Jacoby GA. Mechanism of plasmid-mediated quinolone resistance. Proc Natl Acad Sci U S A. 2002;99:5638–42.

115. Trecarichi EM, Pagano L, Candoni A, et al. Current epidemiology and antimicrobial resistance data for bacterial bloodstream infections in

patients with hematologic malignancies: an Italian multicentre prospective survey. Clin Microbiol Infect. 2015;21:337–43.

116. Trecarichi EM, Tumbarello M. Antimicrobial-resistant Gram-negative bacteria in febrile neutropenic patients with cancer: current epidemiology and clinical impact. Curr Opin Infect Dis. 2014;27:200–10.

117. Trias J, Nikaido H. Outer membrane protein D2 catalyzes facilitated diffusion of carbapenems and penems through the outer membrane of Pseudomonas aeruginosa. Antimicrob Agents Chemother. 1990;34:52–7.

118. Paul M, Bishara J, Yahav D, Goldberg E, Neuberger A, Ghanem-Zoubi N, Dickstein Y, Nseir W, Dan M, Leibovici L. Trimethoprim-sulfamethoxazole versus vancomycin for severe infections caused by meticillin resistant *Staphylococcus aureus*: randomised controlled trial. BMJ. 2015;350:h2219.

119. Tumbarello M, Viale P, Bassetti M, et al. Infections caused by KPC-producing *Klebsiella pneumoniae*: differences in therapy and mortality in a multicentre study–authors' response. J Antimicrob Chemother. 2015;70:2922.

120. Tumbarello M, Viale P, Viscoli C, et al. Predictors of mortality in bloodstream infections caused by *Klebsiella pneumoniae* carbapenemase-producing *K. pneumoniae*: importance of combination therapy. Clin Infect Dis. 2012;55:943–50.

121. Vydra J, Shanley RM, Geroge I, Ustun C, Smith AR, Weisdorf DJ, Young JAH. Enterococcal bacteraemia is associated with increased risk of mortality in recipients of allogenic hematopoietic stem cell transplantation. Clin Infect Dis. 2012;55:764–70.

122. Warrilow AG, Parker JE, Kelly DE, Kelly SL. Azole affinity of sterol 14α-demethylase (CYP51) enzymes from *Candida albicans* and *Homo sapiens*. Antimicrob Agents Chemother. 2013;57(3):1352–60.

123. Weinstock DM, Conlon M, Iovino C, Aubrey T, Gudiol C, Riedel E, Young JW, Kiehn TE, Zuccotti G. Colonization, bloodstream infection and mortality caused by vancomycin resistant enterococcus early after allogenic hematopoietic stem cell transplant. Biol Blood Marrow Transplant. 2007;13:615–62.

124. Werner G, Coque TM, Hammerum AM, Hope R, Hryniewicz W, Johnson A, et al. Emergence and spread of vancomycin resistance among enterococci in Europe. Euro Surveill. 2008;13(47):1–11.

125. White PL, Posso RB, Barnes RA. Analytical and clinical evaluation of the PathoNostics AsperGenius assay for detection of invasive aspergillosis and resistance to azole antifungal drugs during testing of serum samples. J Clin Microbiol. 2015;53(7):2115–21.

126. Wingard, Wingard JR, Eldjerou L, Leather H. Use of antibacterial prophylaxis in patients with chemotherapy-induced neutropenia. Curr Opin Hematol. 2012;19(1):21.

127. Wolfson JS, Hooper DC. The fluoroquinolones: structures, mechanisms of action and resistance, and spectra of activity in vitro. Antimicrob Agents Chemother. 1985;28:581–5861985.

128. Yamane K, Wachino J, Doi Y, et al. Global spread of aminoglycoside resistance genes. Emerg Infect Dis. 2005;11:951–3.

129. Yemisen M, Balkan İİ, Salihoglu A, et al. The changing epidemiology of blood stream infections and resistance in haematopoietic stem cell transplantation recipients. Turk J Haematol. 2015. [Epub ahead of print]. https://doi.org/10.4274/tjh.2014.0378.

130. Yokoyama K, Doi Y, Yamane K, et al. Acquisition of 16S rRNA methylase gene in Pseudomonas aeruginosa. Lancet. 2003;362:1888–93.

131. Zapun A, Contreras-Martel C, Vernet T. Penicillin-binding proteins and β-lactam resistance. FEMS Microbiol Rev. 2008;32:361–85.

132. Zhao Y, Nagasaki Y, Kordalewska M, Press EG, Shields RK, Nguyen MH, et al. Rapid detection of FKS-associated echinocandin resistance in Candida glabrata. Antimicrob Agents Chemother. 2016;60:6573–7.

133. Zhou Y, Yu H, Guo Q, et al. Distribution of 16S rRNA methylases among different species of gram-negative bacilli with high-level resistance to aminoglycosides. Eur J Clin Microbiol Infect Dis. 2010;29:1349–53.

Ella J. Ariza-Heredia, Firas El Chaer,
and Roy F. Chemaly

Introduction

Management of viral infections is challenging because viruses are intracellular parasites that use many of the host's own pathways to replicate and propagate, and therefore antiviral agents need to target specific viral components, for example, thymidine kinase for herpes simplex viruses, to avoid potential damage to the host cell [1]. Viral infections are common and have the potential for severe morbidity and mortality in immunocompromised patients; thus, ample knowledge of their diagnosis, management, and treatment is of utmost importance for the clinician. This chapter will provide an overview of the main antiviral agents that are used for immunocompromised patients, including patients with cancer and stem cell and solid organ transplant recipients, focusing on their clinical indications.

E. J. Ariza-Heredia · F. El Chaer · R. F. Chemaly (✉)
Department of Infectious Diseases, Infection Control
and Employee Health, The University of Texas MD
Anderson Cancer Center, Houston, TX, USA
e-mail: eariza@mdanderson.org; rfchemaly@
mdanderson.org

Antiviral Agents for *Herpesviridae*

Commonly Used Antiviral Agents

Acyclovir

Acyclovir (ACV) acts through the function of two herpesvirus enzymes: thymidine kinase and DNA polymerase. As acyclovir is a nucleoside analog (9-[2-hydroxymethyl] guanine) of guanosine, after its intracellular uptake, this drug is converted to acyclovir monophosphate by virally encoded thymidine kinase (the first involved enzyme) and subsequently converted to acyclovir triphosphate in the cell. Acyclovir triphosphate competitively inhibits viral DNA polymerase (the second involved enzyme) by acting as an analog to deoxyguanosine triphosphate (dGTP). The incorporation of acyclovir triphosphate into DNA results in premature chain termination of the viral DNA since the absence of a 3′ hydroxyl group prevents the attachment of additional nucleosides [2]. Acyclovir is active against herpes simplex virus types 1 (HSV-1) and 2 (HSV-2) and varicella-zoster virus (VZV), although it is ten times more potent against HSV-1 and -2 than VZV. Cytomegalovirus (CMV), which does not encode for thymidine kinase, is resistant to acyclovir at clinically achievable blood levels of the drug. In addition, acyclovir inhibits the replication of Epstein-Barr virus (EBV) in the lytic phase, but it has no effect on EBV infections in the latent or persistent phases [3]. Valacyclovir, which is a prodrug of acyclovir, has 55% more oral bioavailability than oral acyclovir and exactly the same mechanism of action.

Clinical Uses The US Food and Drug Administration (FDA) approved acyclovir in 1982 and valacyclovir in 1995. The FDA indications for the oral formulations include cold sores (herpes labialis), genital herpes (initial or recurrent episode), and reduction of transmission of genital herpes, as well as herpes zoster. In stem cell and solid organ transplant recipients, acyclovir has been used for prophylaxis in patients with positive IgG antibodies to HSV [4, 5]. The use of acyclovir for herpes simplex infections or eruptions in immunocompromised patients has been associated with shorter duration of virus shedding, less pain at the site of eruption, and faster scabbing and healing of the lesions, as well as prevention of recurrent HSV infections [6]. Table 16.1 describes dosing of acyclovir for its most common clinical indications.

Prophylaxis with acyclovir is recommended for patients after hematopoietic cell transplantation and is seropositive for HSV or VZV [11],

hematological malignancies who are undergoing chemotherapy with purine analogs, second-line chemotherapy or treatment containing corticosteroids, and those with CD4 counts <50 cells/mm^3 or prolonged grade III or IV neutropenia [12, 13]. In addition, prophylaxis is strongly recommended for patients receiving alemtuzumab, but not for patients receiving rituximab [12, 13].

For hematopoietic stem cell transplant (HCT) recipients, acyclovir is started immediately after transplantation for the prevention of mucocutaneous HSV reactivation. The intravenous route is preferred (5 mg/kg intravenously every 12 h, for patients with normal renal function) when significant chemotherapy-induced mucositis is present [14, 15]. Long-term prophylaxis is preferred to decrease the frequency of HSV and varicella-zoster virus (VZV) reactivation [11, 16]. Most centers continue prophylaxis up to 6 months or beyond if patients continue to require systemic immunosuppression [11]. In contrast, in solid organ transplant recipients, prophylaxis for HSV reactivation is most effective in the first 4 weeks after transplantation [5], and prophylaxis for VZV is not offered regularly. Disseminated and complicated HSV or

Table 16.1 Dosing recommendations for acyclovir* [7–10, 23]

	Mucocutaneous HSV	Genital HSV	VZV	Encephalitis	Prophylactic dose
Acyclovir oral	400 mg every 8 h or 200 mg every 4 h for 7–10 days	200 mg every 4 h or 400 mg every 8 h recurrence 400 mg every 12 h	800 mg every 4 h for 7–10 days (not recommended for immunocompromised host)	Not recommended	400 mg twice daily or 200 mg 3–5 times daily
Acyclovir IV	5 mg/kg every 8 h for 7–10 days	If severe, 5 mg/kg every 8 h for 7–10 days	10 mg/kg every 8 h (when improvement is noted, can transition to oral route)	10 mg/kg every 8 h for 2–3 weeks	
Valacyclovir oral	1000 mg every 12 h for 5 to 10 days or 2 g twice daily for 1 day	For first episode, 1000 mg every 12 h; for recurrent infection, 500 mg every 12 h for 5 to 10 days	1000 mg every 8 h for 7–10 days (may need longer treatment)	Not recommended	500 to 1000 mg daily

HSV herpes simplex virus, *VZV* varicella-zoster virus, *IV* intravenous
*For intravenous use, maintain adequate hydration prior to and during the treatment. The doses in this table are for adult patients with normal kidney function. Doses need to be adjusted in patients with renal impairment

VZV infections, including encephalitis, should be treated with high-dose intravenous acyclovir (10 mg/kg/ every 8 h, renally adjusted).

Pharmacokinetics Oral bioavailability of acyclovir is about 20–30%, decreasing with higher doses; therefore, the intravenous formulation should be used for serious infections such as HSV encephalitis and may be considered in certain cases of disseminated varicella infection [16, 17]. Excretion is predominantly renal, both by glomerular filtration and tubular secretion, and dosage modifications are required in the presence of renal insufficiency [18]. In contrast, valacyclovir has better bioavailability than oral acyclovir, with serum bioavailability of 54–70% [19].

In obese patients (e.g., BMI ≥ 30 kg/m^2), weight-based dosing should be scaled to ideal body weight rather than actual body weight to avoid an increased risk of toxicity as acyclovir is hydrophilic, is not highly bound to plasma proteins, and distributes mainly into body fluids and non-adipose tissue [20].

Adverse Effects Acyclovir is remarkably well tolerated in most patients. There are, however, several important potential adverse effects.

Acute Renal Failure Acute renal failure, produced by the precipitation of relatively insoluble acyclovir crystals in the renal tubules, is an occasional complication of intravenous therapy [7, 8]; rarely, interstitial nephritis may occur. The risk can be minimized by prior hydration (with the urine output maintained above 75 mL/h) and slow drug infusion (over a 1- to 2-h period) [21].

Neurologic Toxicities Rare reports of neurologic toxicity, particularly in patients with chronic kidney disease, include headaches, agitation, tremors, delirium, and hallucinations. Severe neurotoxicity, characterized by delirium and coma, has been described at doses as low as 800 mg twice daily in patients requiring dialysis. The potential for this complication is greater in patients treated with peritoneal dialysis, which is associated with minimal removal of acyclovir [22].

Mechanism of Resistance Concern for acyclovir resistance associated with long-term use has been raised, and reports of resistant isolates to acyclovir in HCT recipients have been published. The incidence of acyclovir-resistant HSV infections in HCT recipients has been reported as between 7% and 36% [24, 25]. Some reports suggest that acyclovir resistance may develop more frequently during short-term prophylaxis or during repeated treatment for recurrent infections than during long-term prophylaxis [26].

Three mechanisms have been shown to confer resistance to acyclovir in HSV: (1) reduced or absent thymidine kinase (the most common), (2) altered thymidine kinase activity resulting in decreased acyclovir phosphorylation, and (3) altered viral DNA polymerase with decreased affinity for acyclovir triphosphate (rare).

Other DNA Polymerase inhibitors
Penciclovir
Penciclovir is a guanosine analog that, after phosphorylation to penciclovir triphosphate, inhibits DNA polymerase, selectively inhibiting herpes viral DNA synthesis and replication. It is poorly absorbed orally, but it is available as a topical agent for local therapy of mucocutaneous herpes infections. Reported side effects of penciclovir include application site reaction, hyperesthesia, and taste changes [27].

Famciclovir
Famciclovir is a guanosine analog prodrug of penciclovir that, like penciclovir, acts through inhibition of the viral DNA polymerase after phosphorylation to penciclovir triphosphate. Famciclovir has excellent oral bioavailability and a prolonged in vitro intracellular half-life, which results in persistent antiviral activity [28, 29]. It is approved by the FDA for the treatment of herpes labialis, herpes zoster, and genital herpes, including recurrent cases [30, 31]. Famciclovir is also eliminated by the kidneys and requires renal adjustment in cases of abnormal renal function [29].

Ganciclovir

Ganciclovir (GCV, 9-[(1,3-dihydroxy-2-propoxy)methyl]guanine, or DHPG) is a synthetic analog of guanosine. It is initially phosphorylated to ganciclovir 5′-monophosphate by a viral kinase, encoded by the CMV gene *UL97*. Ganciclovir monophosphate is phosphorylated by cellular kinases in cells infected by CMV and HSV; this phosphorylation yields ganciclovir diphosphate and ganciclovir triphosphate. The triphosphorylated ganciclovir is a competitive inhibitor of dGTP, blocking its incorporation into DNA, inhibiting viral DNA polymerase, and also serving as a poor substrate for DNA chain elongation [32].

Clinical Use Due to the poor bioavailability of oral ganciclovir (<5%) [28], the most commonly used products are intravenous ganciclovir or its oral prodrug valganciclovir [33, 34]. Ganciclovir is mainly used for the management of CMV infection, but it also inhibits the replication of other herpes viruses in vitro, including HSV-1, HSV-2, EBV, VZV, and human herpes viruses 6 and 7 (HHV-6 and HHV-7), but not human herpes virus 8 (HHV-8) [1].

Intravenous ganciclovir is recommended for induction treatment of severe CMV infection, including CMV reactivation, retinitis, colitis, esophagitis, and pneumonia, in solid organ and HCT recipients [35]. Oral valganciclovir is FDA approved for the treatment of CMV retinitis in patients with acquired immunodeficiency syndrome (AIDS) and for prevention of CMV disease in kidney, heart, and kidney-pancreas transplant patients at risk for CMV disease (see below) [36].

In solid organ transplant recipients, ganciclovir and valganciclovir have been used for CMV prophylaxis, depending on the type of transplant and patient and donor CMV sero-status. High-risk patients, defined according to seropositivity of the recipient (R) and/or donor (D) for CMV antibodies (R+ or D+/R−), receive prophylaxis for 3–6 months after most solid organ transplants, except for lung transplants, where patients receive 6–12 months of posttransplant prophylaxis [5]. On the other hand, D−/R− solid organ transplant recipients receive preemptive therapy in which antiviral therapy is begun following diagnosis of CMV reactivation (described below) [37]. The good bioavailability of valganciclovir and lessen pill burden compared with oral ganciclovir make it the preferred drug for prophylaxis, even in liver transplant recipients [38, 39]. Interestingly, the implementation of these prophylaxis recommendations has shifted the peak incidence of CMV disease in solid organ transplant recipients from the first 3–6 months after transplantation, when prophylaxis is usually discontinued [40].

On the other hand, for HCT recipients, due mostly to adverse effects of ganciclovir, including bone marrow suppression [41], preemptive strategies are widely preferred as a prevention method by most transplant centers. In most institutions, CMV preemptive strategy consists of close monitoring of CMV by either antigenemia or by PCR, with therapy initiated at a certain threshold of CMV viral load; however, its success depends largely on structured standard-of-care practices and close monitoring [40, 42, 43].

Pharmacokinetics Ganciclovir is excreted, unmodified, in the urine; therefore, dosage adjustment is required in patients with impaired renal function [44, 45].

Valganciclovir has an oral bioavailability of around 60% and thus is an excellent option for the outpatient management of CMV [28, 46].

Adverse Effects Bone marrow toxicity is a frequent side effect of ganciclovir. Neutropenia in ganciclovir recipients is dose-dependent and results from the inhibition of DNA polymerase in hematopoietic progenitor cells [47]. The incidence of neutropenia defined by a neutrophil count of less than 1000/μL, associated with ganciclovir, ranges between 21% and 31% in HCT recipients [48] and around 10% in solid organ transplant patients [49]. Furthermore, thrombocytopenia and anemia have been described in 19% and 2% of patients, respectively [50]. Other more rare side effects are fever, ataxia, confusion, and elevation of liver enzymes.

Mechanisms of Resistance Ganciclovir resistance can occur in patients receiving prolonged therapy with either intravenous ganciclovir or oral valganciclovir. Depending on the transplanted organ, the incidence of ganciclovir-resistant virus in transplant recipients could vary between 5% and 10% [51].

Mutations in the *UL97*-encoded CMV phosphotransferase have been associated with resistance [13], as have alterations in *UL54*-encoded viral DNA polymerase. It has been postulated that *UL97* mutations arise first and confer moderate resistance to ganciclovir but not to other CMV-directed antivirals, such as cidofovir or foscarnet. With continued therapy, DNA polymerase mutations may subsequently appear, leading to high-level resistance to ganciclovir with cross-resistance to cidofovir and, sometimes, to foscarnet [52].

Foscarnet

Foscarnet (FCN) is a pyrophosphate analog whose mechanism of action is noncompetitive inhibition of the pyrophosphate-binding site of DNA viral polymerase, preventing the cleavage of the pyrophosphate from deoxynucleotide triphosphates and blocking DNA chain elongation. Foscarnet inhibition of viral polymerase does not require previous phosphorylation or activation by a viral kinase [53].

Clinical Use Foscarnet is usually used as second-line therapy, mainly for CMV when ganciclovir is contraindicated or not well tolerated, for acyclovir-resistant HSV, for HHV-6 viremia and/or encephalitis, and occasionally for VZV infections [53]. Its use is limited because of significant toxic effects, including renal dysfunction (see Adverse Effects, below). In our institution, because of concerns of myelosuppression that could be related to ganciclovir, foscarnet is frequently used, especially during the first few weeks after stem cell transplantation for the management of CMV infections [43].

Pharmacokinetics Foscarnet has poor oral bioavailability and is therefore administered intravenously. It is excreted solely by the kidneys. Clearance decreases with impaired renal function, and doses must be adjusted in patients with renal insufficiency. Renal toxicity can be minimized with hydration; therefore, it is recommended to use 0.5–1 L of normal saline at 0.9% with each infusion. This infusion should be used with caution in patients with impaired cardiac function. Due to its toxicity profile, foscarnet is not recommended for prophylaxis.

Adverse Effects Specific toxic effects are somewhat difficult to measure, given that foscarnet is used mainly in patients with significant underlying illnesses who are often receiving multiple medications. The most important adverse effects of foscarnet are decreased renal function, electrolyte abnormalities, and infusion-related nausea. Genital ulcerations and neurotoxicity, including seizures, have also been documented [53, 54].

Renal Toxicity Foscarnet appears to be directly toxic to renal tubular cells. Although tubular damage is probably the principal factor underlying foscarnet-induced renal dysfunction, the finding of crystals in the glomerular capillaries of three patients suggests that other mechanisms may contribute to renal injury [55]. In one case report, a patient developed crystal nephropathy and multiorgan failure after the use of foscarnet [56].

Electrolyte Abnormalities Hypocalcemia is a well-established side effect of foscarnet, possibly the result of complex formation between the drug and free calcium. Hypomagnesemia is also commonly found and may contribute to the development of both hypocalcemia and hypokalemia [53].

Genital Ulcerations Genital ulcerations have been associated with foscarnet therapy and are possibly caused by a topical toxic effect of the drug when concentrated in urine [1]. These genital lesions are reversible and potentially preventable with careful urinary hygiene [56].

Mechanism of Resistance Foscarnet resistance can result from mutations in the CMV *UL54* gene, which encodes the DNA polymerase required for viral replication. Mutations in this gene reduce antiviral affinity [57]. *UL54* mutations can emerge during therapy with foscarnet and can also emerge in the presence of prolonged ganciclovir exposure, after the development of *UL97* mutations (which confers resistance to ganciclovir but not to foscarnet) [57] (Table 16.2).

Cidofovir

Cidofovir (CDV) is a monophosphate nucleotide analog that inhibits viral synthesis after undergoing cellular phosphorylation to its diphosphate form [2]. It competitively inhibits the incorporation of deoxycytidine triphosphate into viral DNA by viral DNA polymerase. Incorporation of the drug disrupts further chain elongation. Similar to foscarnet, cidofovir does not require phosphorylation (and hence activation) by a viral kinase [59, 60].

Clinical Use The clinical importance of cidofovir relies on its activity against herpesviruses, adenovirus, and polyomavirus. Its clinical efficacy has been mainly demonstrated in HIV-positive patients with CMV retinitis where intravenous cidofovir is approved at a dosing of 5 mg/kg intravenously once weekly for 2 weeks and then every other week [2, 61]. Few case reports on cidofovir use in HCT recipients with CMV retinitis have been published, mostly in

patients with resistance to ganciclovir, with good clinical response [62, 63].

In HCT recipients, a small pilot study was done to determine the efficacy and toxicity of cidofovir as preemptive therapy for CMV. Cidofovir was given at 5 mg/kg with probenecid and hydration, weekly for a maximum of 4 weeks. Twenty patients received treatment for CMV disease (mostly pneumonia), with half of them experiencing good response to cidofovir; but adverse events, including severe vomiting, renal dysfunction, and uveitis, were common [64, 65]. Preemptive therapy has not been further studied. Cidofovir is mostly used as salvage therapy for the treatment of complicated CMV and HSV infections especially when ganciclovir- and/or foscarnet-resistant CMV is documented or suspected as cidofovir retains activity against resistant thymidine kinase-negative HSV strains and resistant CMV strains with mutations in the *UL97* gene [28, 60]. Cidofovir use is however limited by its adverse effects (see below). Other uses include therapy for adenovirus infection (with a dose of 1 mg/kg three times per week used to try to avoid nephrotoxicity) [66, 67] and BK virus infection (at doses of 0.25– to 5 mg/kg with and without oral probenecid g 3 h before and 1 g 3 h and 9 h after cidofovir administration) [68–71]. In small case series, low dose of cidofovir without probenecid achieved higher urinary concentration and reduce nephrotoxicity, representing a safe and probably efficacious option

Table 16.2 Dosing recommendations for ganciclovir and foscarnet* [58]

	HSV reactivation	CMV treatment	Maintenance therapy or prophylaxis for CMV
Ganciclovir	Not indicated	5 mg/kg IV every 12 h for 2–3 weeks	5 mg/kg IV daily is used after treatment or for prophylaxis in intestinal transplant or patients for whom the oral route is not an option (e.g., severe mucositis)
		IV therapy is preferred for organ disease	
Valganciclovir	Not indicated	900 mg oral twice daily for 2–3 weeks	900 mg oral daily
Foscarnet	40 mg/kg every 8–12 h for 10–14 days or until improvement	60 mg/kg every 8–12 h OR 90 mg/kg IV every 12 h for 2–3 weeks, followed by maintenance dosing	Between 90 and 120 mg/kg daily

For intravenous use, maintain adequate hydration prior to and during the treatment. The above doses are for adult patients with normal renal function. Dose adjustment is required in patients with renal impairment
*Recommend consultation with a clinical pharmacy specialist for dosing and monitoring
HSV herpes simplex virus, *CMV* cytomegalovirus, *IV* intravenous

[70, 71]. The use of cidofovir is most commonly once a week for 2 weeks and then two injections at 2-week interval [69]. Further studies are still needed to determine and standardized doses and frequency of cidofovir therapy for BK in HCT patients.

Pharmacokinetics Over 80% of cidofovir is excreted unchanged in the urine within 24 h of administration, with a half-life of 2.4–3.2 h; however, cidofovir diphosphate, an active metabolite, is eliminated more slowly, with first- and second-phase intracellular half-lives of 24 and 65 h, respectively. This property permits the drug to be dosed every 2 weeks. Patients should receive around a liter of normal saline (0.9%) over 1–2 h immediately preceding cidofovir and, if they can tolerate the fluid load, a second liter either during or immediately following cidofovir administration. The volume of administered normal saline (0.9%) may require modification in patients with cardiac dysfunction. Patients must also receive probenecid (2 g orally 3 h prior to cidofovir and 1 g orally 2 and 8 h following cidofovir), which may prevent damage to proximal renal tubular epithelial cells by preventing the uptake of cidofovir into these cells [1, 72, 73].

Adverse Effects The most significant toxic effect of cidofovir is renal dysfunction, which has been reported in approximately 24% of patients receiving the medication in clinical trials [74]. Renal toxicity can be reduced by co-administration with hydration with normal saline and probenecid as described above [72]. Serum creatinine and urine protein (the dipstick method is acceptable) should be checked within 48 h before each dose of cidofovir, and dose reduction or discontinuation may be required when there is evidence of renal dysfunction. This adverse event is usually reversible with discontinuation of the drug; however, a few cases of end-stage renal disease associated with the use of cidofovir in HIV-positive individuals have been reported [73]. Cidofovir has also been rarely associated with the emergence of a Fanconi-type syndrome, with proteinuria, glycosuria, and bicarbonate wasting [75].

Topical or intralesional use of cidofovir may also be associated with renal dysfunction, although this is rare; monitoring of renal function is advised [61]. The systemic absorption of cidofovir after topical application is probably higher if it is applied to non-intact skin. At MD Anderson, we evaluated the pharmacokinetics of intravesicular cidofovir in six patients; intravesicular instillation of cidofovir resulted in systemic exposure as high as 74% in some patients. Only two of six patients were able to tolerate the treatment. The primary cause of non-tolerance was lower abdominal pain, and one patient had a significant increase in serum creatinine [76].

Ophthalmic Side Effects Anterior uveitis secondary to low-dose cidofovir has been reported and is associated with renal dysfunction (creatinine clearance <30 mL/min) [77, 78].

Gastrointestinal Side Effects Nausea and vomiting are common side effects of probenecid and may be reduced by administering the drug with food and/or an antiemetic.

Rare side effects include neutropenia and rash, which could be managed with an antihistamine if appropriate [1].

Mechanism of Resistance Based on cidofovir mechanism of action, resistance to the drug is related to mutations in the viral DNA polymerase gene *UL54* [60]. A report of patients with CMV retinitis described development of reduced susceptibility to cidofovir with long-term use (mean of 17 weeks); however, there was no difference in the clinical outcome in terms of progression of retinitis [79].

Brivudin

Brivudin is a 5′-halogenated thymidine nucleoside analog that is highly active against HSV-1 and VZV. Its mechanism of action involves competitive inhibition of the viral DNA polymerase [28]. It is available in some countries, but not in the United States, for the treatment of herpes zoster and herpes simplex [80].

Other Antivirals and Investigational Drugs

Leflunomide

Leflunomide belongs to a family of drugs called malonitrilamides and is an isoxazole derivative used for the treatment of rheumatoid arthritis. Leflunomide is structurally unrelated to other immunomodulatory disease-modifying anti-rheumatic drugs. Its antiviral activity is a result of its inhibition of phosphorylation of one or more viral structural phosphoproteins, thus leading to an inhibition of the assembly of the mature infectious virion [81, 82]. As adjuvant antiviral therapy, leflunomide has been used to treat CMV infection in renal allograft recipients, patients undergoing allogeneic HCT, and patients suffering from BK virus nephropathy [83–85].

Brincidofovir

Brincidofovir (CMX001, Chimerix, Durham, NC, USA), an investigational antiviral agent, is a hexadecyloxypropyl-cidofovir with broad-spectrum activity against dsDNA viruses. The lipid conjugate of cidofovir is converted intracellularly into the active antiviral cidofovir diphosphate. The lipid conjugation results in oral bioavailability, higher intracellular concentrations of active drug, lower plasma concentrations of cidofovir, and increased antiviral potency against dsDNA viruses [86]. In a phase 2 trials, the incidence of CMV events was lower among allogeneic HCT recipients who received brincidofovir when compared with placebo (10% vs. 37%; $P = 0.002$). In December 2015, the company reported the results from the phase 3 SUPPRESS trial, in which brincidofovir did not reach its primary endpoint for the prevention of clinically significant CMV infection through week 24 after transplantation. Diarrhea was the most common adverse event in patients receiving the medication. The dose used in these two trials was 100 mg twice weekly. Neither myelosuppression [87] nor nephrotoxicity has been reported, as brincidofovir is not concentrated in the renal proximal tubules [75].

Maribavir

Maribavir (Shire, Lexington, MA, USA) is an investigational benzimidazole nucleoside that prevents viral DNA synthesis by inhibition of UL97 (CMV-encoded protein kinase). UL97 kinase is an early viral gene product involved in viral DNA elongation, DNA packaging, and egress or shedding of capsids from viral nuclei. Maribavir, unlike ganciclovir, does not require phosphorylation for antiviral activity. It is more potent than ganciclovir against CMV and is effective against ganciclovir-resistant CMV strains [88]. Maribavir showed promise in a phase 2 clinical trials and was granted "fast-track" status by the FDA, but in a phase 3 trial, it failed to meet the primary endpoint of prevention of CMV disease when the medication was initiated after engraftment. The low dose used in the trials for maribavir prophylaxis, 100 mg twice daily, has been considered in part responsible for the lack of efficacy [89, 90]. In a phase 2 trial of maribavir for refractory CMV cases, four of six patients had no detectable CMV DNAemia within 6 weeks of starting maribavir therapy. One patient developed maribavir-resistance mutations. The results of a phase 2, double-blind-dose ranging study for the treatment with maribavir of CMV resistant or refractory to ganciclovir or foscarnet in HCT or solid transplant recipients were recently presented at the American Society of Bone Marrow Transplant meeting in 2017 [91]. Maribavir up to 1200 mg twice a day was effective for treatment of CMV infection resistant or refractory to prior therapy on HCT and SOT recipients and supported the safety of maribavir administered for up to 24 weeks [91]. No nephrotoxicity or hematological toxicity has been reported to date [92].

Letermovir

Letermovir (Merck, Kenilworth, NJ, USA) is a new antiviral that is under investigation. Its mechanism of action involves the viral terminase subunit pUL56 (exclusive to virus), which is a component of the terminase complex involved in viral DNA cleavage and packaging. Because of its novel mechanism of action, letermovir is promising as a potential new treatment option for patients infected with CMV strains with *UL97* and *UL54* mutations. Initial clinical data on the use of letermovir in a patient infected with a multidrug-resistant CMV strain who had multi-organ CMV disease appear to support the in vitro data [93]. Letermovir is highly specific for human CMV, as it has no activity against other herpesviruses or any other virus. In a phase 2 trial, letermovir, when compared to placebo, was effective in reducing the incidence of CMV infection in recipients of allogeneic HCT. The higher letermovir dose used in that study was 240 mg per day, with minimal adverse events [94]. The results of the phase 3 randomized, double-blind, placebo-controlled trial of letermovir for prevention of CMV infection in adult CMV-seropositive recipients of allogeneic HCT in over 500 patients were recently reported at the American Society of Bone Marrow Transplant meeting, and letermovir prophylaxis was effective in reducing clinically significant CMV infection and was overall well tolerated [95]. Based on these findings, in November 2017 the FDA approved Letermovir for prophylaxis of CMV infection in adult CMV-seropositive recipients of an allogeneic hematopoietic stem cell transplant. https://www.accessdata.fda.gov/drugsatfda_docs/nda/2017/209939Orig1s000,209940Orig1s000Approv.pdf. Accessed April 6, 2018.

Antiviral Agents for Respiratory Viruses

Commercially Available Antiviral Agents

M2 Inhibitors Amantadine and Rimantadine

The mechanism of action of M2 inhibitors is inhibition of the ion channel function of the M2 protein of influenza A viruses; these drugs act by blocking penetration, uncoating, and assembly of the virus [96].

Clinical Use Both M2 inhibitors are effective against influenza A; however, the development of resistance and lack of effects against influenza B have limited their use, and they are no longer recommended as first-line therapy for influenza A [97].

Pharmacokinetics Amantadine has good bioavailability, 86–90% with a half-life of 17 h (longer, 29 h, in adults 60 years of age or older). It is dosed at 100 mg orally twice a day in adults younger than 60 years or daily in adults older than 60 years. Dose adjustment is required for renal impairment, and the same dosing is used for treatment and prophylaxis.

Adverse Effects The most common adverse effects are gastrointestinal symptoms, including nausea and anorexia, and central nervous systems symptoms, such as nervousness, anxiety, and difficulty concentrating [96].

Mechanisms of Resistance Due to the high incidence of resistance to M2 inhibitors, these drugs should not be used as first-line therapy or chemoprophylaxis for currently circulating influenza A viruses, in immunocompromised patients in particular [97, 98]. The mechanism of resistance to this drug class is mutations to the pore-lining residues of the ion channel, leading to the inability of amantadine and rimantadine to enter the channel in their usual way. Resistance of influenza 2009 H1N1 and H3N2 strains to the M2 inhibitors is usually recognized early during outbreaks and frequently develops over the course of treatment, particularly in immunocompromised patients [99].

Neuraminidase Inhibitors

Neuraminidase inhibitors (NAIs) interfere with the release of progeny influenza virus from infected cells, thereby preventing new rounds of replication. The main NAIs are oseltamivir, zanamivir, and peramivir. Oseltamivir is administered orally. In immunocompromised patients, increased doses of oseltamivir (150 mg twice daily, adjusted to renal function) have been evaluated compared with standard doses; however, a beneficial impact on clinical outcomes of high-dose oseltamivir has not been conclusively demonstrated [100]. Zanamivir is most commonly given in inhaled form, but intravenous zanamivir has undergone evaluation in a phase 3 trial and is available for compassionate use from its manufacturer via an FDA emergent investigational new drug application in the United States [101] and the compassionate use program in Europe [102]. Peramivir is available in Japan and South Korea and was recently approved in the United States. It is active against influenza A and B and is indicated for the treatment of influenza infection in adults. Peramivir is the first NAI that is FDA approved for intravenous use and is administered as a single intravenous dose; however, longer duration may be considered for severe disease [86]. It should be considered for patients who are unable to tolerate oral or enteric administration of drugs. However, further studies are needed to determine the efficacy and safety of peramivir in immunocompromised patients [103].

Clinical Use Zanamivir, oseltamivir, and peramivir have activity against influenza A and B. For optimal effect, therapy should be initiated as close to the onset of symptoms as possible. Initiating therapy during the first 48 h of onset of symptoms is recommended as it decreases complications, including intensive care unit (ICU) admission [101]; prompt initiation of therapy, preferably within 24–48 h of onset of symptoms, is essential to prevent complications in patients with cancer, including HCT recipients [104]. However, in immunocompromised patients, including patients with hematological malignancies and transplant recipients, even late initiation has been associated with improved outcomes [101, 105]. Furthermore, prophylaxis for 10 days is recommended for immunocompromised patients in close contact with influenza.

Mechanism of Resistance Resistance to NAIs among the influenza viruses is an emerging problem of serious epidemiological and clinical implications. A specific mutation in the seasonal influenza A/H1N1 virus strains, H275Y (histidine-to-tyrosine substitution in the neuraminidase), has been reported worldwide [106–108], including in immunocompromised patients

[109, 110]. Of note, this specific mutation (H275Y) confers resistance to oseltamivir and peramivir as well [111, 112]. A recent meta-analysis including 19 studies reported a pooled incidence rate of 2.6% for oseltamivir resistance [113]. However, higher rates of resistance (up to 68%) were found in Europe for influenza A/H1N1 related to the H275Y mutation in the neuraminidase during the 2007–2008 winter season [114]. Furthermore, although rare, some instances of oseltamivir-resistant H3N2 strains have been detected worldwide [96].

The treatment of choice for oseltamivir-resistant influenza with the H275Y mutation is zanamivir, and a few reports of good outcomes with the use of zanamivir in HCT recipients can be found in the literature [115, 116]. Nonetheless, it is important to note that zanamivir resistance has also been described, including nine strains with a mutation in the neuraminidase gene of a substitution of glutamine for lysine at position 136 (Q136K), and the presence of resistance was not associated with exposure to zanamivir [117]. Consequently, suboptimal clinical response within 3–5 days of antiviral therapy initiation and/or worsening infection despite ongoing therapy in patients with influenza infection should raise suspicion of an oseltamivir-resistant strain and consideration for resistance testing as well as change of therapy to zanamivir with or without rimantadine [118, 119].

Adverse Effects Oseltamivir is administered orally, and its most common side effects are gastrointestinal (mainly nausea, so it is better tolerated with food), behavioral disturbance, and delirium.

Zanamivir, because it is administered by inhalation, is not well tolerated in patients with chronic obstructive pulmonary disease and asthma (i.e., underlying airway disease).

Peramivir, administered intravenously, has also been associated with neurological side effects (including delirium and behavioral disturbance), as well as neutropenia and elevation of creatinine kinase and liver function test results [96].

Ribavirin

Ribavirin is a nucleoside analog that resembles guanosine. As a monophosphate, ribavirin inhibits dehydrogenase enzyme, which is essential for the synthesis of guanosine triphosphate, and results in a drop of the cellular deposits of guanidine necessary for viral growth. It also inhibits mRNA, affecting the production of viral proteins.

Clinical Use Ribavirin is active against respiratory syncytial virus (RSV), among other respiratory viruses in vitro including human metapneumovirus [120] and parainfluenza [121] . The only FDA-approved indication for aerosolized ribavirin is the treatment of RSV infection in hospitalized high-risk infants and young children [122, 123].

As infections due to RSV are a significant cause of morbidity and mortality in HCT recipients, ribavirin-based antiviral therapy has been used on this population for treatment of lower tract respiratory infection and high-risk patients at the upper respiratory tract infection stage [124]. Ribavirin is not FDA-approved for this indication. Risk factors for progression to lower tract respiratory infection have been identified from multiple studies and include infection during pre-engraftment or within 30 days of the conditioning regimen, lymphopenia, age older than 40 years, low lymphocyte and neutrophil counts, as well as graft-versus-host disease and/or corticosteroid usage [124, 125]. At MD Anderson Cancer Center, an immunodeficiency scoring index has been developed with the aim of stratifying patients into low, moderate, or high risk for worse outcomes and thereby determining the need for ribavirin-based therapy, and this scoring index is systematically used at our institution for HCT recipients [126].

The effect of aerosolized ribavirin for the treatment of RSV in the HCT setting was evaluated in a systematic review by Chemaly et al., concluding that among patients whose infection progressed to lower tract respiratory infection, those treated with aerosolized ribavirin and an immunomodulator (either palivizumab or intravenous immunoglobulins) had a lower mortality rate (24%) than those treated with aerosolized ribavirin alone (50%) or with intravenous or oral ribavirin with or without an immunomodulator (54%; $P < 0.001$) [125].

Whether these benefits are clinically relevant and cost-effective remains a subject of continued controversy, especially recently with the major price increase of aerosolized ribavirin. As an alternative, several studies have evaluated the use of oral ribavirin instead [127]. Khanna et al. in 2004 reported that oral ribavirin had a good safety profile in 34 patients, but could not draw a strong conclusion in terms of its efficacy [128]. Furthermore, a recent study by the Mayo Clinic concluded that oral ribavirin therapy might not improve clinical outcomes in hematologic malignancies [129]. Thus, the effect of oral ribavirin on RSV infection, optimal dosing and length of therapy, and the patient population who may benefit from it require further study. For intravenous formulation of ribavirin, a few case series have been published with good results; however, further trials are needed [130, 131]. The recent NCCN guidelines acknowledge the lack of standard for the treatment of RSV infection and designated the oral or aerosolized route of ribavirin as category 3 [132].

Pharmacokinetics For the oral formulation, the dose commonly used at least at our center is between 10 and 20 mg/kg/day divided into three doses. The dosing has to be renally adjusted [125, 133].

Aerosolized ribavirin can be administered using two different schedules. Standard therapy consists of 6 g of the drug administered continuously with a small-particle aerosol generator over 12–18 h daily, for 3–7 days. Particles of 1–2 μm in diameter are generated and are small enough to reach the lower airways. Alternatively, another schedule of 6 g administered over 2–3 h every 8 h has been used and is probably preferred because it was shown to be equally effective as the standard therapy but may reduce environmental contamination and allows more patient-care time [134, 135].

Adverse Events For the aerosolized formulation, the most common side effects are cough and bronchospasm. Other reported side effects are eye redness; blurred vision; chest pain or discomfort; decreased pulmonary function; bluish color of fingernails, lips, skin, palms, or nail beds; confusion; dizziness; or faintness. Ribavirin has demonstrated significant teratogenic and/or embryocidal potential in all animal species. The National Institute of Occupational Safety and Health recommends avoiding unnecessary occupational exposure to such drugs wherever possible. Hospitals are encouraged to conduct training programs to minimize potential occupational exposure to aerosolized ribavirin. Health-care workers who are pregnant should consider avoiding direct care of patients receiving this drug.

For the oral and IV formulations of ribavirin, the main side effects are hemolytic anemia, which may require dose reduction or discontinuation of the medication, leukopenia, and hypocalcemia.

Ribavirin is contraindicated in pregnant women, and a negative pregnancy test should precede its use in women of childbearing age. Given the long half-life of ribavirin, it is also recommended that women who receive ribavirin and the female partners of men who receive ribavirin avoid pregnancy for 6 months after completion of treatment.

New Investigational Drugs

DAS181

DAS181 (Ansun BioPharma, Inc., San Diego, CA) is a recombinant fusion protein containing a sialidase catalytic domain that cleaves sialic acid receptors that are recognized by human and influenza strains, and a respiratory epithelium anchoring domain amphiregulin, which prolongs DAS181 retention on epithelial surfaces. This mechanism of action differs from that of neuraminidase inhibitors that prevent the virus from binding to and cleaving this receptor [136]. DAS 181 is administered through inhalation and has shown preclinical activity against numerous strains of influenza and parainfluenza viruses [137]. Parainfluenza and influenza viral shedding are reduced by the compound, and in phase 1 clinical trials, DAS181 was well tolerated for up

to 7 days when 20 mg was administered daily for 5–7 days [138]. A phase 2 trial and an open-label trial in immunocompromised patients are currently under way [4].

Clinical Use Although not FDA approved, DAS181 has been studied in influenza and parainfluenza infections. Case reports have been published about its use in immunocompromised hosts with good results [139].

Adverse Effects Administration of DAS 181 for over 5 days was associated with the drug being absorbed and inducing antibodies that can precipitate respiratory symptoms, hypersensitivity, pneumonitis, and decreases in FEV1 [138]. Thrombocytopenia and liver test abnormalities have also been associated with DAS181 administration [140].

GS-5806

GS-5806 (Gilead Science, Foster City, CA, USA) is an oral small-molecule antiviral fusion inhibitor being evaluated for the treatment of RSV. GS-5806 is believed to block RSV replication by inhibiting RSV F-mediated fusion of RSV RNA. The results of a phase 2a trial in healthy adult volunteers infected with RSV showed that the medication achieved its primary and secondary endpoints of lower viral load and better symptom-diary scores when compared to placebo [141].

Favipiravir

Favipiravir (T705, Toyama Chemical, Tokyo, Japan) is an investigational antiviral drug that functions as a nucleotide analog and inhibitor of the viral RNA polymerase of influenza types A, B, and C, including oseltamivir-resistant strains [96]. Synergy with oseltamivir has been demonstrated in preclinical models [142, 143], and favipiravir is currently undergoing phase 3 clinical trials in the United States, Europe, and Latin America.

Laninamivir

Laninamivir (CS-8958; Biota pharma, Alpharetta, GA, USA) is a long-acting neuraminidase inhibitor administered via a dry-powder inhaler and was as effective as oseltamivir in a large double-blinded randomized study for what kind of infection. The drug is potentially effective against oseltamivir-resistant influenza A virus and is currently available in Japan [96].

Antivirals for Hepatitis B and C

Antiviral Agents for Hepatitis B

The morbidity and mortality in patients with chronic hepatitis B who have immune suppression are high; therefore, it is recommended that all such patients (including those undergoing chemotherapy for hematological or oncological malignancies, solid organ transplant recipients, and bone marrow or stem cell recipients) have their hepatitis B virus (HBV) status assessed by testing for serum hepatitis B surface antigen (HBsAg) and hepatitis B core (HBc) antibodies. The risk of reactivation in HBsAg-positive patients undergoing chemotherapy for hematological malignancies is between 33% and 67%. This risk is increased significantly in regimens containing high doses of steroids and/or rituximab [144, 145].

Therapy is indicated for patients with active hepatitis, and prophylaxis is indicated for HBsAg positive. For patients that are anti-HBc antibody carriers, especially if they are undergoing immunosuppressive therapies including stem cell transplant and myelosuppressive chemotherapy, prophylaxis with antivirals is the preferred option. For patients with hematological malignancies, autoimmune diseases, solid tumors, or HIV and for HCT recipients, therapy should be limited to the periods of immunosuppression and subsequent immune-reconstitution. Individuals with HBV anti-core antibodies not undergoing prophylaxis should be closely monitored (i.e., monthly and/or when evidence of new transaminitis) with HBV DNA by PCR in blood and for HBsAg with the aim of starting antiviral therapy if reactivation occurs [145]. Antiviral agents approved for the treatment of chronic hepatitis B include entecavir, lamivudine, tenofovir, and adefovir.

As complete eradication of hepatitis B virus is an exceedingly rare, patient with chronic hepatitis B infection who undergo solid organ or hematopoietic cell transplantation should be evaluated by a liver specialist to determine the long-term need for antiviral therapy (ref).

Entecavir

Entecavir, a nucleoside analog of guanosine, inhibits reverse transcriptase and incorporates into viral DNA (nucleoside reverse transcriptase inhibitor). The dose of entecavir varies if it is used for nucleoside-naïve patients (0.5 mg orally once daily) or if the patient is nucleoside refractory or has decompensated liver disease (1 mg orally once daily) [28]. Entecavir has a higher barrier to resistance than lamivudine and requires at least three mutations for phenotypic resistance. The rate of resistance in nucleoside-naive patients is very low (less than 1% after 5 years); however, patients with preexisting mutations (i.e., rtM204V/I) have a higher rate of entecavir resistance (up to 51% after 5 years) [28, 146].

Adverse effects of entecavir include headache, fatigue, nausea, and diarrhea; however, more complicated events such as lactic acidosis have been reported in patients with renal dysfunction.

Lamivudine

Lamivudine is a nucleoside analog of cytosine, which is phosphorylated into lamivudine triphosphate (active metabolite), and is then integrated into the viral DNA by a HBV polymerase, causing DNA chain termination [28]. Lamivudine has the lowest barrier to resistance, which develops with one mutation (rtM204V). After 4 years of lamivudine monotherapy, rtM204V/I develops in up to 70% of patients [28, 147]. Lamivudine is excreted renally, requiring dose adjustment for patients with creatinine clearance <50 mL/min.

Adverse events for lamivudine include hepatic steatosis, lactic acidosis, and hepatic flares after discontinuation of drug.

Acyclic Diphosphonates

The three drugs in this class are adefovir dipivoxil (adefovir), tenofovir disoproxil fumarate (TDF), and the new approved prodrug tenofovir alafenamide (TAF) [148]. They are analogs of adenosine monophosphate that undergo intracellular phosphorylation to their active metabolite, which inhibits the HBV polymerase competitively with deoxyadenosine 5-triphosphate, resulting in DNA chain termination [28]. TDF is the most potent antiviral for the treatment of hepatitis B and is the preferred agent in cases of lamivudine resistant where entecavir mutations are unknown [149]. TAF has not been studied in HCT or solid organ transplant recipients yet; however, in two phase 3 studies, once daily 25 mg of TAF was non-inferior to TDF in treatment naïve and experienced patients with chronic hepatitis B infection. Adefovir is the least potent agent against hepatitis B.

The major adverse effect of this class of drugs is nephrotoxicity. When compared to TDF, TAF has shown to be associated with less renal toxicities, which makes it a safer option.

Antiviral Agents for Hepatitis C

The treatment of hepatitis C has evolved rapidly in recent years with new regimens; the previous standard therapy (peginterferon-α in combination with ribavirin) has been replaced with the use of direct-acting antiviral agents (DAAs) and interferon-free regimens. Few studies have been carried out in immunocompromised patients. The review of new hepatitis C antiviral agents is beyond the scope of this chapter, and it has grown exponentially over the last few years (Table 16.3) [150–152]. Choice of regimen is based on genotype, study results on optimal efficacy, favorable tolerability and toxicity profiles, and duration. A recent publication reviews the clinical perspective of hepatitis C burden in oncological patients and presents a great outline of antiviral treatment, drug-drug interactions, and side effects [153]. It is important to remember initial evaluation for hepatitis B coinfection and monitoring for hepatitis B reactivation on those patients with coinfection that are not on hepatitis B therapy. Trials in patients before and after liver transplantation are underway [154]. Guidelines for the diagnosis and management of HCV are updated on a continuous basis, as new medications are

Table 16.3 Direct antiviral (DAA) treatment – medication class

NS3/NS4A (protease inhibitors)
Hepatitis C NS3 protease is a nonstructural protein responsible for polyprotein processing of viral replication proteins, such as grazoprevir (combined with elbasvir [NS5A] – Zepatier, Merck, New Jersey, USA)
NS5A polymerase inhibitors
The nonstructural (NS) 5A protein controls phosphorylation/hyperphosphorylation and plays a vital role in HCV viral replication. NS5A inhibitors limit viral replication such as ledipasvir (combined with sofosbuvir – Harvoni, Gilead Sciences, Inc., Foster City, CA, USA), velpatasvir (combined with sofosbuvir – Epclusa, Gilead Sciences, Inc., Foster City, CA, USA)
NS5B polymerase inhibitors
Nonstructural protein 5B RNA-dependent RNA polymerase synthesizes the HCV RNA template directly. NS5B inhibitors terminate viral replication; such as sofosbuvir (Sovaldi, Gilead Sciences, Inc., Foster City, CA, USA)

validated in clinical trials, and can be accessed at www.hcvguidelines.org. Limited data are available for treatment of HCV infection in HCT recipients; recommendations for screening, follow-up, and management of hepatitis C in HCT and solid organ recipients have been published [155, 156].

Conclusions and Future Perspectives

Viral infections continue to be an important cause of morbidity and mortality in immunocompromised patients. In-depth understanding of the indications for prophylaxis and treatment of these viral infections is of utmost importance for clinicians caring for immunocompromised patients.

The testing of new antiviral agents in clinical trials continues to expand. We are currently witnessing the rapid development of new drugs for hepatitis C virus and at a lower-scale for CMV and respiratory viruses. Due to the compromised status of the host and risk for invasive viral infections, in addition to prolonged exposure to antiviral agents in many instances, development of viral resistance may become problematic in these patients. Further research is needed for the development of new antivirals that improve outcomes and combat resistance. Finally, evaluating novel strategies including monoclonal antibodies, viral-specific T-cell infusions, and strategies focusing on attacking viral reservoirs for latent viruses such as HPV and EBV – similar to the "kick-and-kill strategies" that have been investigated in HIV – may be on the frontier of the antiviral treatment for immunocompromised patients at high risk for opportunistic viral infections.

References

1. De Clercq E. Antiviral drugs in current clinical use. J Clin Virol: Off Publ Pan Am Soc Clin Virol. 2004;30:115–33.
2. De Clercq E. Therapeutic potential of cidofovir (hpmpc, vistide) for the treatment of DNA virus (i.e. Herpes-, papova-, pox- and adenovirus) infections. Verh – K Acad Geneeskd Belg. 1996;58:19–47. discussion -9.
3. De Clercq E, Andrei G, Snoeck R, De Bolle L, Naesens L, Degreve B, et al. Acyclic/carbocyclic guanosine analogues as anti-herpesvirus agents. Nucleosides Nucleotides Nucleic Acids. 2001;20:271–85.
4. Saral R, Burns WH, Laskin OL, Santos GW, Lietman PS. Acyclovir prophylaxis of herpes-simplex-virus infections. N Engl J Med. 1981;305:63–7.
5. Slifkin M, Doron S, Snydman DR. Viral prophylaxis in organ transplant patients. Drugs. 2004;64:2763–92.
6. Engelhard D, Morag A, Or R, Naparstek E, Cividalli G, Ruchlemer R, et al. Prevention of herpes simplex virus (hsv) infection in recipients of hla-matched t-lymphocyte-depleted bone marrow allografts. Isr J Med Sci. 1988;24:145–50.
7. Wald A, Carrell D, Remington M, Kexel E, Zeh J, Corey L. Two-day regimen of acyclovir for treatment of recurrent genital herpes simplex virus type 2 infection. Clin Infect Dis: Off Publ Infect Dis Soc Am. 2002;34:944–8.
8. Spruance SL, Tyring SK, DeGregorio B, Miller C, Beutner K. A large-scale, placebo-controlled, dose-ranging trial of peroral valaciclovir for episodic treatment of recurrent herpes genitalis. Valaciclovir hsv study group. Arch Intern Med. 1996;156:1729–35.
9. Wald A, Corey L, Cone R, Hobson A, Davis G, Zeh J. Frequent genital herpes simplex virus 2 shedding in immunocompetent women. Effect of acyclovir treatment. J Clin Invest. 1997;99:1092–7.
10. Tyler KL. Herpes simplex virus infections of the central nervous system: encephalitis and meningitis, including Mollaret's. Herpes: J IHMF. 2004;11(Suppl 2):57A–64A.
11. Tomblyn M, Chiller T, Einsele H, Gress R, Sepkowitz K, Storek J, et al. Guidelines for preventing infectious complications among hematopoietic cell transplantation recipients: a global perspective. Biol Blood Marrow Transplant: J Am Soc Blood Marrow Transplant. 2009;15:1143–238.
12. Bow EJ. Infection risk and cancer chemotherapy: the impact of the chemotherapeutic regimen in patients with lymphoma and solid tissue malignancies. J Antimicrob Chemother. 1998;41(Suppl D):1–5.
13. Sandherr M, Einsele H, Hebart H, Kahl C, Kern W, Kiehl M, et al. Antiviral prophylaxis in patients with haematological malignancies and solid tumours: guidelines of the Infectious Diseases Working Party (agiho) of the German Society for Hematology and Oncology (dgho). Ann Oncol: Off J Eur Soc Med Oncol/ESMO. 2006;17:1051–9.
14. Gluckman E, Lotsberg J, Devergie A, Zhao XM, Melo R, Gomez-Morales M, et al. Oral acyclovir prophylactic treatment of herpes simplex infection after bone marrow transplantation. J Antimicrob Chemother. 1983;12(Suppl B):161–7.
15. Shepp DH, Dandliker PS, Flournoy N, Meyers JD. Sequential intravenous and twice-daily oral acyclovir for extended prophylaxis of herpes simplex virus infection in marrow transplant patients. Transplantation. 1987;43:654–8.
16. Gnann JW Jr, Barton NH, Whitley RJ. Acyclovir: mechanism of action, pharmacokinetics, safety and clinical applications. Pharmacotherapy. 1983;3:275–83.
17. Brigden D, Bye A, Fowle AS, Rogers H. Human pharmacokinetics of acyclovir (an antiviral agent) following rapid intravenous injection. J Antimicrob Chemother. 1981;7:399–404.
18. de Miranda P, Blum MR. Pharmacokinetics of acyclovir after intravenous and oral administration. J Antimicrob Chemother. 1983;12(Suppl B):29–37.
19. Bras AP, Sitar DS, Aoki FY. Comparative bioavailability of acyclovir from oral valacyclovir and acyclovir in patients treated for recurrent genital herpes simplex virus infection. Can J Clin Pharmacol: J Can Pharmacol Clin. 2001;8:207–11.
20. Wurtz R, Itokazu G, Rodvold K. Antimicrobial dosing in obese patients. Clin Infect Dis: Off Publ Infect Dis Soc Am. 1997;25:112–8.
21. Sawyer MH, Webb DE, Balow JE. Straus SE acyclovir-induced renal failure. Clinical course and histology. Am J Med. 1988;84:1067–71.
22. Adair JC, Gold M, Bond RE. Acyclovir neurotoxicity: clinical experience and review of the literature. South Med J. 1994;87:1227–31.
23. Valencia I, Miles DK, Melvin J, Khurana D, Kothare S, Hardison H, et al. Relapse of herpes encephalitis after acyclovir therapy: report of two new cases and review of the literature. Neuropediatrics. 2004;35:371–6.
24. Darville JM, Ley BE, Roome AP, Foot AB. Acyclovir-resistant herpes simplex virus infections in a bone marrow transplant population. Bone Marrow Transplant. 1998;22:587–9.

25. Langston AA, Redei I, Caliendo AM, Somani J, Hutcherson D, Lonial S, et al. Development of drug-resistant herpes simplex virus infection after haploidentical hematopoietic progenitor cell transplantation. Blood. 2002;99:1085–8.

26. Wade JC, Newton B, McLaren C, Flournoy N, Keeney RE, Meyers JD. Intravenous acyclovir to treat mucocutaneous herpes simplex virus infection after marrow transplantation: a double-blind trial. Ann Intern Med. 1982;96:265–9.

27. Schmid-Wendtner MH, Korting HC. Penciclovir cream – improved topical treatment for herpes simplex infections. Skin Pharmacol Physiol. 2004;17:214–8.

28. Razonable RR. Antiviral drugs for viruses other than human immunodeficiency virus. Mayo Clin Proc. 2011;86:1009–26.

29. Crumpacker C. The pharmacological profile of famciclovir. Semin Dermatol. 1996;15:14–26.

30. Chakrabarty A, Tyring SK, Beutner K, Rauser M. Recent clinical experience with famciclovir – a "third generation" nucleoside prodrug. Antivir Chem Chemother. 2004;15:251–3.

31. Sacks SL. Famciclovir suppression of asymptomatic and symptomatic recurrent anogenital herpes simplex virus shedding in women: a randomized, double-blind, double-dummy, placebo-controlled, parallel-group, single-center trial. J Infect Dis. 2004;189:1341–7.

32. Faulds D, Heel RC. Ganciclovir. A review of its antiviral activity, pharmacokinetic properties and therapeutic efficacy in cytomegalovirus infections. Drugs. 1990;39:597–638.

33. Scott JC, Partovi N, Ensom MH. Ganciclovir in solid organ transplant recipients: is there a role for clinical pharmacokinetic monitoring? Ther Drug Monit. 2004;26:68–77.

34. Sommadossi JP, Bevan R, Ling T, Lee F, Mastre B, Chaplin MD, et al. Clinical pharmacokinetics of ganciclovir in patients with normal and impaired renal function. Rev Infect Dis. 1988;10(Suppl 3):S507–14.

35. Caldes A, Gil-Vernet S, Armendariz Y, Colom H, Pou L, Niubo J, et al. Sequential treatment of cytomegalovirus infection or disease with a short course of intravenous ganciclovir followed by oral valganciclovir: efficacy, safety, and pharmacokinetics. Transplant Infect Dis: Off J Transplant Soc. 2010;12:204–12.

36. FDA USFaDA. Valacyclovir. Label and approval history. 2015. http://www.accessdata.fda.gov/scripts/cder/drugsatfda/index.cfm?fuseaction=Search.Label_ApprovalHistory#apphistcited. 28 Mar 2016.

37. Razonable RR, Humar A. Practice ASTIDCo Cytomegalovirus in solid organ transplantation. Am J Transplant: Off J Am Soc Transplant Am Soc Transplant Surg. 2013;13(Suppl 4):93–106.

38. Paya C, Humar A, Dominguez E, Washburn K, Blumberg E, Alexander B, et al. Efficacy and safety of valganciclovir vs. oral ganciclovir for prevention of cytomegalovirus disease in solid organ transplant recipients. Am J Transplant: Off J Am Soc Transplant Am Soc Transplant Surg. 2004;4:611–20.

39. Kalil AC, Levitsky J, Lyden E, Stoner J, Freifeld AG. Meta-analysis: the efficacy of strategies to prevent organ disease by cytomegalovirus in solid organ transplant recipients. Ann Intern Med. 2005;143:870–80.

40. Small LN, Lau J, Snydman DR. Preventing post-organ transplantation cytomegalovirus disease with ganciclovir: a meta-analysis comparing prophylactic and preemptive therapies. Clin Infect Dis: Off Publ Infect Dis Soc Am. 2006;43:869–80.

41. Nichols WG, Corey L, Gooley T, Davis C, Boeckh M. High risk of death due to bacterial and fungal infection among cytomegalovirus (cmv)-seronegative recipients of stem cell transplants from seropositive donors: evidence for indirect effects of primary cmv infection. J Infect Dis. 2002;185:273–82.

42. Ljungman P, Hakki M, Boeckh M. Cytomegalovirus in hematopoietic stem cell transplant recipients. Hematol Oncol Clin North Am. 2011;25:151–69.

43. Ariza-Heredia EJ, Nesher L, Chemaly RF. Cytomegalovirus diseases after hematopoietic stem cell transplantation: a mini-review. Cancer Lett. 2014;342:1–8.

44. Lake KD, Fletcher CV, Love KR, Brown DC, Joyce LD, Pritzker MR. Ganciclovir pharmacokinetics during renal impairment. Antimicrob Agents Chemother. 1988;32:1899–900.

45. Perrottet N, Decosterd LA, Meylan P, Pascual M, Biollaz J, Buclin T. Valganciclovir in adult solid organ transplant recipients: pharmacokinetic and pharmacodynamic characteristics and clinical interpretation of plasma concentration measurements. Clin Pharmacokinet. 2009;48:399–418.

46. Brown F, Banken L, Saywell K, Arum I. Pharmacokinetics of valganciclovir and ganciclovir following multiple oral dosages of valganciclovir in hiv- and cmv-seropositive volunteers. Clin Pharmacokinet. 1999;37:167–76.

47. Sommadossi JP, Carlisle R. Toxicity of 3′-azido-3′-deoxythymidine and 9-(1,3-dihydroxy-2-propoxymethyl)guanine for normal human hematopoietic progenitor cells in vitro. Antimicrob Agents Chemother. 1987;31:452–4.

48. Salzberger B, Bowden RA, Hackman RC, Davis C, Boeckh M. Neutropenia in allogeneic marrow transplant recipients receiving ganciclovir for prevention of cytomegalovirus disease: risk factors and outcome. Blood. 1997;90:2502–8.

49. Merigan TC, Renlund DG, Keay S, Bristow MR, Starnes V, O'Connell JB, et al. A controlled trial of ganciclovir to prevent cytomegalovirus disease after heart transplantation. N Engl J Med. 1992;326:1182–6.

50. Reines ED, Gross PA. Antiviral agents. Med Clin North Am. 1988;72:691–715.

51. Lurain NS, Chou S. Antiviral drug resistance of human cytomegalovirus. Clin Microbiol Rev. 2010;23:689–712.

52. Drew WL, Miner R, Saleh E. Antiviral susceptibility testing of cytomegalovirus: criteria for detecting resistance to antivirals. Clin Diagn Virol. 1993;1:179–85.

53. Wagstaff AJ, Bryson HM. Foscarnet. A reappraisal of its antiviral activity, pharmacokinetic properties and therapeutic use in immunocompromised patients with viral infections. Drugs. 1994;48:199–226.

54. Deray G, Martinez F, Katlama C, Levaltier B, Beaufils H, Danis M, et al. Foscarnet nephrotoxicity: mechanism, incidence and prevention. Am J Nephrol. 1989;9:316–21.

55. Trifillis AL, Cui X, Drusano GL. Use of human renal proximal tubule cell cultures for studying foscarnet-induced nephrotoxicity in vitro. Antimicrob Agents Chemother. 1993;37:2496–9.

56. Torres T, Fernandes I, Sanches M, Selores M. Foscarnet-induced penile ulceration. Acta Dermatovenerol Alpina Pannonica Adriat. 2011;20:39–40.

57. Product Information. FOSCAVIR(R) IV injection, foscarnet sodium IV injection. Lake Forest: AstraZeneca; 2005.

58. Centers for Disease Control and Prevention, National Institutes of Health, HIV Medicine Association of the Infectious Diseases Society of America, et al. Guidelines for Prevention and Treatment of Opportunistic Infections in HIV-Infected Adults and Adolescents: Recommendations from the CDC, the National Institutes of Health, and the HIV Medicine Association of the Infectious Diseases Society of America. MMWR Recomm Rep. 2009;58(RR4):1–207.

59. Lea AP, Bryson HM. Cidofovir. Drugs. 1996;52:225–30. discussion 31.

60. Rodriguez MZK. Cidofovir: an overview. 2015. http://www.uptodate.com/contents/cidofovir-an-ove rview?source=machineLearning&search=cidofovir &selectedTitle=5%7E60&sectionRank=1&anchor= H8#H2. Accessed 13 Mar 2016.

61. Safrin S, Cherrington J, Jaffe HS. Cidofovir. Review of current and potential clinical uses. Adv Exp Med Biol. 1999;458:111–20.

62. Crippa F, Corey L, Chuang EL, Sale G, Boeckh M. Virological, clinical, and ophthalmologic features of cytomegalovirus retinitis after hematopoietic stem cell transplantation. Clin Infect Dis: Off Publ Infect Dis Soc Am. 2001;32:214–9.

63. Hubacek P, Keslova P, Formankova R, Pochop P, Cinek O, Zajac M, et al. Cytomegalovirus encephalitis/retinitis in allogeneic haematopoietic stem cell transplant recipient treated successfully with combination of cidofovir and foscarnet. Pediatr Transplant. 2009;13:919–22.

64. Chakrabarti S, Collingham KE, Osman H, Fegan CD, Milligan DW. Cidofovir as primary pre-emptive therapy for post-transplant cytomegalovirus infections. Bone Marrow Transplant. 2001;28:879–81.

65. Ljungman P, Deliliers GL, Platzbecker U, Matthes-Martin S, Bacigalupo A, Einsele H, et al. Cidofovir for cytomegalovirus infection and disease in allogeneic stem cell transplant recipients. The infectious diseases working party of the European group for blood and marrow transplantation. Blood. 2001;97:388–92.

66. Ljungman P, Ribaud P, Eyrich M, Matthes-Martin S, Einsele H, Bleakley M, et al. Cidofovir for adenovirus infections after allogeneic hematopoietic stem cell transplantation: a survey by the infectious diseases working party of the European group for blood and marrow transplantation. Bone Marrow Transplant. 2003;31:481–6.

67. Hoffman JA, Shah AJ, Ross LA, Kapoor N. Adenoviral infections and a prospective trial of cidofovir in pediatric hematopoietic stem cell transplantation. Biol Blood Marrow Transplant: J Am Soc Blood Marrow Transplant. 2001;7:388–94.

68. Ganguly N, Clough LA, Dubois LK, McGuirk JP, Abhyankar S, Aljitawi OS, et al. Low-dose cidofovir in the treatment of symptomatic bk virus infection in patients undergoing allogeneic hematopoietic stem cell transplantation: a retrospective analysis of an algorithmic approach. Transplant Infect Dis: Off J Transplant Soc. 2010;12:406–11.

69. Philippe M, Ranchon F, Gilis L, Schwiertz V, Vantard N, Ader F, et al. Cidofovir in the treatment of bk virus-associated hemorrhagic cystitis after allogeneic hematopoietic stem cell transplantation. Biol Blood Marrow Transplant: J Am Soc Blood Marrow Transplant. 2016;22:723–30.

70. Savona MR, Newton D, Frame D, Levine JE, Mineishi S, Kaul DR. Low-dose cidofovir treatment of bk virus-associated hemorrhagic cystitis in recipients of hematopoietic stem cell transplant. Bone Marrow Transplant. 2007;39:783–7.

71. Araya CE, Lew JF, Fennell RS, Neiberger RE, Dharnidharka VR. Intermediate dose cidofovir does not cause additive nephrotoxicity in bk virus allograft nephropathy. Pediatr Transplant. 2008;12:790–5.

72. Lacy SA, Hitchcock MJ, Lee WA, Tellier P, Cundy KC. Effect of oral probenecid coadministration on the chronic toxicity and pharmacokinetics of intravenous cidofovir in cynomolgus monkeys. Toxicol Sci: Off J Soc Toxicol. 1998;44:97–106.

73. Meier P, Dautheville-Guibal S, Ronco PM, Rossert J. Cidofovir-induced end-stage renal failure. Nephrol Dial Transplant: Off Publ Eur Dial Transplant Assoc – Eur Ren Assoc. 2002;17:148–9.

74. Lalezari JP, Holland GN, Kramer F, McKinley GF, Kemper CA, Ives DV, et al. Randomized, controlled study of the safety and efficacy of intravenous cidofovir for the treatment of relapsing cytomegalovirus retinitis in patients with aids. J Acquir Immune Defic Syndr Human Retrovirol: Off Publ Int Retrovirol Assoc. 1998;17:339–44.

75. Ortiz A, Justo P, Sanz A, Melero R, Caramelo C, Guerrero MF, et al. Tubular cell apoptosis and cidofovir-induced acute renal failure. Antivir Ther. 2005;10:185–90.

76. Aitken SL, Zhou J, Ghantoji SS, Kontoyiannis DP, Jones RB, Tam VH, et al. Pharmacokinetics and safety of intravesicular cidofovir in allogeneic hsct recipients. J Antimicrob Chemother. 2016;71:727–30.

77. Tseng AL, Mortimer CB, Salit IE. Iritis associated with intravenous cidofovir. Ann Pharmacother. 1999;33:167–71.

78. Akler ME, Johnson DW, Burman WJ, Johnson SC. Anterior uveitis and hypotony after intravenous cidofovir for the treatment of cytomegalovirus retinitis. Ophthalmology. 1998;105:651–7.

79. Cherrington JM, Fuller MD, Lamy PD, Miner R, Lalezari JP, Nuessle S, et al. In vitro antiviral susceptibilities of isolates from cytomegalovirus retinitis patients receiving first- or second-line cidofovir therapy: relationship to clinical outcome. J Infect Dis. 1998;178:1821–5.

80. Wutzler P, De Clercq E, Wutke K, Farber I. Oral brivudin vs. intravenous acyclovir in the treatment of herpes zoster in immunocompromised patients: a randomized double-blind trial. J Med Virol. 1995;46:252–7.

81. Farasati NA, Shapiro R, Vats A, Randhawa P. Effect of leflunomide and cidofovir on replication of bk virus in an in vitro culture system. Transplantation. 2005;79:116–8.

82. Waldman WJ, Knight DA, Lurain NS, Miller DM, Sedmak DD, Williams JW, et al. Novel mechanism of inhibition of cytomegalovirus by the experimental immunosuppressive agent leflunomide. Transplantation. 1999;68:814–25.

83. Chacko B, John GT. Leflunomide for cytomegalovirus: bench to bedside. Transplant Infect Dis: Off J Transplant Soc. 2012;14:111–20.

84. Chon WJ, Kadambi PV, Xu C, Becker YT, Witkowski P, Pursell K, et al. Use of leflunomide in renal transplant recipients with ganciclovir-resistant/refractory cytomegalovirus infection: a case series from the university of Chicago. Case Rep Nephrol Dial. 2015;5:96–105.

85. Battiwalla M, Paplham P, Almyroudis NG, McCarthy A, Abdelhalim A, Elefante A, et al. Leflunomide failure to control recurrent cytomegalovirus infection in the setting of renal failure after allogeneic stem cell transplantation. Transplant Infect Dis: Off J Transplant Soc. 2007;9:28–32.

86. Florescu DF, Keck MA. Development of cmx001 (brincidofovir) for the treatment of serious diseases or conditions caused by dsdna viruses. Expert Rev Anti-Infect Ther. 2014;12:1171–8.

87. Marty FM, Winston DJ, Rowley SD, Vance E, Papanicolaou GA, Mullane KM, et al. Cmx001 to prevent cytomegalovirus disease in hematopoietic-cell transplantation. N Engl J Med. 2013;369:1227–36.

88. Trofe J, Pote L, Wade E, Blumberg E, Bloom RD. Maribavir: a novel antiviral agent with activity against cytomegalovirus. Ann Pharmacother. 2008;42:1447–57.

89. Marty FM, Ljungman P, Papanicolaou GA, Winston DJ, Chemaly RF, Strasfeld L, et al. Maribavir prophylaxis for prevention of cytomegalovirus disease in recipients of allogeneic stem-cell transplants: a phase 3, double-blind, placebo-controlled, randomised trial. Lancet Infect Dis. 2011;11:284–92.

90. Marty FM, Boeckh M. Maribavir and human cytomegalovirus-what happened in the clinical trials and why might the drug have failed? Curr Opin Virol. 2011;1:555–62.

91. Papanicolaou GSF, Langston F, Pereira M, Avery R, Wijatyk A et al. Maribavir for treatment of cytomegalovirus infections resistant or refractory to ganciclovir or foscarnet in hematopoietic stem cell transplant or solid organ transplant recipients: a randomized, dose-ranging, double-blind, phase 2 study. The 2017 BMT Meeting; Orlando, Florida. Biol Blood Marrow Transplant. 2017. S18–S391.

92. Avery RK, Marty FM, Strasfeld L, Lee I, Arrieta A, Chou S, et al. Oral maribavir for treatment of refractory or resistant cytomegalovirus infections in transplant recipients. Transplant Infect Dis: Off J Transplant Soc. 2010;12:489–96.

93. Goldner T, Hewlett G, Ettischer N, Ruebsamen-Schaeff H, Zimmermann H, Lischka P. The novel anticytomegalovirus compound aic246 (letermovir) inhibits human cytomegalovirus replication through a specific antiviral mechanism that involves the viral terminase. J Virol. 2011;85:10884–93.

94. Chemaly RF, Ullmann AJ, Stoelben S, Richard MP, Bornhauser M, Groth C, et al. Letermovir for cytomegalovirus prophylaxis in hematopoietic-cell transplantation. N Engl J Med. 2014;370:1781–9.

95. Marty FM, Ljungman P, Chemaly RF, et al. Letermovir prophylaxis for cytomegalovirus in hematopoietic-cell transplantation. N Engl J Med. 2017;377:2433–44. https://www.accessdata.fda. gov/drugsatfda_docs/nda/2017/209939Orig1s000,2 09940Orig1s000Approv.pdf.

96. Ison MG. Antivirals and resistance: influenza virus. Curr Opin Virol. 2011;1:563–73.

97. Dong G, Peng C, Luo J, Wang C, Han L, Wu B, et al. Adamantane-resistant influenza a viruses in the world (1902–2013): frequency and distribution of m2 gene mutations. PLoS One. 2015;10:e0119115.

98. Baranovich T, Bahl J, Marathe BM, Culhane M, Stigger-Rosser E, Darnell D, et al. Influenza a viruses of swine circulating in the United States during 2009–2014 are susceptible to neuraminidase inhibitors but show lineage-dependent resistance to adamantanes. Antivir Res. 2015;117:10–9.

99. Abed Y, Goyette N, Boivin G. Generation and characterization of recombinant influenza a (h1n1) viruses harboring amantadine resistance mutations. Antimicrob Agents Chemother. 2005;49:556–9.

100. Watcharananan SP, Suwatanapongched T, Wacharawanichkul P, Chantratitaya W, Mavichak V, Mossad SB. Influenza a/h1n1 2009 pneumonia in kidney transplant recipients: characteristics and outcomes following high-dose oseltamivir exposure. Transplant Infect Dis: Off J Transplant Soc. 2010;12:127–31.

101. Chemaly RF, Shah DP, Boeckh MJ. Management of respiratory viral infections in hematopoietic cell transplant recipients and patients with hematologic malignancies. Clin Infect Dis: Off Publ Infect Dis Soc Am. 2014;59(Suppl 5):S344–51.

102. Conditions of use, conditions for distribution and patients targeted and conditions for safety monitoring addressed to member states for iv zanamivir available for compassionate use. 2011. http://www.ema.europa.eu/docs/en_GB/document_library/Other/2010/02/WC500074124.pdfcited. 28 Aug 2015.

103. Ison MG, Fraiz J, Heller B, Jauregui L, Mills G, O'Riordan W, et al. Intravenous peramivir for treatment of influenza in hospitalized patients. Antivir Ther. 2014;19:349–61.

104. Shah DP, El Taoum KK, Shah JN, Vigil KJ, Adachi JA, Granwehr BP, et al. Characteristics and outcomes of pandemic 2009/h1n1 versus seasonal influenza in children with cancer. Pediatr Infect Dis J. 2012;31:373–8.

105. Kumar D, Michaels MG, Morris MI, Green M, Avery RK, Liu C, et al. Outcomes from pandemic influenza a h1n1 infection in recipients of solid-organ transplants: a multicentre cohort study. Lancet Infect Dis. 2010;10:521–6.

106. Lackenby A, Hungnes O, Dudman SG, Meijer A, Paget WJ, Hay AJ, et al. Emergence of resistance to oseltamivir among influenza a(h1n1) viruses in Europe. Euro Surveill: Bull Eur Mal Transmissibles Eur Commun Dis Bull. 2008;13.

107. Baz M, Abed Y, Simon P, Hamelin ME, Boivin G. Effect of the neuraminidase mutation h274y conferring resistance to oseltamivir on the replicative capacity and virulence of old and recent human influenza a(h1n1) viruses. J Infect Dis. 2010;201:740–5.

108. Takashita E, Meijer A, Lackenby A, Gubareva L, Rebelo-de-Andrade H, Besselaar T, et al. Global update on the susceptibility of human influenza viruses to neuraminidase inhibitors, 2013–2014. Antivir Res. 2015;117:27–38.

109. Gooskens J, Jonges M, Claas EC, Meijer A, Kroes AC. Prolonged influenza virus infection during lymphocytopenia and frequent detection of drug-resistant viruses. J Infect Dis. 2009;199:1435–41.

110. Weinstock DM, Gubareva LV, Zuccotti G. Prolonged shedding of multidrug-resistant influenza a virus in an immunocompromised patient. N Engl J Med. 2003;348:867–8.

111. Renaud C, Boudreault AA, Kuypers J, Lofy KH, Corey L, Boeckh MJ, et al. H275y mutant pandemic (h1n1) 2009 virus in immunocompromised patients. Emerg Infect Dis. 2011;17:653–60. quiz 765.

112. Takashita E, Fujisaki S, Kishida N, Xu H, Imai M, Tashiro M, et al. Characterization of neuraminidase inhibitor-resistant influenza a(h1n1)pdm09 viruses isolated in four seasons during pandemic and post-pandemic periods in Japan. Influenza Other Respir Viruses. 2013;7:1390–9.

113. Thorlund K, Awad T, Boivin G. Thabane L systematic review of influenza resistance to the neuraminidase inhibitors. BMC Infect Dis. 2011;11:134.

114. Meijer A, Lackenby A, Hungnes O, Lina B, van der Werf S, Schweiger B, et al. Oseltamivir-resistant influenza virus a (h1n1), europe, 2007–08 season. Emerg Infect Dis. 2009;15:552–60.

115. Johny AA, Clark A, Price N, Carrington D, Oakhill A, Marks DI. The use of zanamivir to treat influenza a and b infection after allogeneic stem cell transplantation. Bone Marrow Transplant. 2002;29:113–5.

116. Harter G, Zimmermann O, Maier L, Schubert A, Mertens T, Kern P, et al. Intravenous zanamivir for patients with pneumonitis due to pandemic (h1n1) 2009 influenza virus. Clin Infect Dis. 2010;50:1249–51.

117. Hurt AC, Holien JK, Parker M, Kelso A, Barr IG. Zanamivir-resistant influenza viruses with a novel neuraminidase mutation. J Virol. 2009;83:10366–73.

118. Tamura D, DeBiasi RL, Okomo-Adhiambo M, Mishin VP, Campbell AP, Loechelt B, et al. Emergence of multidrug-resistant influenza a(h1n1) pdm09 virus variants in an immunocompromised child treated with oseltamivir and zanamivir. J Infect Dis. 2015;212(8):1209–13.

119. Nguyen HT, Fry AM, Loveless PA, Klimov AI, Gubareva LV. Recovery of a multidrug-resistant strain of pandemic influenza a 2009 (h1n1) virus carrying a dual h275y/i223r mutation from a child after prolonged treatment with oseltamivir. Clin Infect Dis. 2010;51:983–4.

120. Wyde PR, Chetty SN, Jewell AM, Boivin G, Piedra PA. Comparison of the inhibition of human metapneumovirus and respiratory syncytial virus by ribavirin and immune serum globulin in vitro. Antivir Res. 2003;60:51–9.

121. Leyssen P, Balzarini J, De Clercq E, Neyts J. The predominant mechanism by which ribavirin exerts its antiviral activity in vitro against flaviviruses and paramyxoviruses is mediated by inhibition of imp dehydrogenase. J Virol. 2005;79:1943–7.

122. Hall CB, Powell KR, MacDonald NE, Gala CL, Menegus ME, Suffin SC, et al. Respiratory syncytial viral infection in children with compromised immune function. N Engl J Med. 1986;315:77–81.

123. Pope JF, Besunder JB, Kumar ML, Super DM. Concerned about ribavirin recommendations. Pediatrics. 1994;94:132–3.

124. Shah DP, Ghantoji SS, Shah JN, El Taoum KK, Jiang Y, Popat U, et al. Impact of aerosolized ribavirin on mortality in 280 allogeneic haematopoietic stem cell transplant recipients with respiratory syncytial virus infections. J Antimicrob Chemother. 2013;68:1872–80.

125. Shah JN, Chemaly RF. Management of rsv infections in adult recipients of hematopoietic stem cell transplantation. Blood. 2011;117:2755–63.

126. Shah DP, Ghantoji SS, Ariza-Heredia EJ, Shah JN, El Taoum KK, Shah PK, et al. Immunodeficiency scoring index to predict poor outcomes in hematopoietic cell transplant recipients with rsv infections. Blood. 2014;123:3263–8.

127. Hirsch HH, Martino R, Ward KN, Boeckh M, Einsele H, Ljungman P. Fourth European conference on infections in leukaemia (ecil-4): guidelines for diagnosis and treatment of human respiratory syncytial virus, parainfluenza virus, metapneumovirus, rhinovirus, and coronavirus. Clin Infect Dis: Off Publ Infect Dis Soc Am. 2013;56:258–66.

128. Khanna N, Widmer AF, Decker M, Steffen I, Halter J, Heim D, et al. Respiratory syncytial virus infection in patients with hematological diseases: single-center study and review of the literature. Clin Infect Dis: Off Publ Infect Dis Soc Am. 2008;46:402–12.

129. Marcelin JR, Wilson JW, Razonable RR, Mayo Clinic HO. Transplant infectious diseases S oral ribavirin therapy for respiratory syncytial virus infections in moderately to severely immunocompromised patients. Transplant Infect Dis: Off J Transplant Soc. 2014;16:242–50.

130. Molinos-Quintana A, Perez-de Soto C, Gomez-Rosa M, Perez-Simon JA, Perez-Hurtado JM. Intravenous ribavirin for respiratory syncytial viral infections in pediatric hematopoietic sct recipients. Bone Marrow Transplant. 2013;48:265–8.

131. Glanville AR, Scott AI, Morton JM, Aboyoun CL, Plit ML, Carter IW, et al. Intravenous ribavirin is a safe and cost-effective treatment for respiratory syncytial virus infection after lung transplantation. J Heart Lung Transplant: Off Publ Int Soc Heart Transplant. 2005;24:2114–9.

132. Baden LR, Swaminathan S, Angarone M, Blouin G, Camins BC, Casper C, et al. Prevention and treatment of cancer-related infections, version 2.2016, nccn clinical practice guidelines in oncology. J Natl Compr Cancer Netw JNCCN. 2016;14:882–913.

133. Nichols WG, Corey L, Gooley T, Davis C, Boeckh M. Parainfluenza virus infections after hematopoietic stem cell transplantation: risk factors, response to antiviral therapy, and effect on transplant outcome. Blood. 2001;98:573–8.

134. Chemaly RF, Torres HA, Munsell MF, Shah DP, Rathod DB, Bodey GP, et al. An adaptive randomized trial of an intermittent dosing schedule of aerosolized ribavirin in patients with cancer and respiratory syncytial virus infection. J Infect Dis. 2012;206:1367–71.

135. Englund JA, Piedra PA, Ahn YM, Gilbert BE, Hiatt P. High-dose, short-duration ribavirin aerosol therapy compared with standard ribavirin therapy in children with suspected respiratory syncytial virus infection. J Pediatr. 1994;125:635–41.

136. Moscona A, Porotto M, Palmer S, Tai C, Aschenbrenner L, Triana-Baltzer G, et al. A recombinant sialidase fusion protein effectively inhibits human parainfluenza viral infection in vitro and in vivo. J Infect Dis. 2010;202:234–41.

137. Nicholls JM, Moss RB, Haslam SM. The use of sialidase therapy for respiratory viral infections. Antivir Res. 2013;98:401–9.

138. Zenilman JM, Fuchs EJ, Hendrix CW, Radebaugh C, Jurao R, Nayak SU, et al. Phase 1 clinical trials of das181, an inhaled sialidase, in healthy adults. Antivir Res. 2015;123:114–9.

139. Waghmare A, Wagner T, Andrews R, Smith S, Kuypers J, Boeckh M, et al. Successful treatment of parainfluenza virus respiratory tract infection with das181 in 4 immunocompromised children. J Pediatr Infect Dis Soc. 2015;4:114–8.

140. https://clinicaltrials.Gov/ct2/show/nct01644877?Term=das181&rank=5. 2012. cited 2016 Feb 2.

141. DeVincenzo JP, Whitley RJ, Mackman RL, Scaglioni-Weinlich C, Harrison L, Farrell E, et al. Oral gs-5806 activity in a respiratory syncytial virus challenge study. N Engl J Med. 2014;371:711–22.

142. Smee DF, Tarbet EB, Furuta Y, Morrey JD, Barnard DL. Synergistic combinations of favipiravir and oseltamivir against wild-type pandemic and oseltamivir-resistant influenza a virus infections in mice. Futur Virol. 2013;8:1085–94.

143. Tarbet EB, Vollmer AH, Hurst BL, Barnard DL, Furuta Y, Smee DF. In vitro activity of favipiravir and neuraminidase inhibitor combinations against oseltamivir-sensitive and oseltamivir-resistant pandemic influenza a (h1n1) virus. Arch Virol. 2014;159:1279–91.

144. Tsutsumi Y, Kawamura T, Saitoh S, Yamada M, Obara S, Miura T, et al. Hepatitis b virus reactivation in a case of non-Hodgkin's lymphoma treated with chemotherapy and rituximab: necessity of prophylaxis for hepatitis b virus reactivation in rituximab therapy. Leuk Lymphoma. 2004;45:627–9.

145. Hwang JP, Somerfield MR, Alston-Johnson DE, Cryer DR, Feld JJ, Kramer BS, et al. Hepatitis b virus screening for patients with cancer before therapy: American society of clinical oncology provisional clinical opinion update. J Clin Oncol: Off J Am Soc Clin Oncol. 2015;33:2212–20.

146. Levine S, Hernandez D, Yamanaka G, Zhang S, Rose R, Weinheimer S, et al. Efficacies of entecavir against lamivudine-resistant hepatitis b virus replication and recombinant polymerases in vitro. Antimicrob Agents Chemother. 2002;46:2525–32.

147. Lai CL, Chien RN, Leung NW, Chang TT, Guan R, Tai DI, et al. A one-year trial of lamivudine for chronic hepatitis b. Asia hepatitis lamivudine study group. N Engl J Med. 1998;339:61–8.

148. Marcellin P, Chang TT, Lim SG, Tong MJ, Sievert W, Shiffman ML, et al. Adefovir dipivoxil for the treatment of hepatitis b e antigen-positive chronic hepatitis b. N Engl J Med. 2003;348:808–16.

149. Marcellin P, Heathcote EJ, Buti M, Gane E, de Man RA, Krastev Z, et al. Tenofovir disoproxil fumarate

versus adefovir dipivoxil for chronic hepatitis b. N Engl J Med. 2008;359:2442–55.

150. Vaisberg VV, Kim V, Ono SK, Mendes LC, Carrilho FJ. Comparison of chronic hepatitis c treatment efficacy in randomized controlled trials and real-life studies – influence of study design in the sustained virological response: a systematic review of published literature. Value Health: J Int Soc Pharmacoeconomics Outcomes Res. 2015;18:A815.

151. Zhang J, Nguyen D, Hu KQ. Chronic hepatitis c virus infection: a review of current direct-acting antiviral treatment strategies. N Am J Med Sci. 2016;9:47–54.

152. Gotte M, Feld JJ. Direct-acting antiviral agents for hepatitis c: structural and mechanistic insights. Nat Rev Gastroenterol Hepatol. 2016;13:338–51.

153. Torres HA, Shigle TL, Hammoudi N, Link JT, Samaniego F, Kaseb A, et al. The oncologic burden of hepatitis c virus infection: a clinical perspective. CA Cancer J Clin. 2017;67:411–31.

154. Curry MP, Forns X, Chung RT, Terrault NA, Brown R Jr, Fenkel JM, et al. Sofosbuvir and ribavirin prevent recurrence of hcv infection after liver transplantation: an open-label study. Gastroenterology. 2015;148:100–7. e1.

155. Torres HA, Chong PP, De Lima M, Friedman MS, Giralt S, Hammond SP, et al. Hepatitis c virus infection among hematopoietic cell transplant donors and recipients: American society for blood and marrow transplantation task force recommendations. Biol Blood Marrow Transplant: J Am Soc Blood Marrow Transplant. 2015;21:1870–82.

156. Levitsky J, Doucette K. Practice ASTIDCo viral hepatitis in solid organ transplantation. Am J Transplant: Off J Am Soc Transplant Am Soc Transplant Surg. 2013;13(Suppl 4):147–68.

Role of Immunoglobulin Therapy to Prevent and Treat Infections

17

Aspasia Katragkou, Emmanuel Roilides, and Thomas J. Walsh

Immunoglobulin Use in Therapeutics and Historical Overview

Immunoglobulin therapy has been used for the prevention and treatment of infectious disease before the introduction of antimicrobial agents into the clinical practice. In the early 1890s, Emil von Behring and Shibasaburo Kitasato set the basis of "serum therapy" showing that antibody preparations derived from the serum of immunized animals have the ability to protect against

A. Katragkou
Transplantation-Oncology Infectious Diseases Program, Division of Infectious Diseases, Department of Medicine, Pediatrics, and Microbiology & Immunology, Weill Cornell Medicine, Henry Schueler Foundation Scholar, New York, NY, USA

E. Roilides
Infectious Disease Unit, 3rd Department of Pediatrics, Faculty of Medicine, Aristotle University School of Health Sciences, Hippokration Hospital, Thessaloniki, Greece

T. J. Walsh (✉)
Transplantation-Oncology Infectious Diseases Program, Division of Infectious Diseases, Department of Medicine, Pediatrics, and Microbiology & Immunology, Weill Cornell Medicine, Henry Schueler Foundation Scholar, New York, NY, USA

Departments of Pediatrics, Microbiology and Immunology Weill Cornell Medicine, New York, NY, USA
e-mail: thw2003@med.cornell.edu

bacterial toxins [115]. Ehrlich's subsequent work contributed to the conception of passive immunity, demonstrating that increasing doses of bacterial toxins could provide immunity against lethal doses of toxin [68]. Cenci first used human serum in 1907 for the prevention of measles and thereafter for the prevention of pertussis and mumps [45]. Systemic administration of "serum therapy" was widely used in the 1930s for the treatment of bacterial and viral infections; however its use was often associated with adverse reactions due to administration of large amounts of animal proteins, ranging from fever and chills to "serum sickness," a form of immune complex disease, characterized by rash, proteinuria, and arthralgias [45]. After improvements in antibody purification methods, which reduced serum toxicity, the role of "serum therapy" was further expanded. In the pre-antibiotic era, serum therapy significantly reduced the mortality in some infectious outbreaks such as meningococcal and *Haemophilus influenzae* meningitis, pneumococcal pneumonia, and diphtheria. The efficacy of serum therapy varied with the type and severity of the infections and the timing of treatment administration in relation to symptom onset [27, 28, 43]. For some infections like whooping cough, anthrax, dysentery (*Shigella dysenteriae*), and gas gangrene, the efficacy of "serum therapy" was uncertain, while for other pathogens like *Staphylococcus*, *Mycobacterium*, and

© Springer International Publishing AG, part of Springer Nature 2018
B. H. Segal (ed.), *Management of Infections in the Immunocompromised Host*,
https://doi.org/10.1007/978-3-319-77674-3_17

Salmonella species, no consistently effective sera were produced [28].

With the discovery of antibiotics in 1940s, the interest in "serum therapy" for the treatment of infectious disease waned. The initial interest in using combination therapies with antibiotics and serum was abandoned, as the potential benefits were marginal. Antimicrobial chemotherapy proved to be less toxic and more effective than serum therapy in the treatment of infections. However, Dr. Cohn's discovery of purified antibodies through cold ethanol fractionation of plasma during the Second World War revived the interest in antibody treatment especially for infections not able to be treated with antibiotics. The fractionation procedure stabilizes the product, denatures most viruses, and assures a more uniform antibody content. Cohn fraction (IgG from plasma after cold alcohol fractionation) was initially used for prophylaxis against prevalent and life-threatening infections, such as measles. It was not until 1952 that Bruton reported for the first time the use of immunoglobulin preparation injected subcutaneously for the treatment of a young boy with agammaglobulinemia [21]. Thereafter, the use of immunoglobulin injected intramuscularly became established as the standard therapy for primary immunodeficiencies, lasting until the development of purer and safer intravenous immunoglobulin preparation in the early 1980s [86].

The advent of hybridoma technology, which allows continuous generation of large quantities of monoclonal antibodies specific to antigens of interest and the generation of humanized antibodies, revolutionized antibody therapeutics [63]. Monoclonal antibody technology offers supply advantage, reduces the risks of adverse events, and decreases lot-to-lot variation. In the mid-1980s a monoclonal antibody (mAb) to CD3 was introduced into clinical practice to prevent organ rejection. Almost a decade later, the humanized mAb palivizumab (Synagis®, a humanized mouse monoclonal antibody to prevent RSV pulmonary infections in high-risk patients, especially infants) was licensed. Palivizumab was 50-fold more potent than the polyclonal product, resulting in reduced volume of administration and intramuscular use [45]. During the last three decades, 30 therapeutic mAbs have been licensed, mainly for treatment of malignancies and rheumatic or autoimmune diseases, but only two were licensed for infectious diseases (palivizumab and raxibacumab: human mAb to anthrax toxin). Although the use of mAbs to treat infectious diseases does not depend on discrimination between self-antigen as there are large antigenic differences between the microorganism and the host, the pace of discovery and development of new mAbs against infectious disease is limited. Currently, the areas of mAbs development have been focused on viral diseases without available vaccines [HIV, Ebola, severe acute respiratory syndrome (SARS), Middle East respiratory syndrome, Marburg virus], viral disease with limited effective antiviral drugs (influenza, rabies), and bacterial toxin-mediated disease (anthrax, *Clostridium difficile* colitis). In the clinical setting, therapeutic mAbs can be used when there are nosocomial/iatrogenic outbreaks. For example, a new approach to the prevention of recurrent *C. difficile* infection is the administration of mAbs against *C. difficile* toxins (in addition to antibiotic therapy) as a form of passive immunity. Actoxumab and bezlotoxumab are fully human monoclonal antibodies that bind and neutralize *C. difficile* toxins A and B, respectively. A double-blind randomized placebo-controlled phase 3 trial showed that a single intravenous dose of bezlotoxumab when given with standard-of-care antibiotics provided protection against recurrent *C. difficile* infection for up to 12 weeks that was superior to that provided by treatment with standard-of-care antibiotics alone [114]. Other therapeutic mAbs can be applied in drug resistance (*Staphylococcus aureus*, VRSA), pandemic outbreaks (Ebola virus), bioterrorism attacks (*Bacillus anthracis*), emerging infectious diseases (Nipah or Hendra virus), and use in high-risk host groups or in severe diseases (respiratory syncytial virus, cytomegalovirus retinitis in HIV patients, hepatitis C virus, influenza virus). Another application of therapeutic mAbs concerns their use as adjunct therapies that have anti-inflammatory or immune modulatory roles (mAbs against TNF-α and other immune mediators) [45, 55].

Immunoglobulins: Types and Characteristics

Immunoglobulins are glycoprotein molecules that are produced by plasma cells in response to antigens or immunogens and which function as antibodies. Serum contains a heterogeneous immunoglobulin pool that reflects the host response to endogenous microbiota and the immunological memory of the host for a variety of acquired microbial agents [26]. Different immunoglobulins can differ structurally; however, they are built from the same basic units.

There are five classes of immunoglobulin, classified according to the type of heavy chain they possess (Table 17.1) [70]. Each class of immunoglobulins has a specific function, and deficiency of each class leads to particular dysfunction of immune system. Serum IgM predominates in the acute immune response to most antigens and is the most efficient complement-fixing immunoglobulin. Immunoglobulin class switching subsequently occurs, leading to a predominance of IgG, which is responsible for protection during the first infectious attack and long-term protection via memory B cells. Secretory IgA, due to its abundance in mucosal secretions, provides primary defense mechanism against some mucosal infections. IgE primarily defends against parasitic invasion [2].

Immunoglobulins together with T cells are the key mediators of adaptive immunity, and deficiencies in either of these two arms of the adaptive immune system can result in higher host susceptibility to bacterial, fungal, or viral infections [76]. Immunoglobulins interact with the

Table 17.1 Properties of human serum immunoglobulin isotypes

	IgG				IgA	IgM	IgE	IgD
	IgG1	IgG2	IgG3	IgG4				
Molecular weight (x1000)	146	146	170	146	320	900	73	70
Heavy chain	γ1	γ2	γ3	γ4	α	μ	ε	δ
In vivo serum half-life (days)	21–23	20–23	7–8	21–23	6	5	2.5	3
Percent of total Ig	66%	23%	7%	4%	13%	6%	0.02%	0.2%
Activate classical complement pathway	+	+/−	++	−	−	+++	−	−
Crosses placenta	+	+/−	+	+	−	−	−	−
Present on membrane of mature B cells	−	−	−	−	−	+	−	+
Bind to Fc receptor of phagocytes	++	+/−	++	+	−	?	−	−
Mucosal transport	−	−	−	−	++	+	−	−
Distribution	Intravascular and extravascular				Intravascular and secretions	Mostly intravascular	Basophils, mast cells in saliva and nasal secretions	Lymphocyte surface
Structure	Monomeric				Dimeric	Pentameric	Monomeric	Monomeric

++, high; +, moderate; +/− minimal; ?, questionable

cellular immune compartment at multiple levels aiming different cells, including dendritic cells, the monocyte/macrophage system, granulocytes, natural killer cells, and various subsets of T cells and B cells [38, 102]. Understanding the mechanisms of interactions between immunoglobulins, immunomodulatory molecules, and cells of the immune system, both innate and adaptive, is the basis for understanding the future therapeutic perspectives of immunoglobulins [38].

Immunoglobulins, upon binding of a specific antigen, stimulate significant direct and indirect "effector functions." Classically, in bacterial disease, immunoglobulins neutralize toxins, facilitate opsonization, and, with complement, promote bacteriolysis. In viral diseases, immunoglobulins block viral entry into uninfected cells, promote antibody-directed cell-mediated cytotoxicity by natural killer cells, and neutralize virus alone or with the participation with the complement [62]. Furthermore, more recent studies have demonstrated the immunomodulatory functions of antibodies, including the potential for antibody therapy to reduce damage from the host inflammatory response to major infections [24, 25].

Notably, IgG can exert pro- and anti-inflammatory activities depending on its concentration. Low dose of IgG has pro-inflammatory activity and requires complement activation or binding of the Fc fragment from IgG to IgG-specific receptors (FcγR) on innate immune effector cells. This results in receptor clustering, recruitment of secondary effector functions, and subsequent activation of signaling pathways, leading to an increase in intracellular calcium levels and cell activation. By comparison, high concentrations of IgG have anti-inflammatory properties. The mechanisms proposed for this mode of action are modulation of the expression and function of FcγRs, interference with activation of the complement cascade and the cytokine network, neutralization of autoantibodies, and regulation of cell proliferation [38].

Immunoglobulin Preparations

The immunoglobulin preparations used in passive immunization are the standard human serum immunoglobulin, which is available in three forms: immune globulin (IG) for intramuscular use (IMIG), intravenous use (IVIG), and subcutaneous use (SCIG). IMIG is used primarily for the prevention of certain infections, such as hepatitis A, measles, and rubella, and less commonly for the treatment of antibody immunodeficiencies. IVIG is used in the treatment of primary and secondary antibody deficiencies, many immunoregulatory disorders (e.g., immune thrombocytopenic purpura, Kawasaki disease), and neurologic disorders (e.g., Guillain-Barré syndrome, peripheral neuritis). IGSC is used exclusively for the antibody deficiencies.

IVIG preparations comprise the pooled fraction of serum from ~3000 to 60,000 donors, which is generated by a cold ethanol precipitation, providing, thus, a broad spectrum of opsonic and neutralizing IgG antibodies. Opsonic and neutralizing IgG antibody content varies with each product batch, primarily due to differences in the local pathogen ecology of donor exposure. IgG and complement proteins are the principal classes of opsonins contributing to bacterial clearance. In addition to IgG, varying amounts of immunoglobulin isotypes, especially IgA, can be found in the IVIG preparation. Regarding the different human IgG subclasses (IgG1-IgG4), IVIG preparations reflect the hierarchy present in the serum, consisting mainly of IgG1 and IgG2 and containing much smaller amounts of the other IgG subclasses. Only the product Pentaglobin® (Biotest, Germany) is IgM-enriched [93]. The clinical use of IVIG can be distinguished by the infused amount [92]. The principal manufacturing process in all current IgG preparations is cold ethanol fractionation with product-specific additional processes for manufacturing. The commonest processes for virus reduction include solvents/detergent, low pH (pH 4), incubation, nanofiltration, and chromatography [93]. Other major quality control practices in the production process, besides viral reduction, include the depletion of blood coagulation factors and the removal of IgG aggregates, since these aggregates could result in a cytokine release syndrome owing to the ubiquitous activation of innate immune effector cells via activating FcγRs. IgG aggregations are absent from the majority of IVIG preparation; however, depending on the provider and batch, up to 1–10% of IgG can be found in dimeric form in most IVIG preparations [92].

Immunoglobulins and Clinical Indications

The two major indications for which immunoglobulins are used are IgG replacement therapy and anti-inflammatory therapy in a variety of acute and chronic autoimmune diseases. Apart from immunoglobulin replacement therapy, currently licensed application of immunoglobulin (IVIG) administration includes Guillain-Barré syndrome, Kawasaki disease, and chronic inflammatory demyelinating polyneuropathy. Licensed indications, however, only account for approximately 40–50% of the worldwide immunoglobulin sales, as most immunoglobulin administrations are "off-label" [76]. The use of immunoglobulins for infectious disease can involve the passive transfer of antibodies for pre-/postexposure prophylaxis or for treatment. Passive immunization provides temporal immunity to unimmunized individuals either prophylactically or therapeutically. The different forms of passive immunotherapies are shown in Table 17.2 [96].

The technology of ethanol fractionation of plasma resulted in products used for the treatment and prophylaxis of infectious diseases (Table 17.3). Human immune sera have fewer adverse effects, but there are concerns about availability, potency, and consistency.

Table 17.4 summarizes the adverse reactions of immunoglobulin used in the prevention and treatment of infectious diseases.

Immunoglobulins to Prevent Infections in Immunodeficiencies

Administration of immunoglobulins is indicated for the majority of patients with primary immune deficiencies and for patients with combined immune deficiencies and for those with secondary immune deficiency with significant antibody deficiency. The benefits of replacement immunoglobulin therapy for the prevention of infections in patients with antibody deficiencies are well established and pertain to the reduction of the incidence and the severity of infections and prevention long-term deterioration in organ function [12, 13].

Primary immune deficiencies (PIDD) are one of the US Food and Drug Administration (FDA)-approved indications for immunoglobulin therapy. Over 80% of all PIDD involve antibody-mediated immunity; however, each individual disorder has a different immunopathogenesis in terms of the number of B cells in the blood and B-cell function. Moreover, any persisting endogenous antibody production varies both between specific conditions and within individual disorders [10, 35, 97]. Table 17.5 describes the PIDD for which immunoglobulin replacement is or may be efficacious. The recommendations for immunoglobulin replacement treatment in primary and secondary immune deficiencies are shown in Table 17.6 [32, 84, 97]. The main indications are primary antibody deficiencies including agammaglobulinemia (autosomal recessive or X-linked) and common variable immunodeficiency disorders. Rarely, other

Table 17.2 Different forms of passive immunotherapy

| Animal antisera and antitoxins (e.g., diphtheria antitoxin) |
| Human immune serum globulins for general use |
| Immunoglobulins for intramuscular use (normal and specific immunoglobulins) |
| Immunoglobulins for intravenous use (human and enriched immunoglobulins) |
| Special human immune serum globulins (e.g., hepatitis B immunoglobulin) |
| Humanized monoclonal antibodies |

Modified from Annals of Internal Medicine 1987; 107: 367–382. Intravenous Immunoglobulins as Therapeutic Agents & Biologicals 2012; 40: 196. "Role of passive immunotherapies in managing infectious outbreaks"

Table 17.3 Summary of the immunoglobulin uses for the prevention and treatment of the infectious diseases

Infection	Prophylaxis	Treatment	Recommendations	Immunoglobulin preparations used
Bacterial infections				
Respiratory infections (streptococcal, *Streptococcus pneumonia, Neisseria meningitidis, Haemophilus influenzae*)	Proven	Proven	For prophylaxis and treatment: recommended for immunodeficient patients	IVIG or IMIG
Diphtheria	Probable benefit	Proven	For prophylaxis: not recommended	Diphtheria antitoxin of equine origin
Pertussis	Unproven	Unproven	For prophylaxis and treatment: not recommended	No agent is available for passive immunity, high titer human IVIG was used
Tetanus	Proven	Proven		Hyperimmune human tetanus immunoglobulin (TIG), human IVIG can be used when TIG is not available, equine tetanus antitoxin is available for veterinary use
Other clostridial infections				
Clostridium botulinum	Proven	Proven		Botulinum antitoxins (heptavalent)
Newborn botulism	Unproven	Proven		Human botulinum intravenous immunoglobulin (BIG)
Clostridium difficile	Unproven	Possible benefit		IVIG, monoclonal antibodies for prevention of recurrence of diarrhea under development
Staphylococcal infections				
Toxic shock syndrome	Unproven	Probable benefit	For prophylaxis: not recommended for toxic shock syndrome	IVIG
Antibiotic resistance	Unproven	Possible benefit	For treatment: not recommended in cases of antibiotic resistance	IVIG
Staphylococcus epidermidis in newborns	Unproven	Possible benefit		IVIG
Toxic shock	Unproven	Probable benefit	For prophylaxis: not recommended	IVIG
Newborn sepsis	Possible benefit	Probable benefit	For prophylaxis: not recommended	IVIG
Shock, intensive care, and trauma	Unproven	Possible benefit	For treatment: not recommended	IVIG

Pseudomonas infections				
Cystic fibrosis	Unproven	No benefit	For prophylaxis and treatment: not recommended	IVIG
Burns	Unproven	No benefit	For prophylaxis and treatment: not recommended	IVIG or IMIG
Viral diseases				
Hepatitis A	Proven	No benefit		IMIG
Hepatitis B	Proven	No benefit		Hepatitis B immune globulin (HBIG) for subcutaneous or intramuscular use
Hepatitis C	Unproven	No benefit	For prophylaxis: not recommended	No passive immune product is available, monoclonal antibodies under development (for prevention for liver transplants)
HIV infection	Unproven	Unproven	For prophylaxis and treatment: not recommended	Monoclonal antibodies under development
RSV infection	Proven	Unproven	For treatment: not recommended	Palivizumab
Herpesvirus infections				
CMV	Proven	Possible benefit		CMV immune globulin
EBV	Unproven	Unproven	For prophylaxis and treatment: not recommended	Rituximab
HSV	Unproven	Unproven	For prophylaxis and treatment: not recommended	IVIG not recommended for the prevention or treatment of HSV
VZV	Proven	Unproven	For treatment: not recommended	Varicella-zoster immune globulin (VZIG) or IVIG
Parvovirus	Possible benefit	Proven	For treatment: not recommended	IVIG
Enterovirus infections				
In newborns	Unproven	Possible benefit		IVIG or IMIG
Encephalomyelitis	Possible benefit	Probable benefit	For treatment: not recommended	IVIG
Poliovirus	Proven	Unproven	For prophylaxis and treatment: not recommended	IMIG
Ebola	Unproven	Unproven		Hyperimmune serum, monoclonal antibodies under development
Rabies	Proven	No benefit		Rabies immune globulin, monoclonal antibodies under development
Measles	Proven	No benefit		IGIM or IVIG
Rubella	Unproven	No benefit	For prophylaxis: not recommended	IGIM

(continued)

Table 17.3 (continued)

Infection	Prophylaxis	Treatment	Recommendations	Immunoglobulin preparations used
Mumps	Unproven	No benefit	For prophylaxis: not recommended	Mumps immune globulin was ineffective, the product no longer manufactured
Tick-borne encephalitis	Possible benefit	No benefit		Hyperimmune human globulin
Vaccinia	Proven	Proven		Vaccinia immune globulin
Variola (smallpox)	Proven	Unproven		Vaccinia immune globulin

Modified from: Stiehm and Keller [120]

CMV cytomegalovirus, *EBV* Epstein-Barr virus, *HIV* human immunodeficiency virus, *HSV* herpes simplex virus, *RSV* respiratory syncytial virus, *VZV* varicella-zoster virus, *IVIG* standard human immune globulin intravenous, *IMIG* immune globulin intramuscular

Table 17.4 Adverse effects due to immunoglobulin therapy

Adverse reaction	Frequency[a]	Severity
Infusion site pain, swelling, erythema	Up to 75% in SCIG	Usually mild
Anxiety	20–40%	
Malaise, fatigue		
Myalgia, arthralgia, back pain		
Fever, chills, flushing		
Tachycardia		
Hypo-/hypertension		
Headache		Mild to moderate
Aseptic meningitis	<5%	Moderate
Hyponatremia		Moderate
Neutropenia		Mild/ transient
Hemolytic anemia		Moderate to severe
Interference with vaccine effectiveness and/or immunodiagnosis		N/A
Eczema		
Renal impairment		
Anaphylactoid reaction	<0.1%	
Severe thrombosis		
Blood-borne infectious diseases		

Modified from: Peter and Chapel [86]
SCIG subcutaneous immunoglobulin, *N/A* not applicable
[a]Frequencies are for patients using long-term therapy

antibody deficiencies, such as IgG subclass deficiency, may be managed by immunoglobulin replacement. In these immunodeficiencies, a trial of 12 months may be indicated if there is a substantial infection burden. On the contrary, for selective IgA deficiency, immunoglobulin replacement is not required or recommended, as anaphylactic reactions may occur during IVIG infusions. Combined immunodeficiencies with antibody deficiency also benefit from immunoglobulin therapy until the defects in cell-mediated immunity are corrected by hematopoietic stem cell transplantation. However, B-cell function is not restored universally after transplantation, and immunoglobulin therapy may be continued [86]. It is important that each patient receives a thorough evaluation before starting immunoglobulin therapy especially those with partial antibody defects.

The American Academy of Allergy, Asthma, and Immunology, based on a 2006 review of evidence, recommends for PIDD the dose of 400–600 mg/kg of IVIG every 4 weeks, titrating the dose and interval between infusions to achieve a trough IgG level at least greater than 500 mg/dl in agammaglobulinemic patients [84]. However, recent evidence suggests that the goal of IgG replacement therapy should be to reduce or prevent serious or recurrent infections instead of aiming to achieve a specific IgG level. The clinicians should identify for each patient with PIDD an individual "biological" IgG level with which the patient achieves the best clinical outcome instead of trying to reach a specific IgG level [16, 17].

The two modes of IgG replacement (IVIG and SCIG) have significant pharmacokinetic differences, which are important to know when choosing the mode of IgG delivery or switching from IVIG to SCIG. SCIG causes sustained release of IgG and thus attains higher IgG trough levels; this mode of delivery may benefit the 10–15% of patients who show increased risk of infection during the 3rd and 4th weeks after receiving IVIG or who experience extreme lethargy during the same period. IVIG achieves higher peak levels (160% higher than that obtained by SC infusion), and this mode of delivery is usually initially preferred for patients with PIDD who are very symptomatic (present with pneumonia or other serious infectious such as sepsis) and who present with pneumonia or for those with other medical problems such as sepsis [16].

IVIG has also been used in a number of diseases that cause secondary humoral immunodeficiency. While for the majority of secondary immunodeficiencies, the use of IVIG was supported only by anecdotal reports, and B-cell chronic lymphocytic leukemia (CLL) and pediatric HIV infection are FDA-approved indications. For both, CLL and HIV, infections are the most common complications. IVIG has been shown to be a useful prophylactic therapy against infections in such patients [29, 53, 54, 72, 95, 110].

Table 17.5 Primary immunodeficiencies and immunoglobulin replacement

Primary immunodeficiency	Immunologic findings	Immunoglobulin replacement	Immunoglobulin cessation
Antibody deficiency			
X-linked or autosomal agammaglobulinemia	<1% normal B cells, agammaglobulinemia, poor specific antibodies	Absolute indication, start immediately	Lifelong replacement
Common variable immunodeficiency disorders (CVID)	Hypogammaglobulinemia, poor specific antibodies, variable T-cell abnormalities	Absolute indication, start immediately	Lifelong replacement
IgG subclass deficiency with IgA deficiency	IgG subclass deficiency (usually IgG2), absent IgA, poor specific antibodies	Replacement only in symptomatic patients (clinically significant infections)	Reassessment for efficacy after 12-month treatment trial
Selective IgG subclass deficiency	Single IgG subclass deficiency, normal total IgG, poor specific antibodies	Replacement may not be necessary	
Specific antibody deficiency with recurrent infections	Normal IgG, IgA, IgM, abnormal IgG antibody responses to protein and/or unconjugated polysaccharide vaccines	Consider replacement if patient has vaccine unresponsiveness and clinically significant infections	Reassessment for efficacy after 12-month treatment trial, watch for development of more severe antibody failure
Transient hypogammaglobulinemia of infancy	Low serum IgG and IgA, poor specific antibodies	Preferable to use prophylactic antibiotics as deficiency is transient, some are given replacement for a period	Replacement stopped after some months to ascertain recovery
Combined immunodeficiencies			
Severe combined immunodeficiencies (SCIDs)	Absent or severely reduced lymphocytes and no antibody production	Replacement is required prior to HSCT	If B-cell reconstitution fails, replacement may still be required after HSCT
NEMO deficiency	Reduced IgG; IgA or IgM may be increased; B cells present	Replacement is required	Cessation inappropriate except after successful HSCT
X-linked lymphoproliferative syndromes	May have reduced B cells and low IgG and IgA levels post EBV infection	Consider replacement	Cessation inappropriate unless HSCT is successful
Hyper-IgE syndromes	IgE elevated, sometimes reduced class switching and low levels of IgA and IgG subclasses with poor antibody responses	Replacement in selected patients	Cessation inappropriate if antibody failure confirmed
Wiskott-Aldrich syndrome	Decreased lymphocytes, variable defects in T-, B-, and NK-cell function, variable IgM, normal or elevated IgA, elevated IgG and IgE, often abnormal IgG antibody response to unconjugated polysaccharide vaccines	Consider replacement	Cessation inappropriate if antibody failure confirmed until successful HSCT

(continued)

Table 17.5 (continued)

Primary immunodeficiency	Immunologic findings	Immunoglobulin replacement	Immunoglobulin cessation
Ataxia-telangiectasia	Partial antibody deficiency in some cases	Replacement in selected patients	Cessation inappropriate if antibody failure confirmed
Hyper-IgM syndromes	Normal or elevated IgM, low or absent IgG, IgA and IgE, poor specific antibodies, variable T-cell abnormalities	Start replacement at the time of diagnosis until successful HSCT	Cessation inappropriate

Modified from Peter and Chapel, Immunotherapy 2014; 6: 853–869, Albin and Cunningham-Rundles, Immunotherapy 2014; 6: 1113–1126

EBV Epstein-Barr virus, *HSCT* human stem cell transplantation, *NEMO* NF-κB essential modulator

Table 17.6 Recommendations for the use of immunoglobulins in immune deficiencies

Benefit	Disease
Definitely beneficial	Primary immune defects with absent B cells
	Primary immune defects with hypogammaglobulinemia and impaired specific antibody production
Probably beneficial	Chronic lymphocytic leukemia with reduced IgG and history of infections
	Prevention of bacterial infections in HIV-infected children
	Primary immune defects with normo-gammaglobulinemia and impaired specific antibody production
Unlikely to be beneficial	Isolated IgA deficiency
	Isolated IgG4 deficiency

The recommendations for immunoglobulin indications according to the Primary Immunodeficiencies Committee of the American Academy of Allergy, Asthma, and Immunology; 2006

Administration of IVIG in CLL patients with hypogammaglobulinemia has been shown to decrease the rate of bacterial infections; however, decision analysis modeling showed that this decrease might not improve the length or quality of treated patients' lives, and, furthermore, it is extraordinarily expensive [110]. The prophylactic administration of IVIG in CLL patients has not been studied extensively, and, thus, there are no guidelines to define the patient population that would benefit from this treatment; also the optimal dosing and timing of IVIG administration remained to be defined. Some experts support the use of IVIG in selected cases, depending on the history of the patient and especially in patients that IVIG has been shown to work in the past.

IVIG therapy together with antiviral therapy was beneficial in infants and children with AIDS and hypogammaglobulinemia or two or more bacterial infections in the previous year. Other indications for IVIG therapy in HIV-infected patients include those with severe parvovirus B19 or measles infection [72, 95, 119]. However, it is important to note that these studies occurred before the era of highly active antiretroviral treatment for HIV [84].

Transplantation

IVIG has been utilized in allogeneic bone marrow transplantation (BMT) in an attempt to decrease the incidence of cytomegalovirus (CMV) infection, infections due to other pathogens, and graft-versus-host disease (GVHD). Immunoglobulin use in the setting of BMT is FDA approved. The rationale for using IVIG in transplantation is that the administration of passive antibodies may prevent infections in these immunocompromised patients and especially infections caused by CMV [84]. Several randomized controlled trials provided the basis to recommend IVIG after allogeneic BMT [19, 31, 46, 87, 98, 116, 117]. Meta-analysis of these trials found significant reduction of fatal CMV infections, CMV pneumonia, non-CMV interstitial pneumonia, and transplant-related mortality among patients receiving prophylactic IVIG [11]. While an improvement in survival was reported in some studies [46, 49, 118], a more recent meta-analysis showed that IVIG or hyperimmune CMV-IVIG had no effect on the reduction of all-cause mortality [90]. Collectively, the data regarding the benefit of prophylactic administration of IVIG after BMT remain controversial and contradictory. In addition, until currently, there is no consensus on the type, schedule, dose, and patients benefiting from IVIG. Subsequent studies suggested that double prophylaxis consisting of high-dose IVIG and ganciclovir was more successful than either treatment alone in reversing CMV pneumonia in patients after BMT [39, 69].

The American Society for Blood and Marrow Transplantation does not recommend the routine use of IVIG to hematopoietic cell transplant recipients for prophylaxis for CMV disease or for bacterial infections within the first 100 days after transplantation. For patients with severe hypogammaglobulinemia (IgG <400 mg/dl), IVIG prophylaxis of bacterial infections may be considered. IVIG dose and frequency for these patients should be individualized to maintain trough serum IgG concentrations >400 mg/dl [103]. Routine use of IVIG appears to offer little benefit to patients with malignancies undergoing HLA-identical sibling BMT [84]. Given that the landscape of patients receiving BMT is evolving, it is likely that the available data are outdated, and more updated randomized trials are warranted to inform clinical practice.

GVHD and infection are major complications of allogeneic BMT. In vitro and in vivo experimental models showed that the prevention of acute GVHD by IVIG is mediated by the induction of apoptosis of activated alloreactive CD4+ expressing CD134+ donor T cells and reducing the amount of IFN-γ produced by donor T cells [22]. IVIG was shown to decrease the severity of acute GVHD in recipients of allogeneic BMT [98, 116, 117]. On the contrary, administration of IVIG prophylaxis has no effect on the incidence or mortality of chronic GVHD on BMT [99]. While there is no consensus on the optimal dose of IVIG, it appears that the incidence of acute GVHD is less in patients receiving higher doses

of IVIG. The benefits of IVIG appear to correlate with IgG trough levels where acute GVHD was less frequent among patients achieving maximum serum IgG levels ≥3000 mg/dl after the administration of IVIG. Trough serum IgG levels >1200 mg/dl were associated with less severe acute GVHD [1, 33, 40].

Over the last decade, IVIG usage in solid organ transplantation has increased significantly. There are encouraging data on the role of IVIG for the treatment of antibody-mediated rejection, desensitization to HLA and/or ABO antigens, as well as prevention and treatment of infectious complications for patients undergoing solid organ transplantation [74, 94]. There is also some evidence that IVIG may be useful for the treatment of autoimmune cytopenias after solid organ transplantation [91]. Dosing of IVIG is empiric although higher than those for replacement therapy. Especially for the treatment of antibody-mediated rejection, the dose is 1–2 gm/kg [23, 38, 58, 60, 61, 76]. The use of higher doses of IVIG is related to higher rates of adverse events. These include aseptic meningitis thrombotic events and bronchospasm [59].

Immunoglobulin Therapy for Sepsis and Septic Shock

Sepsis is the systemic inflammatory response of the host to an infectious insult. Severe sepsis is characterized by acute organ dysfunction, while septic shock is characterized by hypotension, which is refractory to fluid replacement, or by hyperlactatemia [9]. Severe sepsis and septic shock represent one of the oldest and most pressing problems in medicine. Care of patients with sepsis has improved over the last decades; however, the incidence of sepsis is increasing along with morbidity and mortality rates especially in critically ill adults. Worldwide, the annual incidence of severe sepsis lies between 100 and 300 cases per 100,000 population, and mortality for severe sepsis and septic shock reaches 30% and 50%, respectively [8, 56, 73, 109]. While our understanding of the underlying biologic features of sepsis has made significant progress, the clinical assessment of several new strategies for implementation for sepsis treatment has led to disappointing results [3, 7, 15, 18, 108]. There have been more than 100 randomized clinical trials of strategies to modify the systemic inflammatory response during sepsis; however, no strategy showed to improve dramatically the survival of patients with sepsis [71].

The development of highly purified human plasma-derived polyclonal IVIGs presented a very compelling therapy for severe infections including sepsis and septic shock. IVIGs have broad and potent activity against microorganisms, their extracellular products, and potent immunomodulatory effects [78]. IVIG preparations, in particular IgM-enriched preparations, contain antibodies against lipopolysaccharides of *Escherichia coli*, *Pseudomonas aeruginosa*, and *Klebsiella* spp. [104]. The effects of IVIGs on the sepsis-induced host response seem to be pleotropic, not yet completely clarified, and are likely to be secondary to both suppression of synthesis and direct scavenging of upstream and downstream mediators of the host response and complex immunomodulatory effects [93].

The cellular effects of immunoglobulins are mediated through the IgG constant fragment (Fc). Immunoglobulin acts as an adaptor between the innate and adaptive immune system by interacting with Fc, which mediate both pro- and anti-inflammatory signals. IVIGs have direct antibacterial effects through pathogen recognition and increased clearance. IVIGs also have anti-inflammatory properties mediated by the scavenging of bacterial toxins and pro-inflammatory cytokines, by immune cell depletion, by the blockade of activating receptors, and by modulating FcγR expression, dendritic cell activity, and T-cell expansion [77, 92, 93].

The challenging pathobiology of sepsis is associated with acquired hypogammaglobulinemia, which seems to prevent optimal pathogen clearance and pathogen toxin scavenging [100, 107, 113]. Furthermore, sepsis, by causing endothelial dysfunction and capillary leak together with the iatrogenic fluid resuscitation-related increase in extravascular volume, eventually causes an alteration in the distribution of immunoglobulins [93]. Consequently, it is logical to predict that the administration of IVIG during sepsis would be of benefit.

In the clinical setting, the role of IVIG as an adjunctive treatment in sepsis has been controversial for years. A number of randomized placebo-controlled clinical trials in adult critical care patients evaluating standard polyclonal IVIG- or IgM-enriched polyclonal adjunctive therapy in severe sepsis as well as the meta-analyses of these trials have been published [5, 65, 67, 75, 88, 105]. Positive findings of controlled trials and anecdotal reports have been criticized for methodological weakness including the small number of the patients and adequacy of blinding. The more recent studies, which were more meticulously designed, have shown much less effect of IVIG than older, smaller, and less well-designed studies [50]. Of note, the studies that used albumin as control showed less benefit of IVIG than those that did not [41]. The Score-Based Immunoglobulin G Treatment in Sepsis (SBITS) study, one carefully designed, large study representing almost half of all the adults studied to date, showed no reduction in mortality by IVIG in patients with score-defined sepsis and sepsis-induced multi-organ failure [113].

The first clinical trial, which evaluated the effect of IgMA-enriched immunoglobulin preparation (7.8 g IgM, 7.8 g IgA, and 49.4 g IgG), which have shown to contain superior antibody content against bacterial lipopolysaccharides, in an appreciable number of neutropenic patients with hematologic malignancies and sepsis or septic shock, showed that immunoglobulins had no beneficial effects [51]. However, as the editor comments, the study, with a high evidence level, demonstrates that neutropenic patients with malignancies and low-grade sepsis with no or only one organ failure will not benefit from adjunctive IVIG treatment [111].

The prophylaxis and treatment of neonatal sepsis has been a major global priority, and large international trials have been carried out testing IVIG ([57, 79–83]; Group et al. 2011). Mortality during hospital stay in infants with clinically suspected infection at trial entry was not significantly different after IVIG treatment [81]. The results of the International Neonatal Immunotherapy Study (INIS) and recent meta-analyses showed that IVIG did not reduce mortality during hospital stay or major disability at 2 years of age in infants with sepsis [48, 83]. Based on the results of the INIS trial (3493 subjects), routine administration of IVIG to prevent mortality in infants with sepsis is not currently recommended [48].

When considering the administration of IVIG during sepsis, important aspects that should be taken into account are the dose, the type, the timing, and pharmacokinetics of IVIG [6, 50]. While dose-ranging studies have not been completed, studies that used high (>1 g/kg body weight) doses of IVIG demonstrated better effects. This seems plausible given the clinical observations in other inflammatory conditions, such as Kawasaki disease, where greater effect was noted with higher doses [52]. The type of IVIG may have an important effect, possibly in favor of a greater pooled effect of IgMA-enriched compared with standard preparations of IVIG. IgMA-enriched preparations are associated with greater complement inactivation and improvement in microvascular perfusion in experimental models [112]. However, collectively, the results from animal models and in vitro experiments show contradictory results and do not allow for a definite conclusion regarding the superiority of one specific immunoglobulin preparation in patients with sepsis. In an efficacy study, administration of polyvalent IgG versus IgMA in selected patients at high risk for sepsis was associated with a comparable improvement in disease severity [89].

Regarding the timing of IVIG administration during sepsis, there is probably a "window of opportunity" in the first days that follow clinical presentation of sepsis [14]. If this window is missed, probabilities of success could be greatly diminished [6]. Pharmacokinetic studies of IVIG in sepsis have not been performed yet. Data for dosage selection in current practice are primarily derived from studies in volunteers and in patients with primary immune deficiencies and other indications for immunomodulation. Existing pharmacokinetic studies also do not address immunoglobulin clearance or area under the curve parameters and target serum immunoglobulin concentrations [64]. In addition, it is still unknown whether the main goal of IVIG in sepsis is to refill low levels of endogenous immunoglobulins or alternatively whether IVIG could exert a beneficial effect regardless of these levels [6].

Most studies evaluating the use of IVIG for sepsis are small; some have methodological flaws and high-quality, large studies showed no effect [48, 113]. Given immunoglobulin high-cost, limited supply and the lack of strong evidence to support their beneficial effect, widely used guidelines either neglect or grade as a weak recommendation the use of polyclonal IVIG in sepsis [36]. While clinical judgment may guide immunoglobulin use in individual cases, particularly those due to Gram-negative etiologies or streptococcal toxic shock syndrome, these practices are based largely on theoretical rationale, anecdotal, and retrospective clinical observations [50, 66, 106].

The effect of monoclonal antibodies against tumor necrosis factor (TNF)-α has been evaluated in a series of trials on different anti-TNF-α-directed therapies [4, 30, 37, 42]. The long-anticipated sepsis trial (MONARCS [Monoclonal Anti-TNF, A Randomized Controlled Sepsis trial]) reported that afelimomab, which is made up of the Fab component of a monoclonal antibody against TNF-α, in patients with severe sepsis and elevated IL-6 levels decreased mortality and had a safety profile similar to placebo [85]. However, combining the results of these studies, a small improvement in mortality can be detected [34, 47]. As sepsis is increasingly being considered as an exaggerated, poorly regulated innate immune response to microbial products, by the time of diagnosis, an entire network of cytokines has already been activated. In this regard, the results of the previous studies would have been anticipated, as it seems unlikely that therapy aimed at only one cytokine would by itself have the highly significantly impact on sepsis mortality [34].

Future Directions

Immunoglobulins have been used widely in medicine for a variety of diseases including infectious diseases. While the two major indications for immunoglobulin use are as replacement and anti-inflammatory therapy in a variety of acute and chronic autoimmune diseases, their use in the prevention and treatment of infectious diseases is emerging as an attractive option especially in the era of multi-antibiotic resistance. Many aspects of immunoglobulin therapy remain controversial and contradictory. Consequently, immunoglobulin use is sometimes determined by clinical judgment or expert opinion, which is based largely on theoretical rationale, anecdotal, and retrospective clinical observations. Gaps of knowledge that need to be addressed are certain categories of patient populations that would benefit from immunoglobulin treatment or prophylaxis, the optimal immunoglobulin dosing, and duration, as well as timing of administration.

Monoclonal antibody technology has opened a new era in antibody therapy. On many occasions, human monoclonal antibodies have better therapeutic properties than immunoglobulins including low toxicity, longer protective immunity, higher than natural protection, and high specificity. Several antibodies for the treatment of bacterial and viral infections have been developed [101]. However, some challenges need to be overcome before they become preferred agents for the treatment and prophylaxis against infectious diseases.

Biofilms are now acknowledged to contribute to a plethora of chronic and recurrent infections. While treatment or eradication of biofilm-related infections is still challenging, there are sufficient in vitro and preclinical data to support the use of antibodies directed against extracellular DNA-binding proteins entrapped into the extracellular biofilm polymeric substance [20, 44]. While still an area of ongoing preclinical and clinical research, this use of antibodies constitutes a novel therapeutic approach for treatment of biofilm-related infections.

References

1. Abdel-Mageed A, Graham-Pole J, Del Rosario ML, Longmate J, Ochoa S, Amylon M, et al. Comparison of two doses of intravenous immunoglobulin after allogeneic bone marrow transplants. Bone Marrow Transplant. 1999;23(9):929–32. https://doi.org/10.1038/sj.bmt.1701742.
2. Abolhassani H, Asgardoon MH, Rezaei N, Hammarstrom L, Aghamohammadi A. Different brands of intravenous immunoglobulin for primary immunodeficiencies: how to choose the best option for the patient? Expert Rev Clin Immunol. 2015;11(11):1229–43. https://doi.org/10.1586/1744666X.2015.1079485.
3. Abraham E, Reinhart K, Opal S, Demeyer I, Doig C, Rodriguez AL, et al. Efficacy and safety of tifacogin (recombinant tissue factor pathway inhibitor) in severe sepsis: a randomized controlled trial. JAMA. 2003;290(2):238–47. https://doi.org/10.1001/jama.290.2.238.
4. Abraham E, Wunderink R, Silverman H, Perl TM, Nasraway S, Levy H, et al. Efficacy and safety of monoclonal antibody to human tumor necrosis factor alpha in patients with sepsis syndrome. A randomized, controlled, double-blind, multicenter clinical trial. TNF-alpha MAb Sepsis Study Group. JAMA. 1995;273(12):934–41.
5. Alejandria MM, Lansang MA, Dans LF, Mantaring JB. Intravenous immunoglobulin for treating sepsis and septic shock. Cochrane Database Syst Rev. 2002;1:CD001090. https://doi.org/10.1002/14651858.CD001090.
6. Almansa R, Tamayo E, Andaluz-Ojeda D, Nogales L, Blanco J, Eiros JM, et al. The original sins of clinical trials with intravenous immunoglobulins in sepsis. Crit Care. 2015;19:90. https://doi.org/10.1186/s13054-015-0793-0.
7. Angus DC, Birmingham MC, Balk RA, Scannon PJ, Collins D, Kruse JA, et al. E5 murine monoclonal antiendotoxin antibody in gram-negative sepsis: a randomized controlled trial. E5 Study Investigators. JAMA. 2000;283(13):1723–30.
8. Angus DC, Linde-Zwirble WT, Lidicker J, Clermont G, Carcillo J, Pinsky MR. Epidemiology of severe sepsis in the United States: analysis of incidence, outcome, and associated costs of care. Crit Care Med. 2001;29(7):1303–10.
9. Angus DC, van der Poll T. Severe sepsis and septic shock. N Engl J Med. 2013;369(9):840–51. https://doi.org/10.1056/NEJMra1208623.
10. Ballow M, Notarangelo L, Grimbacher B, Cunningham-Rundles C, Stein M, Helbert M, et al. Immunodeficiencies. Clin Exp Immunol. 2009;158(Suppl 1):14–22. https://doi.org/10.1111/j.1365-2249.2009.04023.x.
11. Bass EB, Powe NR, Goodman SN, Graziano SL, Griffiths RI, Kickler TS, et al. Efficacy of immune globulin in preventing complications of bone mar-

row transplantation: a meta-analysis. Bone Marrow Transplant. 1993;12(3):273–82.

12. Berger M. Goals of therapy in antibody deficiency syndromes. J Allergy Clin Immunol. 1999;104(5):911–3.

13. Berger M. Principles of and advances in immunoglobulin replacement therapy for primary immunodeficiency. Immunol Allergy Clin N Am. 2008;28(2):413–37., x. https://doi.org/10.1016/j.iac.2008.01.008.

14. Berlot G, Vassallo MC, Busetto N, Bianchi M, Zornada F, Rosato I, et al. Relationship between the timing of administration of IgM and IgA enriched immunoglobulins in patients with severe sepsis and septic shock and the outcome: a retrospective analysis. J Crit Care. 2012;27(2):167–71. https://doi.org/10.1016/j.jcrc.2011.05.012.

15. Bernard GR, Wheeler AP, Russell JA, Schein R, Summer WR, Steinberg KP, et al. The effects of ibuprofen on the physiology and survival of patients with sepsis. The Ibuprofen in Sepsis Study Group. N Engl J Med. 1997;336(13):912–8. https://doi.org/10.1056/NEJM199703273361303.

16. Bonagura VR. Using intravenous immunoglobulin (IVIG) to treat patients with primary immune deficiency disease. J Clin Immunol. 2013;33(Suppl 2):S90–4. https://doi.org/10.1007/s10875-012-9838-1.

17. Bonagura VR, Marchlewski R, Cox A, Rosenthal DW. Biologic IgG level in primary immunodeficiency disease: the IgG level that protects against recurrent infection. J Allergy Clin Immunol. 2008;122(1):210–2. https://doi.org/10.1016/j.jaci.2008.04.044.

18. Bone RC, Fisher CJ Jr, Clemmer TP, Slotman GJ, Metz CA, Balk RA. A controlled clinical trial of high-dose methylprednisolone in the treatment of severe sepsis and septic shock. N Engl J Med. 1987;317(11):653–8. https://doi.org/10.1056/NEJM198709103171101.

19. Bowden RA, Sayers M, Flournoy N, Newton B, Banaji M, Thomas ED, et al. Cytomegalovirus immune globulin and seronegative blood products to prevent primary cytomegalovirus infection after marrow transplantation. N Engl J Med. 1986;314(16):1006–10. https://doi.org/10.1056/NEJM198604173141602.

20. Brockson ME, Novotny LA, Mokrzan EM, Malhotra S, Jurcisek JA, Akbar R, et al. Evaluation of the kinetics and mechanism of action of anti-integration host factor-mediated disruption of bacterial biofilms. Mol Microbiol. 2014;93(6):1246–58. https://doi.org/10.1111/mmi.12735.

21. Bruton OC. Agammaglobulinemia. Pediatrics. 1952;9(6):722–8.

22. Caccavelli L, Field AC, Betin V, Dreillard L, Belair MF, Bloch MF, et al. Normal IgG protects against acute graft-versus-host disease by targeting CD4(+)CD134(+) donor alloreactive T cells. Eur J Immunol. 2001;31(9):2781–90. https://doi.

23. Casadei DH, CRM D, Opelz G, Golberg JC, Argento JA, Greco G, et al. A randomized and prospective study comparing treatment with high-dose intravenous immunoglobulin with monoclonal antibodies for rescue of kidney grafts with steroid-resistant rejection. Transplantation. 2001;71(1):53–8.

24. Casadevall A, Dadachova E, Pirofski LA. Passive antibody therapy for infectious diseases. Nat Rev Microbiol. 2004;2(9):695–703. https://doi.org/10.1038/nrmicro974.

25. Casadevall A, Pirofski LA. Antibody-mediated regulation of cellular immunity and the inflammatory response. Trends Immunol. 2003;24(9):474–8.

26. Casadevall A, Pirofski LA. A reappraisal of humoral immunity based on mechanisms of antibody-mediated protection against intracellular pathogens. Adv Immunol. 2006;91:1–44. https://doi.org/10.1016/S0065-2776(06)91001-3.

27. Casadevall A, Scharff MD. Serum therapy revisited: animal models of infection and development of passive antibody therapy. Antimicrob Agents Chemother. 1994;38(8):1695–702.

28. Casadevall A, Scharff MD. Return to the past: the case for antibody-based therapies in infectious diseases. Clin Infect Dis. 1995;21(1):150–61.

29. Chapel H, Dicato M, Gamm H, Brennan V, Ries F, Bunch C, et al. Immunoglobulin replacement in patients with chronic lymphocytic leukaemia: a comparison of two dose regimes. Br J Haematol. 1994;88(1):209–12.

30. Cohen J, Carlet J. INTERSEPT: an international, multicenter, placebo-controlled trial of monoclonal antibody to human tumor necrosis factor-alpha in patients with sepsis. International Sepsis Trial Study Group. Crit Care Med. 1996;24(9):1431–40.

31. Condie RM, O'Reilly RJ. Prevention of cytomegalovirus infection by prophylaxis with an intravenous, hyperimmune, native, unmodified cytomegalovirus globulin. Randomized trial in bone marrow transplant recipients. Am J Med. 1984;76(3A):134–41.

32. Condino-Neto A, Costa-Carvalho BT, Grumach AS, King A, Bezrodnik L, Oleastro M, et al. Guidelines for the use of human immunoglobulin therapy in patients with primary immunodeficiencies in Latin America. Allergol Immunopathol (Madr). 2014;42(3):245–60. https://doi.org/10.1016/j.aller.2012.09.006.

33. Cottler-Fox M, Lynch M, Pickle LW, Cahill R, Spitzer TR, Deeg HJ. Some but not all benefits of intravenous immunoglobulin therapy after marrow transplantation appear to correlate with IgG trough levels. Bone Marrow Transplant. 1991;8(1):27–33.

34. Cross AS, Opal SM. A new paradigm for the treatment of sepsis: is it time to consider combination therapy? Ann Intern Med. 2003;138(6):502–5.

35. Cunningham-Rundles C. Key aspects for successful immunoglobulin therapy of primary immunodeficiencies. Clin Exp Immunol.

2011;164(Suppl 2):16–9. https://doi.org/10.1111/j.1365-2249.2011.04390.x.

36. Dellinger RP, Levy MM, Rhodes A, Annane D, Gerlach H, Opal SM, et al. Surviving Sepsis Campaign: international guidelines for management of severe sepsis and septic shock, 2012. Intensive Care Med. 2013;39(2):165–228. https://doi.org/10.1007/s00134-012-2769-8.

37. Dhainaut JF, Vincent JL, Richard C, Lejeune P, Martin C, Fierobe L, et al. CDP571, a humanized antibody to human tumor necrosis factor-alpha: safety, pharmacokinetics, immune response, and influence of the antibody on cytokine concentrations in patients with septic shock. CPD571 Sepsis Study Group. Crit Care Med. 1995;23(9):1461–9.

38. Durandy A, Kaveri SV, Kuijpers TW, Basta M, Miescher S, Ravetch JV, et al. Intravenous immunoglobulins – understanding properties and mechanisms. Clin Exp Immunol. 2009;158(Suppl 1):2–13. https://doi.org/10.1111/j.1365-2249.2009.04022.x.

39. Emanuel D, Cunningham I, Jules-Elysee K, Brochstein JA, Kernan NA, Laver J, et al. Cytomegalovirus pneumonia after bone marrow transplantation successfully treated with the combination of ganciclovir and high-dose intravenous immune globulin. Ann Intern Med. 1988;109(10):777–82.

40. Feinstein LC, Seidel K, Jocum J, Bowden RA, Anasetti C, Deeg HJ, et al. Reduced dose intravenous immunoglobulin does not decrease transplant-related complications in adults given related donor marrow allografts. Biol Blood Marrow Transplant. 1999;5(6):369–78.

41. Finfer S, Bellomo R, Boyce N, French J, Myburgh J, Norton R, et al. A comparison of albumin and saline for fluid resuscitation in the intensive care unit. N Engl J Med. 2004;350(22):2247–56. https://doi.org/10.1056/NEJMoa040232.

42. Fisher CJ Jr, Opal SM, Dhainaut JF, Stephens S, Zimmerman JL, Nightingale P, et al. Influence of an anti-tumor necrosis factor monoclonal antibody on cytokine levels in patients with sepsis. The CB0006 Sepsis Syndrome Study Group. Crit Care Med. 1993;21(3):318–27.

43. Flexner S. The results of the serum treatment in thirteen hundred cases of epidemic meningitis. J Exp Med. 1913;17(5):553–76.

44. Goodman SD, Obergfell KP, Jurcisek JA, Novotny LA, Downey JS, Ayala EA, et al. Biofilms can be dispersed by focusing the immune system on a common family of bacterial nucleoid-associated proteins. Mucosal Immunol. 2011;4(6):625–37. https://doi.org/10.1038/mi.2011.27.

45. Graham BS, Ambrosino DM. History of passive antibody administration for prevention and treatment of infectious diseases. Curr Opin HIV AIDS. 2015;10(3):129–34. https://doi.org/10.1097/COH.0000000000000154.

46. Graham-Pole J, Camitta B, Casper J, Elfenbein G, Gross S, Herzig R, et al. Intravenous immuno-globulin may lessen all forms of infection in patients receiving allogeneic bone marrow transplantation for acute lymphoblastic leukemia: a pediatric oncology group study. Bone Marrow Transplant. 1988;3(6):559–66.

47. Grass G, Neugebauer EA. Afelimomab-another therapeutic option in sepsis therapy? Crit Care Med. 2004;32(11):2343–4.

48. Group IC, Brocklehurst P, Farrell B, King A, Juszczak E, Darlow B, et al. Treatment of neonatal sepsis with intravenous immune globulin. N Engl J Med. 2011;365(13):1201–11. https://doi.org/10.1056/NEJMoa1100441.

49. Guglielmo BJ, Wong-Beringer A, Linker CA. Immune globulin therapy in allogeneic bone marrow transplant: a critical review. Bone Marrow Transplant. 1994;13(5):499–510.

50. Hartung HP, Mouthon L, Ahmed R, Jordan S, Laupland KB, Jolles S. Clinical applications of intravenous immunoglobulins (IVIg) – beyond immunodeficiencies and neurology. Clin Exp Immunol. 2009;158(Suppl 1):23–33. https://doi.org/10.1111/j.1365-2249.2009.04024.x.

51. Hentrich M, Fehnle K, Ostermann H, Kienast J, Cornely O, Salat C, et al. IgMA-enriched immunoglobulin in neutropenic patients with sepsis syndrome and septic shock: a randomized, controlled, multiple-center trial. Crit Care Med. 2006;34(5):1319–25. https://doi.org/10.1097/01.CCM.0000215452.84291.C6.

52. Imbach P, Barandun S, d'Apuzzo V, Baumgartner C, Hirt A, Morell A, et al. High-dose intravenous gammaglobulin for idiopathic thrombocytopenic purpura in childhood. Lancet. 1981;1(8232):1228–31.

53. The National Institute of Child Health and Human Developments Intravenous Immunoglobulin Study Group. Intravenous immune globulin for the prevention of bacterial infections in children with symptomatic human immunodeficiency virus infection. N Engl J Med. 1991;325(2):73–80. https://doi.org/10.1056/NEJM199107113250201.

54. Cooperative Group for the Study of Immunoglobulin in Chronic Lymphocytic Leukemia. Intravenous immunoglobulin for the prevention of infection in chronic lymphocytic leukemia. A randomized, controlled clinical trial. N Engl J Med. 1988;319(14):902–7. https://doi.org/10.1056/NEJM198810063191403.

55. Irani V, Guy AJ, Andrew D, Beeson JG, Ramsland PA, Richards JS. Molecular properties of human IgG subclasses and their implications for designing therapeutic monoclonal antibodies against infectious diseases. Mol Immunol. 2015;67(2 Pt A):171–82. https://doi.org/10.1016/j.molimm.2015.03.255.

56. Iwashyna TJ, Ely EW, Smith DM, Langa KM. Long-term cognitive impairment and functional disability among survivors of severe sepsis. JAMA. 2010;304(16):1787–94. https://doi.org/10.1001/jama.2010.1553.

57. Jenson HB, Pollock BH. The role of intravenous immunoglobulin for the prevention and treatment of neonatal sepsis. Semin Perinatol. 1998;22(1):50–63.

58. Jordan SC, Quartel AW, Czer LS, Admon D, Chen G, Fishbein MC, et al. Posttransplant therapy using high-dose human immunoglobulin (intravenous gammaglobulin) to control acute humoral rejection in renal and cardiac allograft recipients and potential mechanism of action. Transplantation. 1998;66(6):800–5.

59. Jordan SC, Toyoda M, Kahwaji J, Vo AA. Clinical aspects of intravenous immunoglobulin use in solid organ transplant recipients. Am J Transplant. 2011;11(2):196–202. https://doi.org/10.1111/j.1600-6143.2010.03400.x.

60. Jordan SC, Toyoda M, Vo AA. Intravenous immunoglobulin a natural regulator of immunity and inflammation. Transplantation. 2009;88(1):1–6. https://doi.org/10.1097/TP.0b013e3181a9e89a.

61. Jordan SC, Tyan D, Stablein D, McIntosh M, Rose S, Vo A, et al. Evaluation of intravenous immunoglobulin as an agent to lower allosensitization and improve transplantation in highly sensitized adult patients with end-stage renal disease: report of the NIH IG02 trial. J Am Soc Nephrol. 2004;15(12):3256–62. https://doi.org/10.1097/01.ASN.0000145878.92906.9F.

62. Keller MA, Stiehm ER. Passive immunity in prevention and treatment of infectious diseases. Clin Microbiol Rev. 2000;13(4):602–14.

63. Kohler G, Milstein C. Continuous cultures of fused cells secreting antibody of predefined specificity. Nature. 1975;256(5517):495–7.

64. Koleba T, Ensom MH. Pharmacokinetics of intravenous immunoglobulin: a systematic review. Pharmacotherapy. 2006;26(6):813–27. https://doi.org/10.1592/phco.26.6.813.

65. Kreymann KG, de Heer G, Nierhaus A, Kluge S. Use of polyclonal immunoglobulins as adjunctive therapy for sepsis or septic shock. Crit Care Med. 2007;35(12):2677–85.

66. Laupland KB, Boucher P, Rotstein C, Cook DJ, Doig CJ. Intravenous immunoglobulin for severe infections: a survey of Canadian specialists. J Crit Care. 2004;19(2):75–81.

67. Laupland KB, Kirkpatrick AW, Delaney A. Polyclonal intravenous immunoglobulin for the treatment of severe sepsis and septic shock in critically ill adults: a systematic review and meta-analysis. Crit Care Med. 2007;35(12):2686–92.

68. Lindenmann J. Origin of the terms 'antibody' and 'antigen'. Scand J Immunol. 1984;19(4):281–5.

69. Ljungman P, Engelhard D, Link H, Biron P, Brandt L, Brunet S, et al. Treatment of interstitial pneumonitis due to cytomegalovirus with ganciclovir and intravenous immune globulin: experience of European Bone Marrow Transplant Group. Clin Infect Dis. 1992;14(4):831–5.

70. Llewelyn MB, Hawkins RE, Russell SJ. Discovery of antibodies. BMJ. 1992;305(6864):1269–72.

71. Marshall JC. Why have clinical trials in sepsis failed? Trends Mol Med. 2014;20(4):195–203. https://doi.org/10.1016/j.molmed.2014.01.007.

72. Mofenson LM, Moye J Jr, Korelitz J, Bethel J, Hirschhorn R, Nugent R. Crossover of placebo patients to intravenous immunoglobulin confirms efficacy for prophylaxis of bacterial infections and reduction of hospitalizations in human immunodeficiency virus-infected children. The National Institute of Child Health and Human Development Intravenous Immunoglobulin Clinical Trial Study Group. Pediatr Infect Dis J. 1994;13(6):477–84.

73. Moss M. Epidemiology of sepsis: race, sex, and chronic alcohol abuse. Clin Infect Dis. 2005;41(Suppl 7):S490–7. https://doi.org/10.1086/432003.

74. Nahirniak S, Hume HA. Guidelines for the use of immunoglobulin therapy for primary immune deficiency and solid organ transplantation. Transfus Med Rev. 2010;24(Suppl 1):S1–6. https://doi.org/10.1016/j.tmrv.2009.09.009.

75. Neilson AR, Burchardi H, Schneider H. Cost-effectiveness of immunoglobulin M-enriched immunoglobulin (Pentaglobin) in the treatment of severe sepsis and septic shock. J Crit Care. 2005;20(3):239–49. https://doi.org/10.1016/j.jcrc.2005.03.003.

76. Nimmerjahn F, Ravetch JV. Anti-inflammatory actions of intravenous immunoglobulin. Annu Rev Immunol. 2008a;26:513–33. https://doi.org/10.1146/annurev.immunol.26.021607.090232.

77. Nimmerjahn F, Ravetch JV. Fcgamma receptors as regulators of immune responses. Nat Rev Immunol. 2008b;8(1):34–47. https://doi.org/10.1038/nri2206.

78. Norrby-Teglund A, Haque KN, Hammarstrom L. Intravenous polyclonal IgM-enriched immunoglobulin therapy in sepsis: a review of clinical efficacy in relation to microbiological aetiology and severity of sepsis. J Intern Med. 2006;260(6):509–16. https://doi.org/10.1111/j.1365-2796.2006.01726.x.

79. Ohlsson A, Lacy JB. Intravenous immunoglobulin for preventing infection in preterm and/or low-birth-weight infants. Cochrane Database Syst Rev. 2004a;1:CD000361. https://doi.org/10.1002/14651858.CD000361.pub2.

80. Ohlsson A, Lacy JB. Intravenous immunoglobulin for suspected or subsequently proven infection in neonates. Cochrane Database Syst Rev. 2004b;1:CD001239. https://doi.org/10.1002/14651858.CD001239.pub2.

81. Ohlsson A, Lacy JB. Intravenous immunoglobulin for preventing infection in preterm and/or low birth weight infants. Cochrane Database Syst Rev. 2013a;7:CD000361. https://doi.org/10.1002/14651858.CD000361.pub3.

82. Ohlsson A, Lacy JB. Intravenous immunoglobulin for suspected or proven infection in neonates. Cochrane Database Syst Rev. 2013b;7:CD001239. https://doi.org/10.1002/14651858.CD001239.pub4.

83. Ohlsson A, Lacy JB. Intravenous immunoglobulin for suspected or proven infection in neonates.

Cochrane Database Syst Rev. 2015;3:CD001239. https://doi.org/10.1002/14651858.CD001239.pub5.

84. Orange JS, Hossny EM, Weiler CR, Ballow M, Berger M, Bonilla FA, et al. Use of intravenous immunoglobulin in human disease: a review of evidence by members of the Primary Immunodeficiency Committee of the American Academy of Allergy, Asthma and Immunology. J Allergy Clin Immunol. 2006;117(4 Suppl):S525–53. https://doi.org/10.1016/j.jaci.2006.01.015.

85. Panacek EA, Marshall JC, Albertson TE, Johnson DH, Johnson S, MacArthur RD, et al. Efficacy and safety of the monoclonal anti-tumor necrosis factor antibody F(ab')2 fragment afelimomab in patients with severe sepsis and elevated interleukin-6 levels. Crit Care Med. 2004;32(11):2173–82.

86. Peter JG, Chapel H. Immunoglobulin replacement therapy for primary immunodeficiencies. Immunotherapy. 2014;6(7):853–69. https://doi.org/10.2217/imt.14.54.

87. Petersen FB, Bowden RA, Thornquist M, Meyers JD, Buckner CD, Counts GW, et al. The effect of prophylactic intravenous immune globulin on the incidence of septicemia in marrow transplant recipients. Bone Marrow Transplant. 1987;2(2):141–7.

88. Pildal J, Gotzsche PC. Polyclonal immunoglobulin for treatment of bacterial sepsis: a systematic review. Clin Infect Dis. 2004;39(1):38–46. https://doi.org/10.1086/421089.

89. Pilz G, Appel R, Kreuzer E, Werdan K. Comparison of early IgM-enriched immunoglobulin vs polyvalent IgG administration in score-identified postcardiac surgical patients at high risk for sepsis. Chest. 1997;111(2):419–26.

90. Raanani P, Gafter-Gvili A, Paul M, Ben-Bassat I, Leibovici L, Shpilberg O. Immunoglobulin prophylaxis in hematological malignancies and hematopoietic stem cell transplantation. Cochrane Database Syst Rev. 2008;4:CD006501. https://doi.org/10.1002/14651858.CD006501.pub2.

91. Riechsteiner G, Speich R, Schanz U, Russi EW, Weder W, Boehler A. Haemolytic anaemia after lung transplantation: an immune-mediated phenomenon? Swiss Med Wkly. 2003;133(9–10):143–7. doi:2003/09/smw-10123

92. Schwab I, Nimmerjahn F. Intravenous immunoglobulin therapy: how does IgG modulate the immune system? Nat Rev Immunol. 2013;13(3):176–89. https://doi.org/10.1038/nri3401.

93. Shankar-Hari M, Spencer J, Sewell WA, Rowan KM, Singer M. Bench-to-bedside review: immunoglobulin therapy for sepsis – biological plausibility from a critical care perspective. Crit Care. 2012;16(2):206. https://doi.org/10.1186/cc10597.

94. Shehata N, Palda VA, Meyer RM, Blydt-Hansen TD, Campbell P, Cardella C, et al. The use of immunoglobulin therapy for patients undergoing solid organ transplantation: an evidence-based practice guideline. Transfus Med Rev. 2010;24(Suppl 1):S7–S27. https://doi.org/10.1016/j.tmrv.2009.09.010.

95. Spector SA, Gelber RD, McGrath N, Wara D, Barzilai A, Abrams E, et al. A controlled trial of intravenous immune globulin for the prevention of serious bacterial infections in children receiving zidovudine for advanced human immunodeficiency virus infection. Pediatric AIDS Clinical Trials Group. N Engl J Med. 1994;331(18):1181–7. https://doi.org/10.1056/NEJM199411033311802.

96. Stiehm ER, Ashida E, Kim KS, Winston DJ, Haas A, Gale RP. Intravenous immunoglobulins as therapeutic agents. Ann Intern Med. 1987;107(3):367–82.

97. Stiehm ER, Orange JS, Ballow M, Lehman H. Therapeutic use of immunoglobulins. Adv Pediatr Infect Dis. 2010;57(1):185–218. https://doi.org/10.1016/j.yapd.2010.08.005.

98. Sullivan KM, Kopecky KJ, Jocom J, Fisher L, Buckner CD, Meyers JD, et al. Immunomodulatory and antimicrobial efficacy of intravenous immunoglobulin in bone marrow transplantation. N Engl J Med. 1990;323(11):705–12. https://doi.org/10.1056/NEJM199009133231103.

99. Sullivan KM, Storek J, Kopecky KJ, Jocom J, Longton G, Flowers M, et al. A controlled trial of long-term administration of intravenous immunoglobulin to prevent late infection and chronic graft-vs.-host disease after marrow transplantation: clinical outcome and effect on subsequent immune recovery. Biol Blood Marrow Transplant. 1996;2(1):44–53.

100. Taccone FS, Stordeur P, De Backer D, Creteur J, Vincent JL. Gamma-globulin levels in patients with community-acquired septic shock. Shock. 2009;32(4):379–85. https://doi.org/10.1097/SHK.0b013e3181a2c0b2.

101. Ter Meulen J. Monoclonal antibodies in infectious diseases: clinical pipeline in 2011. Infect Dis Clin N Am. 2011;25(4):789–802. https://doi.org/10.1016/j.idc.2011.07.006.

102. Tha-In T, Bayry J, Metselaar HJ, Kaveri SV, Kwekkeboom J. Modulation of the cellular immune system by intravenous immunoglobulin. Trends Immunol. 2008;29(12):608–15. https://doi.org/10.1016/j.it.2008.08.004.

103. Tomblyn M, Chiller T, Einsele H, Gress R, Sepkowitz K, Storek J, et al. Guidelines for preventing infectious complications among hematopoietic cell transplantation recipients: a global perspective. Biol Blood Marrow Transplant. 2009;15(10):1143–238. https://doi.org/10.1016/j.bbmt.2009.06.019.

104. Trautmann M, Held TK, Susa M, Karajan MA, Wulf A, Cross AS, et al. Bacterial lipopolysaccharide (LPS)-specific antibodies in commercial human immunoglobulin preparations: superior antibody content of an IgM-enriched product. Clin Exp Immunol. 1998;111(1):81–90.

105. Turgeon AF, Hutton B, Fergusson DA, McIntyre L, Tinmouth AA, Cameron DW, et al. Meta-analysis: intravenous immunoglobulin in critically ill adult patients with sepsis. Ann Intern Med. 2007;146(3):193–203.

106. Valiquette L, Low DE, Chow R, McGeer AJ. A survey of physician's attitudes regarding management of severe group a streptococcal infections. Scand J Infect Dis. 2006;38(11–12):977–82. https://doi.org/10.1080/00365540600786499.

107. Venet F, Gebeile R, Bancel J, Guignant C, Poitevin-Later F, Malcus C, et al. Assessment of plasmatic immunoglobulin G, A and M levels in septic shock patients. Int Immunopharmacol. 2011;11(12):2086–90. https://doi.org/10.1016/j.intimp.2011.08.024.

108. Veterans Administration Systemic Sepsis Cooperative Study, G. Effect of high-dose glucocorticoid therapy on mortality in patients with clinical signs of systemic sepsis. N Engl J Med. 1987;317(11):659–65. https://doi.org/10.1056/NEJM198709103171102.

109. Vincent JL, Rello J, Marshall J, Silva E, Anzueto A, Martin CD, et al. International study of the prevalence and outcomes of infection in intensive care units. JAMA. 2009;302(21):2323–9. https://doi.org/10.1001/jama.2009.1754.

110. Weeks JC, Tierney MR, Weinstein MC. Cost effectiveness of prophylactic intravenous immune globulin in chronic lymphocytic leukemia. N Engl J Med. 1991;325(2):81–6. https://doi.org/10.1056/NEJM199107113250202.

111. Werdan K. Immunoglobulin treatment in sepsis – is the answer "no"? Crit Care Med. 2006;34(5):1542–4. https://doi.org/10.1097/01.CCM.0000216189.80613.BB.

112. Werdan K. Mirror, mirror on the wall, which is the fairest meta-analysis of all? Crit Care Med. 2007;35(12):2852–4. https://doi.org/10.1097/01.CCM.0000297164.40980.F0.

113. Werdan K, Pilz G, Bujdoso O, Fraunberger P, Neeser G, Schmieder RE, et al. Score-based immunoglobulin G therapy of patients with sepsis: the SBITS study. Crit Care Med. 2007;35(12):2693–701.

114. Wilcox MH, Gerding DN, Poxton IR, Kelly C, Nathan R, Birch T, et al. Bezlotoxumab for prevention of recurrent clostridium difficile infection. N Engl J Med. 2017;376(4):305–17. https://doi.org/10.1056/NEJMoa1602615.

115. Winau F, Winau R. Emil von Behring and serum therapy. Microbes Infect. 2002;4(2):185–8.

116. Winston DJ, Ho WG, Bartoni K, Champlin RE. Intravenous immunoglobulin and CMV-seronegative blood products for prevention of CMV infection and disease in bone marrow transplant recipients. Bone Marrow Transplant. 1993;12(3):283–8.

117. Winston DJ, Ho WG, Lin CH, Bartoni K, Budinger MD, Gale RP, et al. Intravenous immune globulin for prevention of cytomegalovirus infection and interstitial pneumonia after bone marrow transplantation. Ann Intern Med. 1987;106(1):12–8.

118. Wolff SN, Fay JW, Herzig RH, Greer JP, Dummer S, Brown RA, et al. High-dose weekly intravenous immunoglobulin to prevent infections in patients undergoing autologous bone marrow transplantation or severe myelosuppressive therapy. A study of the American Bone Marrow Transplant Group. Ann Intern Med. 1993;118(12):937–42.

119. Yap PL. Does intravenous immune globulin have a role in HIV-infected patients? Clin Exp Immunol. 1994;97(Suppl 1):59–67.

120. Stiehm EM, Keller MA. Passive immunization. In: Feigin RD, Cherry JD, Demmler-Harrison GJ, et al., editors. Textbook of pediatric infectious diseases. 6th ed. Philadelphia: Saunders/Elsevier; 2009. p. 3412–47.

Vaccines in the Immunocompromised Hosts

18

Paratosh Prasad and John Treanor

Introduction

Vaccination remains the single most effective means available to prevent infectious diseases and mitigate their impact on the health of individuals. However, conditions that result in impairment of adaptive immunity both increase the risk and severity of these infections, as well as decreasing the efficacy of immunizations, posing unique challenges to medical care of these vulnerable patients. In addition, the complex relationships between the immunity of the subject and the mechanisms by which vaccines stimulate the immune system raise safety concerns as well, particularly related to the safety of live vaccines in this population, and the possibility that non-specific stimulation of the immune system could precipitate transplant rejection or increasing autoimmunity.

In this brief review, we will discuss the evidence supporting safety, immunogenicity, and efficacy of selected commonly used vaccines specifically in immunocompromised patient populations. Although the prevalence of immunocompromising conditions and treatments is steadily increasing, in many cases relatively little data are available regarding vaccine performance in specific populations. Where available, existing guidelines for immunization of specific populations will also be referenced.

The term "immunocompromised" can be used to describe a wide variety of patient populations with both intrinsic and iatrogenic mechanisms of altered immunity. Consequently, the safety and immunogenicity of vaccines can vary widely according to the severity and mechanism of the immune compromising condition. This review will focus on two of the most common types of immunocompromise in the United States and other developed countries, infection with human immunodeficiency virus (HIV), and medical immunosuppression designed to combat organ rejection after solid organ transplantation (SOT) and graft-versus-host disease (GVHD) after allogeneic hematopoietic stem cell transplantation (HSCT).

Influenza Vaccine

Influenza has been shown to result in more severe disease and increased rates of complications in a variety of immunocompromising conditions, including transplantation and HIV. Although current influenza vaccines are primarily designed to induce neutralizing antibodies, the greatest impact of immunocompromising conditions is typically in those cases where T cell immunity is impaired. Such individuals can exhibit extremely prolonged viral shedding and frequent

P. Prasad · J. Treanor (✉)
Division of Infectious Diseases, University of Rochester Medical Center, Rochester, NY, USA
e-mail: John_Treanor@urmc.rochester.edu

© Springer International Publishing AG, part of Springer Nature 2018
B. H. Segal (ed.), *Management of Infections in the Immunocompromised Host*,
https://doi.org/10.1007/978-3-319-77674-3_18

development of antiviral resistance when treated with antiviral agents.

Available Vaccines

Both live attenuated influenza vaccines (LAIV) and inactivated influenza vaccines (IIV) have been developed, although LAIV is not generally recommended for use in immunocompromised patients. Recent years have seen a substantial expansion in the number of different approaches to generation of inactivated influenza vaccines, and there are multiple options currently licensed for use in the United States and other countries. Traditional inactivated vaccines are generated by propagation of the target viruses in eggs, purification and chemical inactivation of the virions, followed by disruption of virions and purification of the hemagglutinin (HA) and neuraminidase (NA) proteins by a variety of means, leading to so-called "subvirion," "split-virus," or "purified subunit" vaccines. The final product is a mixture of antigens of influenza A (H1N1), A (H3N2), and B viruses, a trivalent formulation referred to as IIV3. Over the last several decades, influenza B viruses have evolved into two antigenically distinct lineages (Yamagata and Victoria), and many recent vaccines are designed to include both B lineages in a quadrivalent formulation or IIV4.

Influenza vaccines can also be produced in mammalian cell culture (ccIIV4) or by expressing the relevant HA proteins in a baculovirus expression system (RIV4). Although most inactivated influenza vaccines are administered intramuscularly, one formulation is designed to be administered intradermally (ID IIV4). Studies in healthy adults have suggested that these alternative formulations and modes of administration result in antibody titers that are not inferior to those seen with standard approaches.

Two approaches have been evaluated in attempts to improve the protective efficacy of vaccination of older adults. The standard dose of inactivated influenza vaccine is a content of not less than 15 mcg of each HA protein, as assessed by single radial immunodiffusion. The use of a higher dose (60 mcg of each HA) is well tolerated and associated with significantly higher levels of antibody response and is licensed in the United States. This vaccine has demonstrated improved protective efficacy in adults over 65 years old in a randomized trial (HD IIV3) [1]. A formulation of inactivated vaccine with the squalene-based adjuvant MF59 (aIIV3) has been used in older adults in Europe for many years [2] and was also recently licensed in the United States based on non-inferiority of the immune response compared to standard vaccine.

Production of current live attenuated influenza vaccine (LAIV) relies on the exchange of gene segments between a well-characterized master donor virus, which contributes the genes governing attenuation of the vaccine virus, and the target strain of influenza, which donates the genes for the HA and NA. In the United States, the licensed LAIV is based on the master donor A/Ann Arbor/6/60 and B/Ann Arbor/6/66 viruses. A different LAIV based on the master donor virus A/Leningrad/66 is licensed in Russia and some other countries.

Safety and Immunogenicity in Immunocompromised Hosts

Because influenza vaccines are recommended for administration annually in all individuals, there have been many opportunities to evaluate vaccine performance in a variety of immunocompromised patient populations. In general, these studies have shown diminished immunogenicity reflective of the degree of immune suppression and a safety profile similar to that in the general population.

Extensive studies have been done to evaluate influenza vaccination in persons living with HIV. Responses to inactivated vaccines in adults and children, as measured by serum titers, generally correlate with CD4 cell count numbers, with better responses seen in those with CD4 counts above 200/μl, and with HIV viral load, with best responses seen in those with undetectable loads. Randomized prospective trials in relatively well-controlled individuals with HIV in the United

States [3] and Africa [4] have demonstrated levels of vaccine efficacy against laboratory confirmed influenza that are similar to those seen in healthy populations.

Studies in stem cell transplant populations have been less extensive but also support the use of vaccine in these individuals. During the 2009 H1N1 pandemic, several studies were done to evaluate pandemic vaccines, which generally showed that the immune response to a single dose was substantially less than that seen in age matched healthy controls for both solid organ transplant as well as stem cell transplant recipients. However, a second dose of pH1N1 vaccine substantially improved the proportion of recipients judged to be seroprotected on the bases of an HAI antibody titer of 40 or greater [5, 6]. Studies using seasonal vaccine formulations have been less extensive but have also demonstrated lower levels of immune response in these patients than healthy controls. In contrast to pH1N1 vaccine, administration of subsequent booster doses of seasonal vaccines to transplant recipients does not appear to substantially improve responses [7]. Several features have been shown to impact the immune response. In HSCT, these have included better responses in autologous compared to allogeneic transplants, and increasing time since transplantation, and worsened responses with the use of myeloablative therapy as opposed to reduced intensity, and the presence of graft-versus-host disease [8], as well as the effects of the specific immunosuppressive chemotherapy being used.

Solid organ transplant recipients have similarly decreased immune responses. In addition to the time since transplantation and the general state of immunosuppression, mycophenolate is associated with decreased responsiveness to influenza vaccine [9, 10]. Sirolimus may associate with relatively better influenza vaccine responses [11] than other forms of immunosuppression.

Given that high-dose and standard-dose seasonal vaccines administered with MF59 are intended to improve the immune response in older recipients, it is logical to ask whether these approaches would also enhance immunity in immunocompromised populations. In many countries, pH1N1 vaccine was administered with the oil-in-water adjuvant AS03. Not all studies have shown significant enhancement of antibody response with AS03 in transplant recipients [12], although the adjuvant did allow substantial dose sparing [13], with equivalent responses seen with lower doses of HA antigen. Small trials of high-dose vaccine in transplant recipients have suggested increases in seroresponses to the high dose [14].

In both allogeneic HSCT recipients and SOT recipients, there is concern regarding whether the immune stimulus of vaccination, with or without an adjuvant, might non-specifically stimulate the immune system to cause increased severity of graft-versus-host disease or organ rejection. Several studies have documented minor and transient increases in allogeneic anti-HLA antibodies following influenza (and other) vaccines. However, the weight of evidence does not support a significant association between vaccination and the development of autoimmune adverse events.

As a live vaccine, LAIV would not normally be recommended for use in immunocompromised subjects in any case. However, there are a number of studies that have evaluated LAIV in adults [15] and children [16] with well-controlled HIV infection, showing that the rate of adverse events and the shedding of the vaccine virus were similar to that observed in healthy adults and children. Similar studies have not been performed in patients with other types of immunosuppression.

The risk of transmission of LAIV from household contacts is low. In the most definitive study of potential transmission of LAIV, children attending day care were randomized to receive LAIV or placebo, and viral shedding was followed in both groups. There was evidence of transmission from child to child in two subjects, for an estimated transmission rate among susceptible contacts under close quarters of less than 2% [17]. Shedding of the vaccine virus by adults is much less frequent [18], and the likelihood of transmission would be predicted to be much lower.

Guidelines for Use

Because immunocompromised individuals are at higher risk for influenza and influenza complications, and with an extensive safety record in both healthy and immunocompromised adults, guidelines from a variety of organizations recommend annual vaccination of immunocompromised subjects and individuals with HIV [19]. Where possible, delaying vaccination until 6 months after transplant can result in improved immune responses, but if the normal timing of influenza vaccine occurs earlier than 6 months, it would still be recommended to administer vaccine.

LAIV is not recommended for use in immunocompromised subjects, although because of the low risk of transmission, use in household contacts was generally considered acceptable except in cases of very severe immunocompromised. Recent observational studies have suggested that the effectiveness of LAIV, particularly against pH1N1 viruses, has declined substantially and is now inferior to that of IIV in comparable populations. The reasons for this are unclear, but at this time, LAIV is not recommended for routine use in the United States [20]. Similar studies of the effectiveness of LAIV based on the Russian master donor viruses are not available.

Hepatitis B Vaccine

Available Vaccines

Hepatitis B vaccines contain the hepatitis B surface antigen (HBsAg), generated by expression of recombinant DNA in yeast or mammalian cells, and are formulated to contain 10 mcg or 40 mcg of HBsAg. Two single antigen vaccines are currently available in the United States, and general guidelines recommend a three-dose schedule at 0, 1, and 6 months, although other schedules have been shown to give similar results.

Safety and Immunogenicity in Immunocompromised Hosts

Generally, the responses of transplant recipients to hepatitis B vaccine are substantially diminished compared to healthy controls. For solid organ transplant recipients, vaccination of the recipient prior to transplant has generally been associated with better responses [21], even though the recipient may have significant compromise related to the conditions requiring transplantation. After transplant, responsiveness is affected by the time posttransplant, with best responses after 2 years, and other features of immune competence [22, 23]. In HIV, responses to HBV vaccination are inversely associated with HIV viral load [24]. Attempts to improve the immune response have included the use of high-dose vaccine, multiple additional doses, and adjuvants such as AS04 [25, 26] and monophosphoryl lipid A (MPL) [27], with limited success.

Transplant recipients with resolved hepatitis B infection (i.e., HBcAb positive but DNA negative), or recipients of livers from donors with resolved hepatitis B, are at high risk of reactivation following transplantation. The standard approach to prophylaxis of recurrent HBV in these patients is the use of long chronic antiviral suppression and the use of hepatitis B immune globulin (HBIG). Vaccination represents a potential alternative approach to prevention [28], especially in HBV-negative recipients of core antibody-positive livers.

Guidelines for Use

Most authorities recommend HBV vaccination of antibody-negative candidates prior to transplantation and for susceptible solid organ transplant recipients after transplantation. HBS antibody titers should be assessed, and if the patient does not achieve a titer of >10 mIU/mL, a second three- or four-dose series should be administered

[29]. For subjects on hemodialysis, the high-dose vaccine should be administered. Although there are limited data in HSCT recipients, antibody-negative subjects should be vaccinated [19]. Because immunogenicity is poor in the immediate posttransplant period, vaccination should be done 6 months or more following transplant [30]. Vaccination should be further delayed in patients receiving rituximab, which can interfere with vaccine responses for many months after administration.

Pneumococcal Vaccine

Patients with immunosuppressive conditions, especially those that affect phagocytic function or the reticulo-epithelial system, are at increased risk for invasive disease due to encapsulated organisms including *Streptococcus pneumoniae*. Invasive pneumococcal disease is recognized as an important problem following HSCT, with patients with chronic GvHD [31] and hyposplenism defining a high-risk group within this population [32].

Available Vaccines

Current pneumococcal vaccines are primarily designed to induce opsonizing antibody against the bacterial capsule, which subsequently mediates opsonophagocytosis of the bacteria by neutrophils and other phagocytic cells and killing of the bacteria. As such, the immunogenicity of pneumococcal vaccines is primarily assessed by the ability to induce functional, opsonophagocytic antibody (OPA). Over 90 antigenically distinct serotypes of pneumococcus are recognized, complicating the process of achieving broad protection. However, the distribution of serotypes associated with invasive disease is more narrow, and current vaccines are formulated to include those serotypes most frequently associated with disease in the target population.

Two types of vaccines are available for prevention of pneumococcal disease. The current pneumococcal polysaccharide vaccine (PPV) contains 23 serotypes of pneumococcal capsule at a dose of approximately 25 mcg per serotype (PPV-23), while the polysaccharide conjugate vaccine (PCV) contains a smaller number of serotypes chemically conjugated to a carrier protein. As an antigen made of repeating subunits, polysaccharides can generally stimulate B cells directly and are referred to as T-independent antigens. However, because polysaccharides do not recruit T cell help, the antibody response does not undergo affinity maturation, and the response generally does not boost with subsequent doses. Importantly, the developing immune system does not gain the ability to respond to these polysaccharides until ages 2–4 years, depending on the serotype. However, if the polysaccharide is chemically linked to a carrier protein, the immune response transitions to a T cell-dependent response, which is boostable and can induce strong immune responses in infants. A disadvantage of this approach is that the valency of the vaccine is more limited, with 13 serotypes being the largest number included in currently available conjugated vaccine (PCV-13). Thus, current strategies for immunization typically use both approaches in sequence to generate the broadest possible response.

Safety and Immunogenicity in Immunocompromised Hosts

Polysaccharide pneumococcal vaccines have been studied extensively in a variety of immunocompromised populations. Studies in patients with HIV have shown a reduced anticapsular antibody response following PPV-23 in HIV patients compared to healthy controls, with a more rapid decline in antibody titers after vaccination as well [33–35]. Responses have not always correlated with CD4 cell counts, but there is a suggestion of improved responses after successful antiretroviral therapy [36, 37]. As is true in healthy individuals [38], revaccination with PPV-23 generally leads to modest increases in antibody, which do not reach the same levels as after primary vaccination [34].

The efficacy of pneumococcal polysaccharide vaccination in HIV-infected adults has been evaluated in one randomized, controlled trial conducted in Uganda, [39] which did not show reduced rates of invasive pneumococcal infection or pneumonia in vaccine recipients. A number of observational studies have also attempted to assess the effectiveness of PPV in this population. In the largest such study, conducted in over 23,000 HIV-infected adults, PPV-23 was associated with an overall lower risk of pneumonia [40]. The effectiveness of the vaccine in this study was inversely associated with viral load at the time of vaccination, with reduced effectiveness with higher viral loads.

Studies in transplant recipients have also shown diminished responses to PPV-23. Antibody responses tend to be less vigorous than in healthy controls, and titers decline more quickly. As is true in other populations, revaccination typically results in modest increases in antibody that do not reach the level achieved after primary vaccine. In hematologic transplant, the response tends to improve with time since vaccination [41–43].

Pneumococcal conjugate vaccines have been shown to generate superior responses in several situations [44, 45]. However, immunocompromised patients may be more likely to be infected with serotypes not covered by the conjugate vaccine [46]. PCV vaccination may be given beginning as early as 3 months after stem cell transplantation [47], with good responses to a subsequent booster dose of PPSV [48]. In solid organ transplant, there may be relatively less benefit to the booster dose, [49] because the effects of immunosuppression time since transplant is predictive of the response to PCV in organ transplant recipients [50]. In liver transplant recipients, administration of PCV-7 followed by PPV-23 8 weeks later was not better than PPV-23 alone, suggesting that in adult transplant recipients, PPV-23 should remain the standard of care [51].

More recently, a randomized, placebo-controlled trial of two doses of a 7-valent pneumococcal conjugate vaccine in predominantly HIV-infected Malawian adolescents and adults who had recovered from documented invasive pneumococcal disease found that the PCV-7 vaccine was associated with a significantly lower risk of subsequent invasive pneumococcal disease due to the vaccine serotypes (plus serotype 6A) [52].

Guidelines for Use

Because immunocompromised patients are at higher risk for invasive pneumococcal infection, they represent an important target group for vaccination. Of the two types of vaccines, conjugated vaccines have the advantage of allowing boosting at the expense of a limited number of serotypes, while the polysaccharide vaccine contains a greater range of serotypes but generates progressively lower responses with subsequent doses as a general finding. Therefore, a strategy using both vaccines, with priming by PCV and subsequent dose of PPV to increase serotype coverage, might be ideal. This strategy has been shown to generate superior responses in healthy older adults [53]. Therefore, most guidelines recommend initial vaccination with PCV followed by PSV in transplant recipients [19].

Recommendations in HIV-infected patients are similar to those for healthy adults, and recommended schedules are based on age [19]. This would include initial vaccination with PCV in childhood, with a booster dose of PPV to increase the number of serotypes in later childhood. For adults with HIV, vaccination with PCV followed by PPV is recommended.

Measles-Mumps-Rubella (MMR) Vaccine

Severe measles is a recognized complication of immunosuppression of various types. Monitoring of antibody levels after allogeneic stem cell transplantation has suggested that there can be a gradual loss of immunity to measles in the months following transplantation, particularly in individuals with vaccine-acquired immunity [54–56].

Available Vaccines

Measles, mumps, and rubella vaccines are all live attenuated vaccines that were generated using traditional methods designed to adapt representative wild-type viruses to growth conditions that resulted in attenuated viruses that maintained their immune characteristics but were unable to cause illness. In the United States, measles vaccine is based on the Edmonston strain of measles virus, further passaged in cell culture to create the Moraten strain, the mumps vaccine is based on the Jeryl Lynn strain (named for the daughter of Maurice Hilleman, from whom the virus was originally obtained), and the rubella vaccine is based on the RA 27/3 isolate. Each of these viruses was extensively passaged and adapted to grow in various cell lines, resulting in relative attenuation in humans. The vaccines are typically formulated as a multivalent preparation (MMR) and administered intramuscularly.

Safety and Immunogenicity in Immunocompromised Hosts

Although live vaccines are generally not recommended for use in individuals with immunosuppression, there is extensive experience with use of MMR in young, HIV-infected children. Generally, HIV-infected children have poor responses to measles vaccine compared to healthy controls [57]. Measles seroprotection rates at age 24 months were lower in HIV-infected than HIV-uninfected children [58]. An early, two-dose schedule at 6 and 9 months was immunogenic in children in Malawi, but response rates were lower among HIV-infected children [59]. However, children on HAART have higher response rates to measles [60] as well as to subsequent doses [61] than untreated children.

Vaccine is well tolerated in HIV-infected children [59]. However, rare serious complications have been reported in severely immunosuppressed patients [62, 63].

MMR vaccine has been used in children awaiting organ transplant with good responses to all three components [64]. However, loss of antibody to MMR is common with chemotherapy or other immunosuppressive treatments [65, 66] or after HSCT [67]. There is limited data on the safety and immunogenicity of MMR post transplantation. Early measles vaccination after BMT has been well tolerated and immunogenic [68]. Immunization of solid organ transplant recipients was safe in children who were not severely immunosuppressed [69].

Guidelines for Use

Most HSCT patients loose immunity to measles following transplantation, and MMR can be considered 2 years after transplantation in patients without chronic GVHD or ongoing immunosuppression [19]. Adults who have natural measles immunity do not loose antibody as readily, and it is recommended that serology can be performed prior to vaccination, and vaccine be administered only to seronegatives. Because of lack of safety and effectiveness data, MMR vaccine is not recommended for use following solid organ transplantation [19, 70].

MMR vaccination is recommended for all asymptomatic HIV-infected persons who do not have evidence of severe immunosuppression (age-specific CD4+ T-lymphocyte percentages of

≥15%) and for whom measles vaccination would otherwise be indicated evidence of severe immunosuppression (age-specific CD4+ T-lymphocyte percentages ≥15%) for whom measles vaccination would otherwise be indicated. Similarly, MMR vaccination should be considered for mildly symptomatic HIV-infected persons for whom measles vaccination would otherwise be indicated who do not have evidence of severe immunosuppression [71].

Varicella and Zoster Vaccines

The varicella-zoster virus (VZV) is an alpha-herpes virus found throughout the human population worldwide. Primary infection with VZV results in varicella (chicken pox), a once common childhood illness presenting with fever and characteristic vesicular eruptions. Reactivation of infection along the latently infected dorsal root ganglia is called zoster and presents with a localized painful vesicular rash [72].

Immunocompromised patients, particularly those with impaired cell-mediated immunity, are unable to control cell-associated viremia and are at risk for severe life-threatening illness both with primary infection and with reactivation [73]. Disseminated disease occurs in up to 36% of immunocompromised patients with primary or reactivation varicella disease. This most commonly involves the lungs, liver, or central nervous system and can be hemorrhagic in presentation [74].

Available Vaccines

There are two live attenuated vaccines available for primary prevention of varicella and one for the prevention of zoster reactivation. All three vaccines contain the Oka strain of the varicella-zoster virus, a clinical isolate passaged repeatedly in guinea pig embryo fibroblasts and used in the first live attenuated varicella vaccine by Takahashi et al. in the 1970s [75]. The two formulations of the varicella vaccine licensed for use in the United States are the monovalent Varivax [76] and the polyvalent ProQuad (MMR-V) [77] which also contains live measles, mumps, and rubella vaccine. Consequently, MMR-V is formulated with a slightly higher concentration of Oka varicella virus (9772 plaque-forming units compared to 1350 for Varivax). Zostavax, which is intended for use in varicella-immune adults, contains 19,400 PFU or approximately 20 times that of Varivax [76].

Safety and Immunogenicity in Immunocompromised Hosts

Live vaccines are generally not recommended for use in individuals with significant immunocompromise. However, the risk of severe illness as a consequence of varicella primary infection or zoster reactivation is highest in these populations, and there has therefore been significant interest in the safety and efficacy of these vaccines in immunocompromised populations.

Many of the early studies of live varicella vaccines were performed in immunosuppressed children. An early study of single dose Varivax (1500 PFU) in 307 children with acute lymphoblastic leukemia in remission for 9 months demonstrated that the vaccine was well tolerated and was associated with a significant decrease in attack rate of primary varicella, conferring approximately 80% protection. These patients had normal cell-mediated immunity prior to vaccination based on response to phytohemagglutinin and skin testing with multiple antigens, and maintenance chemotherapy was held for a week before and a week after vaccination. Breakthrough varicella was mild, and the major side effect in leukemic children receiving maintenance chemotherapy was development of vaccine-associated rash [78]. Efficacy in smaller studies of patients with lymphoma and solid tumors was 90% and 90.7%, respectively [79].

In a subsequent study of acute leukemic children also in remission, seroconversion was noted in 88% of patients after the first dose of Varivax and in 98% of patients after one or two doses. Loss of antibody was noted in 20% at 1 year, 25% at 3 years, and 30% at 5 years. Of the 437 children vaccinated, 8% developed mild varicella. Two doses of vaccine were no more effective than one dose in preventing varicella disease. Three hundred seventy two patients studied were receiving maintenance chemotherapy when they were immunized, and 40% of these patients developed post-vaccination rash [80, 81]. Rates of zoster in acute leukemic children who received Varivax were also lower (9.1–15.4%) compared to rates in acute leukemic children with history of natural infection (17.5–21.6%) [79]. This same finding was confirmed in a later study [82].

Several small studies also support the safety of varicella vaccination in select patients after bone marrow transplantation. In one study, 15 rigorously selected children were vaccinated with 2000 PFU of live attenuated Oka strain 12–23 months following bone marrow transplant. Seven were autologous transplants and eight were allogenic. All had lymphocyte counts >1000 µL, T cell counts >700/µL, and positive skin test to candida, tuberculin, streptokinase, or tetanus, IgG blood level >5 g/L. In addition, their last administration of intravenous immunoglobulin was at least 6 weeks prior with no immunosuppressive therapy for 3 months and no evidence of infection or fever for at least 4 weeks prior to vaccination. In these patients, there were no cases of primary varicella or zoster reactivation observed for 2 years following immunization and 88.8% seroconverted. The vaccine was well tolerated. The incidence of VZV disease in non-immunized children following bone marrow transplant was 26.3% [83]. A subsequent study of 46 VZV seronegative allogeneic HSCT recipients who had CD4 counts ≥200/µL were off immunosuppression and responded to ≥1 post-transplant vaccine which demonstrated a 64% seroconversion rate. Seven percent developed a self-limited varicella-like rash within 2.5 weeks of vaccination, but no subsequent cases of varicella or zoster reactivation were noted over 2.5 years of follow-up [84]. A study of 68 children 24 months following HSCT who had no active GVHD, and were off immunosuppressive therapies, and who also had demonstrated serologic responses to inactivated vaccines, and normal in vitro lymphocyte proliferation to tetanus,

showed no severe reactions following live attenuated varicella vaccine administration, with mild post-vaccination rash in three subjects (4.4%). In a subset of 28 subjects with negative prevaccination antibody titers, seroconversion was demonstrated in 18 (64.3%) [85].

Evaluation of zoster vaccine in immunocompromised patients has been less extensive. Immunization preceding immunosuppression has been demonstrated to be effective in providing subsequent protection in a cohort study of patients receiving Zostavax per the CDC-ACIP schedule who subsequently underwent chemotherapy. The adjusted HR for herpes zoster was 0.58 with an incidence of 3.28% in the vaccinated patients compared to 5.34% in the unvaccinated group. Of interest, the rate of herpes zoster remained elevated in a subset of patients who underwent vaccination within 60 days before chemotherapy [86].

There are inadequate data to support the use of Zostavax following bone marrow transplant and no data on its efficacy or safety. In one small study of 62 patients with hematologic malignancy, 31 patients were post stem cell transplant (26 autologous and 5 allogeneic) [86]. The mean time to vaccination posttransplant was over 1 year for autologous transplants and over 3.5 years for allogeneic transplants. Twenty three of the 31 patients were in complete remission, and eight that were not in complete remission all had myeloma and were on a range of chemotherapies. One patient developed zoster 5.5 months after vaccination, although virus was not cultured, and it was unknown whether this represented wild type or live attenuated virus.

In bone marrow transplantation, donor immunity can be transferred through transplantation [87, 88]. Unfortunately, antibody levels fall after transplantation and continue to fall for years despite engraftment and immune reconstitution. As such, post-bone marrow transplantation patients are considered "never" vaccinated regardless of donor immunity [89].

Zostavax has been studied in a large cohort of patients with end-stage renal disease on dialysis. Vaccination was associated with a reduced risk of herpes zoster with HR 0.49. Three-year cumulative risk of herpes zoster in unvaccinated patients was 6.6% compared to 4.1% in vaccinated patients [90]. It is unclear what percentage of these patients went on to renal transplantation and, as such, the efficacy of pretransplantation vaccination on posttransplant risk of herpes zoster remains unknown.

Recently, a subunit vaccine has been developed for prevention of zoster in adults. The vaccine consists of recombinant varicella-zoster virus glycoprotein E and the $AS01_B$ adjuvant system, a liposome-based adjuvant containing monophosphoryl lipid A (MPL) and fraction 21 of the bark of the *Quillaja saponaria* tree, or so-called QS21. This vaccine was initially demonstrated to have an overall efficacy of 97% in prevention of zoster in a study involving 15,400 subjects 50 years of age and older [91]. In a follow-on study performed in 13,900 adults 70 and older, a two-dose schedule of vaccine demonstrated almost 90% efficacy in prevention of confirmed cases of zoster over the 30 months of post-vaccination observation [92]. This vaccine has shown promising results in HSCT recipients [93] and may emerge as an important intervention for immunosuppressed patients.

Guidelines for Use

In 2013, the Infectious Disease Society of America published guidelines for vaccine administration in the immunocompromised host which provide a framework for use of these vaccines to maximize preventative care in this population. The use of Varivax and Zostavax per these guidelines remains contraindicated in highly immunocompromised individuals, but this group was more stringently delineated. High-level immune compromise was defined as patients with combined primary immunodeficiency; those receiving cancer chemotherapy; patients within 2 months of solid organ transplantation; those receiving daily corticosteroid therapy (≥ 20 mg of prednisone for ≥ 14 days), tumor necrosis factor alpha-blockers, or rituximab; and HIV patients with CD4 count <200cells/mm^3. Hematopoietic stem cell transplantation was included as well;

however, it was noted that duration of high-level immune compromise following stem cell transplant depended on the type of transplant (autologous vs. allogeneic), the type of stem cell source, and the presence or absence of posttransplant complications such as GVHD [19].

Emphasis is placed on completing vaccine schedules before initiation of immunosuppression when possible and defining when vaccine administration is safe after immunosuppressive therapy [19]. When vaccination is indicated per these guidelines, recommendations are for use of single-agent vaccines such as Varivax and Zostavax only. It is recommended that vaccinations should not be initiated within the first 2–6 months following transplant to avoid impaired efficacy due to the high-dose immunosuppression used following transplantation [19].

Individuals living with immunocompromised patients and lacking immunity to varicella should receive Varivax and Zoster based on the standard CDC-ACIP schedule as acquisition of primary varicella or zoster reinfection presents a greater risk for transmission than vaccination [94]. If the vaccinated individual develops skin lesions following vaccination with Varivax or Zoster vaccine, then immunocompromised individuals should avoid contact with the vaccinee until lesions have resolved [95].

Varicella Vaccine

In patients with cancer, varicella vaccine should not be administered during chemotherapy but can be administered 3–6 months after cessation of chemotherapy. Patients with leukemia should be in remission and should not be on maintenance chemotherapy (despite the fact that most early studies were in leukemic patients in remission on maintenance chemotherapy held for 1 week prior to and 1 week after vaccination). For patients lacking evidence of immunity to varicella, if vaccination can be provided at least 4 weeks prior to immunosuppression, vaccination with Varivax should be provided. Current recommendations are for a two-dose series of Varivax separated by 28 days in patients over the age of 13 and separated by ≥ 3 months in those aged 12 months to 12 years.

Data to guide vaccination practices in hematopoietic stem cell transplant are limited. Because pre-existing recipient antibody titers are sustained for several months following transplantation, vaccination of patients lacking immunity prior to conditioning is recommended if adequate time is available [54]. A two-dose series is recommended if it can be completed ≥4 weeks prior to conditioning for transplant, but a single dose is acceptable if time is insufficient. Vaccination should not be pursued in allogeneic stem cell transplant patients with active graft-versus-host disease or in those receiving immunosuppressive therapy [19]. However, a two-dose series of varicella vaccine is recommended for those who have 2-year post-bone marrow transplant without ongoing immunosuppressive therapy or active GVHD and who have not received intravenous immunoglobulin for 8–11 months [19].

Morbidity and mortality in the varicella non-immune solid organ transplant population is extremely high, with 50 % of patients developing visceral involvement and a mortality rate of 25% despite maximal medical therapy [96]. As such, live attenuated varicella vaccination is recommended prior to transplant in all solid organ transplant candidates who lack varicella immunity and who are neither expected to undergo transplantation within the following 2 months nor have high-level immune compromise (e.g., combined primary immunodeficiency; those receiving cancer chemotherapy, daily corticosteroid therapy, tumor necrosis factor alpha-blockers, or rituximab; and HIV patients with CD4 count <200cells/mm^3). Based primarily on the time necessary to achieve adequate immunologic response, vaccination is only pursued if the time between completion of the series and planned transplantation is ≥4 weeks [19]. Safety and efficacy data for use of live attenuated vaccines in the posttransplant period are limited, and they are not generally administered. Varicella vaccine should only be considered in pediatric renal or liver transplant recipients without evidence of immunity to varicella and who are receiving minimal or no immunosuppression and no recent graft rejection [19].

Zoster Vaccine

Though Zoster vaccine is contraindicated in patients receiving chemotherapy, it is recommended patients ≥60 years of age who have ≥4 weeks until the onset of highly immunosuppressive therapy receive the vaccine. This approach can also be considered in patients 50–59 years or age as well. The primary method of prophylaxis against reactivation of varicella-zoster virus following solid organ transplantation is the use of prophylactic antiviral therapy such as acyclovir. There are inadequate data to support the use of Zostavax following solid organ transplantation and no data on its efficacy or safety. Zostavax is recommended in patients ≥60 years of age who have ≥4 weeks before transplantation, and this approach can also be considered in patients 50–59 years of age. However, for patients awaiting liver transplantation, it should be noted that there are no studies of Zostavax safety and efficacy in the cirrhotic population. In the initial studies of Zostavax for FDA approval, the only death occurring in the initial safety phase of the Zostavax arm was in a 56-year-old male with cirrhosis and cardiovascular disease who died after a fall at home [97].

Travel-Related Vaccines

In general, vaccines recommended for organ transplant, HIV, and other immunocompromised patients who are traveling to international destinations follow the general recommendations for all travelers [98–100]. However, the likely reduced efficacy of many vaccines in immunocompromised hosts must be taken into consideration when advising such travelers. Although there is relatively little data on which to base recommendations, travel should generally be avoided if possible in persons with substantial immunosuppression. Solid organ transplants are advised not to travel in the immediate posttransplant period, and travel should generally be avoided in all immunocompromised patients during intense immunocompromise.

As detailed earlier, live vaccines are generally contraindicated in individuals with significant immunocompromise. In the case of travel-related vaccines, this particularly pertains to vaccination against yellow fever, which is required for travel in some countries. Yellow fever vaccine is a live attenuated vaccine created by over 230 serial passages of the virus in cell culture [101]. Multiple mutations in the virus probably contribute to attenuation, and there is an excellent track record of safety in healthy adults. However, vaccination is associated with transient viremia in healthy recipients. More frequent serious or severe adverse reactions have been noted in elderly recipients [102].

Relatively little data is available regarding the safety of yellow fever vaccine in immunocompromised recipients. Cases of fatal encephalitis have been reported after administration of yellow fever vaccine to immunocompromised hosts [103]. However, other case series have suggested that the vaccine can be administered safely to SOT recipients several years after transplantation [104]. Successful vaccination after bone marrow transplantation has been reported as well [105, 106]. If YF vaccine can be administered prior to SOT, serologic data suggests that protection can be long-lived following transplant [107].

In general, YF vaccine should be avoided in HIV patients with CD4 less than 200 but can be used in those with well-controlled disease [19]. Vaccine should be avoided in those with significant immunosuppression. If travel to an area where YF vaccine is required is necessary, the traveler can be given a letter on physician letterhead explaining the medical exemption to vaccination [99]. It can be helpful for the traveler to carry documentation of requirements for waivers obtained from the destination country.

Conclusions and Future Directions

Both underlying conditions, such as solid organ or hematologic malignancies, underlying chronic liver or renal diseases, and autoimmune or immune deficiency diseases, and the treatments for those diseases such as chemotherapy, immunosuppression, and transplantation increase the risk and severity of common vaccine-preventable infections. However, these same conditions can reduce the immunogenicity and efficacy of vaccination and increase the risks of live attenuated vaccine particularly. Thus, decisions regarding the choice and timing of individual vaccines must weigh the risk of the disease, the degree of immunosuppression, and the expected course of treatment. Although modifications to the vaccine schedule are often required, in most cases the benefits of vaccination outweigh the potential risks.

Continued research to develop more effective and selective approaches to modulation of the immune system will undoubtedly contribute to enhanced vaccine safety and efficacy in these populations. In addition, there is a need for more detailed understanding of the effects of immune modulation on the response to vaccines and development of vaccines that can be targeted to these unique patient populations. The recent development of an inactivated zoster vaccine may be an example of such a project, and others will certainly follow.

References

1. DiazGranados CA, Dunning AJ, Kimmel M, et al. Efficacy of high-dose versus standard-dose influenza vaccine in older adults. N Engl J Med. 2014;371:635–45.
2. Iob A, Brianti G, Zamparo E, Gallo T. Evidence of increased clinical protection of an MF59-adjuvant influenza vaccine compared to a non-adjuvant vaccine among elderly residents of long-term care facilities in Italy. Epidemiol Infect. 2005;133(4):687–93.
3. Tasker SA, O'Brien WA, Treanor JJ, et al. Effects of influenza vaccination in HIV-infected adults: a double-blind, placebo-controlled trial. Vaccine. 1998;16:1039–42.
4. Madhi SA, Maskew M, Koen A, et al. Trivalent inactivated influenza vaccine in African adults infected with human immunodeficient virus: double blind, randomized clinical trial of efficacy, immunogenicity, and safety. Clin Infect Dis. 2011;52(1):128–37.
5. de Lavallade H, Garland P, Sekine T, et al. Repeated vaccination is required to optimize seroprotection against H1N1 in the immunocompromised host. Haematologica. 2011;96(2):307–14.
6. Le Corre N, Thibault F, Pouteil Noble C, et al. Effect of two injections of non-adjuvanted influenza A H1N1pdm2009 vaccine in renal transplant

recipients: INSERM C09-32 TRANSFLUVAC trial. Vaccine. 2012;30(52):7522–8.

7. Karras NA, Weeres M, Sessions W, et al. A randomized trial of one versus two doses of influenza vaccine after allogeneic transplantation. Biol Blood Marrow Transplant. 2013;19(1):109–16.

8. Mohty B, Bel M, Vukicevic M, et al. Graft-versus-host disease is the major determinant of humoral responses to the AS03-adjuvanted influenza A/09/H1N1 vaccine in allogeneic hematopoietic stem cell transplant recipients. Haematologica. 2011;96(6):896–904.

9. Siegrist CA, Ambrosioni J, Bel M, et al. Responses of solid organ transplant recipients to the AS03-adjuvanted pandemic influenza vaccine. Antivir Ther. 2012;17(5):893–903.

10. Salles MJ, Sens YA, Boas LS, Machado CM. Influenza virus vaccination in kidney transplant recipients: serum antibody response to different immunosuppressive drugs. Clin Transpl. 2010;24(1):E17–23.

11. Azevedo LS, Gerhard J, Miraglia JL, et al. Seroconversion of 2009 pandemic influenza A (H1N1) vaccination in kidney transplant patients and the influence of different risk factors. Transpl Infect Dis. 2013;15(6):612–8.

12. Engelhard D, Zakay-Rones Z, Shapira MY, et al. The humoral immune response of hematopoietic stem cell transplantation recipients to AS03-adjuvanted A/California/7/2009 (H1N1)v-like virus vaccine during the 2009 pandemic. Vaccine. 2011;29(9):1777–82.

13. Manuel O, Pascual M, Hoschler K, et al. Humoral response to the influenza A H1N1/09 monovalent AS03-adjuvanted vaccine in immunocompromised patients. Clin Infect Dis. 2011;52(2):248–56.

14. GiaQuinta S, Michaels MG, McCullers JA, et al. Randomized, double-blind comparison of standard-dose vs. high-dose trivalent inactivated influenza vaccine in pediatric solid organ transplant patients. Pediatr Transplant. 2015;19(2):219–28.

15. King JC, Treanor J, Fast PE, et al. Comparison of the safety, vaccine virus shedding, and immunogenicity of influenza virus vaccine, trivalent, types A and B, live cold-adapted, administered to human immunodeficiency virus (HIV)-infected and non-HIV-infected adults. J Infect Dis. 2000;181(2):725–8.

16. King JC Jr, Fast PE, Zangwill KM, et al. Safety, vaccine virus shedding and immunogenicity of trivalent, cold-adapted, live attenuated influenza vaccine administered to human immunodeficiency virus-infected and noninfected children. Pediatr Infect Dis J. 2001;20:1124–31.

17. Vesikari T, Karvonen A, Korhonen T, et al. A randomized, double-blind study of the safety, transmissibility, and phenotypic and genotypic stability of cold-adapted influenza virus vaccine. Pediatr Infect Dis J. 2006;25:590–7.

18. Talbot TR, Crocker DD, Peters J, et al. Duration of virus shedding after trivalent intranasal live attenuated influenza vaccination in adults. Infect Control Hosp Epidemiol. 2005;26:494–500.

19. Rubin LG, Levin MJ, Ljungman P, et al. 2013 IDSA clinical practice guideline for vaccination of the immunocompromised host. Clin Infect Dis. 2014;58(3):309–18.

20. Grohskopf LA, Sokolow LZ, Broder KR, et al. Prevention and control of seasonal influenza with vaccines: recommendations of the advisory committee on immunization practices – United States, 2016–17 influenza season. MMWR Recomm Rep. 2016;65(5):1–52.

21. Gutierrez Domingo I, Pascasio Acevedo JM, Alcalde Vargas A, et al. Response to vaccination against hepatitis B virus with a schedule of four 40-mug doses in cirrhotic patients evaluated for liver transplantation: factors associated with a response. Transplant Proc. 2012;44(6):1499–501.

22. Leung DH, Ton-That M, Economides JM, Healy CM. High prevalence of hepatitis B nonimmunity in vaccinated pediatric liver transplant recipients. Am J Transplant. 2015;15(2):535–40.

23. Jaffe D, Papadopoulos EB, Young JW, et al. Immunogenicity of recombinant hepatitis B vaccine (rHBV) in recipients of unrelated or related allogeneic hematopoietic cell (HC) transplants. Blood. 2006;108(7):2470–5.

24. O'Bryan TA, Rini EA, Okulicz J, et al. HIV viraemia during hepatitis B vaccination shortens the duration of protective antibody levels. HIV Med. 2015;16(3):161–7.

25. Nevens F, Zuckerman JN, Burroughs AK, et al. Immunogenicity and safety of an experimental adjuvanted hepatitis B candidate vaccine in liver transplant patients. Liver Transpl. 2006;12(10):1489–95.

26. Beran J. Safety and immunogenicity of a new hepatitis B vaccine for the protection of patients with renal insufficiency including pre-haemodialysis and haemodialysis patients. Expert Opin Biol Ther. 2008;8(2):235–47.

27. Di Paolo D, Lenci I, Cerocchi C, et al. One-year vaccination against hepatitis B virus with a MPL-vaccine in liver transplant patients for HBV-related cirrhosis. Transpl Int. 2010;23(11):1105–12.

28. Ishigami M, Kamei H, Nakamura T, et al. Different effect of HBV vaccine after liver transplantation between chronic HBV carriers and non-HBV patients who received HBcAb-positive grafts. J Gastroenterol. 2011;46(3):367–77.

29. Chow J, Golan Y. Vaccination of solid-organ transplantation candidates. Clin Infect Dis. 2009;49(10):1550–6.

30. Wilck MB, Baden LR. Vaccination after stem cell transplant: a review of recent developments and implications for current practice. Curr Opin Infect Dis. 2008;21(4):399–408.

31. Kulkarni S, Powles R, Treleaven J, et al. Chronic graft versus host disease is associated with long-term risk for pneumococcal infections in recipients of bone marrow transplants. Blood. 2000;95(12):3683–6.

32. Torda A, Chong Q, Lee A, et al. Invasive pneumo-coccal disease following adult allogeneic hemato-poietic stem cell transplantation. Transpl Infect Dis. 2014;16(5):751–9.

33. Nielsen H, Kvinesdal B, Benfield TL, Lundgren JD, Kondradsen HB. Rapid loss of specific antibod-ies after pneumococcal vaccination in patients with human immunodeficiency virus-1 infection. Scand J Infect Dis. 1998;30(6):597–601.

34. Rodriguez-Barradas MC, Groover JE, Lacke CE, et al. IgG antibody to pneumococcal capsular polysaccharide in human immunodeficiency virus-infected subjects: persistence of antibody in respond-ers, revaccination in nonresponders, and relationship of immunoglobulin allotype to response. J Infect Dis. 1996;173(6):1347–53.

35. Kroon FP, van Dissel JT, Ravensbergen E, Nibbering PH, van Furth R. Antibodies against pneumococcal polysaccharides after vaccination in HIV-infected individuals: 5-year follow-up of antibody concentra-tions. Vaccine. 1999;18(5–6):524–30.

36. Tangsinmankong N, Kamchaisatian W, Day NK, Sleasman J, Emmanuel PJ. Immunogenicity of 23-valent pneumococcal polysaccharide vaccine in children with human immunodeficiency virus undergoing highly active antiretroviral therapy. Ann Allergy Asthma Immunol. 2004;92:558–64.

37. Falcó V, Jordano Q, Cruz MJ, et al. Serological response to pneumococcal vaccination in HAART-treated HIV-infected patients: one year follow-up study. Vaccine. 2006;24(14):2567–74.

38. Musher DM, Manoff SB, Liss C, et al. Safety and antibody response, including antibody persistence for 5 years, after primary vaccination or revac-cination with pneumococcal polysaccharide vac-cine in middle-aged and older adults. J Infect Dis. 2010;201(4):516–24.

39. French N, Nakiyingi J, Carpenter LM, et al. 23-valent pneumococcal polysaccharide vaccine in HIV-1-infected Ugandan adults: double-blind, randomised and placebo controlled trial. Lancet. 2000;355(9221):2106–11.

40. Teshale EH, Hanson D, Flannery B, et al. Effectiveness of 23-valent polysaccharide pneu-mococcal vaccine on pneumonia in HIV-infected adults in the United States, 1998–2003. Vaccine. 2008;26(46):5830–4.

41. Winston DJ, Ho WG, Schiffman G, Champlin RE, Feig SA, Gale R. Pneumococcal vaccination of recipients of bone marrow transplants. Arch Intern Med. 1983;143(9):1735–7.

42. Avanzini MA, Carra AM, Maccario R, et al. Antibody response to pneumococcal vaccine in chil-dren receiving bone marrow transplantation. J Clin Immunol. 1995;15(3):137–44.

43. Spoulou V, Victoratos P, Ioannidis JPA, Grafakos S. Kinetics of antibody concentration and avidity for the assessment of immune response to pneumococ-cal vaccine among children with bone marrow trans-plants. J Infect Dis. 2000;182(3):965–9.

44. Pao M, Papadopoulos EB, Chou J, et al. Response to pneumococcal (PNCRM7) and *Haemophilus influenzae* conjugate vaccines (HIB) in pediat-ric and adult recipients of an allogeneic hemato-poietic cell transplantation (alloHCT).(Erratum appears in Biol Blood Marrow Transplant. 2008 Nov;14(11):1319). Biol Blood Marrow Transplant. 2008;14(9):1022–1030.

45. Meisel R, Kuypers L, Dirksen U, et al. Pneumococcal conjugate vaccine provides early protective antibody responses in children after related and unrelated allogeneic hematopoietic stem cell transplantation. Blood. 2007;109(6):2322–6.

46. Lujan M, Burgos J, Gallego M, et al. Effects of immunocompromise and comorbidities on pneumo-coccal serotypes causing invasive respiratory infec-tion in adults: implications for vaccine strategies. Clin Infect Dis. 2013;57(12):1722–30.

47. Cordonnier C, Labopin M, Chesnel V, et al. Randomized study of early versus late immuniza-tion with pneumococcal conjugate vaccine after allogeneic stem cell transplantation. Clin Infect Dis. 2009;48(10):1392–401.

48. Cordonnier C, Labopin M, Chesnel V, et al. Immune response to the 23-valent polysaccharide pneumo-coccal vaccine after the 7-valent conjugate vac-cine in allogeneic stem cell transplant recipients: results from the EBMT IDWP01 trial. Vaccine. 2010;28(15):2730–4.

49. Gattringer R, Winkler H, Roedler S, Jaksch P, Herkner H, Burgmann H. Immunogenicity of a com-bined schedule of 7-valent pneumococcal conjugate vaccine followed by a 23-valent polysaccharide vac-cine in adult recipients of heart or lung transplants. Transpl Infect Dis. 2011;13(5):540–4.

50. Barton M, Wasfy S, Dipchand AI, et al. Seven-valent pneumococcal conjugate vaccine in pediatric solid organ transplant recipients: a prospective study of safety and immunogenicity. Pediatr Infect Dis J. 2009;28(8):688–92.

51. Kumar D, Chen MH, Wong G, et al. A randomized, double-blind, placebo-controlled trial to evaluate the prime-boost strategy for pneumococcal vaccination in adult liver transplant recipients. Clin Infect Dis. 2008;47(7):885–92.

52. French N, Gordon SB, Mwalukomo T, et al. A trial of a 7-valent pneumococcal conjugate vaccine in HIV-infected adults. N Engl J Med. 2010;362(9):812–22.

53. Jackson LA, Gurtman A, van Cleeff M, et al. Influence of initial vaccination with 13-valent pneu-mococcal conjugate vaccine or 23-valent pneumo-coccal polysaccharide vaccine on anti-pneumococcal responses following subsequent pneumococcal vaccination in adults 50 years and older. Vaccine. 2013;31:3594–602.

54. Ljungman P, Lewensohn-Fuchs I, Hammarstrom V, et al. Long-term immunity to measles, mumps, and rubella after allogeneic bone marrow transplanta-tion. Blood. 1994;84(2):657–63.

55. Machado CM, Gonçalves FB, Pannuti CS, Dulley FL, de Souza VAUF. Measles in bone marrow transplant recipients during an outbreak in São Paulo Brazil. Blood. 2002;99(1):83–7.

56. Ljungman P, Aschan J, Barkholt L, et al. Measles immunity after allogeneic stem cell transplantation; influence of donor type, graft type, intensity of conditioning, and graft-versus host disease. Bone Marrow Transplant. 2004;34(7):589–93.

57. Krasinski K, Borkowsky W. Measles and measles immunity in children infected with human immunodeficiency virus. JAMA. 1989;261(17):2512–6.

58. Fowlkes A, Witte D, Beeler J, et al. Persistence of vaccine-induced measles antibody beyond age 12 months: a comparison of response to one and two doses of Edmonston-Zagreb measles vaccine among HIV-infected and uninfected children in Malawi. J Infect Dis. 2011;204(Suppl 1):S149–57.

59. Helfand RF, Witte D, Fowlkes A, et al. Evaluation of the immune response to a 2-dose measles vaccination schedule administered at 6 and 9 months of age to HIV-infected and HIV-uninfected children in Malawi. J Infect Dis. 2008;198(10):1457–65.

60. Pensieroso S, Cagigi A, Palma P, et al. Timing of HAART defines the integrity of memory B cells and the longevity of humoral responses in HIV-1 vertically-infected children. Proc Natl Acad Sci. 2009;106(19):7939–44.

61. Berkelhamer S, Borock E, Elsen C, Englund J, Johnson D. Effect of highly active antiretroviral therapy on the serological response to additional measles vaccinations in human immunodeficiency virus-infected children. Clin Infect Dis. 2001;32(7):1090–4.

62. Angel JB, Walpita P, Lerch RA, et al. Vaccine-associated measles pneumonitis in an adult with aids. Ann Intern Med. 1998;129(2):104–6.

63. Goon P, Cohen B, Jin L, Watkins R, Tudor-Williams G. MMR vaccine in HIV-infected children—potential hazards? Vaccine. 2001;19(28–29):3816–9.

64. Mori K, Kawamura K, Honda M, Sasaki N. Responses in children to measles vaccination associated with perirenal transplantation. Pediatr Int. 2009;51(5):617–20.

65. Zignol M, Peracchi M, Tridello G, et al. Assessment of humoral immunity to poliomyelitis, tetanus, hepatitis B, measles, rubella, and mumps in children after chemotherapy. Cancer. 2004;101(3):635–41.

66. Cheng FWT, Leung TF, Chan PKS, et al. Recovery of humoral and cellular immunities to vaccine-preventable infectious diseases in pediatric oncology patients. Pediatr Hematol Oncol. 2010;27(3):195–204.

67. Kawamura K, Yamazaki R, Akahoshi Y, et al. Evaluation of the immune status against measles, mumps, and rubella in adult allogeneic hematopoietic stem cell transplantation recipients. Hematology. 2015;20(2):77–82.

68. Machado CM, de Souza VA, Sumita LM, da Rocha IF, Dulley FL, Pannuti CS. Early measles vaccination in bone marrow transplant recipients. Bone Marrow Transplant. 2005;35(8):787–91.

69. Shinjoh M, Hoshino K, Takahashi T, Nakayama T. Updated data on effective and safe immunizations with live-attenuated vaccines for children after living donor liver transplantation. Vaccine. 2015;33(5):701–7.

70. Kumar D. Immunizations following solid-organ transplantation. Curr Opin Infect Dis. 2014;27(4):329–35.

71. Control CD. General recommendations on immunization. Morbid Mortal Wkly Rep – Rep Recomm. 2011;60:RR2:1–61.

72. Arvin AM. Varicella-zoster virus. Clin Microbiol Rev. 1996;9(3):361–81.

73. Myers MG. Viremia caused by varicella-zoster virus: association with malignant progressive varicella. J Infect Dis. 1979;140(2):229–33.

74. Hamborsky J, Kroger A, Wolfe S. Epidemiology and prevention of vaccine-preventable diseases. 13th ed. Washington, DC: Public Health Foundation; 2015.

75. Takahashi M. Current status and prospects of live varicella vaccine. Vaccine. 1992;10(14):1007–14.

76. Merck. VARIVAX prescriber information. 2013. Accessed 1/6/2017.

77. Merck. ProQuad prescriber information. 2016. Accessed 1/6/17.

78. Gershon AA, Steinberg SP, Gelb L. Live attenuated varicella vaccine use in immunocompromised children and adults. Pediatrics. 1986;78(4 Pt 2):757–62.

79. Takahashi M. Clinical overview of varicella vaccine: development and early studies. Pediatrics. 1986;78(4 Pt 2):736–41.

80. Gershon AA, Steinberg SP, Gelb L, et al. Live attenuated varicella vaccine. Efficacy for children with leukemia in remission. JAMA. 1984;252(3):355–62.

81. Gershon AA, Steinberg SP. Persistence of immunity to varicella in children with leukemia immunized with live attenuated varicella vaccine. N Engl J Med. 1989;320(14):892–7.

82. Hardy I, Gershon AA, Steinberg SP, LaRussa P. The incidence of zoster after immunization with live attenuated varicella vaccine. A study in children with leukemia. Varicella Vaccine Collaborative Study Group. N Engl J Med. 1991;325(22):1545–50.

83. Sauerbrei A, Prager J, Hengst U, Zintl F, Wutzler P. Varicella vaccination in children after bone marrow transplantation. Bone Marrow Transplant. 1997;20(5):381–3.

84. Chou JF, Kernan NA, Prockop S, et al. Safety and immunogenicity of the live attenuated varicella vaccine following T replete or T cell-depleted related and unrelated allogeneic hematopoietic cell transplantation (alloHCT). Biol Blood Marrow Transplant. 2011;17(11):1708–13.

85. Kussmaul SC, Horn BN, Dvorak CC, Abramovitz L, Cowan MJ, Weintrub PS. Safety of the live, attenuated varicella vaccine in pediatric recipients of hematopoietic SCTs. Bone Marrow Transplant. 2010;45(11):1602–6.

86. Naidus E, Damon L, Schwartz BS, Breed C, Liu C. Experience with use of Zostavax((R)) in patients with hematologic malignancy and hematopoietic cell transplant recipients. Am J Hematol. 2012;87(1):123–5.

87. Lum LG, Munn NA, Schanfield MS, Storb R. The detection of specific antibody formation to recall antigens after human bone marrow transplantation. Blood. 1986;67(3):582–7.

88. Lum LG, Seigneuret MC, Storb R. The transfer of antigen-specific humoral immunity from marrow donors to marrow recipients. J Clin Immunol. 1986;6(5):389–96.

89. Johnston BL, Conly JM. Immunization for bone marrow transplant recipients. Can J Infect Dis. 2002;13(6):353–7.

90. Tseng HF, Luo Y, Shi J, et al. Effectiveness of herpes zoster vaccine in patients 60 years and older with end-stage renal disease. Clin Infect Dis. 2016;62(4):462–7.

91. Lal H, Cunningham AL, Godeaux O, et al. Efficacy of an adjuvanted herpes zoster subunit vaccine in older adults. N Engl J Med. 2015;372(22):2087–96.

92. Cunningham AL, Lal H, Kovac M, et al. Efficacy of the herpes zoster subunit vaccine in adults 70 years of age or older. N Engl J Med. 2016;375(11):1019–32.

93. Stadtmauer EA, Sullivan KM, Marty FM, et al. A phase 1/2 study of an adjuvanted varicella-zoster virus subunit vaccine in autologous hematopoietic cell transplant recipients. Blood. 2014;124(19):2921–9.

94. Diaz PS, Au D, Smith S, Amylon M, Link M, Arvin AM. Lack of transmission of the live attenuated varicella vaccine virus to immunocompromised children after immunization of their siblings. Pediatrics. 1991;87(2):166–70.

95. Sharrar RG, LaRussa P, Galea SA, et al. The postmarketing safety profile of varicella vaccine. Vaccine. 2000;19(7–8):916–23.

96. Lynfield R, Herrin JT, Rubin RH. Varicella in pediatric renal transplant recipients. Pediatrics. 1992;90(2 Pt 1):216–20.

97. Agger PE. Summary basis for regulatory action. 2011. Accessed 1/8/17.

98. Visser LG. The immunosuppressed traveler. Infect Dis Clin N Am. 2012;26(3):609–24.

99. Rosen J. Travel medicine and the solid-organ transplant recipient. Infect Dis Clin N Am. 2013;27(2):429–57.

100. Aung AK, Trubiano JA, Spelman DW. Travel risk assessment, advice and vaccinations in immunocompromised travellers (HIV, solid organ transplant and haematopoeitic stem cell transplant recipients): a review. Travel Med Infect Dis. 2015;13(1):31–47.

101. Staples JE, Monath TP, Gershman MD, Barrett ADT. Yellow fever vaccines. In: Plotkin SA, Orenstein WA, Offit PA, Edwards KM, editors. Plotkin's vaccines. Philadelphia: Elsevier; 2017.

102. Rafferty E, Duclos P, Yactayo S, Schuster M. Risk of yellow fever vaccine-associated viscerotropic disease among the elderly: a systematic review. Vaccine. 2013;31(49):5798–805.

103. Kengsakul K, Sathirapongsasuti K, PUnyagupta S. Fatal myeloencephalitis following yellow fever vacation in a case with HIV infection. J Med Assoc Thail. 2002;85:131–4.

104. Azevedo LS, Lasmar EP, Contieri FL, et al. Yellow fever vaccination in organ transplanted patients: is it safe? A multicenter study. Transpl Infect Dis. 2012;14(3):237–41.

105. Gowda R, Cartwright K, Bremner JA, Green ST. Yellow fever vaccine: a successful vaccination of an immunocompromised patient. Eur J Haematol. 2004;72(4):299–301.

106. Yax JA, Farnon EC, Cary Engleberg N. Successful immunization of an allogeneic bone marrow transplant recipient with live, attenuated yellow fever vaccine. J Travel Med. 2009;16(5):365–7.

107. Wyplosz B, Burdet C, Francois H, et al. Persistence of yellow fever vaccine-induced antibodies after solid organ transplantation. Am J Transplant. 2013;13(9):2458–61.

Stem Cell Transplantation for Primary Immunodeficiency

19

Juliana Silva, Claire Booth, and Paul Veys

Abbreviations

ADA	Adenosine deaminase
APDS	Activated PI3Kδ syndrome
ATG	Anti-thymocyte globulin
CGD	Chronic granulomatous disease
CTLs	Cytotoxic T lymphocytes
DLI	Donor lymphocyte infusion
DOCK8	Dedicator of cytokinesis 8
EBV	Epstein-Barr virus
FHLH	Familial haemophagocytic lymphohistiocytosis
GvHD	Graft versus host disease
HLA	Human leukocyte antigen
HLH	Haemophagocytic lymphohistiocytosis
HSCT	Haematopoietic stem cell transplant
iC9-T	Inducible human caspase 9
LAD	Leukocyte adhesion deficiency type 1
MAC	Myeloablative conditioning
MHC class II	Major histocompatibility complex class II
MIC	Minimal intensity conditioning
MMFD	Mismatched family donor
MRD	Matched related donor
MSD	Matched sibling donor
mTOR	Mammalian target of rapamycin
MUD	Matched unrelated donor
NBS	Newborn screening
NKT	NK+ T cells
OS	Overall survival
PBSC	Peripheral blood stem cells
PEG-ADA	Polyethylene glycol-conjugated adenosine deaminase
PI3K	Phosphatidylinositol-3 kinase
PID	Primary immunodeficiency diseases
RIC	Reduced intensity conditioning
SCETIDE	Stem cell transplant for immunodeficiencies in Europe
SCID	Severe combined immunodeficiency
TCR	T-cell receptor
TRECs	T-cell receptor excision circles
TRM	Transplant-related mortality
UCBT	Umbilical cord blood stem cell transplantation
WAS	Wiskott-Aldrich syndrome
XIAP	X-linked inhibitor of apoptosis
XLP	X-linked lymphoproliferative disease

J. Silva · P. Veys (✉)
Department of Bone Marrow Transplantation, Great Ormond Street Hospital, London, UK
e-mail: Paul.Veys@gosh.nhs.uk

C. Booth
Department of Paediatric Immunology, Great Ormond Street Hospital, London, UK

© Springer International Publishing AG, part of Springer Nature 2018
B. H. Segal (ed.), *Management of Infections in the Immunocompromised Host*,
https://doi.org/10.1007/978-3-319-77674-3_19

Introduction

Primary immunodeficiency diseases (PID) are a group of rare heterogeneous disorders that can affect the development and/or function of T and B lymphocytes, natural killer cells, phagocytes and proteins of the complement pathway. For the majority of these conditions, haematopoietic stem cell transplant (HSCT), and in some cases gene therapy, offers the only curative approach. Transplant procedures in many of these conditions may entail significant morbidity and mortality risk, as many patients referred for transplantation have established complications including previous or active infections, autoimmunity and rarely malignancy. Newborn screening policies are being introduced in a number of countries with the aim of diagnosing severe combined immune deficiencies (SCIDs) prior to the onset of potentially fatal infections, enabling early referral for a definitive procedure while the child remains infection free, thereby reducing the risk associated with HSCT or gene therapy procedures.

Current indications for HSCT in PID are shown in Table 19.1 [1, 2]. Recent advances in the field of genetics and molecular diagnostics, such as high-throughput next-generation sequencing and whole genome sequencing, have led to the characterization of an increasing number of newly described PIDs. Case series of the disease progression and management of these new disorders are emerging, and although some patients have proceeded to HSCT, the indication and timing of HSCT for several of these PIDs remain unclear.

Over the past two decades, novel treatment options such as gene therapy and thymic transplantation have also been developed to cure specific PIDs, with clinical trials demonstrating encouraging results. Alongside these advances, adjuvant cellular therapies, including virus-specific cytotoxic T lymphocytes (CTLs) and graft manipulation techniques, are also in clinical use, helping to improve the outcome for patients with devastating immune disorders. Some of these advances will be discussed at length in other chapters, but here we focus on the current state of play of HSCT in treating these conditions and improving survival for many diseases.

SCIDs

Severe combined immunodeficiencies (SCIDs) represent a group of genetic disorders leading to abnormal development and function of lymphocytes with impairment of both cellular and humoral immunity. T-cell development is invariably affected, but the presence or absence of B and/or NK cells varies with the molecular abnormality and level of maturational arrest Fig. 19.1 [3]. Affected infants have increased susceptibility to severe or recurrent opportunistic infections, which often prove fatal if immunity is not restored within the first years of life. Although supportive measures such as prophylactic antimicrobials, replacement immunoglobulin, nutritional support and close monitoring for infection have certainly reduced morbidity associated with these conditions, a definitive procedure is required to cure patients with SCID.

The outcome of HSCT for SCID patients as a whole has improved significantly over the last 20 years with survival rates of more than 90% in the matched sibling donor (MSD) setting, which remains the donor source of choice [4]. Recently, data from the Stem Cell Transplant for Immunodeficiencies in Europe (SCETIDE) registry has shown that the outcomes following matched unrelated donor (MUD) transplants are comparable to sibling donor transplants with overall survival (OS) of approximately 82%, while OS following mismatched unrelated donors and haploidentical stem cell transplants have been lower (62% and 58%, respectively) (A Gennery, personal communication), Fig. 19.2. With the very recent introduction of new methodologies, such as T-cell receptor (TCR) αβ depletion, the outcome of haploidentical grafts has improved further (see below).

Table 19.1 Indications for HSCT in PID, based on IUIS classification (1) and modification by Westhafen International BMT group (2) and British Society of Blood and Marrow Transplantation (www.bsbmt.org)

I. Combined immunodeficiency (CID)	
SCID	ADA, reticular dysgenesis, RAG 1/2, DCLREC1C, Cernunnos, DNA ligase 4, DNA PKcs, X-linked, Jak 3 kinase, IL7Rα, CD3γδε, CD45, Zap70 kinase, coronin 1A
CID	CD40 ligand deficiency, CD4 lymphopaenia, MHC class II, PNP, Omenn syndrome, leaky SCID, MALT1, LCK, STK4, CTPS1

II. CID with associated features
WAS, DiGeorge, CHARGE, CID with skeletal dysplasia, RMRP, Nijmegen breakage syndrome*, DOCK 8, Tyk2, ICF, DKC, PI3Kδ activating mutant, LRBA, ORAI-1, STIM1

III. Antibody deficiencies
CIVD, MDS with hypogammaglobulinaemia

IV. Immune dysregulation	
Haemophagocytic disorders	Familial HLH with genetic diagnosis (PRF1, UNC13D, MUNC 18-2, STX11); HLH without genetic diagnosis but with recurrent/refractory disease, affected sibling, absent NK function, CNS disease; Griscelli syndrome type 2 (RAB27A); Chediak-Higashi syndrome (LYST)
Lymphoproliferative disorders*	XLP1 (SH2D1A) and 2 (XIAP), chronic active EBV (with or without lymphoma or HLH)*, ITK, CD27, MAGT1
Autoimmune	ALPS (homozygotes) STAT3 GOF, CTLA4, JIA, SLE, SS, Evans
Intractable colitis	IPEX syndrome, IL-10, IL-10 receptor, immune deficiency with multiple intestinal atresias (TTC7a)

V. Phagocytic cell disorders
Immunodeficiency with partial albinism, severe congenital neutropaenia, Shwachman-Diamond syndrome, LAD 1–3, X-linked CGD, AR CGD, GATA2

VI. Innate defects
NEMO, STAT1, STAT5, IFN-γ receptor, IL-12 receptor

Abbreviations: MHC class II major histocompatibility complex class II, *MALT1* mucosa-associated lymphoid tissue lymphoma translocation protein 1, *LCK* lymphocyte-specific protein tyrosine kinase deficiency, *STK4* serine threonine kinase 4 deficiency, *CTPS1* cytidine triphosphate synthase 1 deficiency, *WAS* Wiskott-Aldrich syndrome, *RMRP* RNA component of the mitochondrial RNA processing mutations causing cartilage-hair hypoplasia, *DOCK8* dedicator of cytokinesis 8 deficiency, *Tyk2* tyrosine kinase 2 deficiency, *ICF* immunodeficiency, centromeric region instability and facial anomalies syndrome, *DKC* dyskeratosis congenita, *PI3Kδ* activating mutant, activated phosphatidylinositol-3 kinase delta syndrome, *LRBA* LPS-responsive beige-like anchor, *ORAI-1* calcium release-activated calcium modulator 1 deficiency, *STIM1* stromal interaction molecule 1 deficiency, *CIVD* common variable immunodeficiency, *MDS* myelodysplastic syndrome, *ITK* interleukin-2-inducible T-cell kinase deficiency, *MAGT1* magnesium transporter 1 deficiency, *XLP* X-linked lymphoproliferative disease, *XIAP* X-linked inhibitor of apoptosis, *ALPS* (homozygotes) autoimmune lymphoproliferative syndrome, *STAT3 GOF* signal transducer and activator of transcription 3 gain of function, *CTLA4* cytotoxic T-lymphocyte-associated protein 4

JIA juvenile idiopathic arthritis, *SLE* systemic lupus erythematosus, *SS* Sjögren's syndrome, *IPEX syndrome* immunodysregulation polyendocrinopathy enteropathy X-linked syndrome, *LAD 1* leukocyte adhesion deficiency type 1, *X-linked CGD* X-linked chronic granulomatous disease

AR CGD autosomal recessive chronic granulomatous disease, *NEMO* nuclear factor-kappa B essential modulator deficiency syndrome, *STAT1* signal transducer and activator of transcription 1

STAT5 signal transducer and activator of transcription 5

*may present as haemophogocytic disorder

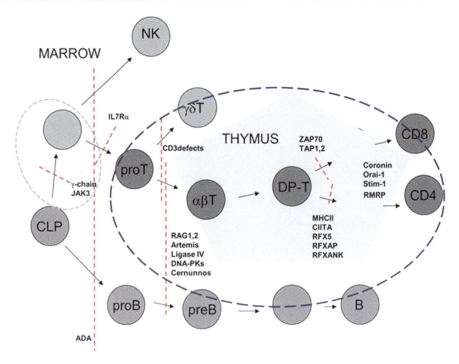

Fig. 19.1 Phenotypic classifications of SCID are based on presence or absence of T, B and NK cells. (Modified from Hassan et al. J Allergy Clin Immunol [3]). *CIITA* class II transactivator, *CLP* common lymphoid progenitor, *DNA-PK* DNA-protein kinases, *DP-T* double-positive T cells, *IL7Rα* IL-7 receptor α, *RAG* recombination-activating gene, *RFX5* regulatory factor X5, *RFXANK* regulatory factor X ankyrin repeat containing, *RFXAP* regulatory factor X5 associated protein, *RMRP* mitochondrial RNA-processing endoribonuclease, *Stim1* stromal interaction molecule 1, *TAP* transporter associated with antigen processing, *ZAP70* ζchain-associated protein of 70 kDa

The outcome of haploidentical and unrelated umbilical cord blood stem cell transplantation (UCBT) was compared by Fernandes et al. in a large cohort of 249 patients [5]. They observed similar 5-year OS between the two groups (62% for haplo vs. 57% for UCBT, $p = 0.68$), despite a higher incidence of chronic graft versus host disease (GvHD) in the UCBT group (22% versus 10%, $p = 0.03$). More patients in the haploidentical group required a second transplant as a result of inferior myeloid engraftment which was more frequently associated with the use of unconditioned grafts or reduced intensity conditioning as compared to more frequent use of myeloablative conditioning in the UCBT group. The use of a myeloablative conditioning regimen in the UCBT group was also associated with improved B-cell engraftment allowing 45% of the patients to stop immunoglobulin replacement compared to 31% of patients in the haploidentical stem cell trans-

plant group [5]. Infection was the commonest cause of death in both groups, 47% in the haploidentical group compared to 30% in the UCBT group. Excellent survival rates of 81% using UCBT for primary immunodeficiency has also been observed in a recent review about the use of this stem cell source in the United Kingdom [6].

The use of chemotherapeutic conditioning prior to HSCT in children with SCID is a controversial area but one that should be addressed, especially in the context of newborn screening where toxicity from conditioning regimens must be balanced against secure engraftment and optimal immune reconstitution. Although it is recognized that a conditioning will lead to improved stem cell engraftment and hence T- and B-cell reconstitution regardless of the donor source, even reduced intensity regimens may be associated with increased transplant-related mortality and as yet undefined long-term risks, such as

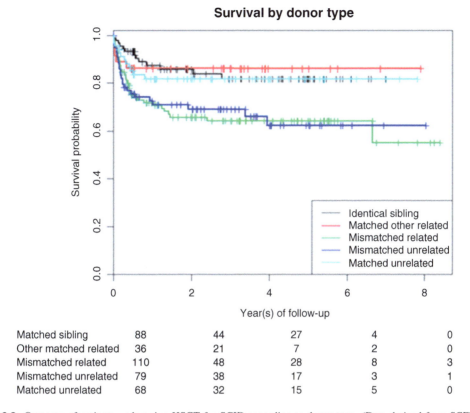

Fig. 19.2 Outcome of patients undergoing HSCT for SCID according to donor type. (Data derived from SCETIDE registry)

infertility. It is important to recognize that some radiation-sensitive SCIDs, such as Artemis and DNA ligase IV deficiency, do not tolerate alkylating therapy or radiation. For these patients there is significant potential for late effects and reduced survival particularly in patients with active infection at the time of transplant and those receiving a mismatched graft [7]. Hassan et al. [3] demonstrated that host NK cells, if present, may compete with donor T cells impairing engraftment and post-thymic T-cell reconstitution. It was observed that NK-cell-deficient SCID (NK-SCID) disorders (such as Janus kinase 3 deficiency, gamma chain-deficient and adenosine deaminase (ADA) SCIDs) are highly permissive and receptive to unconditioned allo-HSCT, and the OS following unconditioned HSCT observed in the context of NK-SCID was 87%, compared to 62% in NK+ SCID. As expected, B-cell reconstitution was suboptimal in both groups. Therefore, in patients with NK+ SCID disorders,

a conditioning regimen should be offered to facilitate engraftment and promote immune recovery with higher T-cell counts and superior thymopoiesis post-transplant, as evidenced by higher numbers of post-transplant T-cell receptor excision circles (TRECs) and naïve T cells [3].

Infusion of unrelated donor cells in SCID patients without the use of conditioning or serotherapy with ATG or alemtuzumab often leads to a high incidence of GVHD, but the use of serotherapy alone has resulted in successful T-cell reconstitution, low rates of GVHD and excellent OS of 100% (compared with OS of 51% in those patients who did not receive serotherapy) [7]. Pai et al. reported [8] recently excellent survival rates associated with young age at transplant (<3.5 months of age, 94% 5-year survival) and absence of infection at the time of transplant (90%), regardless of donor type, cell source or conditioning. Infants with active infections lacking a MSD achieved the best survival using unconditioned grafts from hap-

Fig. 19.3 Outcome of HSCT for SCID according to age and infection status. Based on 5-year survival rates published by Pai et al. [8]

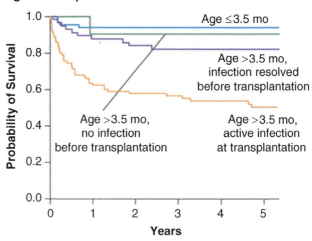

Age at Transplantation and Infection Status

loidentical T-cell-depleted grafts (65% vs. 53% survival rates in recipients of other unrelated donor grafts) (Fig. 19.3). Although immunophenotype did not affect survival per se, patients with B+ and NK− SCIDs achieved better T-cell reconstitution. Conditioned grafts were also associated with improved T-cell count and a higher probability of freedom from immunoglobulin replacement (84% vs. 41% in unconditioned transplants, $p < 0.001$) [8].

In addition to HSCT, gene therapy is available for specific SCID subtypes, such as adenosine deaminase-deficient SCID and X-linked SCID, and this therapeutic option is discussed in detail elsewhere. Figure 19.4 gives an illustration of the approach taken in our centre for ADA-SCID and X-SCID (gamma chain-deficient SCID). Patients affected by ADA-SCID are commenced on enzyme replacement with PEG-ADA at diagnosis to allow metabolic detoxification prior to any procedure. Patients who lack a matched family donor are eligible to be treated with lentiviral gene therapy (phase I/II clinical trial). However, if gene therapy is not available, a 10/10 matched unrelated adult donor (MUD) or 10/10 cord blood unit would be sought [9]. Patients with X-SCID are considered candidates for gene therapy only when no matched related or unrelated donor is available due to the risk of insertional leukaemogenesis following earlier clinical trials in X-SCID patients using a gammaretroviral vector [10].

In the absence of a matched donor or availability of gene therapy, our approach in SCID patients is to consider single antigen mismatched adult unrelated donors or 8–9/10 HLA-matched unrelated cord blood units. The choice between the adult and cord blood donor relies mainly on the presence of viral infections in the patient, and CMV status of the patient and donor is crucial. If the patient has active viral infection, in particular CMV infection detected by PCR, and the donor is CMV seronegative, a cord blood unit is selected and transplanted without anti-thymocyte globulin (ATG)/alemtuzumab in the conditioning regimen. Previous studies showed good engraftment rates (96%) and low mortality associated with infections using this approach (7%) [11]. Other centres consider the use of haploidentical related donors when no matched donor is available. This is due to the emergence of two new approaches to improve immune reconstitution following haploidentical HSCT: the first is the use of T-cell receptor (TCR) αβ depletion, which retains the benefits of both NK+ cells and γδ+ cells to secure engraftment and combat infection without increased risk of GvHD [12]. Bertaina et al. reported an incidence of transplant-related mortality of 9% and graft failure of 16.2% following this approach in 23 children with non-malignant disorders [13]. Particularly good results have been achieved when this technique was combined with the use of donor lymphocyte infusions

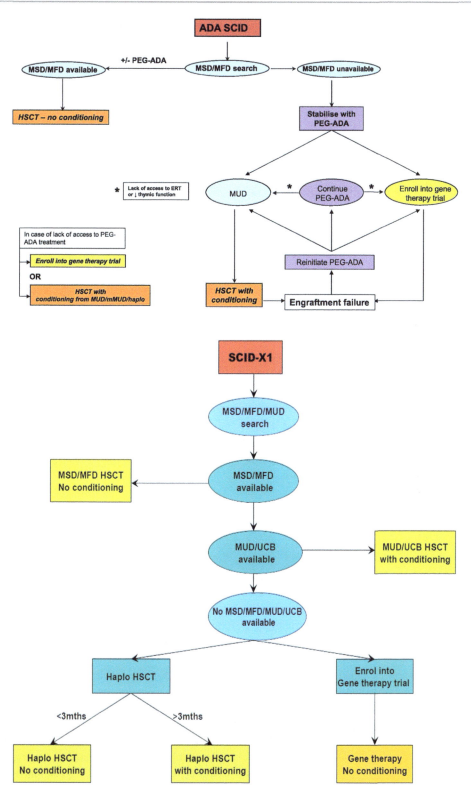

Fig. 19.4 Diagram of donor choice for adenosine deaminase SCID and X-linked SCID based on EBMT/ESID (European Group for Blood and Marrow Transplantation/ European Society for Immunodeficiencies) guidelines for HSCT for PID

genetically modified with an inducible human caspase 9 (iC9-T) suicide switch to reduce the risk of GvHD. Zhou et al. recently described rapid resolution of acute GvHD in four of ten patients following a single administration of AP1903, the dimerizing, bio-inert drug, which can activate the iCaspase-9 transgene. Interestingly the iC9-T cells reactive to CMV, adenovirus, EBV or BK virus persisted for months after AP1903 administration [14].

The second approach utilizes a T-replete graft and in vivo allodepletion with cyclophosphamide post-transplant to improve outcome following mismatched related donor transplantation with low transplant-related mortality, ranging from 4% to 15% in previous studies [15–17]. Although this approach has been mainly used in the context of haematological malignancy, this might also be a feasible strategy in haploidentical transplantation in PID [18].

In conclusion a number of different strategies now exist for the definitive treatment of SCID in patients lacking a matched sibling donor. The outcome from each of these approaches is improving and should now be compared in prospective randomized studies. Such studies would need to be adapted following the early diagnosis of SCID with the introduction of newborn screening programmes.

Newborn Screening

Early diagnosis of SCID has been shown to significantly improve outcomes for children affected by this disorder, allowing early referral for curative treatment prior to infectious complications which are highly correlated with poor outcome [8, 19]. Population-based SCID screening programmes are now established in several countries around the world including the USA, Brazil and Taiwan, and a number of European countries are undertaking preparatory studies to support introduction of the scheme, but it is generally acknowledged that NBS is a cost-effective intervention [20–25]. Screening is performed on dried blood spot tests using a qPCR assay to quantify T-cell receptor excision circles (TRECs), and this

technique is both highly specific and well validated. In order to generate a wide repertoire of T-cell receptors capable of recognizing specific antigens, T cells undergo TCR gene splicing and recombination during development. TRECs are produced as a by-product of this process and therefore serve as a biomarker of thymopoiesis. Very low or absent TREC levels are indicative of SCID but can also be found in conditions causing lymphopaenia such as cardiac abnormalities and prematurity. If abnormal TREC levels are identified, the presence of lymphopaenia will be confirmed using flow cytometric immunophenotyping of lymphocyte subsets, and further relevant immunological testing can be undertaken to identify a molecular diagnosis and allow progression to a curative procedure in as short a time as possible [26, 27]. The best approach to manage presymptomatic patients identified through NBS will need to be determined based on best evidence and experience, but a consensus in the field on how to provide an effective procedure with minimal toxicity is yet to be reached.

HSCT in Non-SCID Primary Immune Deficiencies

In recent years the number of patients diagnosed with PID other than SCID has increased, and consequently, the number of HSCTs for these conditions has also been greater. Survival rates for patients with non-SCID PIDs have also increased [4]. The approach to HSCT has changed with more patients undergoing reduced intensity conditioning with better survival rates. Rao et al. analysed the outcome of 52 patients with inherited immune disorders who underwent HSCT [28]. They compared the survival rates and immune reconstitution between patients receiving reduced intensity conditioning (RIC), mainly with fludarabine and melphalan, to patients receiving myeloablative conditioning (MAC) with busulfan and cyclophosphamide. They demonstrated higher survival rates in the RIC group (94% vs. 53%) and comparable immune recovery [28]. Further RIC combinations have been developed, and their use prior to HSCT in PID has

Table 19.2 A hierarchy of commonly used MIC, RIC and MAC regimens in PID patients

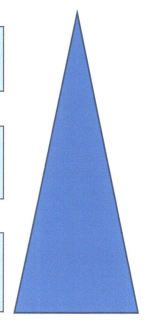

Minimal intensity conditioning (MIC)

Fludarabine/melphalan
Fludarabine/treosulfan
Fludarabine/busulfan (AUC: 45–65 mg/L × h)
+/– ATG or alemtuzumab

Reduced intensity conditioning (RIC)

Fludarabine/TBI2 Gy
Fludarabine/cyclophosphamide (120 mg/kg)
Fludarabine/cyclophosphamide (120 mg/kg)/ Anti-CD45
antibody
+/– ATG or alemtuzumab

Myeloablative intensity conditioning (MAC)

Busulfan (AUC: 80–100 mg/L × h)/cyclophosphamide
(120–200mg/kg)
TBI 12Gy/cyclophosphamide (120 mg/kg)
Fludarabine/treosulfan/thiotepa
+/– ATG or alemtuzumab

Modified from Satwani et al. [30]
TBI total-body irradiation, *Gy* grey, *ATG* anti-thymocyte globulin

been extensively reviewed by Veys and Chiesa [29]. The different combinations of chemotherapeutic agents are shown in Table 19.2 [30].

HSCT in Combined Immunodeficiencies

CD40 Ligand Deficiency

Mutations in the gene encoding CD40 ligand protein cause X-linked hyper-IgM syndrome, more commonly known as CD40 ligand deficiency. CD40L is up-regulated by activated T cells. Its absence causes defective interactions between CD40 (found on B cells) and CD40L, essential for successful immunoglobulin isotype class switch from IgM to IgG, IgA and IgE in B cells and generation of long-term humoral immunity [31, 32]. Patients affected by the disorder usually present with recurrent sinopulmonary infections or *Pneumocystis jiroveci* pneumonia, often when maternal IgG levels are waning. *Cryptosporidium* infection can also occur, lead-

ing to sclerosing cholangitis and cirrhosis, which has significant implications for transplant. Enterovirus encephalitis has also been described despite adequate immunoglobulin replacement therapy [33]. Neutropaenia is also a well-described feature and, more rarely, autoimmune disorder. Conservative management includes immunoglobulin replacement, cotrimoxazole prophylaxis and measures to avoid cryptosporidium exposure (e.g. drinking boiled or filtered water and avoiding swimming). HSCT is a potentially curative approach for CD40 ligand deficiency, although historical outcomes show only a 58% cure rate [34]. Challenges associated with HSCT were illustrated in a European retrospective study analysing data of 38 patients undergoing HSCT. In this cohort, 12 out of 38 patients did not survive and all succumbed to infections. A significant proportion of patients in this study (52%) experienced hepatic disease associated with cryptosporidium [34]. Therefore questions remain surrounding the optimal time to transplant affected children and the most suitable conditioning regimen to use in view of the well-documented hepatic or lung disease in the majority of patients.

We recently reviewed the natural history of 19 patients in our centre managed conservatively from diagnosis with no reports of persistent neutropenia, chronic lung disease or liver disease. Mortality was 10% in this group and was associated with an undefined neurodegenerative condition. The majority of the patients remained free of infection, and a conservative approach should be considered in the first instance in the absence of a fully matched donor, although those patients who present with or develop complications may warrant progression to transplant (Booth C/Davies G, personal communication).

Activated PI3 Kinase Delta Syndrome

Phosphatidylinositol-3 kinase (PI3K) proteins are essential for the production of phosphoinositides which act as second messengers for intracellular signalling transduction cascades that control cell division, survival, metabolism and reorganization of the actin cytoskeleton and cell migration in B- and T-lymphoid cells. A dominant gain-of-function mutation in the PIK3CD gene encoding p110δ protein is associated with a primary immunodeficiency causing hyper-IgM named activated PI3Kδ syndrome (APDS) [35, 36]. Clinical manifestations include recurrent respiratory infections, bronchiectasis, severe human herpes virus infections, autoimmunity and malignancies.

The immunological phenotype includes variable lymphopaenia, increased IgM levels and impaired vaccine responses but also reduced naïve T lymphocytes. PI3K leads to activation of downstream AKT and mammalian target of rapamycin (mTOR). mTOR inhibitors such as sirolimus have been used in patients with APDS, and reports have demonstrated reduction in CD8+ T-cell counts to normal numbers, an increase in percentage of naïve T cells and subsequent restoration of IL-2 secretion and proliferative responses and symptomatic improvement, although a durable remission was variable [37]. A recent multicentre study reported the outcome

of 11 patients who underwent HSCT for APDS. They observed that the use of steroids with and without sirolimus pre-HSCT failed to prevent in many cases recurrent infections and in one case was associated with malignant lymphoma pre-transplant. Patients underwent transplant with various different conditioning regimens including reduced intensity with fludarabine/melphalan and myeloablative conditioning with busulfan/cyclophosphamide. The overall survival was 81%, similar to that for other PIDs [38]. The role of sirolimus or other inhibitors of PI3Kinase such as GS-1101 is still being investigated [36]. As the number of patients diagnosed with this disorder remains limited, questions remain such as which patients would benefit from HSCT and which from immunotherapy.

MHC Class II Deficiency

MHC class II deficiency is a rare form of combined immunodeficiency and is characterized by the absence of major histocompatibility complex II in antigen-presenting cells which results in CD4+ lymphopaenia, absence of antigen-specific responses and thus increased susceptibility of these patients to potentially fatal infections. Curative treatment is limited to HSCT. Previous studies have shown that residual host CD8+T cells can affect engraftment with rates of graft rejection between 13% and 32% despite the use of myeloablative conditioning using busulfan and cyclophosphamide [39, 40]. Another challenge is impaired or delayed immune reconstitution post-transplant, as some patients have persistent CD4+ lymphopaenia consistent with impaired thymic maturation due to lack of HLA class II expression on thymic epithelia [41]. Many patients remain on antimicrobial prophylaxis and immunoglobulin replacement for prolonged periods after transplantation. Recently, the outcomes after HSCT have been improving even in unrelated donor setting. Small et al. [39] reported overall survival of 68.7% when using alternative donors for MHC class II deficiency. Three of 16 patients developed grade II–IV GvHD, and 1 of 11 developed extensive chronic GvHD following a secondary graft [39]. Our experience of T-cell replete cord blood transplantation in this condition is of improved immune reconstitution with 5/6 patients having CD4+ T-cell count of more than 300 μ/L at 6 months post-transplant and relatively rapid clearance of existing chronic infections although two of six patients developed chronic GvHD [42]. It is preferential that patients should be referred for transplant prior to developing severe infection or organ damage, but the optimal donor and conditioning regimen to prevent rejection and hasten immune reconstitution remains unclear.

DOCK 8

Dedicator of cytokinesis 8 (DOCK8) deficiency is a combined immunodeficiency characterized by hypereosinophilia, increased IgE levels and T-cell lymphopaenia. Clinical manifestations include recurrent respiratory infections and viral infections (affecting mainly the skin) and eczema. Previous retrospective studies of the natural history of the disease observed that affected patients are also at high risk of developing autoimmunity, cerebral events and malignancies with incidences of 13%, 14% and 17%, respectively [43]. HSCT should be considered for children before life-threatening infections and organ damage such as hepatic disease or bronchiectasis develop [44]. Recent reports showed good overall survival of 82% after HSCT with the main factors favourably impacting outcome identified as treosulfan-based conditioning and early age at transplantation (<8 years) [45].

HSCT in Wiskott-Aldrich Syndrome

Wiskott-Aldrich syndrome (WAS) is an X-linked immunodeficiency characterized by microthrombocytopaenia, eczema, recurrent infection, autoimmunity and an increased risk of lymphoproliferative malignancy. It is caused by mutations in the WAS gene, encoding the WAS protein and the spectrum of disease severity

correlates to some extent with the amount of residual protein expression [46]. As with other PIDs, it is important to stabilize disease and treat complications of the condition prior to embarking on stem cell transplantation in order to achieve a good outcome, but, in general, patients with WAS have historically experienced improved outcome post-HSCT compared to other non-SCID immunodeficiencies in a matched donor setting. Indeed, over the past two decades, the survival rates for patients with WAS after HSCT have improved significantly with an overall survival of 83% in one large cohort study and 89% for those transplanted after 2000 [47]. This is likely due to improved monitoring, accuracy of HLA-typing and lower rates of graft rejection, thanks to the use of more immunosuppressive chemotherapeutic agents such as fludarabine. Even in the mismatched donor setting, survival has dramatically increased from 52% to 92% [47].

Optimal timing of HSCT in WAS has been well characterized, and undertaking a transplant procedure before the age of 5 years affords significantly better outcome, preventing mortality associated with bleeding, infection and malignancy [47–49]. HSCT prior to the development of autoimmune complications is also beneficial. However, most centres would prefer to wait until a child is over 1 year of age before proceeding to transplant, provided that the child was clinically stable, in order to avoid what can be unpredictable toxicity related to conditioning regimes in infancy. Choice of conditioning regimen is an important consideration in WAS patients as mixed chimerism and graft rejection is not an uncommon finding. Moratto et al. reported that stable full donor chimerism was achieved in only 72% of transplanted patients, and despite 88% of boys receiving a myeloablative conditioning regimen, the rate of graft failure was still 7% (including 8 of 13 patients receiving T-cell-depleted grafts from MMFD) [47]. Results in HSCT for PID using treosulfan conditioning are promising with high-level donor chimerism achieved in a recent series [50], and we would suggest that a fludarabine- and treosulfan- or busulfan-based regime offers low TRM and incidence of GvHD together with a high rate of engraftment when PBSCs are used as a stem cell source. The presence of mixed donor chimerism appears to affect post-transplant course, correlating with a higher risk of incomplete lymphocyte reconstitution, persistent thrombocytopaenia and autoimmune complications (although the data on this point is controversial [49].

Complications were seen in 46% patients in the first year after transplant, and even at the time of last follow-up, the rate remained high at 29% with more frequent complications developing in those receiving an UCB transplant and those entering transplant with more severe disease [47]. The predominant manifestations of autoimmunity, which affected 14% of patients, were cytopaenias and endocrinopathies, often responsive to steroids and rituximab, and in some patients, developed over a year post-HSCT. These phenomena appear to be independent of GvHD and may be related to residual host autoantibodies or recipient Tregs and NKT cells [51]. In patients with mixed chimerism, the highest chimerism tends to be seen in the T-cell compartment, but it is the myeloid chimerism that is crucial in determining post-transplant platelet count. Up to a quarter of transplanted patients have a platelet count below the normal range ($<150 \times 10^9$/l) with some experiencing severe thrombocytopaenia requiring stem cell boosts, repeated platelet transfusion and splenectomy [47]. Other post-HSCT complications included fatal post-transplant lymphoproliferative disease and lymphoma as well as three late deaths related to sepsis with encapsulated organisms (pneumococcus and meningococcus) in patients who underwent splenectomy, highlighting the importance of lifelong antibiotic prophylaxis in this group of patients.

Patients with WAS lacking an HLA-matched donor for HSCT may also benefit from autologous stem cell gene therapy. Although patients treated in early gammaretroviral trials developed myelodysplasia linked to vector design [52, 53], subsequent trials using a safer lentiviral vector design have shown encouraging results [54, 55].

HSCT in Phagocytic Cell Defects

HSCT offers a curative treatment approach for a number of phagocytic disorders, and the increasing experience of transplanting patients with these conditions improves our understanding of the impact of existing infection and inflammation, donor choice and conditioning regimes on the outcome post-transplant. Chronic granulomatous disease (CGD) remains the most common phagocytic disorder encountered by transplant physicians and will be discussed here in detail, but we will also consider the role of HSCT in the management of leukocyte adhesion deficiency (LAD) type 1 and GATA2 deficiency.

Chronic Granulomatous Disease

CGD is an inherited immune deficiency caused by mutations in any of the genes encoding the protein components of the NADPH oxidase complex. The most common and severe form is inherited in an X-linked manner and associated with mutations in the *CYBB* gene encoding the gp91^{phox} protein. An autosomal recessive form affecting the p47^{phox} protein is also considered a transplantable condition, although patients may have a less aggressive phenotype. Abnormalities in the NADPH complex affect phagocytes' ability to kill bacterial and fungal pathogens leading to severe and uncontrolled infection, granuloma formation and often chronic autoinflammation with resultant organ damage. The advent of improved antimicrobial prophylaxis and azoles to both treat and prevent fungal infections has certainly improved survival for patient with CGD who are managed conservatively, but nonetheless they remain at risk of life-threatening infections and inflammatory complications which can severely reduce quality of life.

Early reports of HSCT in CGD demonstrated the negative effect on morbidity and mortality of active infection or inflammation at the time of transplant. Seger et al. described a cohort of 27 patients treated between 1985 and 2000 in which all patients with active fungal infections died, but those who were free of severe infection or colitis did well [56]. Prominent inflammatory symptoms were also associated with the development of severe GvHD. They advocated aggressive investigation and management of infection and discouraged the use of non-genoidentical donors for HSCT. Subsequent series documented improved survival rates up to 100% following HSCT using HLA-matched donors (both related and unrelated) and myeloablative conditioning regimes to secure stable myeloid engraftment [57–62]. Importantly, the data describes disease-free survival with resolution of inflammatory complications including colitis. This evidence supported the use of HSCT as a first-line treatment option for patients with CGD who had a matched donor available for transplant. Studies comparing outcome of patients treated conservatively or with HSCT also support this approach with results suggesting improved quality of life post-transplant [60, 61]. Those patients (both adults and children) managed conservatively experienced more severe infections, hospitalizations and surgical intervention compared to patients receiving a stem cell transplant.

In 2014, Gungor et al. published results of a prospective study involving 56 paediatric and adult patients undergoing HSCT for CGD using a busulfan-based reduced intensity (submyeloablative) conditioning regime [63]. The results were impressive not only for the high survival rates, low incidence of GvHD and stable myeloid engraftment in high risk patients but also outstanding results using mismatched unrelated donors. The conditioning regimen consisted of fludarabine, low dose or targeted busulfan (targeting an AUC of 45–65 mg/l/h) plus either alemtuzumab (in the unrelated donor setting) or ATG (for matched sibling donors). Overall survival for this cohort was 93% irrespective of the use of MRD or MUD. Despite concerns over the use of a RIC regimen, graft failure was only seen in three patients with >90% stable donor chimerism in the surviving patients and a low incidence of GvHD.

Patients with CGD may have a high burden of infection prior to HSCT, and many receive immunosuppressive treatment to control inflammatory complications and colitis further increasing the risk of invasive fungal disease and sepsis.

Anti-TNFα blockade (i.e. g., infliximab) together with steroids can successfully treat inflammatory bowel complications in CGD but has been associated with a predisposition to severe and occasionally fatal infection with typical CGD pathogens [64]. In the case of invasive fungal disease or other deep-seated infection at the time of transplant, granulocyte infusions (in addition to appropriate antimicrobial and antifungal cover) during the period of neutropaenia can improve survival and are generally well tolerated [65].

The management of patients lacking an HLA-matched donor (10/10 or 9/10) remains challenging as the best approach for alternative donors has not been determined. The use of haploidentical donors for HSCT in patients with primary immunodeficiencies is increasing, but published data relating to CGD patients is scarce. Parta et al. report the use of post-transplant cyclophosphamide in a patient with active fungal infection undergoing a haploidentical HSCT achieving full donor chimerism and resolution of infection [66]. Gene therapy may also offer an alternative management strategy for patient lacking a suitable donor and is discussed elsewhere.

Leukocyte Adhesion Deficiency Type 1

LAD type 1 is an autosomal recessive immune disorder caused by disabling mutations in CD18, the common subunit of the β2 integrin family. The β2 integrins contain an alpha chain (CD11a, CD11b or CD11c) non-covalently bound to CD18, and CD18 is required for expression of the heterodimer. CD11b/CD18 is expressed on myeloid cells and mediates leukocyte adhesion to endothelial cells required for trafficking to sites of infection. Patients tend to present in infancy with severe bacterial and fungal infections, often associated with necrotizing lesions and poor wound healing. The clinical phenotype relates to the level of CD18 expression with <1% CD18 expression correlating to the most severely affected patients. Although the condition is extremely rare, a number of multicentre case series have been published providing evidence of the curative nature of the procedure and associated complications. As with many other primary immunodeficiencies, increased transplant-related mortality was seen following myeloablative conditioning, but interestingly for LAD-1, the success rate was comparable between matched related and matched unrelated donors.

Qasim et al. reported a multicentre, retrospective analysis of 36 children with LAD-1 receiving HSCT between 1993 and 2007 and were able to demonstrate long-term benefit for patients in an HLA-matched donor setting and an overall survival rate of 75% [67]. Patients receiving a haploidentical graft (T-cell-depleted) fared significantly worse with graft rejection despite myeloablative conditioning, and all four patients required a second transplant procedure. A RIC regimen was better tolerated with no deaths seen in this group of patients, and although mixed chimerism was a common feature regardless of conditioning type, this was not associated with recurrence of symptoms. A more recent single-centre study reports ten patients treated with a RIC regimen with favourable results and similar survival rates (80%) [68]. Again mixed donor chimerism was seen but was not associated with graft rejection or recurrence of clinical symptoms. The incidence of GvHD was higher in this cohort of patients but likely relates to the use of PBSC as stem cell source rather than bone marrow. In both case series, the majority of deaths were caused by infection and occurred in both the early (<3 m) and late transplant period.

Given the suboptimal survival in this group of patients following mismatched donor transplant, autologous gene therapy strategies have been developed. Following the unsuccessful treatment of two patients in 1999 in the USA using a gammaretroviral vector [69], proof of concept has now been demonstrated through correction of canine and murine disease models using both self-inactivating lentiviral [70–72] and foamy virus vectors [73].

GATA2 Deficiency

GATA2 deficiency is a recently described immune deficiency with a spectrum of clinical manifestations including severe bacterial and viral infections, cytopaenias, aplastic anaemia, myelodysplasia and haematological malignancy, pulmonary alveolar proteinosis and lymphoedema [74]. Multiple haematopoietic lineages are affected in this condition, but HSCT can ameliorate haematopoietic, immunological and pulmonary features of the disease [75]. Given our limited experience of treating patients with GATA2 deficiency, the most appropriate timing and type of transplant is yet to be determined, particularly with respect to conditioning regime balancing the need for a myeloablative regime to achieve high-level engraftment and eradication of any malignant clones with severe infection and lung damage. Grossman et al. published recently results from 14 patients (mainly adult, median age at transplant 33 years) receiving HSCT following non-myeloablative conditioning with the exact regime dependent on donor type [75]. The overall survival rate was 57% reflecting the significant pre-existing morbidities in this group of patients. All had a significant burden of chronic infection (including disseminated non-tuberculous mycobacteria, human papilloma virus, varicella zoster virus and invasive aspergillosis) as well as pulmonary complications and evidence of dysplasia on bone marrow examination. Patients receiving MRD or MUD transplants fared better with survival rates of 75% in both groups, but the outcome following UCB was poor where delayed immune reconstitution contributed heavily to 25% overall survival in this group (one of four patients survived). It is highly likely that in the future, greater awareness and earlier recognition of the diagnosis will improve outcome for this patient group, and multicentre reports will be invaluable to help understand the optimal method and timing of transplant.

Stem Cell Transplant for Primary Haemophagocytic Lymphohistiocytosis

HLH is a life-threatening syndrome of severe hyper-inflammation due to the uncontrolled proliferation of activated lymphocytes and macrophages. Clinical symptoms include fever, cytopaenias, splenomegaly, coagulopathy and haemophagocytosis with specific diagnostic criteria available [76]. Primary HLH refers to genetically determined familial HLH (FHLH) syndromes caused by mutations in proteins involved in the cytotoxic pathway (*PRF1*, *UNC13D*, *STX11* and *STXBP2*) or in association with specific immune deficiencies where HLH is a recognized clinical phenotype such as X-linked lymphoproliferative disease (XLP) and X-linked inhibitor of apoptosis (XIAP) deficiency. Although it is critically important to treat HLH according to standard chemotherapeutic protocols involving heavy immunosuppression (HLH 94 and 2004 protocols), the vast majority of patients with primary HLH will progress to HSCT as a curative procedure, and an absence of disease activity at the time of transplant is paramount to successful outcome. EBV is a common trigger for HLH in these patients. EBV-associated HLH isn't treated with antiviral drugs. Since EBV resides in B lymphocytes, nti-CD20 monoclonal antibodies (rituximab) are routinely used to eliminate B cells harbouring the virus [77]. This may also reduce the incidence of post-transplant EBV reactivation. In clinical situations where EBV viraemia detected by PCR is uncontrolled despite treatment, and, for example, if the central nervous system is affected, EBV-specific CTLs may offer a useful treatment adjunct. In such cases an EBV-positive donor for transplant would be preferentially chosen.

Patients with HLH can be some of the most challenging patients to transplant, and even if remission is induced before HSCT, ongoing infections due to immunosuppression and multi-organ dysfunction may increase transplant-related mortality. Over the past decade, evidence suggests that RIC regimes are well tolerated in this group of patients and can lead to successful outcome even in the face of active disease at the time of transplant [78, 79]. Marsh et al. compared outcome for 40 paediatric patients with FHL and XIAP deficiency receiving either myeloablative busulfan-based regime or a RIC regimen consisting of fludarabine, melphalan and alemtuzumab [79]. Patients treated with a RIC HSCT had a significantly better survival (89% vs. 43% at time of analysis) despite similar disease severity, prior treatment, graft characteristics (including comparable numbers of 7/8 HLA mismatched donors in each group) and incidence of GvHD. Unsurprisingly, the use of a RIC regime led to an increased incidence of mixed chimerism (65% vs. 18%), but this was managed in the majority of cases with reduced immunosuppression, DLI or CD34+ stem cell boost, with only one patient suffering disease relapse. UCB HSCT has also been used in the RIC setting, again with encouraging results described in a single-centre series of infants with FHL [80].

XIAP deficiency, although initially described as XLP type 2, is increasingly recognized as a separate disease entity with features of immune dysregulation and recurrent, often insidious HLH. Patients with XIAP deficiency were noted to have a particularly poor outcome following HSCT, although again survival improved when RIC regimes were employed compared to those children receiving MAC (55% vs. 14%) [81]. Due to the apoptotic defect in XIAP-deficient cells, patients appear to be exquisitely sensitive to chemotherapy and suffer severe transplant-related toxicities. In an attempt to overcome this, we have used an anti-CD45 monoclonal antibody approach (termed minimal intensity conditioning) with some success in this patient group with low TRM, full donor chimerism and good immune reconstitution [82].

Thymic Transplantation

In recent years, thymic transplant has been successfully used to treat patients with athymic conditions, namely, DiGeorge syndrome, allowing reconstitution of functional T cells following transplant of allogeneic thymic tissue obtained from patients undergoing cardiac surgery. Although the immune defects in DiGeorge syndrome are variable, a small percentage present with a SCID phenotype. HSCT has been performed; however, results have been unfavourable compared to other types of SCID with a survival of 60% in the MSD setting [83]. Immune recovery following HSCT is also poor with continued CD4+ lymphopaenia, low numbers of naïve T cells and diminished T-cell repertoire.

Given that the bone marrow compartment in athymic patients is functional, it was postulated that providing normal thymic tissue from an immunocompetent donor would allow normal development and education of T cells capable of normal function. Thymic tissue from suitable donors is cultured in the laboratory to remove donor lymphocytes and screened for infection prior to surgical placement in the quadriceps muscles of recipients. Once implanted, the thymic tissue becomes vascularized, and thymopoiesis can commence with naïve lymphocytes detectable by 3–6 months. Currently donors are matched only for blood group, and recipients do not receive any prior conditioning with ATG unless they exhibit an Omenn's phenotype with oligoclonal expansions of T-cell populations. In this situation ongoing immunosuppression with ciclosporine may be required.

Programmes of thymic transplantation are currently underway in Duke University, North Carolina, and Great Ormond Street Hospital, London. Results from 60 patients published by the Duke group show a survival of 72% with production of naïve T cells, normal T-cell repertoire and ability to make antigen-specific responses [84]. Deaths were related to pre-existing complications such as viral infections and chronic lung disease. Often the T lymphocyte and naïve T-cell count do not reach the normal ranges but are sufficient that patients no longer require prophylactic antibiotics or immunoglobulin therapy. Autoimmunity has been recognized as complication of the procedure, manifesting mainly as hypothyroidism and cytopaenias. Nonetheless, results are promising, and refinements to existing protocols will likely improve results further.

Conclusions and Future Directions

HSCT offers a curative treatment for the majority of PIDs with significantly improved survival even in the non-genoidentical donor setting. The challenges which remain to further improve outcomes are being addressed by early diagnosis with newborn screening, and the use of novel approaches to mismatched grafts to hasten immune reconstitution. Alternative approaches including gene therapy, thymus transplantation and small molecule therapies are now available for certain conditions and may replace HSCT in certain situations. Next-generation sequencing techniques are identifying a number of novel PID conditions, but as yet there is little evidence to guide the use of HSCT in these patients.

References

1. Schultz RK, Baker KS, Boelens JJ, Bollard CM, Egeler RM, Cowan M, et al. Challenges and opportunities for international cooperative studies in pediatric hematopoeitic cell transplantation: priorities of the Westhafen Intercontinental Group. Biol Blood Marrow Transplant. 2013;19(9):1279–87.
2. Al-Herz W, Bousfiha A, Casanova JL, Chatila T, Conley ME, Cunningham-Rundles C, et al. Primary immunodeficiency diseases: an update on the classification from the international union of immunological societies expert committee for primary immunodeficiency. Front Immunol. 2014;5:162.
3. Hassan A, Lee P, Maggina P, Xu JH, Moreira D, Slatter M, et al. Host natural killer immunity is a key indicator of permissiveness for donor cell engraftment in patients with severe combined immunodeficiency. J Allergy Clin Immunol. 2014;133(6):1660–6.
4. Gennery AR, Slatter MA, Grandin L, Taupin P, Cant AJ, Veys P, et al. Transplantation of hematopoietic stem cells and long-term survival for primary immunodeficiencies in Europe: entering a new century, do we do better? J Allergy Clin Immunol. 2010;126(3):602–10. e1–11
5. Fernandes JF, Rocha V, Labopin M, Neven B, Moshous D, Gennery AR, et al. Transplantation in patients with SCID: mismatched related stem cells or unrelated cord blood? Blood. 2012;119(12):2949–55.
6. Veys P, Danby R, Vora A, Slatter M, Wynn R, Lawson S, et al. UK experience of unrelated cord blood transplantation in paediatric patients. Br J Haematol. 2016;172(3):482–6.
7. Dvorak CC, Hassan A, Slatter MA, Honig M, Lankester AC, Buckley RH, et al. Comparison of outcomes of hematopoietic stem cell transplantation without chemotherapy conditioning by using matched sibling and unrelated donors for treatment of severe combined immunodeficiency. J Allergy Clin Immunol. 2014;134(4):935–43. e15
8. Pai SY, Logan BR, Griffith LM, Buckley RH, Parrott RE, Dvorak CC, et al. Transplantation outcomes for severe combined immunodeficiency, 2000–2009. N Engl J Med. 2014;371(5):434–46.
9. Gaspar HB, Qasim W, Davies EG, Rao K, Amrolia PJ, Veys P. How I treat severe combined immunodeficiency. Blood. 2013;122(23):3749–58.

10. Howe SJ, Mansour MR, Schwarzwaelder K, Bartholomae C, Hubank M, Kempski H, et al. Insertional mutagenesis combined with acquired somatic mutations causes leukemogenesis following gene therapy of SCID-X1 patients. J Clin Invest. 2008;118(9):3143–50.

11. Chiesa R, Gilmour K, Qasim W, Adams S, Worth AJ, Zhan H, et al. Omission of in vivo T-cell depletion promotes rapid expansion of naive CD4+ cord blood lymphocytes and restores adaptive immunity within 2 months after unrelated cord blood transplant. Br J Haematol. 2012;156(5):656–66.

12. Locatelli F, Bauquet A, Palumbo G, Moretta F, Bertaina A. Negative depletion of alpha/beta+ T cells and of CD19+ B lymphocytes: a novel frontier to optimize the effect of innate immunity in HLA-mismatched hematopoietic stem cell transplantation. Immunol Lett. 2013;155(1–2):21–3.

13. Bertaina A, Merli P, Rutella S, Pagliara D, Bernardo ME, Masetti R, et al. HLA-haploidentical stem cell transplantation after removal of alphabeta+ T and B cells in children with nonmalignant disorders. Blood. 2014;124(5):822–6.

14. Zhou X, Di Stasi A, Tey SK, Krance RA, Martinez C, Leung KS, et al. Long-term outcome after haploidentical stem cell transplant and infusion of T cells expressing the inducible caspase 9 safety transgene. Blood. 2014;123(25):3895–905.

15. Grosso D, Carabasi M, Filicko-O'Hara J, Kasner M, Wagner JL, Colombe B, et al. A 2-step approach to myeloablative haploidentical stem cell transplantation: a phase 1/2 trial performed with optimized T-cell dosing. Blood. 2011;118(17):4732–9.

16. McCurdy SR, Kanakry JA, Showel MM, Tsai HL, Bolanos-Meade J, Rosner GL, et al. Risk-stratified outcomes of nonmyeloablative HLA-haploidentical BMT with high-dose posttransplantation cyclophosphamide. Blood. 2015;125(19):3024–31.

17. Robinson TM, O'Donnell PV, Fuchs EJ, Luznik L. Haploidentical bone marrow and stem cell transplantation: experience with post-transplantation cyclophosphamide. Semin Hematol. 2016;53(2):90–7.

18. Ouederni M, Mellouli F, Khaled MB, Kaabi H, Picard C, Bejaoui M. Successful haploidentical stem cell transplantation with post-transplant cyclophosphamide in a severe combined immune deficiency patient: a first report. J Clin Immunol. 2016;36:437–40.

19. Brown L, Xu-Bayford J, Allwood Z, Slatter M, Cant A, Davies EG, et al. Neonatal diagnosis of severe combined immunodeficiency leads to significantly improved survival outcome: the case for newborn screening. Blood. 2011;117(11):3243–6.

20. Kobrynski L. Newborn screening for severe combined immune deficiency (technical and political aspects). Curr Opin Allergy Clin Immunol. 2015;15(6):539–46.

21. Gaspar HB, Hammarstrom L, Mahlaoui N, Borte M, Borte S. The case for mandatory newborn screening for severe combined immunodeficiency (SCID). J Clin Immunol. 2014;34(4):393–7.

22. Clement MC, Mahlaoui N, Mignot C, Le Bihan C, Rabetrano H, Hoang L, et al. Systematic neonatal screening for severe combined immunodeficiency and severe T-cell lymphopenia: analysis of cost-effectiveness based on French real field data. J Allergy Clin Immunol. 2015;135(6):1589–93.

23. de Felipe B, Olbrich P, Lucenas JM, Delgado-Pecellin C, Pavon-Delgado A, Marquez J, et al. Prospective neonatal screening for severe T- and B-lymphocyte deficiencies in Seville. Pediatr Allergy Immunol. 2016;27(1):70–7.

24. de Pagter AP, Bredius RG, Kuijpers TW, Tramper J, van der Burg M, van Montfrans J, et al. Overview of 15-year severe combined immunodeficiency in the Netherlands: towards newborn blood spot screening. Eur J Pediatr. 2015;174(9):1183–8.

25. Kwan A, Abraham RS, Currier R, Brower A, Andruszewski K, Abbott JK, et al. Newborn screening for severe combined immunodeficiency in 11 screening programs in the United States. JAMA. 2014;312(7):729–38.

26. van der Spek J, Groenwold RH, van der Burg M, van Montfrans JM. TREC based newborn screening for severe combined immunodeficiency disease: a systematic review. J Clin Immunol. 2015;35(4):416–30.

27. Chan K, Puck JM. Development of population-based newborn screening for severe combined immunodeficiency. J Allergy Clin Immunol. 2005;115(2):391–8.

28. Rao K, Amrolia PJ, Jones A, Cale CM, Naik P, King D, et al. Improved survival after unrelated donor bone marrow transplantation in children with primary immunodeficiency using a reduced-intensity conditioning regimen. Blood. 2005;105(2):879–85.

29. Chiesa R, Veys P. Reduced-intensity conditioning for allogeneic stem cell transplant in primary immune deficiencies. Expert Rev Clin Immunol. 2012;8(3):255–66. quiz 67

30. Satwani P, Cooper N, Rao K, Veys P, Amrolia P. Reduced intensity conditioning and allogeneic stem cell transplantation in childhood malignant and nonmalignant diseases. Bone Marrow Transplant. 2007;41(2):173–82.

31. DiSanto JP, Bonnefoy JY, Gauchat JF, Fischer A, de Saint Basile G. CD40 ligand mutations in x-linked immunodeficiency with hyper-IgM. Nature. 1993;361(6412):541–3.

32. Korthauer U, Graf D, Mages HW, Briere F, Padayachee M, Malcolm S, et al. Defective expression of T-cell CD40 ligand causes X-linked immunodeficiency with hyper-IgM. Nature. 1993;361(6412):539–41.

33. Cunningham CK, Bonville CA, Ochs HD, Seyama K, John PA, Rotbart HA, et al. Enteroviral meningoencephalitis as a complication of X-linked hyper IgM syndrome. J Pediatr. 1999;134(5):584–8.

34. Gennery AR, Khawaja K, Veys P, Bredius RG, Notarangelo LD, Mazzolari E, et al. Treatment of CD40 ligand deficiency by hematopoietic stem cell transplantation: a survey of the European experience, 1993–2002. Blood. 2004;103(3):1152–7.

35. Deau MC, Heurtier L, Frange P, Suarez F, Bole-Feysot C, Nitschke P, et al. A human immunodeficiency caused by mutations in the PIK3R1 gene. J Clin Invest. 2014;124(9):3923–8.

36. Angulo I, Vadas O, Garcon F, Banham-Hall E, Plagnol V, Leahy TR, et al. Phosphoinositide 3-kinase delta gene mutation predisposes to respiratory infection and airway damage. Science. 2013;342(6160):866–71.

37. Lucas CL, Kuehn HS, Zhao F, Niemela JE, Deenick EK, Palendira U, et al. Dominant-activating germline mutations in the gene encoding the PI(3)K catalytic subunit p110delta result in T cell senescence and human immunodeficiency. Nat Immunol. 2014;15(1):88–97.

38. Nademi Z, Slatter MA, Dvorak CC, Neven B, Fischer A, Suarez F, et al. Hematopoietic stem cell transplant in patients with activated PI3K delta syndrome. J Allergy Clin Immunol. 2017;139(3):1046–9.

39. Small TN, Qasim W, Friedrich W, Chiesa R, Bleesing JJ, Scurlock A, et al. Alternative donor SCT for the treatment of MHC class II deficiency. Bone Marrow Transplant. 2013;48(2):226–32.

40. Ouederni M, Vincent QB, Frange P, Touzot F, Scerra S, Bejaoui M, et al. Major histocompatibility complex class II expression deficiency caused by a RFXANK founder mutation: a survey of 35 patients. Blood. 2011;118(19):5108–18.

41. Saleem MA, Arkwright PD, Davies EG, Cant AJ, Veys PA. Clinical course of patients with major histocompatibility complex class II deficiency. Arch Dis Child. 2000;83(4):356–9.

42. J Allergy Clin Immunol. 2018 Jan 31. pii: S0091-6749(18)30083-6. doi: https://doi.org/10.1016/j.jaci.2017.10.051. [Epub ahead of print]

43. Aydin SE, Kilic SS, Aytekin C, Kumar A, Porras O, Kainulainen L, et al. DOCK8 deficiency: clinical and immunological phenotype and treatment options – a review of 136 patients. J Clin Immunol. 2015;35(2):189–98.

44. Al-Herz W, Chu JI, van der Spek J, Raghupathy R, Massaad MJ, Keles S, et al. Hematopoietic stem cell transplantation outcomes for 11 patients with dedicator of cytokinesis 8 deficiency. J Allergy Clin Immunol. 2016;138:852–9.

45. Aydin S, Freeman AF, Su H, Hickstein D, Pai S-Y, Geha R, et al. HSCT for DOCK8 deficiency – an international study on 74 patients. Biol Blood Marrow Transplant. 2016;22(3, Supplement):S103–S4.

46. Jin Y, Mazza C, Christie JR, Giliani S, Fiorini M, Mella P, et al. Mutations of the Wiskott-Aldrich syndrome protein (WASP): hotspots, effect on transcription, and translation and phenotype/genotype correlation. Blood. 2004;104(13):4010–9.

47. Moratto D, Giliani S, Bonfim C, Mazzolari E, Fischer A, Ochs HD, et al. Long-term outcome and lineage-specific chimerism in 194 patients with Wiskott-Aldrich syndrome treated by hematopoietic cell transplantation in the period 1980–2009: an international collaborative study. Blood. 2011;118(6):1675–84.

48. Ozsahin H, Cavazzana-Calvo M, Notarangelo LD, Schulz A, Thrasher AJ, Mazzolari E, et al. Long-term outcome following hematopoietic stem-cell transplantation in Wiskott-Aldrich syndrome: collaborative study of the European Society for Immunodeficiencies and European Group for blood and marrow transplantation. Blood. 2008;111(1):439–45.

49. Shin CR, Kim MO, Li D, Bleesing JJ, Harris R, Mehta P, et al. Outcomes following hematopoietic cell transplantation for Wiskott-Aldrich syndrome. Bone Marrow Transplant. 2012;47(11):1428–35.

50. Slatter MA, Rao K, Amrolia P, Flood T, Abinun M, Hambleton S, et al. Treosulfan-based conditioning regimens for hematopoietic stem cell transplantation in children with primary immunodeficiency: United Kingdom experience. Blood. 2011;117(16):4367–75.

51. Worth AJ, Thrasher AJ. Current and emerging treatment options for Wiskott-Aldrich syndrome. Expert Rev Clin Immunol. 2015;11(9):1015–32.

52. Boztug K, Schmidt M, Schwarzer A, Banerjee PP, Diez IA, Dewey RA, et al. Stem-cell gene therapy for the Wiskott-Aldrich syndrome. N Engl J Med. 2010;363(20):1918–27.

53. Braun CJ, Boztug K, Paruzynski A, Witzel M, Schwarzer A, Rothe M, et al. Gene therapy for Wiskott-Aldrich syndrome – long-term efficacy and genotoxicity. Sci Transl Med. 2014;6(227):227ra33.

54. Aiuti A, Biasco L, Scaramuzza S, Ferrua F, Cicalese MP, Baricordi C, et al. Lentiviral hematopoietic stem cell gene therapy in patients with Wiskott-Aldrich syndrome. Science. 2013;341(6148):1233151.

55. Hacein-Bey Abina S, Gaspar HB, Blondeau J, Caccavelli L, Charrier S, Buckland K, et al. Outcomes following gene therapy in patients with severe Wiskott-Aldrich syndrome. JAMA. 2015;313(15):1550–63.

56. Seger RA, Gungor T, Belohradsky BH, Blanche S, Bordigoni P, Di Bartolomeo P, et al. Treatment of chronic granulomatous disease with myeloablative conditioning and an unmodified hemopoietic allograft: a survey of the European experience, 1985–2000. Blood. 2002;100(13):4344–50.

57. Soncini E, Slatter MA, Jones LB, Hughes S, Hodges S, Flood TJ, et al. Unrelated donor and HLA-identical sibling haematopoietic stem cell transplantation cure chronic granulomatous disease with good long-term outcome and growth. Br J Haematol. 2009;145(1):73–83.

58. Schuetz C, Hoenig M, Gatz S, Speth F, Benninghoff U, Schulz A, et al. Hematopoietic stem cell transplantation from matched unrelated donors in chronic granulomatous disease. Immunol Res. 2009;44(1–3):35–41.

59. Tewari P, Martin PL, Mendizabal A, Parikh SH, Page KM, Driscoll TA, et al. Myeloablative transplantation using either cord blood or bone marrow leads to immune recovery, high long-term donor chimerism and excellent survival in chronic granulomatous disease. Biol Blood Marrow Transplant. 2012;18(9):1368–77.

60. Ahlin A, Fugelang J, de Boer M, Ringden O, Fasth A, Winiarski J. Chronic granulomatous

disease-haematopoietic stem cell transplantation versus conventional treatment. Acta Paediatr. 2013;102(11):1087–94.

61. Cole T, Pearce MS, Cant AJ, Cale CM, Goldblatt D, Gennery AR. Clinical outcome in children with chronic granulomatous disease managed conservatively or with hematopoietic stem cell transplantation. J Allergy Clin Immunol. 2013;132(5):1150–5.

62. Martinez CA, Shah S, Shearer WT, Rosenblatt HM, Paul ME, Chinen J, et al. Excellent survival after sibling or unrelated donor stem cell transplantation for chronic granulomatous disease. J Allergy Clin Immunol. 2012;129(1):176–83.

63. Gungor T, Teira P, Slatter M, Stussi G, Stepensky P, Moshous D, et al. Reduced-intensity conditioning and HLA-matched haemopoietic stem-cell transplantation in patients with chronic granulomatous disease: a prospective multicentre study. Lancet (London, England). 2014;383(9915):436–48.

64. Uzel G, Orange JS, Poliak N, Marciano BE, Heller T, Holland SM. Complications of tumor necrosis factor-alpha blockade in chronic granulomatous disease-related colitis. Clin Infect Dis. 2010;51(12):1429–34.

65. Nikolajeva O, Mijovic A, Hess D, Tatam E, Amrolia P, Chiesa R, et al. Single-donor granulocyte transfusions for improving the outcome of high-risk pediatric patients with known bacterial and fungal infections undergoing stem cell transplantation: a 10-year single-center experience. Bone Marrow Transplant. 2015;50(6):846–9.

66. Parta M, Hilligoss D, Kelly C, Kwatemaa N, Theobald N, Malech H, et al. Haploidentical hematopoietic cell transplantation with post-transplant cyclophosphamide in a patient with chronic granulomatous disease and active infection: a first report. J Clin Immunol. 2015;35(7):675–80.

67. Qasim W, Cavazzana-Calvo M, Davies EG, Davis J, Duval M, Eames G, et al. Allogeneic hematopoietic stem-cell transplantation for leukocyte adhesion deficiency. Pediatrics. 2009;123(3):836–40.

68. Hamidieh AA, Pourpak Z, Hosseinzadeh M, Fazlollahi MR, Alimoghaddam K, Movahedi M, et al. Reduced-intensity conditioning hematopoietic SCT for pediatric patients with LAD-1: clinical efficacy and importance of chimerism. Bone Marrow Transplant. 2012;47(5):646–50.

69. Bauer TR Jr, Hickstein DD. Gene therapy for leukocyte adhesion deficiency. Curr Opin Mol Ther. 2000;2(4):383–8.

70. Hunter MJ, Tuschong LM, Fowler CJ, Bauer TR Jr, Burkholder TH, Hickstein DD. Gene therapy of canine leukocyte adhesion deficiency using lentiviral vectors with human CD11b and CD18 promoters driving canine CD18 expression. Mol Ther. 2011;19(1):113–21.

71. Nelson EJ, Tuschong LM, Hunter MJ, Bauer TR Jr, Burkholder TH, Hickstein DD. Lentiviral vectors incorporating a human elongation factor 1alpha promoter for the treatment of canine leukocyte adhesion deficiency. Gene Ther. 2010;17(5):672–7.

72. Leon-Rico D, Aldea M, Sanchez-Baltasar R, Mesa-Nunez C, Record J, Burns SO, et al. Lentiviral vector-mediated correction of a mouse model of leukocyte adhesion deficiency type I. Hum Gene Ther. 2016;27:668–78.

73. Bauer TR Jr, Allen JM, Hai M, Tuschong LM, Khan IF, Olson EM, et al. Successful treatment of canine leukocyte adhesion deficiency by foamy virus vectors. Nat Med. 2008;14(1):93–7.

74. Hsu AP, McReynolds LJ, Holland SM. GATA2 deficiency. Curr Opin Allergy Clin Immunol. 2015;15(1):104–9.

75. Grossman J, Cuellar-Rodriguez J, Gea-Banacloche J, Zerbe C, Calvo K, Hughes T, et al. Nonmyeloablative allogeneic hematopoietic stem cell transplantation for GATA2 deficiency. Biol Blood Marrow Transplant. 2014;20(12):1940–8.

76. Henter JI, Horne A, Arico M, Egeler RM, Filipovich AH, Imashuku S, et al. HLH-2004: diagnostic and therapeutic guidelines for hemophagocytic lymphohistiocytosis. Pediatr Blood Cancer. 2007;48(2):124–31.

77. Chellapandian D, Das R, Zelley K, Wiener SJ, Zhao H, Teachey DT, et al. Treatment of Epstein Barr virus-induced haemophagocytic lymphohistiocytosis with rituximab-containing chemo-immunotherapeutic regimens. Br J Haematol. 2013;162(3):376–82.

78. Cooper N, Rao K, Gilmour K, Hadad L, Adams S, Cale C, et al. Stem cell transplantation with reduced-intensity conditioning for hemophagocytic lymphohistiocytosis. Blood. 2006;107(3):1233–6.

79. Marsh RA, Vaughn G, Kim MO, Li D, Jodele S, Joshi S, et al. Reduced-intensity conditioning significantly improves survival of patients with hemophagocytic lymphohistiocytosis undergoing allogeneic hematopoietic cell transplantation. Blood. 2010;116(26):5824–31.

80. Nishi M, Nishimura R, Suzuki N, Sawada A, Okamura T, Fujita N, et al. Reduced-intensity conditioning in unrelated donor cord blood transplantation for familial hemophagocytic lymphohistiocytosis. Am J Hematol. 2012;87(6):637–9.

81. Marsh RA, Rao K, Satwani P, Lehmberg K, Muller I, Li D, et al. Allogeneic hematopoietic cell transplantation for XIAP deficiency: an international survey reveals poor outcomes. Blood. 2013;121(6):877–83.

82. Worth AJ, Nikolajeva O, Chiesa R, Rao K, Veys P, Amrolia PJ. Successful stem cell transplant with antibody-based conditioning for XIAP deficiency with refractory hemophagocytic lymphohistiocytosis. Blood. 2013;121(24):4966–8.

83. Janda A, Sedlacek P, Honig M, Friedrich W, Champagne M, Matsumoto T, et al. Multicenter survey on the outcome of transplantation of hematopoietic cells in patients with the complete form of DiGeorge anomaly. Blood. 2010;116(13):2229–36.

84. Markert ML, Devlin BH, McCarthy EA. Thymus transplantation. Clin Immunol. 2010;135(2):236–46.

Specific Adoptive T-Cell Therapy for Viral and Fungal Infections

20

Lawrence G. Lum and Catherine M. Bollard

Introduction

Infections remain the leading cause of mortality and morbidity during the first 3 months after hematopoietic stem cell transplantation (HSCT) [1–4]. Despite advances in prophylactic viral and fungal therapy to minimize the viral and fungal burden early after HSCT, breakthrough viral and fungal infections remain life-threatening, and for some viral and fungal infections, there are no effective therapies [5–9]. Vaccine strategies to induce immunity to CMV began in the 1970s but have been limited in their success [10–12]. The conditioning regimens for HSCT that vary from non-myeloablative to myeloablative create an immunodeficiency that leaves the allogeneic HSCT recipient susceptible to viral and fungal infections while immune reconstitution occurs during the first 6–9 months after HSCT. Immune reconstitution is further abrogated by intensive immunosuppression used to prevent and/or control

GVHD. It is clearly established that the kinetics and rate of T-cell reconstitution are critical to controlling viral infections. Factors that speed T-cell recovery will decrease the risk of viral infection during the first 3 months after HSCT [2, 3, 13]. Early studies showed that donor lymphocyte infusions (DLI) given before T-cell reconstitution from the stem cell donor were effective for treating viral infections in HSCT recipients but were associated with a high risk of GVHD [14]. Since the early 1990s, investigators began to develop virus-specific cytotoxic T lymphocyte (vCTL) for adoptive immunotherapy against specific targets early during immune reconstitution after HSCT [15, 16].

Advances in vCTL therapy have benefited from (1) advances in understanding of immune responses to conserved T-cell epitopes for various pathogens [17–19], (2) technological advances in ex vivo expansion of T cells and advances in the preparation of antigen-presenting cells [20–22], and (3) assays that evaluate vCTL activity and the MHC restriction of vCTL [23, 24].

In this chapter, we review the following areas of how: (1) T cells have been expanded to target multiple pathogens; (2) vCTL production no longer requires viral infection or viral vector transduction of antigen-presenting cells (APCs); (3) The source of lymphocytes is no longer restricted to donors who are immune to the pathogens; (4) Naive T cells have been redirected with chimeric antigen receptor T cells (CARTs) to target pathogen-infected cells; (5) Bispecific antibody

L. G. Lum (✉)
Cellular Therapy and Stem Cell Transplant Program, Emily Couric Cancer Center, University of Virginia, Charlottesville, VA, USA
e-mail: lgl4f@hscmail.mcc.virginia.edu

C. M. Bollard
Program for Cell Enhancement and Technologies for Immunotherapy, Sheikh Zayed Institute for Pediatric Surgical Innovation, and Center for Cancer and Immunology Research, Children's National Health System, Washington, DC, USA

© Springer International Publishing AG, part of Springer Nature 2018
B. H. Segal (ed.), *Management of Infections in the Immunocompromised Host*,
https://doi.org/10.1007/978-3-319-77674-3_20

(BiAb)-armed T cells (BATs) can mediate vCTL activity; and (6) Pathogen-specific T-cell products can be manufactured by third parties and banked for "off-the-shelf" use post-HSCT.

We summarized the methodological approaches, clinical trials using vCTL, promising preclinical studies, and early clinical trials of anti-pathogen CTLs that have promise. These advances provide the rationale and impetus for future vCTL adoptive immunotherapy.

Production of vCTL As a guiding principle to decrease the risk of GVHD in allogeneic HSCT recipients, strategies excluded alloreactive T cells by selecting virus-specific T cells. Four major approaches were used: (1) stimulation with viral antigen(s) during ex vivo culture of donor T cells from peripheral blood mononuclear cells (PBMC), (2) direct selection of donor cells, (3) genetic modification of T cells to confer specific recognition of pathogen or pathogen-infected cells, or (4) arming of ex vivo expanded T cells with bispecific antibody to target the viral antigen (Fig. 20.1).

Antigen Stimulated Expansion Numerous ex vivo culture approaches have been used to produce cytomegalovirus (CMV)-specific CTL or Epstein-Barr virus (EBV)-specific CTL [15, 16, 25–30]. CMV viral- or peptide-specific stimulation in vitro expands single or multiple pathogen-specific vCTL. The advantages of culture over cell selection are the generation and expansion of polyclonal vCTL to clinically useful quantities of vCTL from small amounts of blood [31]. However, the major disadvantages of this strategy is the daunting task of culturing and processing after stimulation to expand the vCTL (up to more than 1 month) and the HLA-histocompatibility requirement of finding a closely matched donor. During these longer-term cultures, the vCTL may lose their capacity to self-renew and to persist in vivo, particularly after prolonged ex vivo culture [32]. It should be noted that clinical trials infusing ex vivo expanded vCTL post-HSCT showed prolonged persistence [33] and that ex vivo expansion using pathogen-specific stimuli decreased alloreactivity [19]. This may be due to selection of virus-specific clones and deselection of alloreactive clones. One study showed that residual alloreactivity seen in vCTL is clinically insignificant [34]. The initial trials of vCTL therapy required CMV lysates on APC, CMV-infected fibroblasts, or EBV-lymphoblastoid cells lines as a stimulant for expansion of donor-derived memory T cells [25, 27, 35]. The discovery of dominant and highly conserved antigens such as CMV-pp65 and adenovirus hexon and penton led to replacement of live viral stimulation with either 15-mer peptide pools spanning viral proteins or DNA plasmid-transduced antigen-presenting cells [36, 37]. The newer approaches to rapidly expand and manipulate APCs enabled use of a less restricted population of donors and the targeting of an increased number of pathogens in a single culture [20, 38]. In a recent rapid vCTL protocol, the addition of IL-4 and IL-7 leads to production of CD4+ T cells with a Th_1 phenotype, whereas IL-2 and IL-15 tended to favor in vitro natural killer (NK) cell expansion [37]. The ideal population to adoptively transfer may be ex vivo expanded central memory T cells with a CD62L and CD45RA phenotype as these cells have a superior ability to persist in vivo after adoptive transfer [39, 40].

Direct Selection via Cell Capture Sorting Direct selection relies on cell sorting of immune donor PBMCs, usually after pulsing them with the antigen(s) of interest, to drive expansion of virus-specific T-cell clones [41]. This approach would not be viable for obtaining immune CTLs from pathogen-naive donors. Multimer selection is achieved by binding of HLA-peptide complexes to T-cell receptors (TCRs) of known antigen specificity, followed by purification of bound cells, e.g., by magnetic column separation. Alternatively, antiviral T cells expressing interferon-γ (IFN-γ) can be isolated using the gamma capture assay. Direct selection methods have the advantage of rapid manufacturing time. Unfortunately, these approaches require apheresis of donors in order to collect sufficient cells for sorting and processing for clinical appli-

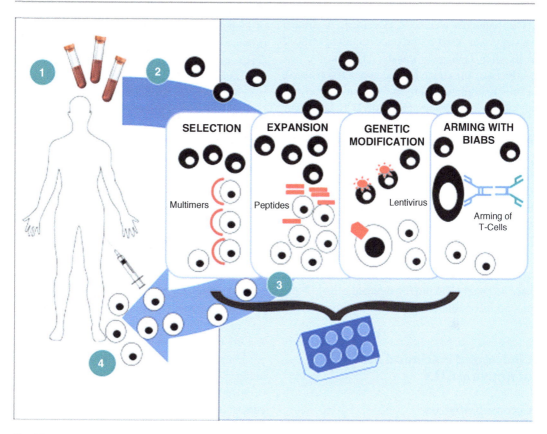

Fig. 20.1 Approaches to produce pathogen-specific CTL. (1) Blood is obtained from donors (autologous, allogeneic, or umbilical cord blood) or is drawn or apheresis is performed to obtain a larger quantity of blood; (2) PBMCs are processed via: (a) cell *selection* panel using multimers with a pathogen-derived peptide associated with a type-I HLA molecule *or* column selection after in vitro stimulation of T cells with antigens followed by binding of IFNγ or CD154-expressing T cells with antibody-coated immu- nomagnetic beads; (b) cell *expansion* by stimulating the PBMC with APCs produced by antigenic peptide pools, viral transduction, or nucleofection; (c) *genetic modifica- tion* that involves the transfer of high-affinity pathogen- specific TCRs or CARs to redirect the specificity of the T cells; and (d) polyclonal expansion of T cells for 8–14 days and arming with BiAbs directed at the pathogen of interest on one hand and the TCR on the other hand; (3) quality control and release testing; and (4) infusion into patients

cations and pre-existing and detectable pathogen- specific T cells in the blood. Multimer selection is major histocompatibility (MHC)-restricted and selects only CD8+ T cells of a limited specificity. This could possibly allow pathogen evasion and impair persistence of vCTL in vivo [42]. Earlier studies suggested that persistent binding of mul- timers to the TCR may impair T-cell function [43]. Recent reversible Streptamer technology for direct selection may overcome the problem of impaired function [44]. IFN-γ positive selection captures polyclonal antigen-specific CD4+ and CD8+ T cells and selects for a wider range of antigen-specific cells. Combining direct selec- tion, culture expansion methods, and cytokine cocktails can optimize the selection of central memory T cells in vCTL products and improve yields on targeted cellular phenotypes [37, 44].

TCR or CAR Gene Modifications T cells can be modified to redirect their specificity with retro- viral and lentiviral vectors to introduce the trans- genes for high-affinity TCRs or chimeric antigen receptors (CARs) consisting of a single-chain variable fragments (scFvs). High-affinity TCR genes can be cloned and transduced into poly- clonal T cells to generate a large population of

TCR pathogen-specific CTLs [45]. A similar strategy was used to produce tumor-specific T cells after TCR gene transfer [18]. In contrast, CARs have an extracellular region that consists of a scFv that binds to antigen, with an intracellular signaling complex composed of TCR zeta chain for first-generation CARs, the TCR zeta chain and the CD28 for second-generation CARs, and TCR zeta and CD28 or 41BB for third-generation CARs [46–48]. The high-affinity TCR-transduced CTLs have been used to target CMV-infected cells [49], HPV-infected cells [50], hepatitis B-infected cells [51], hepatitis C-infected cells [52], tuberculosis-infected cells [53], SARS-infected cells [54], chlamydia-infected cells [55], and HIV-infected cells [56]. CAR T cells were used to target CD4 in HIV-infected cells [57–60] and for recognition of β-glucans in fungi [61].

Clinical and Preclinical Studies of Antiviral CTLs

Cytomegalovirus

Ex vivo CTL expansion is the most common method for producing clinical CTLs for most clinical trials (Table 20.1). Walter et al. were first to demonstrate that CMV stimulation of donor PBMC expanded CMV-specific CTLs and the expanded T cells lost alloreactivity after several weeks of ex vivo culture while retaining antiviral cytotoxicity [25].

CMV has been the primary focus of the first virus targeted therapy trials and remains a primary focus in subsequent studies (Table 20.1). The first clinical report in which CD8[+] CMV-specific CTLs were isolated via tetramer selection [62] generated complete or partial clinical responses in nine patients, but there was limited data on long-term persistence of the infused CMV-specific CTLs.

IFN-γ column selection (Gamma capture, Miltenyi) to produce CMV-CTLs was associated with partial and complete responses in 15 of 18 patients who were given one dose of CMV-CTLs [63]. IFN-γ selection after stimulation with recombinant pp65 or an overlapping peptide pool

of 15-mers covering the pp65 protein was used to produce CMV-CTL [64]. Infusions of CMV-CTLs administered prophylactically after stem cell transplantation successfully protected seven patients from the development of viral reactivation and disease. Further, in vivo expansion of CMV-CTLs was detected in 11 patients [64]. CMV-CTLs from HSCT donors using reversible Streptamers with MHC-restricted pp65 peptides were used to successfully treat two patients with CMV reactivation after HCT [44].

Bispecific Antibody-Armed T Cells Targeting CMV

The strategy for using bispecific antibodies (BiAbs) to target cancer was nearly abandoned due to cytokine storm reactions. However, the last 10 years has seen a resurrection of interest particularly for targeting T cells to various cancer antigens. Studies using retargeted T cells have been reported for HER2 in breast and prostate cancer using anti-CD3 x anti-Her2 BiAb ATC [89, 90]; EGFR in colorectal, pancreatic, and lung cancer using anti-CD3 x anti-EGFR BiAb ATC [91]; and CD20 in non-Hodgkin's lymphoma using anti-CD3 x anti-CD20 BiAb ATC [92–94]. Since chemical or molecularly engineered constructs could be used to target the TCR on one hand and tumor-associated antigen (TAA) on the other hand, we reasoned that CMV could be targeted by chemically heteroconjugating OKT3 (anti-CD3, anti-TCR) with Cytogam® (polyclonal donor-derived anti-CMV IgG, designated CMVBi) to kill CMV-infected fibroblasts [95]. In this strategy shown in Fig. 20.1, anti-CD3 monoclonal antibody-activated T cells (ATC) which expanded in low-dose IL-2 were the T effector cells. ATC alone do not kill CMV-infected targets. Arming doses of CMVBi ranging from as low as 0.01 ng/10[6] ATC to 50 ng/10[6]ATC exhibited high levels of specific anti-CMV cytotoxicity in targets infected with CMV at multiplicities of CMV infection (MOI) ranging from 0.01 to 1. The polyclonal nature of the Cytogam may provide multiple antibody clones directed at multiple CMV epitopes on the

Table 20.1 Previous clinical trials of virus-specific T-cell therapy

Methodology	Pathogen specificity	Setting	Donor	Patient accrual	Number of centers	Methodology
Tetramer selection	CMV	HSCT	HCT donor or third-party	9	1	Cobbold [62]
IFN-γ column selection	CMV	HSCT	HCT donor or third-party	18	1	Feuchtinger [63]
IFN-γ column selection	CMV	HSCT	HCT donor	18	1	Peggs [64]
EBV-LCL stimulation	EBV	SOT	Autologous	3	1	Haque [65]
Irradiated EBV-LCL	EBV	SOT	Third-party	1	1	Haque [66]
Irradiated EBV-LCL	EBV	SOT	Third party	8	1	Haque [67]
Irradiated EBV-LCL	EBV	SOT	Third party	33	1	Haque [68]
Multimer selection	EBV	HSCT	Related haploidentical donor	1	1	Uhlin [69]
IFN-γ column selection	EBV	HSCT	HCT donor	6	1	Moosman [70]
EBV-LCL stimulation	EBV	HSCT	Third-party donor	2	1	Barker [71]
Irradiated EBV-LCL stimulation	EBV	HSCT	HCT donor	114	3	Heslop [33]
EBV-LCL stimulation	EBV	HSCT	Autologous	1	1	Basso [72]
IFN-γ column selection	Adv	HSCT	Third party	1	1	Qasim [73]
IFN-γ column selection	Adv	HSCT	HCT donor	9	1	Feuchtinger [74]
CD8+ HIV-specific ex vivo expanded	HIV	N/A	Autologous	6	1	Lieberman [75]
CD4-ɣ CAR transduction	HIV	N/A	Autologous	24	1	Mitsuyasu [76]
CD4-ɣ CAR transduction	HIV	N/A	Autologous	40	5	Deeks [77]
Transduction with antisense gene to HIV env	HIV	N/A	Autologous CD4-T cells	17	1	Tebas [78]
CCR5 gene editing via ZFN	HIV	N/A	Autologous CD4-enriched	12	1	Tebas [79]
PepMix-pulsed PBMC	JCV	HSCT	HSCT donor	1	1	Balduzzi [80]
Pentamer selection	CMV/EBV/Adv	HSCT	HSCT donor or third-party	8	1	Uhlin [81]
Stimulation of PBMC with CMV antigen or inactivated conidia	CMV or *Aspergillus*	HSCT	HSCT donor	10	1	Perruccio [82]
Ad5f35pp65 transduced LCL	CMV/EBV/Adv	HSCT	HSCT donor	26	3	Leen [83]
Ad5f35pp65 transduced DC	CMV/Adv	HSCT	HSCT donor	12	1	Mickelwaite [84]
Ad5f35null transduced LCL	EBV/Adv	HSCT	HCT donor	13	3	Leen [21]
Ad5f35pp65 transduced LCL	CMV/EBV/Adv	HSCT	Third-party donor	47	8	Leen [85]
Nucleofection of DCs	CMV/EBV/Adv	HSCT	HSCT donor	12	3	Gerdemann [86]
NLV-peptide pulsing or Ad5f35pp65 transduction of DCs	CMV or CMV/Adv	HSCT	HSCT donor	50	2	Blyth [87]
Rapidly generated EBV, adenovirus, CMV, BK virus, HHV6-specific T cells following stimulation with peptide mixes	Adv, EBV, CMV, BKV, HHV6	HSCT	HSCT donor	11	1	Papadopoulou [88]

CMV-infected targets leading to the increased potency at a low arming dose of CMVBi. Cytotoxicity was evident at effector-to-target ratios (E:T) of 25:1, 13:1, 6:1, and 3:1 compared to unarmed ATC alone. At an MOI of 1.0, the mean % specific anti-CMV-specific cytotoxicities at E:T of 3, 6, and 13 were 79%, 81%, and 82%, respectively, whereas unarmed ATC at the same E:Ts killed <20%. Unarmed ATC, Cytogam®, or CMVBi alone did not exhibit significant killing of uninfected or CMV-infected fibroblasts. Furthermore, cultures of CMVBi-armed ATC with CMV-infected targets induced cytokine and chemokine release from CMVBi-armed ATC. This simple targeting strategy bypasses MHC-restricted cytotoxicity for treating viral disease in organ transplant and HSCT recipients. It was shown that CMVBi ATC do not react to alloantigens in vitro in a mixed lymphocyte culture, and they can be frozen and reinfused at different time points as an "off-the-shelf" drug. Although promising, it is not clear from these data whether targeting CMV or other disease agents using this approach will be clinically effective.

Epstein-Barr Virus

EBV-CTLs have been used for prevention and treatment of post-HSCT lymphoproliferative disease (PTLD) as well as EBV+ lymphoma. Irradiated EBV-lymphoblastoid cells (EBV-LCL) were used to generate EBV-specific CTLs in vitro for prophylaxis or treatment for EBV-PTLD in 114 patients [27, 33]. Remarkably, the first 26 patients received gene-marked CTLs, and follow-up studies showed the gene-marked cells persisted up to 105 months after HSCT (Table 20.1).

HLA-A2-specific pentamers and IFN-γ selection procedures were used to produce EBV-CTLs. HLA-A2 specific pentamers were used to produce EBV-CTLs from the haploidentical mother of a patient with EBV-PTLD who had received a cord blood transplantation [69]. A complete clinical response was obtained following two infusions of EBV-CTLs. Three of six patients with early EBV-induced PTLD treated

with EBV-CTLs produced by IFN-γ selection achieved complete responses whereas three patients with advanced, multiorgan disease did not respond [70]. The latest strategy is to target EBV with multiviral CTL products (below) or third-party-derived EBV-CTLs.

Adenovirus

Most studies targeting adenovirus (Adv) use multiviral CTLs [21, 81, 83, 84]. A few exclusively target Adv by selection technology. Adv-CTLs produced by IFN-γ selection was used for treatment of nine patients with drug-refractory Adv infections [74]. There was in vivo CTL expansion in five of six patients and four patients cleared their disease. In all studies using cell selection, clinical benefit was observed in spite of very low doses of vCTLs infused (<5 × 10^4 cells/kg in most studies) [73, 74].

Multiviral CTL Trials

Recent antiviral CTL therapy trials target multiple viruses (CMV, EBV, and Adv as primary targets). CMV, EBV, and Adv are the three leading causes of viral-associated mortality after allogeneic HSCT. Clinical-grade Adv vector Ad5f35pp65 contains the immunodominant CMV antigen pp65, providing a unique opportunity to transduce donor-derived dendritic cells or EBV-LCL to serve as APCs for the CTL cultures. Triviral (CMV, EBV, and Adv-specific) CTLs were tested in a dose-escalation trial involving 26 patients [83]. There were no adverse effects at doses ranging from 5 × 10^6 to 1 × 10^8 cells/m^2, and all patients were effectively protected against CMV, EBV, and Adv. Interestingly, although EBV- and CMV-specific CTLs were detected by IFN-γ ELISpots, Adv-CTLs were not detectable except during infection. In a follow-up trial using Ad5f35-transduced EBV-LCL to produce EBV- and Adv-CTLs, 13 patients received prophylaxis or treatment for EBV and Adv infections after HSCT [21]. Although the CTLs provided protection in vivo, the Adv-CTLs could not be detected except in the setting of Adv infection; these data suggest that levels of specific vCTLs below the limits of detection by IFN-γ ELISpots provide protection and infection induces clonal expansion. Similarly, Ad5f35pp65 transduced dendritic cells (DC) used to produce CMV- and Adv-CTLs were clinically effective in 12 patients after allogeneic HSCT [84]. There were a few cases of CMV reactivation in the setting of low-dose prednisone. This approach was applied to 50 patients after allogeneic HSCT with triviral (CMV, EBV, Adv-specific) CTLs using two methods: 10 were produced by pulsing donor DCs with the HLA-A2 restricted CMV peptide NLVPMVATV and 40 were produced using Ad5f35pp65-transduced donor DCs [87]. Only 5 of 50 patients had CMV reactivation after CTL infusions and only 1 of 5 patients required antiviral drug therapy after steroid treatment for acute GVHD.

Advances in processing protocols have validated 5-mer peptide pools that include immuno-dominant viral antigens that replace viral transduction of APC thereby removing safety and regulatory barriers associated use of viral vectors [36]. The use of gas-permeable rapid-expansion (G-Rex) bioreactors has simplified CTL culture [96]. These advances in technology led to the development of a rapid manufacturing protocol for expanding virus-specific T-cell products (VSTs) that yield clinically relevant numbers of VSTs in 10–12 days. Further, VST products targeting multiple viral antigens have been shown to provide effective antiviral protection (against CNV, EBV and Ad) in ten patients after HSCT [37]. This rapid manufacturing protocol was subsequently adapted to produce five virus-specific CTLs targeting EBV, CMV, Adv, HHV6, and BK virus infections in a single T-cell product for patients following allogeneic HSCT [88]. Fourteen of 48 VST products manufactured from HSCT donors recognized all 5 viral components while 35 (73%) recognized 3 or more by IFN-γ ELISpots. Unexpectedly 22 of the donors were CMV seronegative and VSTs produced predictably lacked CMV specificity. These VSTs were used to treat 11 patients after HSCT. The 3 patients treated prophylactically remained free of

viral infections and 8 patients with 18 viral reactivations received VSTs, with all experiencing partial or complete responses in their CMV, EBV, Adv, or HHV6 infections.

CTL Therapy for Human Immunodeficiency Virus

Although there was intense interest in the use of CTL therapy for HIV, there was only limited success to date [97]. Attempts to expand and reinfuse autologous HIV-specific CTLs resulted in only transient improvements in viral load [75]. A larger number of clinical trials focused on genetically modified CTL to target HIV using transduction of a modified TCR or CARs. These trials established safety, but exhibited limited antiviral efficacy [76, 77]. A major challenge for this approach is the outgrowth of escape mutants expressing alterations of the target epitope so the infected cell can no longer be targeted by the effector cells. A more successful approach has been inserting genes that would provide HIV resistance. This approach was clinically tested when antisense gene complementary to HIV *env* was transduced into T cells from 17 patients using lentiviral vectors [78]. The CTLs persisted for 5 weeks, homed to gut-associated lymphoid tissue, and were well-tolerated with clinical toxicities. Infusions of CTLs in two of eight patients who underwent antiviral treatment interruption keep the viral load u

ndetectable for 4 and 14 weeks. When CCR5-delta32 mutations were introduced to CD4-enriched T cells through the use of a zinc-finger nuclease [79], the CCR5-edited T cells were subsequently infused in 12 patients, and engineered T cells were detectable in the peripheral blood for up to 42 months post infusion. In six patients who underwent antiviral treatment interruption, the absolute number of gene modified CD4+ T cells decreased at a lower rate than non-modified T cells. Recent studies showed that dual gene editing of CXCR4 and CCR5 via zinc-finger nucleases was successful in a T-cell line, and preclinical studies show that the T cells were highly resistant to HIV infection [98]. It is not clear whether this approach could prevent primary infection or have a clinical impact as an HIV cure strategy.

CTL Therapy for Other Viruses

There are a few studies that target other viruses with adoptive immunotherapy. The John Cunningham virus (JCV) is a ubiquitous polyoma virus which can cause progressive multifocal leukoencephalopathy (PML), which occurs in immunocompromised individuals such as acquired immunodeficiency syndrome (AIDS), recipients of HSCT or solid organ transplants, or primary immunodeficiency disorders. Donor-derived JCV-specific CTLs were used in a 14-year-old patient with PML after prolonged steroid treatment for GVHD following HSCT. Cells were manufactured using 15-mer peptide pools that included JC antigens VP1 and LT and infused twice leading to clearance of JV-DNA from the cerebrospinal fluid with improvements in neurologic status [80].

Human papillomavirus (HPV) disease can be a late complication of HSCT. Peptide pools spanning the HPV E6 and E7 proteins were used to generate HPV-specific CTLs from patients with oropharyngeal or cervical cancer that arise after HPV16 infection [99]. The CTLs exhibited specific activity directed at HPV E6 and E7 and anti-tumor activity against the HPV16 cervical cancer cell line CaSki.

Adverse Events in Antigen-Specific CTL Therapy

Adverse events after 381 infusions for 180 patients on 18 protocols by the groups at Baylor College of Medicine were reported [100]. Side effects were limited to 24 mild adverse events observed within 6 h of infusion; nausea and vomiting were most common with 22 nonserious adverse events (fever, chills, nausea) that occurred within 24 h. No significant GVHD was attributed to CTL infusions. The only significant complications were rare reports of systemic inflammatory responses in patients with bulky EBV+ lymphomas following EBV-CTL therapy. Seven cases of acute GVHD occurred in patients who had a greater degree of HLA mismatch than controls after infusions of EBV-CTL. Some of the cases of GVHD were attributable to reducing the corticosteroid dose prior to the CMV-CTL infusions [87].

Third-Party CTL

For years, the selection or culture of anti-pathogen CTLs was dependent on the presence of pathogen-specific memory T cells in the blood of donors, and, therefore, the approach could not help allograft recipients of pathogen-naive hematopoietic cell products after HSCT. One strategy to address this problem is to provide "off-the-shelf" pathogen-specific CTLs derived from third-party donors. This strategy was first validated in a phase I trial involving 8 patients who received partially matched EBV-CTLs for PTLD that developed after solid organ transplantation [66, 67] and confirmed in a cohort of 33 patients in a phase II trial [68]. The latter trial showed a response rate of 64% at 5 weeks and 52% at 6 months; the outcomes correlated with the degree of HLA matching between the CTL donor and recipient. In the HSCT patients, two patients with refractory EBV-PTLD after cord blood transplantation (CBT) with third-party EBV-specific CTLs [71]. A bank of 32 CTL lines with characterized activity against EBV, CMV, and Adv were used to match for 50 patients with refractory viral infections. This strategy resulted in partial or complete antiviral responses in 74%, 78%, and 67% of those with CMV, Adv, and EBV, respectively [85]. This is a marked improvement from standard therapy response rate of 13% in eight patients for whom a matched line could not be identified. Despite partial HLA matching at one to four loci, there were only two patients who developed grade I GVHD. Clones that are responsible for GVHD have been selected against in the expansion culture and may exist at such low precursor frequencies after culture that they do not expand enough to cause clinically significant GVHD. The lower rate of response against EBV relative to CMV and Adv may reflect selective expansion of T cells against immunodominant epitopes of the latter two viruses, thereby complicating the selection of an ideal third-party pathogen-specific line that fulfills the requirements of antiviral activity and MHC-restriction against multiple pathogens. The methods for producing third-party-virus-specific CTL include pentamer selection for Ad, CMV, EBV [81], and IFN-γ selection for Adv-CTL [73].

TCR Gene Transfer

A few studies reported transducing CTLs with a virus-specific TCR [49, 101, 102]. A trial of transgenic CTLs using a retroviral vector that expresses a CMV-specific TCR is ongoing in the United Kingdom (Morris E. et al. MRC# G0701703). Alternatively, Kumaresan et al. transduced T cells with the β-glucan receptor dectin [61]. Since the carbohydrate β-glucan is found in the cell wall of most fungi [103], investigators used its natural receptor, dectin-1, as a recognition receptor coupled to a CD28 (a key co-stimulatory molecule) and CD3-zeta transgene to initiate signaling and killing in T cells. The same group showed that the antifungal CARTs could mediate damage to hyphae in vitro and in vivo [61]. These novel approaches would allow creation of specific CTLs from pathogen-naive donors; however, they are subject to the regulatory challenges in gene transfer technology. Furthermore, use of a single antifungal TCR allows for antigenic escape.

Production of CTL from Pathogen-Naive Donors

A major advance in adoptive viral CTL therapy was development of virus-specific CTLs from virus-naive donors. CTL could be produced from a 20% fraction from cord blood using donor-derived DCs and EBV-lymphoblastoid cell line (LCL) as APC and Ad5f35pp65 transduction as a source of CMV and Adv antigens [20]. The resulting viral CTLs exhibited specific anti-CMV,

EBV, and Adv IFN-γ ELISpots responses as well as specific ^{51}Cr cytotoxicity with no alloreactivity. Epitope mapping showed that the immunodominant epitopes recognized by cord blood-derived CTLs were different from the immunodominant epitopes recognized by the CMV and EBV seropositive adult donors. The HLA-A2-restricted epitope NLVPMVATV was notably absent in the cord blood-derived lines. CTLs derived from cord blood were successfully infused in 12 CBT recipients in the ongoing ACT-CAT trial (Safety, Toxicity and MTD of One Intravenous IV Injection of Donor CTLs Specific for CMV and Adenovirus, # NCT00880789).

Recently, multiviral CTLs were produced from CMV-naive adult donors using column-selected CD45RA+ naive T cells stimulated by donor DCs pulsed with CMV 15-mer peptide pools [38]. Preclinical studies suggest that multiviral CTLs will exhibit similar anti-CMV activity to DCs pulsed with CMV 15-mer peptide pools. The current MUSTAT trial (Multivirus-Specific Cytotoxic T-Lymphocytes for the Prophylaxis and Treatment of EBV, CMV, and Adenovirus Infections Post Allogeneic Stem Cell Transplant, # NCT01945814) compares the clinical efficacy of CTLs derived from CMV-seropositive vs. CMV-naive donors.

CTL for Solid Organ Transplant Recipients

EBV-PTLD is a significant long-term risk in solid organ transplant recipients. Rituximab can be effective, but treatment often requires reduction of immunosuppression which can lead to graft rejection. Autologous EBV-CTLs have been used in this setting [72]. Several prophylactic infusions of autologous EBV-CTLs reduced the EBV viral load without adverse reactions despite ongoing treatment with calcineurin inhibitors [65]. A heart transplant recipient who developed Hodgkin's lymphoma-type PTLD 8 years after transplant had remission after being treated with autologous EBV-CTLs in combination with chemotherapy without alterations in his immunosuppression [72]. This observation supports the prior observations that calcineurin inhibitors block proliferation, but do not impair CTL activity.

Fungal-Specific CTLs

Fungal infections are a major cause of morbidity and mortality in allogeneic HSCT recipients, with GVHD being the major risk factor. Candidal infections can range from mucocutaneous colonization of the skin and mouth to life-threatening systemic infections. *Aspergillus* species are ubiquitous molds that cause invasive pulmonary infections as well as widespread infection including central nervous system dissemination in highly immunocompromised patients [104]. Patients with inherited immunodeficiencies (e.g., chronic granulomatous disease), patients with prolonged neutropenia after repeated rounds of chemotherapy (e.g., for acute leukemia), and those receiving immunosuppression after lung transplant or allogeneic HSCT are at the highest risk for mycoses [105]. The importance of T-cell immunity in defense against invasive aspergillosis and other filamentous fungi is not clear, since patients with these invasive fungal diseases usually have severe deficiencies in multiple components of the immune system. In patients with advanced AIDS, invasive aspergillosis is an uncommon complication and generally occurs when other forms of immune impairment (e.g., neutropenia and use of corticosteroids) are present. Despite these unknowns, it may be clinically useful to target fungal infections with fungus-specific T cells after HSCT.

The adaptive immune response against invasive aspergillosis is believed to be orchestrated by CD4+ T cells. Table 20.2 summarizes preclinical studies that developed fungal-specific CTLs against *Candida*, *Aspergillus*, and *Rhizopus* (a member of the *Mucorales* group) species. *Aspergillus*-specific CTLs were produced by stimulation of PBMC with antigens from aspergillus extracts, selection with IFN-γ secretion, and culture [106]. The CTLs were predominantly CD4+, CD45R0+ memory cells that secrete IFN-γ in response to *Aspergillus* and *Penicillium*. The fungal-specific CTL enhanced hyphal damage by neutrophils and APCs. IFN-γ selection and stimulation with *Candida albicans*, *Aspergillus fumigatus*, and *Rhizopus oryzae* extracts were used to produce multifungal-specific CTL lines, which were also nearly all CD4+ CD45RO+ HLA-DR+ that exhibited activation markers of IFN-γ, CD154, and TNFα and enhanced oxidative activity of neutrophils when co-incubated with antigen and APCs [108]. Several studies target the *Candida* MP65 and *Aspergillus* CRF1 antigens. To produce multi-pathogen-specific T cells that secrete IFN-γ, proliferate, and kill CMV, EBV, Adv, *Candida*, and *Aspergillus*, donor PBMCs were incubated with peptide libraries from CMV-pp65, EBV-LMP2, Adv-Hexon, *Candida* MP65, and a 15-mer peptide from aspergillus CRF1 [107]. However, it remains unclear what the significance of MP65 and CRF1 is in antifungal immunity [117] [113]. Expanded memory/effector Th1 cells following stimulation with *Rhizopus* extracts were used to generate memory/effector Th1 cells for mucormycosis, and the product exhibited specificity to the original *Rhizopus oryzae* extract as well as other *Mucorales* species [118]. *Candida*-specific T cells generated with cellular extracts of *Candida albicans* released cytokines that caused hyphal damage and increased neutrophil activity against hyphae [111].

CTLs produced by stimulation with inactivated conidia (spores) from *Aspergillus fumigatus* resulted in clonal CD4+ CTLs with anti-*Aspergillus* activity by IFN-γ ELISpots [82]. These donor T-cell clones specific for *Aspergillus* antigens were then infused in patients following haploidentical HSCT. Of 23 patients who developed invasive aspergillosis, 10 patients received anti-aspergillus CTLs, while 13 patients did not. Nine of 10 treated patients cleared their infections whereas only 7 of 13 untreated patients cleared their infections. *Aspergillus*-specific CTLs were detected in high frequencies in patients who received immunotherapy while they were barely detectable in untreated patients [82].

Table 20.2 Preclinical studies of T-cell therapy against nonviral infections

Methodology	Pathogen specificity	Donor	Investigator
IFN-γ selection after stimulation of PBMCs with aspergillus extracts	*Aspergillus*	Healthy donors	Beck [106]
CD154 selection after stimulation of PBMCs with fungal extracts	*Aspergillus, Candida, Rhinopus*	Healthy donors	Khanna [107]
IFN-γ selection after stimulation of PBMCs with fungal extracts	*Aspergillus, Candida, Rhinopus*	Healthy donors	Tramsen [108]
Transduction of CTL with chimeric antigen receptor directed against B-glucans	*Aspergillus* (potentially other pathogens	Healthy donors	Kumaresan [61]
Expansion of anti-*Aspergillus* T cell using *Aspergillus* extracts	*Aspergillus*	Healthy donors	Tramsen [109]
Expansion of fungus-specific T cells using a lysate from *A. fumigatus*	*Aspergillus, Candida, Penicillium*	Healthy donors	Gaundar [110]
IFN-γ capture of T cells following stimulation with *C. albicans* cellular extract	*Candida*	Healthy donors	Tramsen [111]
Crf1-stimulated T cells	*Candida* and *Aspergillus*	Murine cells	Stuehler [112]
CD137 selection following stimulation with Crf1 and catalase 1	*Aspergillus*	Healthy donors	Jolink [113]
Transgenic TCR-transduced cells	Tuberculosis	Murine cells	Feng [114]
MHC-Streptamer-enriched antigen-specific T cells	*Listeria*	Murine cells	Stemberger [115]
(Proof of principle) – targeting of OVA-expressing parasites	*Leishmania*	Murine cells	Polley [116]
Transgenic TRC-transduced cells	*Chlamydia*	Murine cells	Roan [55]

Despite notable advances in antifungal CTLs, a better understanding of the immunodominant T-cell targets that should be selected for various fungal species is needed, and standardized clinical-grade cGMP fungal antigen sources are needed to provide consistency between trials.

Controversies and Challenges

Although there have been major advances in producing pathogen-specific CTLs, important questions remain regarding methods that affect potency and efficacy of the T-cell products. It is unclear whether manufacturing CTLs to include more pathogens in a single culture will affect potency and specificity in the CTL cultures. Although the proportions of virus-specific CTLs for each virus decrease as the number of antigens increases, these effects have not seemed to impact clinical trials. CTLs specific for 7 viruses (CMV, EBV, Adv, BK, HHV6, RSV, and influenza) pro-

duced using peptide pools for 15 antigens exhibited specific activity against all targeted viruses [37]. The question remains as to whether adding additional viral targets will skew specific cytotoxicity, alter potency for each target, induce alloreactive T cells, or compromise in vivo responses.

A major challenge is achieving consistent and optimal culture conditions for generating the most effective CTL product. Although multiple rounds of stimulation with antigen select and expand the specific antiviral clones, prolonged culture may lead to T-cell exhaustion. Some groups have decreased production time using newer bioreactors [96]. Identification of the "correct" subset of T cells for clinical use (however selected) will require well-designed randomized phase II trials using a specific CTL product made by the same group or a common standard operating procedure (SOP) in a homogeneous group of HSCT patients. Assays for measuring IFN-γ ELISpots and cytotoxicity need to be standardized and the timing of the studies needs to be the same. Recently, a new population of "stem cell memory T cells" has been putatively identified – which possess characteristics ideal for use in adoptive immunotherapy. Unfortunately, there are no randomized phase II trials to date to support continued development and commercialization of clinically effective CTLs.

The presence of immunosuppression remains a barrier for optimal immunotherapy after allogeneic HSCT and solid organ transplantation since most agents also suppress CTL functions. Nearly all protocols require recipients to be receiving less than 0.5 mg/kg/day of prednisone and wait at least 30 days after anti-T-cell serotherapy to be eligible to receive CTL therapy. Virtually all of the calcineurin inhibitors (cyclosporin A, tacrolimus, or sirolimus) at therapeutic doses impair CTL activity. EBV-specific CTLs can be made resistant to tacrolimus by knockdown of FKBP12 via a retrovirally transduced specific siRNA and exhibit anti-EBV lymphoma activity in the presence of tacrolimus [119]. Similarly, EBV-specific CTLs can be made resistant to both cyclosporine A and tacrolimus by mutating calcineurin [120]. The mutation does not alter the phenotype or antiviral activity of the CTLs and mutated cells have a growth advantage in calcineurin inhibitors. Although they have not been applied clinically, they have great potential for treating HSCT and solid organ transplant recipients.

There is one preclinical report of T cells used to target bacterial and parasitic infections [116], but there are no clinical trials evaluating T-cell immunotherapy for bacterial and parasitic infections. Despite numerous studies evaluating in vitro T-cell responses, there is no consensus on the role of T cells in defense against aspergillosis.

Conclusion

Infusions of anti-pathogen CTLs in several hundred patients over the past several decades have been established as a safe and highly effective therapy following allogeneic HCT. Identifying preserved viral T-cell epitopes, probing the antigen limits in CTL monoculture, testing the clinical efficacy of immunosuppressive-resistant CTLs, and improving conditions for rapid and specific expansion will further broaden the usefulness of this treatment strategy. As advances in protocols and methods for manufacture achieve acceptable clinical standards that can be supported commercially, CTL therapy may become an integral component of care offered to allogeneic HSCT or immunodeficiency patients.

Acknowledgments Special thanks to the clinical coordinators for dedicating their efforts to serve the immunotherapy patients. We thank Manley Huang for his thoughtful reading of the chapter. The studies were supported in part by R01 CA140314 (LGL) and R01 CA182526 (LGL), Translational Grants #6092-09 (LGL) and #6066-06 (LGL) from the Leukemia & Lymphoma Society, and UVA Cancer Center Support Grant NCI 5P30CA044579-24. LGL is a founder of Transtarget, Inc. CMB is supported in part by the NICHD K12-HD-001399 award to MDK and CPRIT R01 RP100469 and NCI P01 CA148600-02 awards to CMB.

References

1. Boeckh M, Leisenring W, Riddell SR, et al. Late cytomegalovirus disease and mortality in recipients of allogeneic hematopoietic stem cell transplants: importance of viral load and T-cell immunity. Blood. 2003;101:407–14.
2. Brunstein CG, Weisdorf DJ, DeFor T, et al. Marked increased risk of Epstein-Barr virus-related complications with the addition of antithymocyte globulin to a nonmyeloablative conditioning prior to unrelated umbilical cord blood transplantation. Blood. 2006;108:2874–80.
3. Myers GD, Krance RA, Weiss H, et al. Adenovirus infection rates in pediatric recipients of alternate donor allogeneic bone marrow transplants receiving either antithymocyte globulin (ATG) or alemtuzumab (Campath). Bone Marrow Transplant. 2005;36:1001–8.
4. Neofytos D, Horn D, Anaissie E, et al. Epidemiology and outcome of invasive fungal infection in adult hematopoietic stem cell transplant recipients: analysis of Multicenter Prospective Antifungal Therapy (PATH) Alliance registry. Clin Infect Dis. 2009;48:265–73.
5. Avery R. Update in management of ganciclovir-resistant cytomegalovirus infection. Curr Opin Infect Dis. 2008;21:433–7.
6. Biron KK. Antiviral drugs for cytomegalovirus diseases. Antivir Res. 2006;71:154–63.
7. Nichols WG, Corey L, Gooley T, et al. Rising pp65 antigenemia during preemptive anticytomegalovirus therapy after allogeneic hematopoietic stem cell

transplantation: risk factors, correlation with DNA load, and outcomes. Blood. 2001;97:867–74.

8. Ljungman P, Deliliers GL, Platzbecker U, et al. Cidofovir for cytomegalovirus infection and disease in allogeneic stem cell transplant recipients. The Infectious Diseases Working Party of the European Group for Blood and Marrow Transplantation. Blood. 2001;97:388–92.

9. Kuehnle I, Huls MH, Liu Z, et al. CD20 monoclonal antibody (rituximab) for therapy of Epstein-Barr virus lymphoma after hemopoietic stem-cell transplantation. Blood. 2000;95:1502–5.

10. Plotkin S. The history of vaccination against cytomegalovirus. Med Microbiol Immunol. 2015;204:247–54.

11. Einsele H, Roosnek E, Rufer N, et al. Infusion of cytomegalovirus (CMV)-specific T cells for the treatment of CMV infection not responding to antiviral chemotherapy. Blood. 2002;99:3916–22.

12. Hebart H, Einsele H. Clinical aspects of CMV infection after stem cell transplantation. Hum Immunol. 2004;65:432–6.

13. Herr W, Plachter B. Cytomegalovirus and varicella-zoster virus vaccines in hematopoietic stem cell transplantation. Expert Rev Vaccines. 2009;8:999–1021.

14. Papadopoulos EB, Ladanyi M, Emanuel D, et al. Infusions of donor leukocytes to treat Epstein-Barr virus-associated lymphoproliferative disorders after allogeneic bone marrow transplantation. N Engl J Med. 1994;330:1185–91.

15. Riddell SR, Greenberg PD. The use of anti-CD3 and anti-CD28 monoclonal antibodies to clone and expand human antigen-specific T cells. J Immunol Methods. 1990;128:189–201.

16. Riddell SR, Watanabe KS, Goodrich JM, et al. Restoration of viral immunity in immunodeficient humans by the adoptive transfer of T cell clones. Science. 1992;257:238–41.

17. Slezak SL, Bettinotti M, Selleri S, et al. CMV pp65 and IE-1 T cell epitopes recognized by healthy subjects. J Transl Med. 2007;5:17.

18. Leen AM, Christin A, Khalil M, et al. Identification of hexon-specific CD4 and CD8 T-cell epitopes for vaccine and immunotherapy. J Virol. 2008;82:546–54.

19. Bollard CM, Rooney CM, Heslop HE. T-cell therapy in the treatment of post-transplant lymphoproliferative disease. Nat Rev Clin Oncol. 2012;9:510–9.

20. Hanley PJ, Cruz CR, Savoldo B, et al. Functionally active virus-specific T cells that target CMV, adenovirus, and EBV can be expanded from naive T-cell populations in cord blood and will target a range of viral epitopes. Blood. 2009;114:1958–67.

21. Leen AM, Christin A, Myers GD, et al. Cytotoxic T lymphocyte therapy with donor T cells prevents and treats adenovirus and Epstein-Barr virus infections after haploidentical and matched unrelated stem cell transplantation. Blood. 2009;114:4283–92.

22. Sili U, Huls MH, Davis AR, et al. Large-scale expansion of dendritic cell-primed polyclonal human cytotoxic T-lymphocyte lines using lymphoblastoid cell lines for adoptive immunotherapy. J Immunother. 2003;26:241–56.

23. Kern F, Faulhaber N, Frommel C, et al. Analysis of CD8 T cell reactivity to cytomegalovirus using protein-spanning pools of overlapping pentadeca-peptides. Eur J Immunol. 2000;30:1676–82.

24. Hanley PJ, Shaffer DR, Cruz CR, et al. Expansion of T cells targeting multiple antigens of cytomegalovirus, Epstein-Barr virus and adenovirus to provide broad antiviral specificity after stem cell transplantation. Cytotherapy. 2011;13:976–86.

25. Walter EA, Greenberg PD, Gilbert MJ, et al. Reconstitution of cellular immunity against cytomegalovirus in recipients of allogeneic bone marrow by transfer of T-cell clones from the donor. N Engl J Med. 1995;333:1038–44.

26. Lucas KG, Sun Q, Burton RL, et al. A phase I-II trial to examine the toxicity of CMV- and EBV-specific cytotoxic T lymphocytes when used for prophylaxis against EBV and CMV disease in recipients of CD34-selected/T cell-depleted stem cell transplants. HumGene Ther. 2000;11:1453–63.

27. Rooney CM, Smith CA, Ng CY, et al. Infusion of cytotoxic T cells for the prevention and treatment of Epstein-Barr virus-induced lymphoma in allogeneic transplant recipients. Blood. 1998;92:1549–55.

28. Heslop HE, Brenner MK, Rooney C, et al. Administration of neomycin-resistance-gene-marked EBV-specific cytotoxic T lymphocytes to recipients of mismatched-related or phenotypically similar unrelated donor marrow grafts. Hum Gene Ther. 1994;5:381–97.

29. Bollard CM, Cooper LJ, Heslop HE. Immunotherapy targeting EBV-expressing lymphoproliferative diseases. Best Pract Res Clin Haematol. 2008;21:405–20.

30. Savoldo B, Huls MH, Liu Z, et al. Autologous Epstein-Barr virus (EBV)-specific cytotoxic T cells for the treatment of persistent active EBV infection. Blood. 2002;100:4059–66.

31. Bollard CM, Kuehnle I, Leen A, et al. Adoptive immunotherapy for posttransplantation viral infections. Biol Blood Marrow Transplant. 2004;10:143–55.

32. Gattinoni L, Klebanoff CA, Palmer DC, et al. Acquisition of full effector function in vitro paradoxically impairs the in vivo antitumor efficacy of adoptively transferred CD8+ T cells. J Clin Invest. 2005;115:1616–26.

33. Heslop HE, Slobod KS, Pule MA, et al. Long-term outcome of EBV-specific T-cell infusions to prevent or treat EBV-related lymphoproliferative disease in transplant recipients. Blood. 2010;115:925–35.

34. Melenhorst JJ, Leen AM, Bollard CM, et al. Allogeneic virus-specific T cells with HLA alloreactivity do not produce GVHD in human subjects. Blood. 2010;116:4700–2.

35. Peggs KS, Verfuerth S, Pizzey A, et al. Adoptive cellular therapy for early cytomegalovirus infection

after allogeneic stem-cell transplantation with virus-specific T-cell lines. Lancet. 2003;362:1375–7.

36. Trivedi D, Williams RY, O'Reilly RJ, et al. Generation of CMV-specific T lymphocytes using protein-spanning pools of pp65-derived overlapping pentadecapeptides for adoptive immunotherapy. Blood. 2005;105:2793–801.

37. Gerdemann U, Keirnan JM, Katari UL, et al. Rapidly generated multivirus-specific cytotoxic T lymphocytes for the prophylaxis and treatment of viral infections. Mol Ther. 2012;20:1622–32.

38. Hanley PJ, Cruz RY, Melenhorst J, Scheinberg P, Blaney J, Savoldo B, Dotti G, Heslop HE, Rooney C, Shpall EJ, Barrett AJ, Rodgers J, Bollard CM. Naïve T-cell-derived CTL recognize atypical epitopes of CMVpp65 with higher avidity than CMV-seropositive donor-derived CTL – a basis for treatment of post-transplant viral infection by adoptive transfer of T-cells from virus-naïve donors. ISCT 2013 annual meeting (Abstract), 2013.

39. Berger C, Jensen MC, Lansdorp PM, et al. Adoptive transfer of effector CD8+ T cells derived from central memory cells establishes persistent T cell memory in primates. J Clin Invest. 2008;118:294–305.

40. Willinger T, Freeman T, Hasegawa H, et al. Molecular signatures distinguish human central memory from effector memory CD8 T cell subsets. J Immunol. 2005;175:5895–903.

41. Sellar RS, Peggs KS. The role of virus-specific adoptive T-cell therapy in hematopoietic transplantation. Cytotherapy. 2012;14:391–400.

42. Hansen SG, Powers CJ, Richards R, et al. Evasion of CD8+ T cells is critical for superinfection by cytomegalovirus. Science. 2010;328:102–6.

43. Neudorfer J, Schmidt B, Huster KM, et al. Reversible HLA multimers (Streptamers) for the isolation of human cytotoxic T lymphocytes functionally active against tumor- and virus-derived antigens. J Immunol Methods. 2007;320:119–31.

44. Schmitt A, Tonn T, Busch DH, et al. Adoptive transfer and selective reconstitution of streptamer-selected cytomegalovirus-specific CD8+ T cells leads to virus clearance in patients after allogeneic peripheral blood stem cell transplantation. Transfusion. 2011;51:591–9.

45. Janeway C. Immunobiology : the immune system in health and disease. 6th ed. New York: Garland Science; 2005.

46. June CH, Riddell SR, Schumacher TN. Adoptive cellular therapy: a race to the finish line. Sci Transl Med. 2015;7:280ps7.

47. Sadelain M, Brentjens R, Riviere I. The promise and potential pitfalls of chimeric antigen receptors. Curr Opin Immunol. 2009;21:215–23.

48. Eshhar Z. Tumor-specific T-bodies: towards clinical application. Cancer Immunol Immunother. 1997;45:131–6.

49. Schub A, Schuster IG, Hammerschmidt W, et al. CMV-specific TCR-transgenic T cells for immunotherapy. J Immunol. 2009;183:6819–30.

50. Scholten KB, Turksma AW, Ruizendaal JJ, et al. Generating HPV specific T helper cells for the treatment of HPV induced malignancies using TCR gene transfer. J Transl Med. 2011;9:147.

51. Gehring AJ, Xue SA, Ho ZZ, et al. Engineering virus-specific T cells that target HBV infected hepatocytes and hepatocellular carcinoma cell lines. J Hepatol. 2011;55:103–10.

52. Zhang Y, Liu Y, Moxley KM, et al. Transduction of human T cells with a novel T-cell receptor confers anti-HCV reactivity. PLoS Pathog. 2010;6:e1001018.

53. Luo W, Zhang XB, Huang YT, et al. Development of genetically engineered CD4+ and CD8+ T cells expressing TCRs specific for a M. tuberculosis 38-kDa antigen. J Mol Med (Berl). 2011;89:903–13.

54. Oh HL, Chia A, Chang CX, et al. Engineering T cells specific for a dominant severe acute respiratory syndrome coronavirus CD8 T cell epitope. J Virol. 2011;85:10464–71.

55. Roan NR, Starnbach MN. Antigen-specific CD8+ T cells respond to Chlamydia trachomatis in the genital mucosa. J Immunol. 2006;177:7974–9.

56. Ueno T, Fujiwara M, Tomiyama H, et al. Reconstitution of anti-HIV effector functions of primary human CD8 T lymphocytes by transfer of HIV-specific alphabeta TCR genes. Eur J Immunol. 2004;34:3379–88.

57. Masiero S, Del Vecchio C, Gavioli R, et al. T-cell engineering by a chimeric T-cell receptor with antibody-type specificity for the HIV-1 gp120. Gene Ther. 2005;12:299–310.

58. Sahu GK, Sango K, Selliah N, et al. Anti-HIV designer T cells progressively eradicate a latently infected cell line by sequentially inducing HIV reactivation then killing the newly gp120-positive cells. Virology. 2013;446:268–75.

59. Bitton N, Verrier F, Debre P, et al. Characterization of T cell-expressed chimeric receptors with antibody-type specificity for the CD4 binding site of HIV-1 gp120. Eur J Immunol. 1998;28:4177–87.

60. Joseph A, Zheng JH, Follenzi A, et al. Lentiviral vectors encoding human immunodeficiency virus type 1 (HIV-1)-specific T-cell receptor genes efficiently convert peripheral blood CD8 T lymphocytes into cytotoxic T lymphocytes with potent in vitro and in vivo HIV-1-specific inhibitory activity. J Virol. 2008;82:3078–89.

61. Kumaresan PR, Manuri PR, Albert ND, et al. Bioengineering T cells to target carbohydrate to treat opportunistic fungal infection. Proc Natl Acad Sci U S A. 2014;111:10660–5.

62. Cobbold M, Khan N, Pourgheysari B, et al. Adoptive transfer of cytomegalovirus-specific CTL to stem

cell transplant patients after selection by HLA-peptide tetramers. J Exp Med. 2005;202:379–86.

63. Feuchtinger T, Opherk K, Bethge WA, et al. Adoptive transfer of pp65-specific T cells for the treatment of chemorefractory cytomegalovirus disease or reactivation after haploidentical and matched unrelated stem cell transplantation. Blood. 2010;116:4360–7.

64. Peggs KS, Thomson K, Samuel E, et al. Directly selected cytomegalovirus-reactive donor T cells confer rapid and safe systemic reconstitution of virus-specific immunity following stem cell transplantation. Clin Infect Dis. 2011;52:49–57.

65. Haque T, Amlot PL, Helling N, et al. Reconstitution of EBV-specific T cell immunity in solid organ transplant recipients. J Immunol. 1998;160:6204–9.

66. Haque T, Taylor C, Wilkie GM, et al. Complete regression of posttransplant lymphoproliferative disease using partially HLA-matched Epstein Barr virus-specific cytotoxic T cells. Transplantation. 2001;72:1399–402.

67. Haque T, Wilkie GM, Taylor C, et al. Treatment of Epstein-Barr-virus-positive post-transplantation lymphoproliferative disease with partly HLA-matched allogeneic cytotoxic T cells. Lancet. 2002;360:436–42.

68. Haque T, Wilkie GM, Jones MM, et al. Allogeneic cytotoxic T-cell therapy for EBV-positive post-transplantation lymphoproliferative disease: results of a phase 2 multicenter clinical trial. Blood. 2007;110:1123–31.

69. Uhlin M, Okas M, Gertow J, et al. A novel haploidentical adoptive CTL therapy as a treatment for EBV-associated lymphoma after stem cell transplantation. Cancer Immunol Immunother. 2010;59:473–7.

70. Moosmann A, Bigalke I, Tischer J, et al. Effective and long-term control of EBV PTLD after transfer of peptide-selected T cells. Blood. 2010;115:2960–70.

71. Barker JN, Doubrovina E, Sauter C, et al. Successful treatment of EBV-associated posttransplantation lymphoma after cord blood transplantation using third-party EBV-specific cytotoxic T lymphocytes. Blood. 2010;116:5045–9.

72. Basso S, Zecca M, Calafiore L, et al. Successful treatment of a classic Hodgkin lymphoma-type post-transplant lymphoproliferative disorder with tailored chemotherapy and Epstein-Barr virus-specific cytotoxic T lymphocytes in a pediatric heart transplant recipient. Pediatr Transplant. 2013;17:E168–73.

73. Qasim W, Derniame S, Gilmour K, et al. Third-party virus-specific T cells eradicate adenoviraemia but trigger bystander graft-versus-host disease. Br J Haematol. 2011;154:150–3.

74. Feuchtinger T, Matthes-Martin S, Richard C, et al. Safe adoptive transfer of virus-specific T-cell immunity for the treatment of systemic adenovirus infection after allogeneic stem cell transplantation. Br J Haematol. 2006;134:64–76.

75. Lieberman J, Skolnik PR, Parkerson GR 3rd, et al. Safety of autologous, ex vivo-expanded human immunodeficiency virus (HIV)-specific cytotoxic T-lymphocyte infusion in HIV-infected patients. Blood. 1997;90:2196–206.

76. Mitsuyasu RT, Anton PA, Deeks SG, et al. Prolonged survival and tissue trafficking following adoptive transfer of CD4zeta gene-modified autologous CD4(+) and CD8(+) T cells in human immunodeficiency virus-infected subjects. Blood. 2000;96:785–93.

77. Deeks SG, Wagner B, Anton PA, et al. A phase II randomized study of HIV-specific T-cell gene therapy in subjects with undetectable plasma viremia on combination antiretroviral therapy. Mol Ther. 2002;5:788–97.

78. Tebas P, Stein D, Binder-Scholl G, et al. Antiviral effects of autologous CD4 T cells genetically modified with a conditionally replicating lentiviral vector expressing long antisense to HIV. Blood. 2013;121:1524–33.

79. Tebas P, Stein D, Tang WW, et al. Gene editing of CCR5 in autologous CD4 T cells of persons infected with HIV. N Engl J Med. 2014;370:901–10.

80. Balduzzi A, Lucchini G, Hirsch HH, et al. Polyomavirus JC-targeted T-cell therapy for progressive multiple leukoencephalopathy in a hematopoietic cell transplantation recipient. Bone Marrow Transplant. 2011;46:987–92.

81. Uhlin M, Gertow J, Uzunel M, et al. Rapid salvage treatment with virus-specific T cells for therapy-resistant disease. Clin Infect Dis. 2012;55:1064–73.

82. Perruccio K, Tosti A, Burchielli E, et al. Transferring functional immune responses to pathogens after haploidentical hematopoietic transplantation. Blood. 2005;106:4397–406.

83. Leen AM, Myers GD, Sili U, et al. Monoculture-derived T lymphocytes specific for multiple viruses expand and produce clinically relevant effects in immunocompromised individuals. Nat Med. 2006;12:1160–6.

84. Micklethwaite KP, Clancy L, Sandher U, et al. Prophylactic infusion of cytomegalovirus-specific cytotoxic T lymphocytes stimulated with Ad5f35pp65 gene-modified dendritic cells after allogeneic hemopoietic stem cell transplantation. Blood. 2008;112:3974–81.

85. Leen AM, Bollard CM, Mendizabal AM, et al. Multicenter study of banked third-party virus-specific T cells to treat severe viral infections after hematopoietic stem cell transplantation. Blood. 2013;121:5113–23.

86. Gerdemann U, Katari UL, Papadopoulou A, et al. Safety and clinical efficacy of rapidly-generated trivirus-directed T cells as treatment for adenovirus, EBV, and CMV infections after allogeneic hematopoietic stem cell transplant. Mol Ther. 2013;21:2113–21.

87. Blyth E, Clancy L, Simms R, et al. Donor-derived CMV-specific T cells reduce the requirement for CMV-directed pharmacotherapy after allogeneic stem cell transplantation. Blood. 2013;121:3745–58.

88. Papadopoulou A, Gerdemann U, Katari UL, et al. Activity of broad-spectrum T cells as treatment for AdV, EBV, CMV, BKV, and HHV6 infections after HSCT. Sci Transl Med. 2014;6:242ra83.

89. Lum LG, Thakur A, Al-Kadhimi Z, et al. Targeted T-cell therapy in stage IV breast cancer: a phase I clinical trial. Clin Cancer Res. 2015;21:2305–14.

90. Vaishampayan UN, Thakur A, Rathore R, et al. Phase I study of anti-CD3 x anti-Her2 bispecific antibody in metastatic castrate resistance prostate cancer patients. Prostate Cancer. 2015;2015:1–10.

91. Reusch U, Sundaram M, Davol PA, et al. Anti-CD3 x anti-EGFR bispecific antibody redirects T cell cytolytic activity to EGFR-positive cancers in vitro and in an animal model. Clin Cancer Res. 2006;12:183–90.

92. Gall JM, Davol PA, Grabert RC, et al. T cells armed with anti-CD3 x anti-CD20 bispecific antibody enhance killing of CD20+ malignant B-cells and bypass complement-mediated Rituximab-resistance in vitro. Exp Hematol. 2005;33:452–9.

93. Lum LG, Thakur A, Liu Q, et al. CD20-targeted T cells after stem cell transplantation for high risk and refractory non-Hodgkin's lymphoma. Biol Blood Marrow Transplant. 2013;19:925–33.

94. Lum LG, Thakur A, Pray C, et al. Multiple infusions of CD20-targeted T cells and low-dose IL-2 after SCT for high-risk non-Hodgkin's lymphoma: a pilot study. Bone Marrow Transplant. 2014;49:73–9.

95. Lum LG, Ramesh M, Thakur A, et al. Targeting cytomegalovirus-infected cells using T cells armed with anti-CD3× anti-CMV bispecific antibody. Biol Blood Marrow Transplant. 2012;18:1012–22.

96. Vera JF, Brenner LJ, Gerdemann U, et al. Accelerated production of antigen-specific T cells for preclinical and clinical applications using gas-permeable rapid expansion cultureware (G-Rex). J Immunother. 2010;33:305–15.

97. Lam S, Bollard C. T-cell therapies for HIV. Immunotherapy. 2013;5:407–14.

98. Didigu CA, Wilen CB, Wang J, et al. Simultaneous zinc-finger nuclease editing of the HIV coreceptors ccr5 and cxcr4 protects CD4+ T cells from HIV-1 infection. Blood. 2014;123:61–9.

99. Ramos CA, Narala N, Vyas GM, et al. Human papillomavirus type 16 E6/E7-specific cytotoxic T lymphocytes for adoptive immunotherapy of HPV-associated malignancies. J Immunother. 2013;36:66–76.

100. Cruz CR, Hanley PJ, Liu H, et al. Adverse events following infusion of T cells for adoptive immunotherapy: a 10-year experience. Cytotherapy. 2010;12:743–9.

101. Xue SA, Gao L, Ahmadi M, et al. Human MHC class I-restricted high avidity CD4 T cells generated by

102. Frumento G, Zheng Y, Aubert G, et al. Cord blood T cells retain early differentiation phenotype suitable for immunotherapy after TCR gene transfer to confer EBV specificity. Am J Transplant. 2013;13:45–55.

103. Goodridge HS, Wolf AJ, Underhill DM. Beta-glucan recognition by the innate immune system. Immunol Rev. 2009;230:38–50.

104. Romani L. Immunity to fungal infections. Nat Rev Immunol. 2004;4:1–23.

105. Groll AH, McNeil Grist L. Current challenges in the diagnosis and management of invasive fungal infections: report from the 15th international symposium on infections in the immunocompromised host: Thessaloniki, Greece, 22–25. Int J Antimicrob Agents. 2008;33:101–4. 2009

106. Beck O, Topp MS, Koehl U, et al. Generation of highly purified and functionally active human TH1 cells against Aspergillus fumigatus. Blood. 2006;107:2562–9.

107. Khanna N, Stuehler C, Conrad B, et al. Generation of a multipathogen-specific T-cell product for adoptive immunotherapy based on activation-dependent expression of CD154. Blood. 2011;118:1121–31.

108. Tramsen L, Schmidt S, Boenig H, et al. Clinical-scale generation of multi-specific anti-fungal T cells targeting Candida, Aspergillus and mucormycetes. Cytotherapy. 2013;15:344–51.

109. Tramsen L, Koehl U, Tonn T, et al. Clinical-scale generation of human anti-Aspergillus T cells for adoptive immunotherapy. Bone Marrow Transplant. 2009;43:13–9.

110. Gaundar SS, Clancy L, Blyth E, et al. Robust polyfunctional T-helper 1 responses to multiple fungal antigens from a cell population generated using an environmental strain of Aspergillus fumigatus. Cytotherapy. 2012;14:1119–30.

111. Tramsen L, Beck O, Schuster FR, et al. Generation and characterization of anti-Candida T cells as potential immunotherapy in patients with Candida infection after allogeneic hematopoietic stem-cell transplant. J Infect Dis. 2007;196:485–92.

112. Stuehler C, Khanna N, Bozza S, et al. Cross-protective TH1 immunity against Aspergillus fumigatus and Candida albicans. Blood. 2011;117:5881–91.

113. Jolink H, Meijssen IC, Hagedoorn RS, et al. Characterization of the T-cell-mediated immune response against the Aspergillus fumigatus proteins Crf1 and catalase 1 in healthy individuals. J Infect Dis. 2013;208:847–56.

114. Feng CG, Britton WJ. CD4+ and CD8+ T cells mediate adoptive immunity to aerosol infection of Mycobacterium bovis bacillus Calmette-Guerin. J Infect Dis. 2000;181:1846–9.

115. Stemberger C, Graef P, Odendahl M, et al. Lowest numbers of primary CD8(+) T cells can reconstitute protective immunity upon adoptive immunotherapy. Blood. 2014;124:628–37.

116. Polley R, Stager S, Prickett S, et al. Adoptive immuno-therapy against experimental visceral leishmaniasis with CD8+ T cells requires the presence of cognate antigen. Infect Immun. 2006;74:773–6.

117. Gomez MJ, Maras B, Barca A, et al. Biochemical and immunological characterization of MP65, a major mannoprotein antigen of the opportunistic human pathogen Candida albicans. Infect Immun. 2000;68:694–701.

118. Schmidt S, Tramsen L, Perkhofer S, et al. Characterization of the cellular immune responses to Rhizopus oryzae with potential impact on immu-notherapeutic strategies in hematopoietic stem cell transplantation. J Infect Dis. 2012;206:135–9.

119. De Angelis B, Dotti G, Quintarelli C, et al. Generation of Epstein-Barr virus-specific cyto-toxic T lymphocytes resistant to the immuno-suppressive drug tacrolimus (FK506). Blood. 2009;114:4784–91.

120. Brewin J, Mancao C, Straathof K, et al. Generation of EBV-specific cytotoxic T cells that are resistant to calcineurin inhibitors for the treatment of post-transplantation lymphoproliferative disease. Blood. 2009;114:4792–803.

Gene Therapy for Primary Immunodeficiencies

Maria Pia Cicalese and Alessandro Aiuti

Introduction

Primary immunodeficiencies (PIDs) represent a large number of heterogeneous, rare, chronic diseases inherited in a Mendelian fashion and resulting from over 300 genetically defined single-gene inborn errors of immunity [1, 2], leading to varying degrees of improper immune cell development and/or function [3]. The reported incidence of specific PIDs ranges from 1 in 600 to 1 in 500,000 live newborns [4, 5]. Recent studies have shown that they may be more common [6] and that as many as 1–2% of the population may be affected with a PID when all types and varieties are considered [7]. Clinical manifestations of PID are highly variable, ranging from life-threatening infections (such as observed in several severe combined immunodeficiency, SCID) to monogenic detriments leading to common infectious diseases such as severe influenza, autoimmune diseases such as cytopenias and systemic lupus erythematosus, and inflammatory diseases, to complete the absence of symptoms [8]. This variability and the lack of awareness among physicians of the broad range of PID manifestations result in many patients with PIDs being undiagnosed, underdiagnosed, or misdiagnosed [9, 10].

The spectrum of PIDs is constantly increasing due to new information on genes affecting the immune system. Next-generation sequencing (NGS), including whole-exome sequencing and whole-genome sequencing (WES and WGS, respectively), has been successful in identifying PIDs with a Mendelian inheritance, even when the condition is seen in a single patient. Indeed, it has been possible to identify single-gene inborn errors in immunodeficient patients by validating the disease-causing role of the genotype through in-depth mechanistic studies demonstrating the structural and functional consequences of mutations [11, 12].

While differing in clinical severity, early diagnosis and treatment is of considerable importance for the majority of PID to prevent organ damage and life-threatening infections and to improve quality of life of affected patients [13–17]. Much effort is currently being put into developing methods for detection of PIDs in the neonatal

M. P. Cicalese
San Raffaele Telethon Institute for Gene Therapy (TIGET), San Raffaele Scientific Institute, Milan, Italy

Pediatric Immunohematology and Bone Marrow Transplantation Unit, IRCCS San Raffaele Scientific Institute, Milan, Italy

A. Aiuti (✉)
San Raffaele Telethon Institute for Gene Therapy (TIGET), San Raffaele Scientific Institute, Milan, Italy

Pediatric Immunohematology and Bone Marrow Transplantation Unit, IRCCS San Raffaele Scientific Institute, Milan, Italy

Vita-Salute San Raffaele University, Milan, Italy
e-mail: aiuti.alessandro@hsr.it

© Springer International Publishing AG, part of Springer Nature 2018
B. H. Segal (ed.), *Management of Infections in the Immunocompromised Host*,
https://doi.org/10.1007/978-3-319-77674-3_21

period, especially for PIDs with lack of functional T or B lymphocytes. PCR-based detection of signal joint T-cell receptor excision circles (TRECs) has proven to be a valuable tool for identifying patients with SCID [15]. Universal newborn screening has been implemented in many states in the USA, facilitating the establishment of the true incidence of SCID in California (1 in 66,250 live births) and leading to early detection and improvement of treatment outcomes of many cases of PIDs [12]. Other countries are considering implementation of newborn screening programs for SCID and other PIDs [13, 14]. A similar method for analysis of k-deleting excision circles (KRECs) has been described for detection of patients with X-linked agammaglobulinemia (XLA). Recently, a robust triplex PCR method for quantitation of TRECs and KRECs, using a single Guthrie card punch, has been developed and validated in a cohort of 2560 anonymized newborn screening cards. Through this method, patients with SCID, XLA, ataxia-telangiectasia, and Nijmegen breakage syndrome have been readily identified, and effective newborn screening for severe immunodeficiency syndromes characterized by the absence of T or B cells has been made easier [15]. Recently, tandem mass spectrometry for analysis of metabolites from dried blood spots has been proposed as an easy and inexpensive method for ADA-SCID and purine nucleoside phosphorylase deficiency screening [16, 17].

For an increasing number of diseases, replacement of the defective recipient immune system with a functioning system from a healthy donor by hematopoietic stem cell transplantation (HSCT) can lead to a permanent cure. The first HSCTs for primary immunodeficiencies (PIDs) were performed in 1968 [18, 19], and so nearly 50 years of experience has led to many significant improvements in technique and outcome among European centers [20–26]. SCIDs are the most profound defects, and HSCT, until recently, has been the only approach to treatment (with the exception of ADA-SCID, for which enzyme replacement is possible). Other PIDs have been managed conservatively or with HSCT at various centers. HSCT is now becoming a more widely

accepted modality of treatment, as long-term outcomes of conservative management are investigated and outcomes improve through earlier diagnosis and safer approaches to transplantation. New conditioning regimens have reduced the risk of HSCT, and new methods of manipulating stem cell sources may provide a donor for almost all patients. Despite this, high-dose chemotherapy and graft-versus-host disease (GvHD) still lead to major risks, as toxicity-related organ dysfunction and infections, in the setting of transplantation from alternative donors, driving a considerable transplant-related mortality [21–26].

For this reason, gene therapy (GT) has been successfully implemented in the last 15 years for the treatment of PID patients who lacked a suitable donor. The main advantages of GT *vs* standard allogeneic transplantation are the use of "low-dose" or "reduced-intensity" conditioning regimens, with consequent low toxicity, based on the evidence that a mixed chimerism is sufficient to improve the clinical phenotype, the absence of GvHD due to the use of an autologous cellular product, the possibility to exploit the selective advantage of transduced cells, and the prompt availability of the stem cells that significantly shortens treatment times. Despite this, in some cases, efficacy of gene therapy has been counterbalanced by the occurrence of insertional oncogenesis. The understanding of the molecular events that led to oncogenesis and improved vector technology has led to progress with safer gene therapy approaches for PID [27, 28]. Here we will give an overview of promising recent clinical trials of gene therapy for SCID-X1, ADA-SCID, Wiskott-Aldrich syndrome (WAS), and chronic granulomatous disease (CGD) and discuss perspectives for new technologies that might be expanded to other diseases.

Gene Therapy for SCID-X1

X-linked SCID represents the most common form of SCID, accounting for 40–50% of SCID cases reported worldwide. It is caused by mutations in the IL2RG gene, leading to defective expression of the common gamma chain, a key subunit of the cytokine receptor complex for interleukin (IL)2, IL4, IL7, IL9, IL15, and IL21, which play a vital role in lymphocyte development and function [2]. Consequently, SCID-X1 patients present profound immunological defects caused by low numbers or complete absence of T and NK cells and presence of nonfunctional B cells. The disease is characterized by common and opportunistic infections that usually occur before 1 year of age and that can be lethal unless allogeneic HSCT is performed [29].

Nonconditioned, allogeneic HSCT has been the gold standard therapy for this disorder since 1968. However, the outcome of HSCT is highly dependent on the availability of a suitable hematopoietic stem cell (HSC) donor: the 3-year overall survival rate is 90–97% when the donor is an HLA-identical sibling, despite partial immune recovery, autoimmunity, and/or retarded growth reported for some patients, but only 66–79% with an alternative donor, for the higher rates of complications, including graft-versus-host disease and lack of B- and NK-cell reconstitution in ~two-thirds of patients, which may ultimately lead to progressive clinical deterioration [21–23]. The presence of an active infection at time of treatment is also strongly associated with a lower survival rate after HSCT, 50% of 5-year survival after HSCT *vs* 80% [30].

The observation of few patients with spontaneous reversion of the mutation and subsequent correction of immune deficiency [31–33] gave rise to the idea that even a small fraction of "naturally" corrected wild-type cells could have a selective advantage over the mutated lymphocytes and therefore led to SCID-X1 being a candidate disease for gene therapy. Since then, gene therapy (GT) via the transduction of a corrected copy of a gene into autologous HSCs has been considered as an attractive approach to overcome the absence of a suitable donor. The efficacy of gamma chain (γc) gene transfer in autologous HSCs from SCID-X1 patients has been confirmed by early clinical trial results. Between 1999 and 2006, 20 subjects with SCID-X1 lacking HLA-identical bone marrow donors underwent GT in 2 European sites, Paris and London. They were infused with autologous CD34+ bone marrow cells transduced with a first-generation Moloney murine leukemia virus vector expressing the γc complementary DNA (MFG-γc) and containing duplicated viral enhancer sequences within the long terminal repeats (LTRs) [34–36]. Seventeen of the 20 subjects treated with ex vivo transduced CD34+ cells without a conditioning regimen are alive and display full (or nearly full) correction of their T-cell immunodeficiency with a median follow-up of 12 years (7–15.5 years) [2]. In most patients, long-term thymopoiesis was demonstrated by the detection of T-cell receptor excision circles and a diverse T-cell receptor Vβ repertoire [37]. However, the transient restoration of NK cells and the limited functional B-cell reconstitution, with a minority of patients able to stop immunoglobulin (IVIG) supplementation, suggest that the lack of a conditioning regimen was probably responsible for insufficient engraftment of gene-modified B cells and that the NK-cell-corrected population was not capable of long-term renewal [38].

Unfortunately, the enthusiasm for the promising results of these studies was dampened by the occurrence of genotoxicity: four patients in the French trial and one patient in the British cohort developed T-cell leukemia [39] between 2 and 5 years after GT: four of them have been in remission after conventional chemotherapy, in one case followed by matched unrelated HCT, and remain in long-term remission, while the remaining patient died despite an allogeneic HSCT from chemotherapy-refractory leukemia [39–41]. In all cases, the adverse event was the result of insertional oncogenesis due to aberrant expression of the LMO2 (LIM domain only 2) or CCND2 (cyclin D2) oncogenes induced by the integration of the γc retroviral vector in the proximity of the gene regulatory regions [2]. Second genome alterations were found in all cases and probably accounted for the advent of overt leukemia [2], favored by the selective advantage conferred to them by the concomitant expression of the γc gene [41–43].

To improve safety while maintaining the efficacy profile for SCID-X1 gene therapy, a new strategy has been developed based on a self-inactivating (SIN) γ-retroviral vector with deleted

Moloney murine leukemia virus LTR U3 enhancer, expressing the IL2RG complementary DNA from the eukaryotic human elongation factor 1α (EF1α) short promoter. This construct was less mutagenic in vitro and effective in a mouse model of SCID-X1 (enhancer-deleted SIN-γc) [41]. The interim results of the first nine patients treated in parallel phase 1/2 trials conducted in London, Paris, Boston, Cincinnati, and Los Angeles have been recently published [30, 34] (ClinicalTrials.gov identifiers, NCT01410019, NCT01175239, NCT01129544). SCID-X1 children were enrolled if a HLA-identical sibling donor was not available or in case of severe ongoing, therapy-resistant infections. Conditioning was not given to most patients, but two patients received fludarabine or anti-thymocyte gobulin due to a large number of maternal blood T cells migrated through the placenta into the fetal circulation, sometimes associated with GvHD. Eight of nine treated patients survived, while a preexisting disseminated adenovirus infection was fatal in one patient 4 months after GT, due to an incomplete T-cell compartment recovery. One patient did not show any gene correction and was successfully transplanted with a mismatched cord blood graft. Up to 48 months of follow-up, immune reconstitution of T-cells occurred in the other seven patients and was comparable to that observed in the previous trials conducted in Paris and London. A significant reduction in infection frequency was observed, and isolation precautions were discontinued. One patient needed a second infusion due to low absolute T-cell numbers. The absence of conditioning in these studies also led to minimal gene marking in B-cell and myeloid lineages, and all patients remain on immunoglobulin replacement therapy. Importantly, integration analysis showed a polyclonal integration profile with reduced numbers of clones near known lymphoid proto-oncogenes and genes implicated in serious adverse events in previous GT trials [30, 38].

Furthermore, five older patients carrying hypomorphic IL2RG mutations, including three from a 2003 initiated trial at the NIH, were treated with G-CSF-mobilized peripheral blood CD34+ cells transduced with γ-retroviral vector. Despite effective transduction, an improvement of T-cell numbers and function occurred only in one subject, the youngest, while no immunological improvement was achieved in the others, probably due to loss of thymic function by the time of gene therapy [44].

A new approach was developed by Sorrentino and colleagues and used in a two-site clinical trial, based on the use of lentiviral vector (LV) (CL20-i4-EF1α-hγc-OPT) containing a 400 bp insulator fragment from the chicken beta-globin locus within the self-inactivating long terminal repeat (LTR), driven by the eukaryotic elongation factor alpha (EF1alpha) promoter to express a codon-optimized gc cDNA [45]. Severe, early-onset SCID-X1 patients (typical SCID-X1) have been enrolled at the St. Jude Children's Research Center in Memphis (ClinicalTrials.gov identifier, NCT01512888), while late-onset SCID-X1 children (atypical SCID-X1) and adolescents between 2 and 20 years of age have been treated at NIH (NCT01306019). Patients enrolled in the latter arm of the trial undergo G-CSF and plerixafor-mobilized peripheral blood apheresis and CD34 isolation and use non-myeloablative conditioning with a total busulfan dose of 6 mg/kg/body weight to improve the efficacy of engraftment of gene-corrected cells [46]. Preliminary results have been reported on the first five patients, age range of 10–24 years, who previously underwent haploidentical HSC transplant without benefit on immune function and IgG supplementation dependence. In the two older patients with longer follow-up (30 and 27 months, respectively), stable engraftment of gamma chain-expressing cells with expansion of gene corrected T, B, and NK cells was observed. Gene marking in the myeloid lineages stabilized by a year following treatment to 8–10% (=0.1 vector genome (vg)/cell), while a continuous increase in B, T, and NK cells was documented. Both patients produced IgG and generated a protective titer response to immunization. (De Ravin SS, Wu X, Moir S, et al. Lentiviral hematopoietic stem cell gene therapy for X-linked severe combined immunodeficiency, personal communication, ASH 57th annual meeting, Orlando, FL, 5–8 Dec 2015).

Recently, a unique clinical retrospective analysis of direct comparison of clinical outcomes and immune reconstitution in 13 consecutive SCID-X1 patients who underwent haploidentical

HSCT and 14 SCID-X1 patients treated with gene therapy at Necker Children's Hospital (Paris, France) over the same period has been performed. The results show a clear advantage in terms of T-cell development of gene therapy over HSCT with a mismatched donor, in particular a faster T-cell reconstitution and a better long-term thymic output in GT-treated patients [38, 47].

Although the more advanced lentivirus vectors [48] have shown improved safety and efficacy, the therapeutic potential of targeted genome editing of HSCs has been recently proven in a subject with SCID X1. Gene-edited HSCs sustained normal hematopoiesis and gave rise to functional lymphoid cells that possess a selective growth advantage over those carrying disruptive IL2RG mutations. These results are expected to open new avenues for treating SCID-X1 and other diseases [49].

Gene Therapy for ADA-SCID

Mutations in *ADA* lead to the intra- and extracellular accumulation of deoxyadenosine and adenosine and through conversion by specific enzymes to the intracellular accumulation of deoxyadenosine triphosphate and adenosine triphosphate. The pathological accumulation of these metabolites in plasma, red blood cells, and tissues gives rise to the phenotype of ADA-SCID, the second most frequent form of SCID, accounting for 15–20% of all cases [50, 51]. In its typical early severe onset form, it is usually fatal in the 1st year of life [52]. Apart from the profound lymphopenia (affecting T, B, and NK cells) and the absence of cellular and humoral immune function [53], diverse non-immunological systemic defects, such as skeletal, gastrointestinal, pulmonary, and neuronal abnormalities, occur [54, 55].

Patients who receive enzyme replacement therapy (ERT) usually have improved immune function, but in the long-term, they develop a decline in T-cell numbers and function and can develop antibodies against bovine ADA and autoimmune manifestations. Moreover, B-cell function defects are not fully repaired, with only 50% of patients able to discontinue immu-

noglobulin replacement therapy [56]. For these reasons, HSCT had been considered as the only definitive treatment, and HLA-matched sibling donor (MSD) or family donor (MFD) transplantation is associated with excellent overall survival (86% for MSD and 83% for MFD), while 67% overall survival (OS) is reported in cases of HLA-matched unrelated donors (MUDs) [57].

Since the early 1990s, genetic modification of autologous lymphocytes with gammaretroviral vectors (γ-RV) was performed while patients were continuing ERT [58–61]. Although this approach was not sufficient to discontinue ERT, the transduced T cells could safely persist for more than 10 years [62, 63]. Importantly, a recently identified population of T cells with stem cell properties was shown to significantly contribute to the pool of long-term living T cells by tracking of insertion sites [63].

The transduction and protocol were improved in order to promote the engraftment of modified stem cells, as well as to provide a selective pressure for the corrected cells that would be turned into a visible clinical benefit for the patients [64]. The inclusion of a mild preconditioning regimen with busulfan (4 mg/kg i.v.) made space for the corrected progenitors and improved the engraftment and safety of the approach [65]. Moreover, the selective pressure for growth of gene-modified cells was promoted by the withdrawal of ERT before GT.

Hence, a subsequent clinical trial in TIGET, Milan, showed in eight of ten treated patients ADA levels sufficient to decrease toxic metabolites and allow functional immune recovery [66]. A recent update in those and eight additional patients treated at median age of 1.7 years (range, 0.5–6.1) showed 100% overall survival, with a median follow-up of 6.9 years (range, 2.3–13.4), and that, among them, 15 no longer received ERT (NCT00598481, enrollment closed). Gene-modified cells were stably present and polyclonal in multiple lineages throughout follow-up, with higher levels in lymphoid cells. ADA expression was increased in lymphocytes, and purine metabolites levels in red blood cells remained low, indicating effective systemic detoxification. GT resulted in a sustained reduction in the severe infection rate, and immune reconstitution was demonstrated by normalization of T-cell subsets (CD3[+], CD4[+], and CD8[+]), evidence of thymopoiesis, and sustained T-cell proliferative capacity. A total of 12 patients discontinued IVIG use (seven of them within 3 years of GT), with stable median serum IgG levels within normal ranges throughout, and protective antibody-forming capacity was demonstrated with detectable antibodies to several vaccines. All 18 patients had infections as adverse events after GT, and no events indicative of leukemic transformation were reported post–treatment [67].

On the basis of these results, a request for marketing authorization of the GT product from GlaxoSmithKline and SR-Tiget was approved by the European Medicines Agency (EMA) in May 2016. The GT product known as Strimvelis will be commercialized to treat ADA-SCID patients, with an indication for all pediatric patients without suitable family-matched, related donors for HSCT [68].

A clinical trial run in London showed results similar to Tiget trial [37] (NCT01279720). In a joint trial between the Children's Hospital Los Angeles and the National Institutes of Health (NIH), the protocol was amended after treating four patients without conditioning. Implementation of a cytoreductive regimen and cessation of ERT prior to gene therapy improved the clinical and immunological outcome in a further six patients [69] (NCT00794508).

Two children with ADA deficiency were further treated in Japan in 2003–2004 by γ-RV-mediated gene transfer to bone marrow CD34+ cells after ERT cessation without a conditioning regimen [70]. This study showed lack of full immune recovery, underlining the need for conditioning for successful gene therapy. Recent murine studies point to cytoreduction of autologous ADA-deficient HSC favoring engraftment of the corrected HSC [71]. Moreover, new observations show that continuation of ERT could significantly increase the levels of gene-modified cells in the thymus [38].

Over 50 patients with ADA-SCID have been treated with γ-RV vectors in Milan, London, and the USA, and all are alive [72], and the majority of them achieved stable ADA enzyme activity in lymphoid cells, persistent immune reconstitution, long-term multilineage engraftment, and sustained systemic detoxification, without needing reintroduction of ERT or subsequent SCT [73]. T-cell reconstitution did not reach normal levels, but in most patients, cellular and humoral responses improved. The application of a mild non-myeloablative regimen also led to significantly improved B and NK lymphocyte and myeloid cell counts.

GammaRV vectors using a similar Moloney murine leukemia virus backbone, but with slightly different envelopes and gene expression systems, have demonstrated clinical and biological efficacy in previous trials, but in some cases hematologic malignancies occurred, as in the SCID-X1 and WAS trials [74–77]. In contrast, there were no genotoxic events in GT-treated SCID patients in an extended follow-up period [5, 67, 69]. Integrations were also found in ADA-SCID patients within and/or near potentially oncogenic loci, but did not result in selection or expansion of malignant cell clones in vivo [73], suggesting that ADA deficiency in itself may create an unfavorable milieu for leukemogenesis. Continuous monitoring of the safety of this treatment is required to evaluate for long-term adverse events.

Given the similarities between the viral backbones, differences in safety profiles between patients with ADA-SCID and patients with Wiskott-Aldrich syndrome and X-linked SCID may involve the nature of the gene of interest or the disease background. In contrast to both WAS protein (WASp) and IL2RG proteins, which are involved in the cellular response to proliferative stimuli, ADA is a metabolic "housekeeping" protein that is constitutively expressed in all cell types [67].

The need for safer vector designs led to the development of two different lentiviral (LV) vectors. Mortellaro et al. showed that self-inactivating (SIN)-LV (deletion of U3 in LTR), driving ADA expression from the phosphoglycerate kinase 1 (PGK1, PGK) promoter, was able to rescue ADA-deficient mice in a preclinical study [78]. The group of Dr. Kohn and Dr. Gaspar designed an LV that included a codon-optimized human cADA gene under the control of the short-form elongation factor-1a promoter (LV EFS ADA) that displayed high-efficiency gene transfer and adequate ADA expression to rescue ADA−/− mice from their lethal phenotype with good T- and B-cell reconstitution [79]. Further modifications involve a Woodchuck hepatitis virus post–transcriptional regulatory element (WPRE) to enhance ADA expression in lentiviruses. In vitro immortalization assays showed a reduced transformation potential of these new lentiviral constructs compared to γ-RV vectors [38]. On this basis, two phase I/II clinical trials of LV EFS ADA have started in the UK and the USA (clinical trials NCT02022696, NCT01852071) for the treatment of ADA-SCID children. Thus far, five patients aged between 1.2 and 4.5 years have been treated with busulfan (at a single dose of 5 mg/kg) conditioning prior to GT. The procedure was well tolerated by all patients. At a mean follow-up of about 1 year, there has been significant immunological recovery, with a rise of total T-cell and CD4 + counts and normalization in mitogen responses [80]. Integration site analysis showed some expansion but no persistence of expanded clones, and there were no clones with genes previously associated with insertional mutagenesis [38].

Gene Therapy for WAS

Wiskott-Aldrich syndrome (WAS) is a rare, complex, X-linked primary immunodeficiency disorder caused by mutations in the WAS gene [81] characterized by recurrent infections, microthrombocytopenia, eczema, and increased risk of autoimmune manifestations and tumors [82]. The prevalence is estimated to be one to ten out of a million male individuals, with an incidence of four out of a million male live births. The WAS protein is a main actin cytoskeleton regulator protein, and mutations affecting WAS protein expression cause functional defects in different leukocyte subsets, including defective function of T and B cells, alteration in NK cell immunological formation synapse, and impaired migra-

tion of all leukocyte subsets [83–86]. Hypomorphic mutations lead to intermediate forms as X-linked thrombocytopenia (XLT), and gain-of-function mutations have been associated with neutropenia [87]. The life expectancy of WAS patients is severely reduced unless they are successfully cured by BMT [24]. HSCT from HLA-identical sibling donor (matched sibling donor, MSD) is the treatment of choice for WAS patients, with a reported 82 to 88% long-term survival in different European and American centers in the past decade [88–90], with a survival close to 100% for patients transplanted after year 2000 [24]. MUD transplant has resulted in survival rates of 85–90%, but better results are obtained when patients are transplanted before the age of 5, and autoimmune complications are more frequent when complete chimerism is not achieved [88]. HSCT from alternative donors (partially HLA-matched relatives or mismatched family donors – MMFD, and umbilical cord blood – UCB) has led to more disappointing results.

Given these results and the evidence of a selective survival advantage of wild-type cells in experiments in mice, and patients with XLT with a low-level expression of WAS protein having a less severe phenotype [24], therapy with WAS gene-transduced autologous HSCs has been considered as a valid alternative approach for patients lacking a suitable donor or older than 5 years [91].

After large preclinical studies performed to evaluate the feasibility and efficacy of gene transfer by means of both γ-retroviral (RV) [92–95] and LV [96, 97] vectors, the first phase I/II study on humans was conducted in 2006 in Hannover, including ten patients, treated with WASp-expressing LTR-driven γ-RV following reduced-intensity busulfan conditioning [77, 87, 98]. Stable engraftment of gene-corrected cells in multiple lineages (HSCs, lymphoid, and myeloid cells) led to restoration of WASp expression, with a proliferative and selective advantage of corrected lymphoid cells over myeloid lineage, in line with the results of preclinical models [99, 100]. Severe infections, bleeding tendency, and autoimmune phenomena impressively decreased in the 1st years of follow-up [77, 98, 100]. However, between 14 months and 5 years after GT, seven out of ten treated patients developed hematologic malignancies [77, 87, 98–100], including four cases of T-cell acute lymphoblastic leukemia (T-ALL), two primary T-ALL with secondary AML, and one acute myeloid leukemia (AML), all LMO-2 related. Despite chemotherapy and secondary allogeneic HSCT, two patients died from leukemia [96]. The analysis of vector common insertion sites (CISs) revealed a marked clustering between patients, with hotspots found within the proto-oncogenes (LMO2 and MDS/Evi1), already known to be associated in other GT trials with the development of leukemia and myelodysplasia [2, 40, 77, 101]. The strong viral promoter in the context of a RV, the relatively high vector copy number per cell (1.7–5.2), and the WAS background might have had a role in the high risk of insertional mutagenesis [77], indicating that LMO2-driven leukemogenesis may occur in several PIDs.

Since then, several groups have developed SIN-LV vectors in which different promoters drive WAS protein expression in various model systems, in order to overcome the risk of leukemia from γ-RV [102–105]. Based on the promising efficacy and long-term safety results in several preclinical studies [103, 105, 106], a lentiviral vector consisting of the endogenous 1.6 kb human WAS promoter has been implemented in clinical trials in Boston, London, Milan, and Paris using different conditioning regimens and enrolling patients with severe clinical score and without a suitable HSCT donor [5]. The short-term results (18-month follow-up) in the Milan study (NCT01515462) in three patients have been published in 2013 [107, 108] and confirmed in a recent update of seven patients, treated at median age 1.9 years (range, 1.1–11.1 years). All patients are alive after a median follow-up of 3.2 years (0.7–5.0). The investigational medicinal product dose ranged between 7.0 and 14.1 × 10^6 CD34+ cells/kg, and the mean vector copy number (VCN)/genome in bulk CD34+ cells was 2.7 ± 0.8. In the first six treated patients with follow-up of more than 2 years, a robust and persistent engraftment of gene-corrected cells was detected in multiple lineages, including bone marrow progenitors, peripheral blood granulocytes, and lymphocytes. WASp expression was restored, and proliferative response to anti-CD3 mAb was in the normal range in all patients, allowing the discontinuation of anti-infective prophylaxis and of restriction measures. All patients became platelet transfusion-independent at a median of 4 months after GT (range, 1.0–8.7). From the 2nd year of follow-up, the number of hospitalizations for infections decreased; four patients stopped immunoglobulin supplementation, and two of them developed specific antibodies after vaccination. No severe bleeding episodes were recorded after treatment. Eczema resolved in four patients and remains mild in two, and no clinical manifestations of autoimmunity were observed. Importantly, no evidence of abnormal clonal proliferations emerged after GT, and the LV integration profile show a polyclonal pattern, with no skewing for proto-oncogenes [109].

An additional seven and four patients have been treated in Paris/London (NCT01347346, NCT01347242) and in Boston (NCT01410825), respectively, and the preliminary results have been recently published. At post–treatment follow-up ranging between 9 and 42 months, six of seven patients in the Paris/London trial show an improved clinical outcome, while one patient unfortunately died 7 months after treatment due to preexisting drug-resistant herpes virus infection. Eczema and susceptibility to infections resolved in all patients. Autoimmunity improved in five of five patients. No severe bleeding episodes were recorded after treatment, and hospitalization days were reduced after treatment. All six surviving patients exhibited high-level, stable engraftment of functionally corrected lymphoid cells. The degree of myeloid cell engraftment and of platelet reconstitution correlated with the dose of gene-corrected cells administered. No evidence of vector-related toxicity was observed clinically or by molecular analysis [110].

Among the second series of patients, all were alive at a median follow-up of 13.5 months (range 9–24 months). Two patients had low WASp expression, while the other two had a null mutation but evidence of somatic reversion in T and/or

NK cells. Busulfan conditioning was myeloablative or near-myeloablative in three patients and sub-myeloablative in one. CD34+ cell doses ranged from 6.3–24.91 × 10^6 cells/kg, while the VCN of the infused cells was variable (range, 0.54–3.37 copies/cell). WASp expression in T cells was increased post-GT over baseline, and the presence of revertants did not appear to interfere with T-cell reconstitution. The patient that received the highest cell dose, the highest VCN, and myeloablative busulfan conditioning had a more robust platelet reconstitution. T- and NK-cell functions were improved post-GT, and the T-cell Vβ repertoire was restored in most of the patients. All patients had improvement in eczema, became platelet transfusion-independent, and had no severe bleeding events after treatment. Integration site analysis showed highly polyclonal reconstitution, with distributions of integration acceptor sites as expected for the lentiviral vector backbone [111].

Another LV vector using a viral MND-derived promoter has also been used to further increase WASp expression in mice, but results indicate that the γ-RV-derived promoter leads to higher transgene expression as compared to the WAS-promoter vector. Moreover, this occurred in association with myeloid clonal expansion and transcriptional dysregulation, highlighting that higher transgene expression may correlate with potential leukemic risk [2, 112].

Gene Therapy for CGD

Chronic granulomatous disease (CGD) is a rare primary immunodeficiency caused by defects in the genes encoding any of the NADPH oxidase components responsible for the respiratory burst of phagocytic leukocytes. CGD is a genetically heterogeneous disease with an X-linked recessive (XR-CGD) form caused by mutations in the *CYBB* gene encoding the gp91^{phox} protein and an autosomal recessive (AR-CGD) form caused by mutations in the *CYBA*, *NCF1*, *NCF2*, or *NCF4* genes encoding p22^{phox}, p47^{phox}, p67^{phox}, and p40^{phox}, respectively. Patients suffering from this disease are susceptible to severe life-threatening bacterial and fungal infections, notably staphylococcus and aspergillus, and excessive inflammation characterized by granuloma formation in any organ, for instance, the gastrointestinal and genitourinary tract. An early diagnosis of and the prompt treatment for these conditions are crucial for an optimal outcome of affected patients.

To prevent infections, CGD patients should receive lifelong antibiotics and antifungal prophylaxis, and anti-inflammatory agents may be required to control inflammatory complications (e.g., inflammatory bowel disease). These measures, as well as newer more effective antimicrobials, have significantly modified the natural history of CGD, resulting in a remarkable change in overall survival. HSCT has recently shown a high success rate as an early intervention in patients with very low superoxide production and in patients with a history of severe invasive fungal infection, organ abscesses, and/or significant inflammatory or autoimmune signs [26, 113–115]. Furthermore, GT could offer a safer alternative, specifically avoiding the risk of GvHD. Early clinical trials performed with γ-RV without conditioning showed only transitory functional correction of ≤0.5% of peripheral blood granulocytes [116, 117]. Since gene-transduced neutrophils have no survival advantage over defective neutrophils and have a life span of only a few days, engraftment of relatively high number of gene-transduced HSCs is required by preparatory conditioning [118]. Additionally, the inflammatory bone marrow milieu could hinder the engraftment of transduced HSCs [74, 76, 118].

The first GT trials were conducted at the NIH in 1995 and 1998 targeting X-linked gp91^{phox} deficiency with a Mo-MLV-based MFG γ-RV. Ten patients underwent harvest and transduction of granulocyte colony-stimulating factor-mobilized CD34+ HSCs that were reinfused without pre-conditioning [117, 119]. In both trials, only a low (≤ 0.5%) and transient population of NADPH oxidase-competent neutrophils was detected, without any long-term clinical benefit [116, 117].

More recent trials for X-CGD were conducted between 2000 and 2010 in five different centers worldwide (Frankfurt, Zurich, London, NIH, Seoul) using γ-RV vector-transduced, mobilized CD34+ cells and non-myeloablative conditioning with low-dose (8–10 mg/kg) busulfan [76, 113, 120, 121] ± fludarabine [122], or melphalan alone (140 mg/m2) [76] in 13 patients. Ten patients showed an initial correction of NADPH activity and 5–25% of the total neutrophils showing gene marking, leading to transient clinical benefit and clearance of severe fungal infections. This was followed by a yet unexplained difficulty in achieving long-term engraftment of significant levels of transduced cells, with loss of the expression of the wild-type gp91^{phox} gene [123]. The methylation of the viral promoter leading to silencing of transgene expression is a hypothesis suggested for loss of engraftment [101]. Alternatively, ectopic gp91^{phox} expression in hematopoietic stem cell and progenitor cells could cause the production of reactive oxygen species that may damage DNA, alter cell growth, or induce apoptosis [124–126]. Moreover, immune-mediated mechanisms against gp91^{phox}-expressing cells could have contributed to the lack of long-term persistence [126].

In three patients (two adults in Frankfurt, one child in Zurich), an increase of gene-marked neutrophils reached 50% of all neutrophils temporarily and led subsequently to the clearance of chronic infections. However, the increase reflected clonal expansion and was found to be caused by insertional mutagenesis due to integration into MECOM (MDS/EVI1 complex) and PRDM16 oncogene loci and transactivation by the viral SFFV LTR similar to that observed in SCID-X1 patients. The adult patients developed myelodysplasia (MDS) with monosomy seven within the next 2.5 years and concomitant loss of oxidase function in the gene-marked cells, probably due to transgene silencing after a series of epigenetic events. Both adult patients died due to complications of MDS [101, 113, 121]. Two children were treated in Zurich with the same SFFV vector and also developed clonal expansion, one with further development to MDS. Both patients are still alive after HSCT [38, 127].

After the failure of the first trials performed with retroviral vectors, some groups have pro-posed the use of regulated SIN-lentiviral vectors targeting gp91^{phox} expression in myeloid cells to increase the safety and efficacy of the GT protocols and using a fully myeloablative conditioning regimen prior to gene therapy (12–16 mg/kg busulfan). A lentiviral vector in which gp91^{phox} is driven by a synthetic chimeric promoter, created by the fusion of cathepsin G and c-Fes minimal 50-flanking regions, has been developed in London and Frankfurt. In these vectors, transgene expression is regulated by the myeloid-specific promoter. Stringent control of gp91^{phox} expression by the miRNA-mediated posttranscriptional control elements in HSCs supports the further development of this microRNA approach as an alternative gene transfer technique for CGD [126, 127]. In vitro and murine in vivo studies showed that this vector is myeloid-specific, restores NADPH oxidase activity, and has a reduced potential regarding insertional mutagenesis [128]. This vector is currently employed in multicenter trials in Europe and in the USA (NCT01906541, NCT01855685, NCT02234934).

Another proposed strategy is based on the use of a gp91^{phox}-encoding vector driven by synthetic chimeric promoter in combination with different myeloid transcription factor binding sites or the A2UCOE element linked to a myeloid promoter driving gp91^{phox} expression in murine myeloid cells [126, 129–131]. However, as A2UCOE protects from promoter methylation, its chromatin remodeling properties could have considerable side effects in HSCs [131, 132], so further studies are needed to proceed to clinical applications [38, 133].

A novel approach based on dual-targeted LV has been developed in Milan, Italy, and represents a promising candidate for further clinical development. This construct targets gp91^{phox} expression to the differentiated myeloid compartment while sparing HSC, to reduce the risk of genotoxicity and potential perturbation of reactive oxygen species levels. Targeting was obtained by a myeloid-specific promoter (MSP) and post–transcriptional, microRNA-mediated regulation. Both components in human bone marrow (BM) HSC and their differentiated progeny in vitro and in a xenotransplantation were optimized to generate therapeutic gp91^{phox}-expressing LVs for CGD gene therapy. All vectors restored gp91^{phox} expression and function in human X-CGD myeloid cell lines, primary monocytes, and differentiated myeloid cells. While unregulated LVs ectopically expressed gp91^{phox} in CD34+ cells, transcriptionally and posttranscriptionally regulated LVs substantially reduced this off-target expression. X-CGD mice transplanted with transduced HSC restored gp91^{phox} expression, and MSP-driven vectors maintained regulation during bone marrow development. Combining transcriptional (SP146.gp91-driven) and posttranscriptional (miR-126-restricted) targeting, high levels of myeloid-specific transgene expression, entirely sparing the CD34+ HSC compartment, were achieved [126]. Recently, the same group set up a mouse model of acute infection closely mimicking the airway infection in CGD patients, involving an intratracheal injection of a methicillin-sensitive reference strain of *S. aureus*. Gene therapy with HSC transduced with regulated LVs restored the functional activity of NADPH oxidase complex (with 20–98% of dihydrorhodamine-positive granulocytes and monocytes) and saved mice from death caused by *S. aureus*, significantly reducing the bacterial load and lung damage similarly to wild-type mice, even at low VCN. When challenged, GT-treated X-CGD mice showed correction of pro-inflammatory cytokines and chemokine imbalance at levels that were comparable to wild type. These results support the clinical development of gene therapy protocols using lentiviral vectors for the protection against infections and inflammation in CGD [134].

New Frontiers and Technologies of Gene Correction for Other Diseases

In recent years, gene therapy of HSCs has proven its efficacy in several genetic diseases, including several PIDs. To address the issue of lymphoid or myeloid proliferation [74] associated with insertional mutagenesis observed in SCID-X1, CGD,

and WAS clinical trials, the γ-RV vectors are being increasingly replaced by SIN vectors, which have shown high efficacy in terms of sustainable transgene expression and reduced risk of insertional mutagenesis in vitro [74] and in vivo.

For several other genetic defects causing PIDs, preclinical studies are already ongoing by SIN-LV vectors or in certain cases of gene editing. Artemis is a single-stranded endonuclease, the deficiency of which results in a radiation-sensitive form of severe combined immunodeficiency (SCID-A). Ex vivo transduction with the APro-Artemis vector supported effective immune reconstitution in a murine model of SCID-A, resulting in fully functional T and B lymphocyte responses. These results demonstrate the importance of regulated Artemis expression in immune reconstitution of Artemis-deficient SCID [135]. As a preclinical model for RAG-SCID, Rag1−/− mice and lentiviral SIN vectors harboring different internal elements to deliver native or codon-optimized human RAG1 sequences were used, resulting in the appearance of peripheral B and T cells and normal serum Ig levels [136]. In another approach, only high vector copy numbers could boost T- and B-cell reconstitution, and mice presented clinical manifestations resembling Omenn syndrome [137]. The development of LVs driving codon-optimized human *RAG2* (*RAG2co*) leads to phenotype amelioration compared to native *RAG2* in *Rag2−/−* mice, with restoration of all immune functions and providing a valid optional vector for clinical implementation [138]. Proof of concept of HSC GT for correction of mutations in the gene encoding SLAM-associated protein (SAP), causing X-linked lymphoproliferative disease (XLP1), has been provided in SAP−/− mice [139]. LVs have been also used in preclinical models to treat familial hemophagocytic lymphohistiocytosis (FHL), with partial recovery of immune cells and normal immune regulation [140]. Other preclinical models of gene therapy are under development and include UNC13D (Munc13-4), CD40LG, BTK, BLNK, and Leucocyte adhesion deficiency [38].

Apart from PIDs, in the last two decades, significant advances have been made in GT for hemoglobinopathies, as beta-thalassemia and sickle-cell disease, with LVs. After some first attempts [141–145], LentiGlobin vector BB305 showed the best preclinical results and was used in 2013 and 2014 in three clinical trials sponsored by the biotechnology company bluebird bio (clinicalTrial.gov identifiers, NCT02151526, NCT01745120, and NCT02140554). Thirteen subjects with transfusion-dependent β-thalassemia and one patient with severe sickle-cell disease have been treated in the context of the studies, and the majority achieved transfusion independence [145–147].

Another clinical trial of GT in adult b-thalassemia major patients was initiated in 2012 in New York, USA, using a non-myeloablative conditioning (clinicalTrial.gov identifier, NCT01639690) [148, 149], that is not currently sufficient to ensure optimal engraftment with transduced stem cells [150].

A more recent trial has also started in 2015 in Milan, Italy, sponsored by Fondazione Telethon [151–153]. Initial data on the first adult patients showed a good yield of HSC collected from peripheral blood, leading to a high number of cells infused, good tolerability of the procedure, and preliminary positive efficacy data.

Metabolic diseases have been another recent field of application of GT, with a big challenge of delivering a sufficient amount of the corrected stem cells and protein beyond the blood-brain barrier. The proof of successful ABCD1 gene transfer to autologous HSCs by a LV was obtained in three patients with X-linked adrenoleukodystrophy [154]. The first clinical trial of GT with LV with ARSA gene recently demonstrated a marked benefit with prevention of disease onset or halted disease progression in 8/9 patients [155, 156]. Various other lysosomal storage disorders are under investigation. Preclinical studies in mucopolysaccharidosis type I (MPS-I), MPS-IIIa, and Pompe disease (glycogen storage disease II) have successfully investigated the efficacy of LV gene correction of HSCs in the murine model with promising results that set the scene for future clinical trials [157–159].

Ultimately, a general shift from the current "gene addition" approaches to "gene editing" strategies will certainly lead to new perspectives

in the treatment of patients affected by PIDs and other genetic diseases. With this approach, genes can be targeted and corrected in situ allowing expression from native regulatory elements. This can be achieved through a number of available platforms including meganucleases, zinc-finger nucleases (ZFN), transcriptor activator-like effector nucleases (TALENs), and clustered regularly interspaced short palindromic repeats (CRISPR)-associated (CRISPR/Cas)-based RNA-guided DNA endonucleases. All of these nucleases combine specific DNA recognition sequences with an endonuclease capable of generating a site-specific double-stranded break (DSB) in the DNA, stimulating homologous recombination (HR) [49, 160]. Several gene-targeting approaches have been recently published, applying ZFN, TALEN, and CRISPR/Cas9 technology to iPSCs from beta-thalassemic, sickle-cell, and CGD patients, with promising results [161–163].

Gene therapy is still at an early stage of development for some diseases, but clinical trials for some PIDs have already provided proof of principle for sustained clinical efficacy with low toxicity in several patients. The experience of ADA-SCID GT has shown that the synergism between the academical institutions and the industry has allowed to produce individualized therapies by gene correction as a standard, approved therapy. This will hopefully open the way to the approval of GT for the treatment of other genetic diseases.

Recent studies indicate that combined gene and cell therapy approaches may exploit the proliferative potential of pluripotent stem cells, but many obstacles to the use of such approaches for the treatment of PIDs and other hematological disorders remain [164–166]. Moreover, although recent gene and cell therapy trials involving LV-mediated gene transfer in HSCs followed by autologous cell transplantation gave excellent outcomes and no observable toxicity, the risk of insertional mutagenesis will need further monitoring in the next years. Finally, if the safety and efficacy results will be persistent in the long term, gene therapy could be considered in the future as a first-line low-risk complication treatment for some diseases.

Authors' Disclosure Statement Dr. Maria Pia Cicalese declares that no competing financial interests do exist.

Prof. Alessandro Aiuti is the PI of clinical trials for ADA-SCID and WAS, which were initially sponsored by Fondazione Telethon/Ospedale San Raffaele and after licensing by GlaxoSmithKline (GSK), in 2010 (ADA) and 2013 (WAS) became GSK-sponsored.

References

1. Locke BA, Dasu T, Verbsky JW. Laboratory diagnosis of primary immunodeficiencies. Clin Rev Allergy Immunol. 2014;46(2):154–68.
2. Fischer A, Hacein-Bey Abina S, Touzot F, et al. Gene therapy for primary immunodeficiencies. Clin Genet. 2015;88:507–15.
3. Al-Herz W, Bousfiha A, Casanova JL, et al. Primary immunodeficiency diseases: an update on the classification from the international union of immunological societies expert committee for primary immunodeficiency. Front Immunol. 2011;8:2–54.
4. Zhang L, Thrasher AJ, Gaspar HB. Current progress on gene therapy for primary immunodeficiencies. Gene Ther. 2013;20:963–9.
5. Mukherjee S, Thrasher AJ. Gene therapy for PIDs: progress, pitfalls and prospects. Gene. 2013;525:174–81.
6. Bousfiha AA, Jeddane L, Ailal F, et al. Primary immunodeficiency diseases worldwide: more common than generally thought. J Clin Immunol. 2013;33(1):1–7.
7. Pachlopnik Schmid J, Gungor T, Seger R. Modern management of primary T-cell immunodeficiencies. Pediatr Allergy Immunol. 2014;25(4):300–13.
8. Griffith LM, Cowan MJ, Notarangelo LD, et al. Primary immune deficiency treatment consortium (PIDTC) report. J Allergy Clin Immunol. 2014;133(2):335–47.
9. Hernandez-Trujillo HS, Chapel H, Lo Re V 3rd, et al. Comparison of American and European practices in the management of patients with primary immunodeficiencies. Clin Exp Immunol. 2012;169(1):57–69.
10. Modell V1, Knaus M, Modell F, et al. Global overview of primary immunodeficiencies: a report from Jeffrey Modell Centers worldwide focused on diagnosis, treatment, and discovery. Immunol Res. 2014;60(1):132–44.
11. Casanova JL, Conley ME, Seligman SJ, et al. Guidelines for genetic studies in single patients: lessons from primary immunodeficiencies. J ExpMed. 2014;211(11):2137–49.

12. Chinen J, Notarangelo LD, Shearer WT. Advances in basic and clinical immunology in 2013. J Allergy Clin Immunol. 2014;133(4):967–76.
13. Somech R, Lev A, Simon AJ, et al. Newborn screening for severe T and B cell immunodeficiency in Israel: a pilot study. Isr Med Assoc J. 2013;15(8):404–9.
14. Audrain M, Thomas C, Mirallie S, et al. Evaluation of the T-cell receptor excision circle assay performances for severe combined immunodeficiency neonatal screening on Guthrie cards in a French single centre study. Clin Immunol. 2014;150(2):137–9.
15. Borte S, von Dobeln U, Fasth A, et al. Neonatal screening for severe primary immunodeficiency diseases using high-throughput triplex real-time PCR. Blood. 2012;119(11):2552–5.
16. la Marca G, Malvagia S, Casetta B, et al. Progress in expanded newborn screening for metabolic conditions by LC–MS/MS in Tuscany: update on methods to reduce false tests. J Inherit Metab Dis. 2008;2:395–404.
17. Azzari C, la Marca G, Resti M. Neonatal screening for severe combined immunodeficiency caused by an adenosine deaminase defect: a reliable and inexpensive method using tandem mass spectrometry. J Allergy Clin Immunol. 2011;127(6):1394–9.
18. Bach FH, Albertini RJ, Joo P, et al. Bone-marrow transplantation in a patient with the Wiskott-Aldrich syndrome. Lancet. 1968;2(7583):1364–6.
19. Gatti RA, Meuwissen HJ, Allen HD, et al. Immunological reconstitution of sex-linked lymphopenic immunological deficiency. Lancet. 1968;2(7583):1366–9.
20. Naik S, Nicholas SK, Martinez CA, et al. Adoptive immunotherapy for primary immunodeficiency disorders with virus-specific T lymphocytes. J Allergy Clin Immunol. 2016;137(5):1498–505.
21. Buckley RH. Transplantation of hematopoietic stem cells in human severe combined immunodeficiency: longterm outcomes. Immunol Res. 2011;49:25–43.
22. Pai SY, Logan BR, Griffith LM, et al. Transplantation outcomes for severe combined immunodeficiency, 2000–2009. N Engl J Med. 2014;371:434–46.
23. Gennery AR, Slatter MA, Grandin L, et al. Transplantation of hematopoietic stem cells and long-term survival for primary immunodeficiencies in Europe: entering a new century, do we do better? J Allergy Clin Immunol. 2010;126:602–10. e601-611
24. Moratto D, Giliani S, Bonfim C, et al. Long-term outcome and lineage-specific chimerism in 194 patients with Wiskott-Aldrich syndrome treated by hematopoietic cell transplantation in the period 1980–2009: an international collaborative study. Blood. 2011;118:1675–84.
25. Bertaina A, Merli P, Rutella S, et al. HLA-haploidentical stem cell transplantation after removal of alphabeta+ T and B cells in children with nonmalignant disorders. Blood. 2014;124:822–6.

26. Gungor T, Teira P, Slatter M, et al. Reduced-intensity conditioning and HLA-matched haemopoietic stem-cell transplantation in patients with chronic granulomatous disease: a prospective multicentre study. Lancet. 2014;383:436–48.

27. Kildebeck E, Checketts J, Porteus M. Gene therapy for primary immunodeficiencies. Curr Opin Pediatr. 2012;24(6):731–8.

28. Rivat C, Santilli G, Gaspar HB, et al. Gene therapy for primary immunodeficiencies. Hum Gene Ther. 2012;23(7):668–75.

29. Fischer A, Cavazzana-Calvo M. Gene therapy of inherited diseases. Lancet. 2008;371(9629):2044–7.

30. Hacein Bey Abina S, Pai SY, Gaspar HB, et al. A modified γ-retrovirus vector for X-linked severe combined immunodeficiency. N Engl J Med. 2014;371(15):1407–17.

31. Gaspar HB, Qasim W, Davies EG, Rao K, Amrolia PJ, Veys P. How I treat severe combined immunodeficiency. Blood. 2013;122(23):3749–58.

32. Stephan V, Wahn V, Le Deist F, Dirksen U, Broker B, Muller-Fleckenstein I, Horneff G, Schroten H, Fischer A, de Saint Basile G. Atypical X-linked severe combined immunodeficiency due to possible spontaneous reversion of the genetic defect in T cells. N Engl J Med. 1996;335:1563–7.

33. Speckmann C, Pannicke U, Wiech E, Schwarz K, Fisch P, Friedrich W, Niehues T, Gilmour K, Buiting K, Schlesier M, Eibel H, Rohr J, Superti-Furga A, Gross-Wieltsch U, Ehl S. Clinical and immunologic consequences of a somatic reversion in a patient with X-linked severe combined immunodeficiency. Blood. 2008;112:4090–7.

34. Touzot F, Moshous D, Creidy R, et al. Faster T-cell development following gene therapy compared with haploidentical HSCT in the treatment of SCID-X1. Blood. 2015;125(23):3563–9.

35. Hacein-Bey-Abina S, Le Deist F, Carlier F, Bouneaud C, Hue C, De Villartay JP, Thrasher AJ, Wulffraat N, Sorensen R, Dupuis-Girod S, Fischer A, Davies EG, Kuis W, Leiva L, Cavazzana-Calvo M. Sustained correction of X-linked severe combined immunodeficiency by ex vivo gene therapy. N Engl J Med. 2002;346:1185–93.

36. Hacein-Bey-Abina S, Hauer J, Lim A, et al. Efficacy of gene therapy for X-linked severe combined immunodeficiency. N Engl J Med. 2010;363(4):355–64.

37. Gaspar HB, Cooray S, Gilmour KC, et al. Long-term persistence of a polyclonal T cell repertoire after gene therapy for X-linked severe combined immunodeficiency. Sci Transl Med. 2011;3(97):97ra79.

38. Ghosh S, Thrasher A, Gaspar B. Gene therapy for monogenic disorders of the bone marrow. Br J Haematol. 2015;171:155–70.

39. Hacein-Bey-Abina S, Garrigue A, Wang GP, et al. Insertional oncogenesis in 4 patients after retrovirus-mediated gene therapy of SCID-X1. J Clin Invest. 2008;118(9):3132–42.

40. Howe SJ, Mansour MR, Schwarzwaelder K, et al. Insertional mutagenesis combined with acquired somatic mutations causes leukemogenesis following gene therapy of SCID-X1 patients. J Clin Invest. 2008;118:3143–50.

41. Candotti F. Gene transfer into hematopoietic stem cells as treatment for primary immunodeficiency diseases. Int J Hematol. 2014;99:383–92.

42. Deichmann A, Hacein-Bey-Abina S, Schmidt M, et al. Vector integration is non random and clustered and influences the fate of lymphopoiesis in SCID-X1 gene therapy. J Clin Invest. 2007;117:2225–32.

43. Schwarzwaelder K, Howe SJ, Schmidt M, et al. Gammaretrovirus-mediated correction of SCID-X1 is associated with skewed vector integration site distribution in vivo. J Clin Invest. 2007;117:2241–9.

44. Chinen J, Davis J, De Ravin SS, Hay BN, Hsu AP, Linton GF, Naumann N, Nomicos EY, Silvin C, Ulrick J, Whiting-Theobald NL, Malech HL, Puck JM. Gene therapy improves immune function in pre-adolescents with X-linked severe combined immunodeficiency. Blood. 2007;110:67–73.

45. Zhou S, Mody D, DeRavin SS, et al. A self-inactivating lentiviral vector for SCID-X1 gene therapy that does not activate LMO2 expression in human T cells. Blood. 2010;116:900–8.

46. De Ravin SS, Choi U, Theobald N, et al. Lentiviral gene transfer for treatment of children 2 years old with x-linked severe combined immunodeficiency. Mol Ther. 2013;21:S118.

47. Kohn DB. Gene therapy outpaces haplo for SCID-X1. Blood. 2015;125(23):3521–2.

48. Naldini L. Ex vivo gene transfer and correction for cell-based therapies. Nat Rev Genet. 2011;12:301–15.

49. Genovese P, Schiroli G, , Escobar G, et al. Targeted genome editing in human repopulating haematopoietic stem cells. Nature 2014;510(7504):235–240.

50. Aiuti A, Brigida I, Ferrua F, et al. Hematopoietic stem cell gene therapy for adenosine deaminase deficient-SCID. Immunol Res. 2009;44:150–9.

51. Gaspar HB, Aiuti A, Porta F, et al. How I treat ADA deficiency. Blood. 2009;114:3524–32.

52. Grunebaum E, Cohen A, Roifman CM. Recent advances in understanding and managing adenosine deaminase and purine nucleoside phosphorylase deficiencies. Curr Opin Allergy Clin Immunol. 2013;13(6):630–8.

53. Hirschhorn, R., Candotti, F. Immunodeficiency due to defects of purine metabolism. in: H.D. Ochs, C.I.E. Smith, J.M. Puck (Eds.) Primary immunodeficiency diseases. A molecular and genetic approach. Oxford University Press, Oxford; 2007:169–196.

54. Honig M, Albert MH, Schulz A, et al. Patients with adenosine deaminase deficiency surviving after hematopoietic stem cell transplantation are at high risk of CNS complications. Blood. 2007;109:3595–602.

55. Sauer AV, Mrak E, Hernandez RJ, et al. ADA-deficient SCID is associated with a specific microenvironment and bone phenotype characterized by RANKL/OPG imbalance and osteoblast insufficiency. Blood. 2009;114:3216–26.

56. Brigida I, Sauer AV, Ferrua F, et al. B-cell development and functions and therapeutic options in adenosine deaminase-deficient patients. J Allergy Clin Immunol. 2014;133:799–806.

57. Hassan A, Booth C, Brightwell A, et al. Outcome of hematopoietic stem cell transplantation for adenosine deaminase-deficient severe combined immunodeficiency. Blood. 2012;120(17):3615–24. quiz 3626

58. Blaese RM, Culver KW, Miller AD, Carter CS, Fleisher T, Clerici M, Shearer G, Chang L, Chiang Y, Tolstoshev P, Greenblatt JJ, B Rosenberg SA, Klein H, Berger M, Mullen CA, Ramsey WJ, Muul L, Morgan RA, Anderson WF. T lymphocyte-directed gene therapy for ADA-SCID: initial trial results after 4 years. Science. 1995;270:475–80.

59. Bordignon C, Notarangelo LD, Nobili N, Ferrari G, Casorati G, Panina P, Mazzolari E, Maggioni D, Rossi C, Servida P, Ugazio AG, Mavilio F. Gene therapy in peripheral blood lymphocytes and bone marrow for ADA-immunodeficient patients. Science. 1995;270:470–5.

60. Onodera M, Ariga T, Kawamura N, Kobayashi I, Ohtsu M, Yamada M, Tame A, Furuta H, Okano M, Matsumoto S, Kotani H, McGarrity GJ, Blaese RM, Sakiyama Y. Successful peripheral T-lymphocyte directed gene transfer for a patient with severe combined immune deficiency caused by adenosine deaminase deficiency. Blood. 1998;91:30–6.

61. Aiuti A, Vai S, Mortellaro A, Casorati G, Ficara F, Andolfi G, Ferrari G, Tabucchi A, Carlucci F, Ochs HD, Notarangelo LD, Roncarolo MG, Bordignon C. Immune reconstitution in ADA-SCID after PBL gene therapy and discontinuation of enzyme replacement. Nat Med. 2002;8:423–5.

62. Muul LM, Tuschong LM, Soenen SL, et al. Persistence and expression of the adenosine deaminase gene for 12 years and immune reaction to gene transfer components: long-term results of the first clinical gene therapy trial. Blood. 2003;101:2563–9. Epub Nov 2002

63. Biasco L, Scala S, Basso Ricci L, et al. In vivo tracking of T cells in humans unveils decadelong survival and activity of genetically modified T memory stem cells. Sci Transl Med. 2015;7(273):273ra13.

64. Montiel-Equihua CA, Thrasher AJ, Gaspar HB. Gene therapy for severe combined immunodeficiency due to adenosine deaminase deficiency. Curr Gene Ther. 2012;12:57–65.

65. Aiuti A, Slavin S, Aker M, et al. Correction of ADA-SCID by stem cell gene therapy combined with nonmyeloablative conditioning. Science. 2002;296(5577):2410–3.

66. Aiuti A, Cattaneo F, Galimberti S, et al. Gene therapy for immunodeficiency due to adenosine deaminase deficiency. N Engl J Med. 2009;360(5):447–58.

67. Cicalese MP, Ferrua F, Castagnaro L, et al. Update on the safety and efficacy of retroviral gene therapy for immunodeficiency due to adenosine deaminase deficiency. Blood. 2016;128:45–54.

68. www.ema.europa.eu

69. Candotti F, Shaw KL, Muul L, et al. Gene therapy for adenosine deaminase-deficient severe combined immune deficiency: clinical comparison of retroviral vectors and treatment plans. Blood. 2012;120:3635–46.

70. Otsu M, Nakajima S, Kida M, et al. Steady ongoing hematological and immunological reconstitution achieved in ADA-deficiency patients treated by stem cell gene therapy with no myelopreparative conditioning. J Gene Med. 2006;8:1436–75.

71. Carbonaro D, Jin X, Wang X, et al. Gene therapy/bone marrow transplantation in ADA-deficient mice: roles of enzyme-replacement therapy and cytoreduction. Blood. 2012;120(18):3677–87.

72. Rivers L, Gaspar HB. Severe combined immunodeficiency: recent developments and guidance on clinical management. Arch Dis Child. 2015;100(7):667–72.

73. Biasco L, Ambrosi A, Pellin D, et al. Integration profile of retroviral vector in gene therapy treated patients is cell-specific according to gene expression and chromatin conformation of target cell. EMBO Mol Med. 2011;3:89–101.

74. Cicalese MP, Aiuti A. Clinical applications of gene therapy for primary immunodeficiencies. Hum Gene Ther. 2015;26(4):210–9.

75. Siler U, Paruzynski A, Holtgreve-Grez H, et al. Successful combination of sequential gene therapy and rescue allo-HSCT in two children with X-CGD—importance of timing. Curr Gene Ther. 2015;15(4):416–27.

76. Grez M, Reichenbach J, Schwäble J, Seger R, Dinauer MC, Thrasher AJ. Gene therapy of chronic granulomatous disease: the engraftment dilemma. Mol Ther. 2011;19(1):28–35.

77. Braun CJ, Boztug K, Paruzynski A, et al. Gene therapy for Wiskott-Aldrich syndrome: long-term efficacy and genotoxicity. Sci Transl Med. 2014;6(227):227ra33.

78. Mortellaro A, Hernandez RJ, Guerrini MM, et al. Ex vivo gene therapy with lentiviral vectors rescues adenosine deaminase (ADA)-deficient mice and corrects their immune and metabolic defects. Blood. 2006;108(9):2979–88.

79. Carbonaro DA, Zhang L, Jin X, et al. Preclinical demonstration of lentiviral vector-mediated correction of immunological and metabolic abnormalities in models of adenosine deaminase deficiency. Mol Ther. 2014;22(3):607–22.

80. Gaspar B, Buckland K, Rivat C, et al. Immunological and metabolic correction after lentiviral vector mediated haematopoietic stem cell gene therapy for ADA deficiency. J Clin Immunol. 2014;34(Suppl 2):S167.

81. Derry JM, Kerns JA, Weinberg KI, et al. WASP gene mutations in Wiskott-Aldrich syndrome and

X-linked thrombocytopenia. Hum Mol Genet. 1995;4(7):1127–35.

82. Catucci M, Castiello MC, Pala F, et al. Autoimmunity in wiskott-Aldrich syndrome: an unsolved enigma. Front Immunol. 2012;3:209.

83. Silvin C, Belisle B, Abo A. A role for Wiskott-Aldrich syndrome protein in T-cell receptor mediated transcriptional activation independent of actin polymerization. J Biol Chem. 2001;276(24):21450–7.

84. Blundell MP, Worth A, Bouma G, Thrasher AJ. The Wiskott-Aldrich syndrome: the actin cytoskeleton and immune cell function. Dis Markers. 2010;29:157–75.

85. Thrasher AJ. New insights into the biology of Wiskott-Aldrich syndrome (WAS). Hematology Am Soc Hematol Educ Program. 2009;2009:132–8.

86. Massaad MJ, Ramesh N, Geha RS. Wiskott-Aldrich syndrome: a comprehensive review. Ann N Y Acad Sci. 2013;1285:26–43.

87. Thrasher AJ, Burns SO. WASP: a key immunological multitasker. Nat Rev Immunol. 2010;10:182–92.

88. Ozsahin H, Cavazzana-Calvo M, Notarangelo LD, et al. Long-term outcome following hematopoietic stem-cell transplantation in Wiskott-Aldrich syndrome: collaborative study of the European Society for Immunodeficiencies and European Group for Blood and Marrow Transplantation. Blood. 2008;111(1):439–45.

89. Filipovich AH, Stone JV, Tomany SC, et al. Impact of donor type on outcome of bone marrow transplantation for Wiskott-Aldrich syndrome: collaborative study of the International Bone Marrow Transplant Registry and the National Marrow Donor Program. Blood. 2001;97(6):1598–603.

90. Kobayashi R, Ariga T, Nonoyama S, et al. Outcome in patients with Wiskott-Aldrich syndrome following stem cell transplantation: an analysis of 57 patients in Japan. Br J Haematol. 2006;135(3):362–6.

91. Fischer A, Hacein-Bey-Abina S, Cavazzana-Calvo M. 20 years of gene therapy for SCID. Nat Immunol. 2010;11(6):457–60.

92. Candotti F, Facchetti F, Blanzuoli L, et al. Retrovirus-mediated WASP gene transfer corrects defective actin polymerization in B cell lines from Wiskott-Aldrich syndrome patients carrying 'null' mutations. Gene Ther. 1999;6(6):1170–4.

93. Wada T, Jagadeesh GJ, Nelson DL, et al. Retrovirus-mediated WASP gene transfer corrects Wiskott-Aldrich syndrome T-cell dysfunction. Hum Gene Ther. 2002;13(9):1039–46.

94. Klein C, Nguyen D, Liu CH, et al. Gene therapy for Wiskott-Aldrich syndrome: rescue of T-cell signaling and amelioration of colitis upon transplantation of retrovirally transduced hematopoietic stem cells in mice. Blood. 2003;101(6):2159–66.

95. Strom TS, Gabbard W, Kelly PF, et al. Functional correction of T cells derived from patients with the Wiskott-Aldrich syndrome (WAS) by transduction with an oncoretroviral vector encoding the WAS protein. Gene Ther. 2003;10(9):803–9.

96. Galy A, Roncarolo MG, Thrasher AJ. Development of lentiviral gene therapy for Wiskott Aldrich syndrome. Expert Opin Biol Ther. 2008;8(2):181–90.

97. Dupré L, Trifari S, Follenzi A, et al. Lentiviral vector-mediated gene transfer in T cells from Wiskott-Aldrich syndrome patients leads to functional correction. Mol Ther. 2004;10(5):903–15.

98. Boztug K, Schmidt M, Schwarzer A, et al. Stem-cell gene therapy for the Wiskott-Aldrich syndrome. N Engl J Med. 2010;363(20):1918–27.

99. Westerberg LS, de la Fuente MA, Wermeling F, et al. WASP confers selective advantage for specific hematopoietic cell populations and serves a unique role in marginal zone B-cell homeostasis and function. Blood. 2008;112(10):4139–47.

100. Paruzynski A, Glimm H, Schmidt M, et al. Analysis of the clonal repertoire of gene-corrected cells in gene therapy. Methods Enzymol. 2012;507:59–87.

101. Stein S, Ott MG, Schultze-Strasser S, et al. Genomic instability and myelodysplasia with monosomy 7 consequent to EVI1 activation after gene therapy for chronic granulomatous disease. Nat Med. 2010;16(2):198–204.

102. Dupré L, Marangoni F, Scaramuzza S, et al. Efficacy of gene therapy for Wiskott-Aldrich syndrome using a WAS promoter/cDNA-containing lentiviral vector and nonlethal irradiation. Hum Gene Ther. 2006;17(3):303–13.

103. Marangoni F, Bosticardo M, Charrier S, et al. Evidence for long-term efficacy and safety of gene therapy for Wiskott-Aldrich syndrome in preclinical models. Mol Ther. 2009;17(6):1073–82.

104. Avedillo Diez I, Zychlinski D, Coci EG, Galla M, Modlich U, Dewey RA, Schwarzer A, Maetzig T, Mpofu N, Jaeckel E, Boztug K, Baum C, Klein C, Schambach A. Development of novel efficient SIN vectors with improved safety features for Wiskott-Aldrich syndrome stem cell based gene therapy. Mol Pharm. 2011;8:1525–37.

105. Bosticardo M, Draghici E, Schena F, Sauer AV, Fontana E, Castiello MC, Catucci M, Locci M, Naldini L, Aiuti A, Roncarolo MG, Poliani PL, Traggiai E, Villa A. Lentiviral-mediated gene therapy leads to improvement of B-cell functionality in a murine model of Wiskott-Aldrich syndrome. J Allergy Clin Immunol. 2011;127:e1375.

106. Scaramuzza S, Biasco L, Ripamonti A, et al. Preclinical safety and efficacy of human CD34(+) cells transduced with lentiviral vector for the treatment of Wiskott-Aldrich syndrome. Mol Ther. 2013;21(1):175–84.

107. Aiuti A, Biasco L, Scaramuzza S, et al. Lentiviral hematopoietic stem cell gene therapy in patients with Wiskott-Aldrich syndrome. Science. 2013;341(6148):1233151.

108. Castiello MC, Scaramuzza S, Pala F, Ferrua F, Uva P, Brigida I, Sereni L, van der Burg M, Ottaviano G, Albert MH, Roncarolo MG, Naldini L, Aiuti A, Villa A, Bosticardo M. B-cell reconstitution after lentiviral vector- mediated gene therapy in patients with

Wiskott-Aldrich syndrome. J Allergy Clin Immunol. 2015. https://doi.org/10.1016/j.jaci.2015.01.035.

109. Ferrua F, Cicalese MP, Galimberti S, et al. Safety and clinical benefit of lentiviral hematopoietic stem cell gene therapy for Wiskott-Aldrich Syndrome. ASH 57th annual meeting, Orlando FL, 5–8 Dec 2015.

110. Hacein-Bey Abina S, Gaspar HB, Blondeau J, Caccavelli L, Charrier S, Buckland K, Picard C, Six E, Himoudi N, Gilmour K, McNicol AM, Hara H, Xu-Bayford J, Rivat C, Touzot F, Mavilio F, Lim A, Treluyer JM, Héritier S, Lefrère F, Magalon J, Pengue-Koyi I, Honnet G, Blanche S, Sherman EA, Male F, Berry C, Malani N, Bushman FD, Fischer A, Thrasher AJ, Galy A, Cavazzana M. Outcomes following gene therapy in patients with severe Wiskott-Aldrich syndrome. JAMA. 2015;313:1550–63.

111. Chu JI, Henderso LA, Armant M et al. Gene therapy using a self-inactivating lentiviral vector improves clinical and laboratory manifestations of Wiskott-Aldrich syndrome. ASH 57th annual meeting, Orlando FL, 5–8 Dec 2015.

112. Astrakhan A, Sather BD, Ryu BY, et al. Ubiquitous high-level gene expression in hematopoietic lineages provides effective lentiviral gene therapy of murine Wiskott-Aldrich syndrome. Blood. 2012;119(19):4395–407.

113. Aiuti A, Bacchetta R, Seger R, et al. Gene therapy for primary immunodeficiencies: part 2. Curr Opin Immunol. 2012;24(5):585–91.

114. Goldblatt D. Recent advances in chronic granulomatous disease. J Inf. 2014;69:S32–5.

115. Holland SM. Chronic granulomatous disease. Hematol Oncol Clin N Am. 2013;27:89–99. viii

116. Sekhsaria S, Fleisher TA, Vowells S, et al. Granulocyte colony-stimulating factor recruitment of CD34+ progenitors to peripheral blood: impaired mobilization in chronic granulomatous disease and adenosine deaminase – deficient severe combined immunodeficiency disease patients. Blood. 1996;88(3):1104–12.

117. Goebel WS, Dinauer MC. Gene therapy for chronic granulomatous disease. Acta Haematol. 2003;110(2–3):86–92.

118. Qasim W, Gennery AR. Gene therapy for primary immunodeficiencies: current status and future prospects. Drugs. 2014;74(9):963–9.

119. Malech HL, Maples PB, Whiting-Theobald N, Linton GF, Sekhsaria S, Vowells SJ, Li F, Miller JA, DeCarlo E, Holland SM, Leitman SF, Carter CS, Butz RE, Read EJ, Fleisher TA, Schneiderman RD, Van Epps DE, Spratt SK, Maack CA, Rokovich JA, Cohen LK, Gallin JI. Prolonged production of NADPH oxidase-corrected granulocytes after gene therapy of chronic granulomatous disease. Proc Natl Acad Sci U S A. 1997;94:12133–8.

120. Kang EM, Choi U, Theobald N, et al. Retrovirus gene therapy for X-linked chronic granulomatous disease can achieve stable long-term correction of

oxidase activity in peripheral blood neutrophils. Blood. 2010;115(4):783–91.

121. Ott MG, Schmidt M, Schwarzwaelder K, et al. Correction of X-linked chronic granulomatous disease by gene therapy, augmented by insertional activation of MDS1-EVI1, PRDM16 or SETBP1. Nat Med. 2006;12(4):401–9.

122. Kang EM, Marciano BE, DeRavin S, et al. Chronic granulomatous disease: overview and hematopoietic stem cell transplantation. J Allergy Clin Immunol. 2011;127(6):1319–26. quiz 1327-8

123. Farinelli G, Capo V, Scaramuzza S, et al. Lentiviral vectors for the treatment of primary immunodeficiencies. J Inherit Metab Dis. 2014;37(4):525–33.

124. Bedard K, Krause KH. The NOX family of ROS-generating NADPH oxidases: physiology and pathophysiology. Physiol Rev. 2007;87(1):245–313.

125. Yahata T, Takanashi T, Muguruma Y, et al. Accumulation of oxidative DNA damage restricts the self-renewal capacity of human hematopoietic stem cells. Blood. 2011;118(11):2941–50.

126. Chiriaco M, Farinelli G, Capo V, et al. Dual-regulated lentiviral vector for gene therapy of X-linked chronic granulomatosis. Mol Ther. 2014;22(8):1472–83.

127. Bianchi M, Hakkim A, Brinkmann V, et al. Restoration of NET formation by gene therapy in CGD controls aspergillosis. Blood. 2009;114(13):2619–22.

128. Santilli G, Almarza E, Brendel C, Choi U, Beilin C, Blundell MP, Haria S, Parsley KL, Kinnon C, Malech HL, Bueren JA, Grez M, Thrasher AJ. Biochemical correction of X-CGD by a novel chimeric promoter regulating high levels of transgene expression in myeloid cells. Mol Ther. 2011;19:122–32.

129. Barde I, Laurenti E, Verp S, et al. Lineage- and stage-restricted lentiviral vectors for the gene therapy of chronic granulomatous disease. Gene Ther. 2011;18(11):1087–97.

130. Brendel C, Müller-Kuller U, Schultze-Strasser S, et al. Physiological regulation of transgene expression by a lentiviral vector containing the A2UCOE linked to a myeloid promoter. Gene Ther. 2012;19(10):1018–29.

131. Sauer AV, Di Lorenzo B, Carriglio N, et al. Progress in gene therapy for primary immunodeficiencies using lentiviral vectors. Curr Opin Allergy Clin Immunol. 2014;14(6):527–34.

132. Williams S, Mustoe T, Mulcahy T, et al. CpG-island fragments from the HNRPA2B1/CBX3 genomic locus reduce silencing and enhance transgene expression from the hCMV promoter/enhancer in mammalian cells. BMC Biotechnol. 2005;5:17.

133. Zhang F, Frost AR, Blundell MP, et al. A ubiquitous chromatin opening element (UCOE) confers resistance to DNA methylation-mediated silencing of lentiviral vectors. Mol Ther. 2010;18(9):1640–9.

134. Farinelli G, Jofra Hernandez R, Rossi A, et al. Lentiviral vector gene therapy protects XCGD mice from acute *Staphylococcus aureus* pneumonia and

inflammatory response. Mol Ther. 2016. https://doi.org/10.1038/mt.2016.150.

135. Multhaup MM, Podetz-Pedersen KM, Karlen AD, et al. Role of transgene regulation in ex vivo lentiviral correction of Artemis deficiency. Hum Gene Ther. 2015;26(4):232–43.

136. Pike-Overzet K, Rodijk M, Ng YY, et al. Correction of murine Rag1 deficiency by self-inactivating lentiviral vector-mediated gene transfer. Leukemia. 2011;25(9):1471–83.

137. van Til NP, Sarwari R, Visser TP, et al. Recombination-activating gene 1 (Rag1)-deficient mice with severe combined immunodeficiency treated with lentiviral gene therapy demonstrate autoimmune Omenn-like syndrome. J Allergy Clin Immunol. 2014;133(4):1116–23.

138. van Til NP, de Boer H, Mashamba N, et al. Correction of murine Rag2 severe combined immunodeficiency by lentiviral gene therapy using a codon-optimized RAG2 therapeutic transgene. Mol Ther. 2012;20(10):1968–80.

139. Rivat C, Booth C, Alonso-Ferrero M, et al. SAP gene transfer restores cellular and humoral immune function in a murine model of X-linked lymphoproliferative disease. Blood. 2013;121(7):1073–6.

140. Carmo M, Risma KA, Arumugam P, et al. Perforin gene transfer into hematopoietic stem cells improves immune dysregulation in murine models of perforin deficiency. Mol Ther. 2015;23(4):737–45.

141. Goettel JA, Biswas S, Lexmond WS, et al. Fatal autoimmunity in mice reconstituted with human hematopoietic stem cells encoding defective FOXP3. Blood. 2015;125(25):3886–95.

142. Cavazzana-Calvo M, Payen E, Negre O, et al. Transfusion independence and HMGA2 activation after gene therapy of human beta-thalassaemia. Nature. 2010;467:318e22.

143. Payen E, Leboulch P. Advances in stem cell transplantation and gene therapy in the beta-hemoglobinopathies. Hematol Am Soc Hematol Educ Progr. 2012;2012:276e83.

144. Cavazzana M, Ribeil JA, Payen E, et al. Outcomes of gene therapy for beta thalassemia major via transplantation of autologous hematopoietic stem cells transduced ex vivo with a lentiviral beta globin vector. Haematologica. 2014;99. abstract:S742.

145. Negre O, Bartholomae C, Beuzard Y, et al. Preclinical evaluation of efficacy and safety of an improved lentiviral vector for the treatment of beta-thalassemia and sickle cell disease. Curr Gene Ther. 2015;15:64e81.

146. Cavazzana M, Ribeil J-A, Payen E, et al. Outcomes of gene therapy for beta-thalassemia major and severe sickle disease via transplantation of autologous hematopoietic stem cells transduced ex vivo with a lentiviral beta globin vector. EHA20, Wien, Jun 11–14 2015.

147. Walters MC, MD1, Rasko J, MBBS, PhD2, Hongeng S, MD3 et al. Update of results from the Northstar study (HGB-204): a phase 1/2 study of gene therapy for beta-thalassemia major via transplantation of autologous hematopoietic stem cells transduced ex-vivo with a lentiviral beta AT87Q-Globin vector (LentiGlobin BB305 Drug Product). ASH 57th annual meeting, Orlando FL, 5–8 Dec 2015.

148. Boulad F, Wang X, Qu J, et al. Safe mobilization of CD34þ cells in adults with betathalassemia and validation of effective globin gene transfer for clinical investigation. Blood. 2014;123:1483e6.

149. Sadelain M, Boulad F, Riviere I, Maggio A, Taher A. Gene therapy. In: Cappellini MD, Cohen A, Porter J, Taher A, Viprakasit V, editors. Guidelines for the management of transfusion dependent thalassaemia (TDT) [internet]. 3rd ed. Nicosia: Thalassaemia International Federation; 2013.

150. Mansilla-Soto J, Riviere I, Boulad F, et al. Cell and gene therapy for the beta-thalassemias: advances and prospects. Hum Gene Ther. 2016;27(4):295–304.

151. Miccio A, Cesari R, Lotti F, et al. In vivo selection of genetically modified erythroblastic progenitors leads to long-term correction of beta-thalassemia. Proc Natl Acad Sci U S A. 2008;105:10547–52.

152. Lidonnici MR, Aprile A, Paleari Y, et al. Update on gene therapy clinical trial for the treatment of beta thalassemia major in Italy [abstract]. Presented at the Tenth Cooley's Anemia Symposium, Chicago, IL, 18–22 Oct 2015.

153. Marktel S Giglio F, Cicalese MP, et al. A phase I/II study of autologous hemapoietic stem cells genetically modified with globe Lentiviral vector for the treatment of transfusion dependent beta-thalassemia. EHA21, Copenhagen, 9–12 Jun 2016.

154. Cartier N, Hacein-Bey-Abina S, Von Kalle C, et al. Gene therapy of x-linked adrenoleukodystrophy using hematopoietic stem cells and a lentiviral vector. Bull Acad Natl Med. 2010;194(2):255–64. discussion 264-8

155. Biffi A, Montini E, Lorioli L, et al. Lentiviral hematopoietic stem cell gene therapy benefits metachromatic leukodystrophy. Science. 2013;341(6148):1233158.

156. Sessa M, Lorioli L, Fumagalli F, et al. Lentiviral haematopoietic stem-cell gene therapy in early-onset metacromatic leukodystrophy: an ad-hoc analysis of a non-randomised, open-label, phase 1 trail. Lancet. 2016:S0140–6736(16). 30374-9

157. van Til NP, Stok M, Aerts Kaya FS, de Waard MC, Farahbakhshian E, Visser TP, Kroos MA, Jacobs EH, Willart MA, van der Wegen P, Scholte BJ, Lambrecht BN, Duncker DJ, van der Ploeg AT, Reuser AJ, Verstegen MM, Wagemaker G. Lentiviral gene therapy of murine hematopoietic stem cells ameliorates the Pompe disease phenotype. Blood. 2010;115:5329–37.

158. Visigalli I, Delai S, Politi LS, Di Domenico C, Cerri F, Mrak E, D'Isa R, Ungaro D, Stok M, Sanvito F, Mariani E, Staszewsky L, Godi C, Russo I, Cecere F, Del Carro U, Rubinacci A, Brambilla R, Quattrini A, Di Natale P, Ponder K, Naldini L, Biffi A. Gene therapy augments the efficacy of

hematopoietic cell transplantation and fully corrects mucopolysaccharidosis type I phenotype in the mouse model. Blood. 2010;116:5130–9.

159. Langford-Smith A, Wilkinson FL, Langford-Smith KJ, Holley RJ, Sergijenko A, Howe SJ, Bennett WR, Jones SA, Wraith J, Merry CL, Wynn RF, Bigger BW. Hematopoietic stem cell and gene therapy corrects primary neuropathology and behavior in mucopolysaccharidosis IIIA mice. Mol Ther. 2012;20:1610–21.

160. Gaj T, Gersbach CA, Barbas CF 3rd. ZFN, TALEN, and CRISPR/Cas-based methods for genome engineering. Trends Biotechnol. 2013;31:397–405.

161. Sun N, Zhao H. Seamless correction of the sickle cell disease mutation of the HBB gene in human induced pluripotent stem cells using TALENs. Biotechnol Bioeng. 2014;111:1048–53.

162. Xie F, Ye L, Chang JC, Beyer AI, Wang J, Muench MO, Kan YW. Seamless gene correction of beta-thalassemia mutations in patient-specific iPSCs using CRISPR/Cas9 and piggyBac. Genome Res. 2014;24:1526–33.

163. De Ravin SS, Li L, Wu X, et al. CRISPR-Cas9 gene repair of hematopoietic stem cells from patients with X-linked chronic granulomatous disease. Sci Transl Med. 2017;9:372.

164. Tubsuwan A, Abed S, Deichmann A, Kardel MD, et al. Parallel assessment of globin lentiviral transfer in induced pluripotent stem cells and adult hematopoietic stem cells derived from the same transplanted beta-thalassemia patient. Stem Cells. 2013;31:1785e94.

165. Papapetrou EP, Lee G, Malani N, et al. Genomic safe harbors permit high beta-globin transgene expression in thalassemia induced pluripotent stem cells. Nat Biotechnol. 2011;29:73e8.

166. de Dreuzy E, Bhukhai K, Leboulch P, et al. Current and future alternative therapies for beta-thalassemia major. Biomed J. 2016;39:24–38.

Index

© Springer International Publishing AG, part of Springer Nature 2018
B. H. Segal (ed.), *Management of Infections in the Immunocompromised Host*,
https://doi.org/10.1007/978-3-319-77674-3

Printed by Printforce, the Netherlands